The Evolution of Forward Surgery in the US Army

FROM THE REVOLUTIONARY WAR TO THE
COMBAT OPERATIONS OF THE 21ST CENTURY

Edited by

LANCE P. STEAHLY, MD
Colonel, Medical Corps
US Army (Retired)

and

DAVID W. CANNON, SR.
Major, Medical Service Corps
US Army (Retired)

BORDEN INSTITUTE
US Army Medical Department Center and School
Health Readiness Center of Excellence
Fort Sam Houston, Texas

Edward A. Lindeke, Colonel (Retired), MS, US Army
Director, Borden Institute

Linette Sparacino
Volume Editor, Borden Institute

Joan Redding
Senior Production Editor, Borden Institute

Christine Gamboa-Onrubia, MBA
Creative Director and Production Manager, Fineline Graphics, LLC

The views expressed are those of the authors and do not necessarily represent those of the US Army, the US Department of Defense, or the United States Government. Use of trade or brand names in this publication does not imply endorsement by the Department of Defense. Partial support for this book was provided by Defense Health Horizons, a policy analysis unit at the Uniformed Services University of the Health Sciences.

CERTAIN PARTS OF THIS PUBLICATION PERTAIN TO COPYRIGHT RESTRICTIONS. ALL RIGHTS RESERVED. NO COPYRIGHTED PARTS OF THIS PUBLICATION MAY BE REPRODUCED OR TRANSMITTED IN ANY FORM OR BY ANY MEANS, ELECTRONIC OR MECHANICAL (INCLUDING PHOTOCOPY, RECORDING, OR ANY INFORMATION STORAGE AND RETRIEVAL SYSTEM), WITHOUT PERMISSION IN WRITING FROM THE PUBLISHER OR COPYRIGHT OWNER.

Published by the
BORDEN INSTITUTE
US Army Medical Department Center and School
Health Readiness Center of Excellence | Fort Sam Houston, Texas

2018

Library of Congress Cataloging-in-Publication Data

Names: Steahly, Lance P., editor. | Cannon, David W., Sr., editor.
Title: The evolution of forward surgery in the US Army : from the
Revolutionary War to the combat operations of the 21st century / edited by
Lance P. Steahly, MD, Colonel, Medical Corps US Army (Retired) and David
W. Cannon, Sr., Major, Medical Service Corps US Army (Retired).
Description: Sam Houston, Texas : Borden Institute, [2018] | Includes
bibliographical references and index.
Identifiers: LCCN 2018047833 (print) | LCCN 2018048270 (ebook) | ISBN
9780160940088 (ebook) | ISBN 9780160940095 (ebook) | ISBN 9780160940101 (ebook) | ISBN
9780160947841 (pbk.).
Subjects: LCSH: Medicine, Military—United States—History. | Surgery,
Military—United States—History. | United States. Army—Medical care—History.
Classification: LCC UH223 (ebook) | LCC UH223 .E94 2018 (print) | DDC
355.3/450973—dc23
LC record available at Caution-https://lccn.loc.gov/2018047833

For sale by the Superintendent of the Documents, U.S. Government Publishing Office
Internet: bookstore.gpo.gov Phone: toll free (866) 512-1800; DC area (202) 512-1800
Fax: (202) 512-2104 Mail: Stop IDCC, Washington, DC 20402-0001
ISBN No. 978-0-16-094784-1

PRINTED IN THE UNITED STATES OF AMERICA

Contents

ACKNOWLEDGMENTS v
ABOUT THE AUTHORS vii
FOREWORD ix
INTRODUCTION..xii

1   Casualty Care From the Revolutionary War to the War of 1812.................1
      Lance P. Steahly

2   Surgery and Medicine in the War of 1812: A New Nation Challenged 33
      Lance P. Steahly

3   The Civil War: Military Medical Care in the War Between the States 65
      Lance P. Steahly

4   Transitions: Army Medicine in the Post-Civil War Period to the
      Start of World War I 107
      Lance P. Steahly

5   Forward Surgery in the Great War: A War of New Technologies.............. 141
      Lance P. Steahly

6   World War II: Army Forward Surgery on a Worldwide Scale 173
      Lance P. Steahly

7   Forward Surgery in the Korean War: The Mobile Army Surgical Hospitals ... 239
      Scott C. Woodard

8   Vietnam: The Rise of Helicopter Medical Evacuation in a
      War Against a New Kind of Enemy 285
      Lance P. Steahly

9   From the Falklands to the Balkans: Toward Formal
    Designation of the Forward Surgical Team 321
    Christopher A. VanFosson

10 Put to the Test: Forward Surgical Teams Challenged
    During the Global War on Terrorism 355
    Jason M. Seery and David W. Cannon, Sr.

11 Homeland Defense, Contingency Operations, and Future Directions......... 429
    David C. Lynn and Jason M. Seery

ACRONYMS AND ABBREVIATIONS..................................... 457

INDEX..461

Acknowledgments

THE AUTHORS HAVE NOTHING BUT PRAISE for our wonderful Borden Institute Volume Editor, Linette Sparacino. Linette has been extremely patient in bringing along the authors. She has provided excellent editing at all levels. Her gracious and kind demeanor has added to our success. Linette and Lieutenant Colonel Daniel Banks, former Director of the Borden Institute, worked well together in the review and editing process, as did Linette and Colonel John Garr, the following Director.

We are indebted to Mary E. Hope, Senior Archivist, and Carlos Alvarado, Archivist, Army Medical Department Center of History and Heritage, Fort Sam Houston, Texas, for their great help in securing artworks and photographs from a number of sources. We appreciate their diligence in researching the copyright status of the illustrations and their pursuit of photographs of museum artifacts. Their help added greatly to the book's coverage of the events.

We would like to recognize the contribution of Second Lieutenant Molly Steahly to the process. She was an Army ROTC Scholarship recipient at Arizona State University. Molly is now enrolled as a second-degree nursing student at George Washington University in Washington, DC. She is a reserve officer in the US Army Reserves. She has assisted us in assembling information, proofreading, and fact checking for many of these chapters. Molly has thereby gained an interest in military medical history of her own and has worked with Dr. Dale Smith, Professor of Medical History at the Uniformed Services University of the Health Sciences.

LANCE P. STEAHLY, MD, FACS
DAVID W. CANNON, SR.
March 2017

About the Authors

DAVID C. LYNN, MD, is a Board-Certified General Surgeon and Fellow of the American College of Surgeons. His first duty assignment as an active duty surgeon was at Womack Army Medical Center at Fort Bragg, North Carolina, in 2009. He deployed to Iraq with the 21st Combat Support Hospital in 2010. He commanded the 759th Forward Surgical Team (Airborne) at Fort Bragg from January 2011 to February 2013, and carried out both Global Response Force and Defense Chemical-Biological-Radiological-Nuclear Response Force missions during this time. He deployed to Afghanistan in 2013 and was honorably discharged from the Army in 2014. He worked at Womack for an additional year as a civilian contractor, while continuing to work on special projects regarding forward surgery for the Department of Defense.

JASON M. SEERY, MD, is a Board-Certified General Surgeon and Fellow of the American College of Surgeons. He is currently serving as the Deputy Commander for Surgical Services at Martin Army Community Hospital, Fort Benning, Georgia. Prior to this assignment, he served for more than three years as the sixth director of the US Army Trauma Training Center, Jackson-Memorial Hospital, Ryder Trauma Center, in Miami, Florida. He deployed to Iraq from October 2003 through July 2004 with the 2d Armor Cavalry Regiment as the Squadron Flight Surgeon and had a 3-year assignment as the commander of the 541st Forward Surgical Team (Airborne) at Fort Bragg, North Carolina. From February 2010 through February 2011 he deployed to combat in Afghanistan with the 541st Forward Surgical Team (Airborne). His unit supported both Global Response Force and Defense Chemical-Biological-Radiological-Nuclear Response Force missions. LTC(P) Seery is a guest lecturer at the Forward Surgical Team Commanders Course and Brigade and Divisions Surgeons Course. He is also a consultant to various special operations forces units on combat trauma management concepts.

LANCE P. STEAHLY, MD, is a Fellow of the American College of Surgeons and board certified by the American Board of Ophthalmology. He is an ophthalmologist who has worked in settings including the military, academia, Veterans Administration, and private practice. He now serves as the Supervisory Physician of the Medical Evaluation Board and Director of the Integrated Disability Evaluation System, San Antonio Military Medical Center, Joint Base San Antonio–Fort Sam Houston, Texas. He is a retired colonel in the US Army. Dr. Steahly has been interested in military history for many years. His interest especially peaked while involved in the Command and General Staff curriculum. COL Steahly has served in many continental US medical facilities, Germany, and Hawaii. He has served as an Army Chief of Surgery and as a Commander of the 900th US Army Hospital Surgical Mobile, a MASH unit.

CHRISTOPHER A. VANFOSSON, MSN/MHA, RN, is an Army nurse with 24 months of service in combat. He deployed with the 28th Combat Support Hospital in support of Operation Iraqi Freedom (2003–2004), where he served as a medical/surgical and critical care nurse. LTC VanFosson also deployed to Afghanistan in support of Operation Enduring Freedom from February 2010 through February 2011, where he served as the chief nurse and critical care nurse on the 541st Medical Detachment, Forward Surgical Team (Airborne). He serves as a subject matter expert for a Department of Defense-level evaluation of the Role 2 medical resources in the Afghanistan Theater of operations. Previously, LTC VanFosson served as the Clinical Nurse Officer in Charge of the Burn Progressive Care Unit at the US Army Burn Center, US Army Institute of Surgical Research, Joint Base San Antonio–Fort Sam Houston, Texas. He also served from 2010 through 2012 as a subject matter expert and reviewer for the Army Medical Department Lessons Learned-developed Forward Surgical Team Guide.

SCOTT C. WOODARD, MA, is a historian in the Office of Medical History at the US Army Medical Department Center of History and Heritage, having previously served in the US Army for over 22 years. He holds a bachelor's in history from The Citadel, The Military College of South Carolina, and a master's in military medical history from the Uniformed Services University of the Health Sciences, Bethesda, Maryland. "Woody" is a certified Military Historian from the US Army Center of Military History. He has traveled in 24 countries and most recently deployed in 2014 to Kuwait and Afghanistan as a Department of the Army Historian.

DAVID W. CANNON, SR., MA, is a retired major in the Medical Service Corps, US Army. He holds both his BA and MA degrees in psychology from the University of Maine, Orono, Maine, and has completed a fellowship in military medical history at the Uniformed Services University of the Health Sciences, Bethesda, Maryland. He served in a variety of assignments while on active duty, including instructor in military medical history at the Academy of Heath Sciences and chief of the Army Medical Department doctrine literature branch, Fort Sam Houston, Texas. He currently works as a Lessons Learned Analyst at the Army Medical Department Center and School, Health Readiness Center of Excellence, Joint Base San Antonio–Fort Sam Houston, Texas.

Foreword

THE PRIMARY MISSION OF ARMY MEDICINE is to support the warfighter. Fundamental to that mission is our ability to provide trauma resuscitation or surgical capabilty on the battlefield. During the most recent era of combat operations in the US Army Central Command area of responsibility, our trained and ready medical providers contributed to a survivability rate of 92%, the highest in the history of warfare. Surgical capability employed far forward was a key component in achieving these survivability rates. To build on these accomplishments, we look to the past, to provide lessons learned and document innovative advances, in order to best prepare for the next conflict. To that end, this book examines the history of forward surgery.

The authors have focused on tracing the evolution of forward surgery in the US Army, but the scope of this book also encompasses the history of the Army Medical Department from the Revolutionary War to the present. The chapters describe the progression of care to wounded, injured, and ill Soldiers from very rudimentary procedures and methods 2 centuries ago, to the advanced medical and surgical technologies now available. The latest in Borden Institute's historical series, this book adds to our knowledge of how military medicine advanced during the nation's history, detailing a new aspect of our medical legacy by examining the changes in forward surgery.

As documented in this volume, the lessons of past conflicts can easily be forgotten, only to be rediscovered during the next war. Today, Army Medicine has made a renewed effort to utilize past experiences and apply historical lessons to develop new and improved combat casualty care capabilities. Newly developed procedures must be responsive to operational needs and effective in a Joint/Combined environment characterized by expeditionary operations and minimal, if any, preestablished health service infrastructure. This volume speaks to the courage, dedication, and selfless service of Army healthcare professionals from this nation's earliest days to the present. In the challenging times faced by our nation and military today, Soldiers and their Families can continue to rely on the Army to provide responsive medical capabilities and the most advanced care to our wounded, injured, and ill Soldiers, Department of the Army civilians, and their Families.

                NADJA Y. WEST
                Lieutenant General, US Army
                The Surgeon General and
                      Commanding General, USAMEDCOM

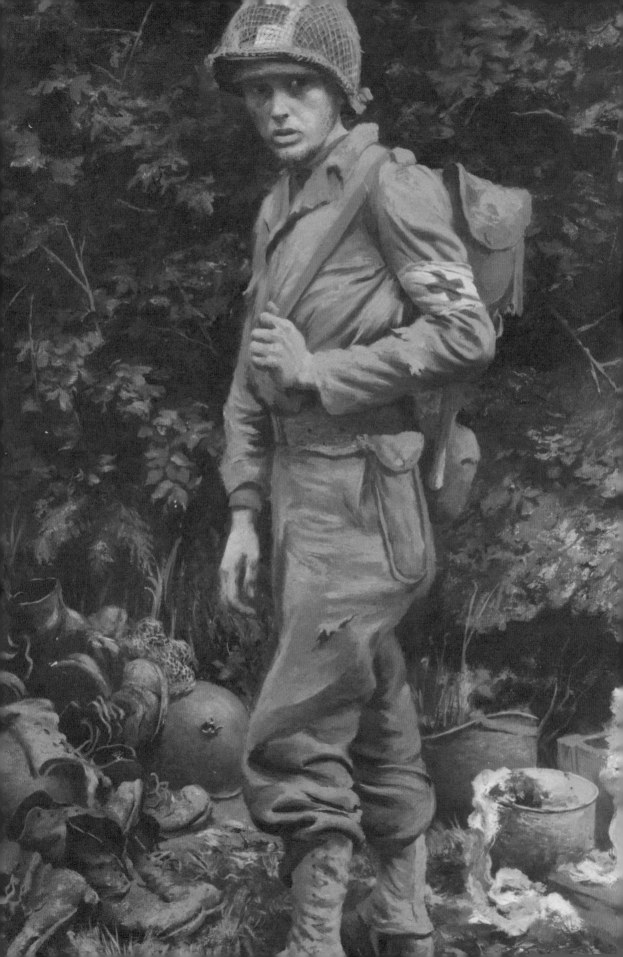

Introduction

THIS BOOK ORIGINALLY WAS CONCEIVED as a history of the evolution of the mobile Army surgical hospital (MASH) into the modern day forward surgical team (FST). Dr Dale Smith, Professor of Medical History and the former Senior Vice President, Uniformed Services University of the Health Sciences, Bethesda, Maryland, wisely suggested that the scope of this writing be expanded to the evolution of forward surgery in the Army in the 20th century and now the 21st century. Once the active editing of the book began, the subject was expanded again to include all the wars fought by the United States from the Revolutionary War onward.

The evolving story of forward surgical care begins during the Revolutionary War. The Medical Department of the Continental Army was created by the Continental Congress in July 1775. At that point there was only a poorly defined organizational structure (largely manned by Massachusetts physicians and surgeons), which had few funds with which to buy basic medicines or supplies. The British medical system was in many ways a role model for the Americans because many of the colonies' senior surgeons had experience with the British during the French and Indian War. Most physicians were trained by the apprentice system or self-trained; only a few American surgeons had attended either a foreign medical college or one of the two in existence in America. The American system had to deal with inadequate manpower, shortage of funds and supplies, and inadequate central administration throughout the entire conflict.

Following the Revolutionary War, the American aversion to standing armies and taxes led to the extreme downsizing of the Army, which was to be replaced by militias and volunteer organizations. Only by 1789 had some semblance of an army returned. The period from 1789 up to the War of 1812 featured a small military organization deployed on the frontier to deal with Indian incursions.

In the War of 1812, there had been little change in field surgery since the Revolutionary War. Surgery was directed to the removal of a bullet or shrapnel. The continued shortage of doctors hindered medical care for the wounded. The many diseases afflicting the troops were treated by the often inadequate methods available at the time. A notable exception was the smallpox menace, which was reduced due to the advent of Jenner's vaccination method.

[Opposite] Lawrence Beall Smith's *The Man Without a Gun, Normandy 1944*, personifies the unselfish service of the medical personnel of all wars to save the lives of other soldiers. Artwork courtesy of the Army Art Collection, Image #13-151-45.

The period between the War of 1812 and the Civil War featured always limited budgets, isolated posts, and a constant battle against Indians and diseases such as typhoid, cholera, malaria, and yellow fever. Indian conflicts included the Blackhawk War, and the First through the Third Seminole Wars. The Mexican-American War required dealing with more illness and casualties due to the increased scale of conflict. After that conflict, Army medicine returned to isolated posts on the frontier keeping the Indians in check.

The Civil War caught the medical departments of both the Union and the Confederacy in an unprepared state. The scale of the troop dispositions and consequent casualties forced change. Doctors William Hammond (as Surgeon General) and Jonathan Letterman brought progress. Hammond advocated improved hospitals and supported Letterman's ideas about the use of ambulances in the evacuation and treatment of the wounded. The medical care of the time included surgical procedures for amputations of more serious extremity wounds, removal of musket balls, dressings for minor wounds, and bandaging and splinting of fractures, along with the use of better analgesics including alcohol, opiates, chloroform, and ether.

The period after the Civil War witnessed shrinkage of the Army and consequent reduction in medical assets available to the smaller Army. Aside from occupation duty in the South and a brief war scare with Mexico in the face of French intervention, Army medicine reverted to the care of small isolated garrisons. The varied Indian wars featured small numbers of casualties, often treated away from permanent medical facilities. Advances in medicine helped Army medicine at the end of the 19th century. The onset of the Spanish-American War and the later challenges of distant warfare in such places as the Philippines and China showed that Army medicine could respond. Army medicine brought advances in infectious disease understanding and treatment through the works of leaders such as Walter Reed, William Gorgas, and George Sternberg.

The period of the new 20th century leading up to World War I featured the 1916 Mexican border incursions and slow preparedness for involvement in the European war, which had started in 1914. Leaders such as Doctors George Crile and Harvey Cushing, as well as liaisons with the British and French, helped awaken America to the challenges ahead.

World War I was the first truly modern war in all of its devastation. The World War I experience with mobile surgical hospitals was noteworthy in a war that quickly became immobile on its fighting fronts. The need for forward surgery was clearly seen in this conflict due to the high-velocity weapons and explosives effects, which produced massive numbers of traumatic injuries. The war's surgical hospitals and relays of surgical teams worked to perform the many operations required under these conditions. Many famous surgeons, such as Cushing and Crile, contributed to US medical readiness and to the care of American and Allied casualties.

The Spanish Civil War proved to be a testing ground for military medical advances, in addition to the obvious trials of advanced weapons and tactics. Tetanus vaccine (introduced in 1931) found use in the war. Sulfonamides found a war use for the first time in the Spanish conflict. The stage was set for World War II.

The US Army in World War II created the portable surgical hospital (PSH) to meet the specific needs of the China-Burma-India (CBI) and Pacific theaters of operations. The PSH was a direct attempt to provide forward surgery as close as possible to the front lines under austere environmental conditions. The PSHs accompanied the troops through jungle terrain, set up in tents and other field expedient shelters, and provided surgical care for patients until they could be evacuated to rear medical treatment facilities. The PSHs could be moved within hours as needed. They were staffed with 37 personnel, consisting of four medical officers and 33 enlisted men, with a 25-bed patient capability. The PSHs worked well and were eventually deployed to all theaters; however, the European PSHs arrived after fighting ended there. The PSHs often had younger and less experienced surgeons than those assigned to the larger hospitals in the rear, despite the lessons from World War I that experienced surgeons should be forward. World War II saw the increased use of antibiotics (especially penicillin), improved blood banking, and enhanced surgical techniques that resulted in a dramatic decrease in died-of-wounds (DOW) rates from the previous wars.

The Korean War MASH was an outgrowth of the field surgical hospital units employed in the European theater and the PSHs in the CBI and Pacific theaters. The concept was to provide high-level surgical care as far forward as possible. The MASH was approved for development in 1945; five MASH units were created on paper between 1948 and 1950. However, they were not ready when war came in 1950. The MASH designation was an early war use; units were officially designated as "Surgical Hospital (Mobile Army)." Advances made in Korea included improvements in anesthesia, management of shock, and vascular surgery. Units were also set up to deal with renal insufficiency.

The success of the MASH in the Korean War led to its use in the Vietnam War. Helicopter medical evacuation, used for the first time toward the end of World War II, saw extensive use during the Korean War and became the norm in Vietnam as medical evacuation helicopters picked wounded soldiers directly from the battlefield and sped them to medical facilities, within minutes in many cases. Advances in wound management along with the proximity of the battlefield to hospitals, improvements in blood banking, and better vascular surgery techniques were a few of the advances that enabled so many soldiers to survive. The Army DOW rate dropped from 3.5% in World War II, to 2.5% in the Korean War, but rose to 3.3% in Vietnam War.[1] The rise in the Vietnam War DOW rate was due in large part to the widespread use of helicopter evacuation. This rapid transportation got the very seriously injured soldiers quickly back to hospitals. These were the men who in previous wars would have died on the battlefield. Unfortunately, some were so gravely wounded that even rapid transport could not save them; thus the slightly higher DOW rate in Vietnam.

The Persian Gulf War saw the first use of the deployable medical systems (DEPMEDS) equipped hospitals that consisted of shelter systems, generators, and environmental control units, along with modular medical and dental materiel sets. Although a vast improvement over the Vietnam-era Medical Unit, Self-Contained, Transportable (MUST) equipment used in combat zone hospitals, the weight and size of the DEPMEDS hospital units limited their mobility in the Persian Gulf War. MASH units could not keep pace with the combat units and were forced to leave much of their surgical and bed capacity behind when they had to move forward. Lessons from Operation Just Cause in 1989 in Panama, and the 1990–1991 Persian Gulf War, led to the development of the forward surgical team (FST) concept to meet the need for a small, easily deployable surgical facility that could perform trauma surgical procedures on US casualties from the moment fighting begins.[2] The first two FSTs were fielded in the early 1990s and consisted of personnel and operating room equipment, generators, and medical supplies capable of being parachuted in at the same time. This delivery system enabled the FSTs to provide wounded paratroopers immediate access to life-saving trauma operations at the start of combat operations. The highly mobile FSTs each consisted of 20 personnel and equipment necessary to perform 30 life-saving operations in 72 hours. This was more robust and capable than the surgical squads and surgical detachments that the rapid deployment divisions and corps of the era had employed during Operation Just Cause and Operation Desert Storm (1990–1991). The new FSTs were initially deployed to various missions in Central and Eastern Europe and throughout Africa before supporting combat brigade-size units during the wars in Iraq and Afghanistan. These units proved their value in saving lives. The FST concepts continue to evolve in the Global War on Terrorism, which continues under different names and in different areas of the world. The ongoing terrorism threat will continue to challenge the Army Medical Department. The challenge of homeland defense and future contingency operations will require new thinking in forward surgery.

Future innovations in the FST design will enhance the mobility, scalability, and flexibility of the Army's forward surgical capability to meet any threat scenario. The goal is to create a forward surgical capability that consists of five key tasks: (1) mission command, (2) advanced trauma management (including damage control resuscitation), (3) surgical services (including damage control surgery), (4) postsurgical/anesthesia and critical care services, and (5) ancillary support services.

This volume chronicles how forward surgery on the battlefield has evolved to this point and the way forward. Just as there will always be wars, there will always be a need and an obligation to provide the most immediate care possible for those who are wounded or injured.

REFERENCES
1. Neel S. Hospitalization and evacuation. In: Neel S. *Vietnam Studies: Medical Support of the US Army in Vietnam 1965–1970*. Washington, DC: Department of the Army; 1991: Chap 4.
2. Thomas RW. *Ensuring Good Medicine in Bad Places: Utilization of Forward Surgical Teams on the Battlefield* [research project]. Carlisle Barracks, PA: US Army War College; 2006: 13–14.

THIS BOOK IS DEDICATED TO THE
FIRST-LINE MEDICAL PERSONNEL WHO FREQUENTLY
PULL THE WOUNDED BACK FROM THE EDGE OF DEATH,
STABILIZE THEM ENOUGH TO TRANSPORT,
AND THEN SEND THEM ON TO THE NEXT ECHELON OR
LEVEL OF CARE WITHOUT EVER KNOWING
IF THEY ULTIMATELY LIVED OR DIED.
THESE ARE THE MEDICAL PERSONNEL
WHO SELFLESSLY SERVE FOR THE BETTERMENT OF
THEIR FELLOW SOLDIERS.

Chapter One

Casualty Care From the Revolutionary War to the War of 1812

LANCE P. STEAHLY, MD

INTRODUCTION

AN OVERVIEW OF THE REVOLUTIONARY WAR will help the reader understand the role of military medicine in the conflict. The American Revolution was the culmination of years of grievances and a growing sense of distance from British rule in the American colonies. As Savas and Dameron point out in their book, *A Guide to the Battles of the American Revolution*,[1] the coalition of states (or colonies) had a common cause in the American Revolution, but had many differences on almost every major topic.[1(pxxv)] While the English were consumed with their own conflicts during the English Civil War of the 1640s, the colonies were left on their own, for the most part.[2(p485)] When the colonists were on their own, their tendency to independent action and mind was reinforced. Years later, the colonists felt that they had contributed to the winning of the French and Indian Wars because they had contributed much manpower and financial aid to bring about victory. The French and Indian Wars were only the North American part of a worldwide conflict. The colonies felt pride in their contributions, but felt that their efforts were not appreciated by the British. The British felt that the colonies should largely pay for their own defense.

EARLY CONFLICT

Antagonisms Increase

The British imposed a series of taxes on the colonists, in part to pay for Colonial defense and to recoup British expenses during the French and Indian War. The Americans were burdened also with the Sugar Act, the Currency Act, and the Quartering Act. In 1767, the Townsend Acts were passed by Parliament and fanned the cry "taxation without representation." The Navigation Acts, and later the Intolerable Acts, were particularly unpopular. The Navigation Acts started in 1651 and were renewed at various intervals.

These acts restricted use of foreign shipping for trade and precluded the colonies from direct trading with foreign countries. The Intolerable Acts (known as the Coercive Acts by the British) were punitive acts passed in 1774 in response to the Boston Tea Party that occurred on 16 December 1773. The Coercive Acts had many punitive consequences for the colonies, which were greatly resented by them. The most egregious sections included the following: (1) appointed Royal officials would not be held accountable locally for criminal misdeeds; (2) Massachusetts governance was suspended and elected officials were replaced with appointed British authorities; (3) British troops were billeted locally in seized private homes; and (4) the Port of Boston was closed until the Crown received restitution for the lost tea.[2(p2)] The Restraining Act in 1775 was yet another grievance. The act, also known as the New England Trade and Fisheries Act, was approved by King George III in March 1775. This act limited Colonial access to the North Atlantic fisheries and restricted New England to trading only with British sources.[2(pp486–487)]

The famous "shot heard 'round the world" happened at Lexington, Massachusetts, on 19 April 1775. The rebellion, which evolved into the Revolutionary War, was a major conflict. The Americans initially relied on ad hoc militias, but soon found it necessary to field their own army to contend with the British. The Americans who fought at Lexington and Concord were New England militia. However, these militia units went on to form the core of the Continental Army. The national army became known as the Continental Line.[1(ppxxiv–xxv)] The nascent army positioned outside occupied Boston had mostly makeshift regimental hospitals available to deal with the wounded. In the Boston area, the only hospitals available were those managed by Massachusetts in Cambridge, Roxbury, and Watertown.[3(p51)]

After the famous encounter at Lexington and Concord, the 1,800 Redcoat troops were harassed by farmers from Lexington to Boston. During the trek, some 273 casualties (73 killed, 174 wounded, and 26 missing) were sustained by the British. The Americans had 49 killed, 41 wounded, and five missing.[1(p5)] The colonists then sealed off Boston, beginning the siege of the city, on 19 April 1775.[1(p6),4(p3)] The British had occupied Dorchester Heights, so the rebels decided to occupy Bunker Hill, and later Breed's Hill, to balance the British move.[4(p4)] Boston was a well-established American city surrounded by a number of small towns including Roxbury, Charlestown, Dorchester Heights, and Cambridge.[1(p7)] Men from Massachusetts, Connecticut, and New Hampshire made up the American contingent. New Hampshire's troops were always short of supplies, especially ammunition. Their commander, Lieutenant Colonel Isaac Wyman, sent to Cambridge where a little powder was found along with lead from the church's organ.[4(p12)] The Americans were given a new confidence after their fighting skills had been amply demonstrated at Breed's Hill. Dr Joseph Warren (Figure 1-1), a physician and leader of the Boston contingent, was killed there. The British left Boston for Halifax on 17 March 1776, ending the siege of Boston.[1(p7)] The army that Washington had for the siege of Boston was composed of soldiers whose enlistment was over at the end of the year. The Continental Congress had selected Washington as the Commander of a Continental Army, which was created on 14 June 1775. Washington pushed Congress to rely on a long-term army with specific periods of enlistment, rather than militia forces. He urged Congress to provide funding and legislation to support a standing army based on the British and European model.[1(p7)]

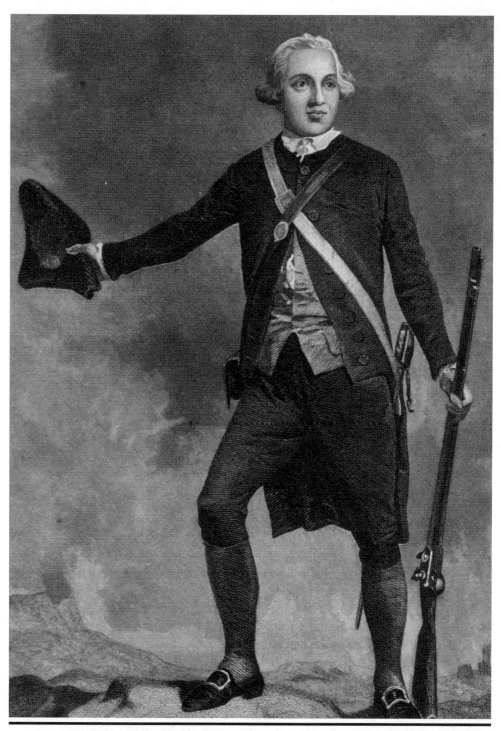

FIGURE 1-1. Joseph Warren. A Boston physician, Dr Warren was a leader of troops in the early Boston conflict with the British at Bunker Hill. Artwork courtesy of the National Library of Medicine, Image #B025354.

Continental Congress Responds

The chronology of the actions of the Continental Congress echoed the rising popular sentiment against Britain. The First Continental Congress convened in Philadelphia, Pennsylvania, on 5 September 1774 and submitted a petition for redress to King George III. After the battles of Lexington and Concord on 19 April 1775, the Second Continental Congress convened in Philadelphia on 10 May 1775. Jefferson and Dickinson produced for Congress on 6 July 1775 "The Declaration of the Causes and Necessity of Taking up Arms."[5(p15)] King George III issued a proclamation on 23 August 1775 declaring the colonies to be in rebellion.[5(p16)] On 26 October 1775, the king addressed Parliament, saying he would seek foreign alliances to suppress the colonists. By 9 November 1775, Congress was informed that the king would not receive its "Olive Branch Petition."[5(p16)] The Declaration of Independence was approved by Congress on 4 July 1776 and then sent to the printers. New York, the sole hold out, voted on 9 July 1776 for independence. The actual signing of the declaration took several months, starting on 2 August 1776. By January 1777, the declaration was fully signed.[5(pp17–19)] There was but one way forward for the colonies.

Continental Army Created

The American Continental Army was created officially by the Continental Congress on 14 June 1775. The following day, George Washington was selected to lead the nascent forces gathered around Boston as the beginnings of the Continental Army.[1(ppx–xvi)] As noted by Wood in his book, *Battles of the Revolutionary War, 1775–1781*,[4] George Washington's contributions to the war effort included brilliant leadership and planning at Trenton and Princeton in the Christmas period of 1776. Wood points out that his good work then was counterbalanced by inept handling at Brandywine only 9 months later (September 1777) when Washington was outmaneuvered by the British and forced to retreat. Howe then moved his Army closer to Philadelphia, which forced the Continental Congress to abandon the city.[4(ppxvi,92–114)] In his evaluation of George Washington (as interpreted by John SD Eisenhower in his Foreword), Wood described an inexperienced officer in the French and Indian War who evolved into a mature and capable officer who learned from his experiences and losses.[4(pxvii)]

Savas and Dameron point out in their book, *A Guide to the Battles of the Revolutionary War*,[1] that the state militias participated together with the Regulars in most conflicts. However, in some battles, such as the 1781 South Carolina battle at Kings Mountain, a combination of militiamen from several southern states were victorious over the British.[1(pxxv)]

In his recent essay in the *Journal of Military History*, Hall speaks to the idea that Washington preferred Regular troops rather than the militia due to the militias' indiscipline, irregular methods of fighting, and being incapable of offensive operations.[6(p970)] Hall notes that Washington utilized his Regulars for training and offensive operations. Washington kept his Regulars just beyond the reach of the British. Hall points out that Washington rarely defended terrain or the people living there. However, the militias' operations did help set the stage for Washington's Princeton and Trenton successes.[6(p979)] Hall notes that Washington did (despite his views) regard the militia as part of his defensive strategy.

He would fault them largely for their inability to wage the grand war (*grande guerre*) as opposed to the small war (*petite guerre*). Hall comments that the "British and their German allies were perhaps more impressed with the militia than was Washington [who was focused on the militias'] inconstancy and indiscipline."[6(p980)] These irregularities made matters of planning for supply and medical facilities/medicines problematic.

The numbers of soldiers in militias varied, but the total numbers of the Continental Line Army reported by Secretary of War Henry Knox in 1789 ranged from a low of 27,443 (1775) to a high of 46,891 (1776). By 1781, only 13,292 were reported.[1(px)] Washington followed the British organization in setting up his forces.[1(ppxlviii–xlix)]

Expanding the Battlefront

The Revolutionary War wasn't just fought on land that would ultimately become part of the new United States. Indeed, the Americans launched an attack on Canada after being emboldened by the capture of Fort Ticonderoga on 10 May 1775 and of Crown Point on 12 May 1775. Washington envisioned the bold plan to capture the British Canadian Capital of Quebec as a way of subduing the interior of Canada. He selected General Benedict Arnold to lead an attack from the Maine area. Montreal was taken and then General Richard Montgomery and Benedict Arnold combined forces to attack Quebec.[7(pp151–152),8(p211)] The attack was carried out in a driving snow storm, during which Arnold was wounded. A year later, in May 1776, the Americans withdrew after an unsuccessful siege attempt, which effectively ended any further Canadian ventures for the duration of the conflict.[1(pp15–16)] The conquest of Canada was for many a way to gain a fourteenth colony.[7(p5)] Anderson, in his book *The Battle for the Fourteenth Colony: America's War of Liberation in Canada, 1774–1776*,[9] believes that the goal of the Continental Congress, which dispatched an ideologically based invitation to the Canadian Quebec Province, was for Quebec to join the American rebels, rather than being a defensive campaign to shore up the colonies' weak border. Anderson feels that this venture was America's "first war of liberation," which he views as anytime when America sought to relieve/liberate an oppressed people.[9(p2)]

Washington's Successes and Failures

Washington's Army was to suffer a number of losses, which imperiled morale and brought up more questions about Washington's leadership skills. The Battle of Long Island, 27–29 August 1776, was a significant loss for the Americans.[1(p55)] After the American Army defeat on Long Island, the British waited to see if negotiations would occur. General Sir William Howe met with John Adams, Benjamin Franklin, and Edmund Rutledge at his headquarters on Staten Island in September 1776. The meeting, called the "Staten Island Peace Conference," did not succeed in ending hostilities.[1(p62)]

General Howe's forces then invaded New York proper, beginning in September 1776. (General Howe's forces had previously taken Staten Island in June 1776.) Additional reinforcements from Halifax arrived for the British, which included German mercenaries (Hessians).[10(p143)] The Americans eventually abandoned Long Island with a rear guard action at White Plains in October 1776.[10(p149)] The American General Nathaniel Greene had to be replaced, due to a high fever, by General Israel Putnam. General Howe's victory sent the American morale to new lows; Washington's fitness to lead was further questioned.[1(pp55–61)] The New York Campaign, from September 1776 to November 1776, involved fighting at Kip's Bay, Harlem Heights, and Fort Washington. Washington was criticized for overextending his forces. The result was that New York was secured as a British stronghold until the end of the conflict. The series of defeats there seemed to show the world that the rebellion was near its end.[1(pp61–68)] The British tactical win at Germantown (part of the Philadelphia Campaign) on 4 October 1777 allowed the British to maintain control of Philadelphia, with the British fleet controlling the Delaware River.

After these successes in the autumn, General Howe placed most of his troops in winter quarters. Howe directed General Charles Cornwallis to continue to pursue Washington, who had escaped to Pennsylvania from New Jersey. Cornwallis placed troops at various points in New Jersey. He also placed Hessians at Trenton and Burlington.[1(p82)] Who were these "Hessian" hired mercenary troops? The Hessian troops actually came from six states in Germany: the majority (12,805) came from Hesse-Cassel. The Regiment *von Knyphausen*, the Regiment *von Lossburg*, and the Regiment *von Rall* were all from Hesse-Cassel and were to play a role in Washington's attack on Trenton.[1(ppxlv–xlvi)] Brunswick (4,300) supplied the next largest number. Anspach-Beyreuth (1,285) followed the two states. Hesse Hanau, Waldeck, and Anhalt Zerbst all supplied much smaller numbers of troops.[1(pxliv)] The German contingent was an important part of the British forces. It should be recalled that the King of England and the prior Hanoverian monarchs were German in origin. At the conclusion of the Revolutionary War, 29,000 German troops had served the British cause. The troops were professionally trained and had a strong tradition of excellent service. The troops provided much needed revenue for themselves and the leaders of the independent German states.[1(pxliv)]

One of Washington's more famous successes occurred when he was able to subdue Hessian regiments at Trenton, New Jersey. The Hessian commander there, Colonel Johann von Rahl, was known to like drink and celebration, as well as bands and parades. Hence Christmas Eve was selected as the date to launch the American attack, hoping the celebrating Germans would let their guard down. Washington formulated a plan involving a water crossing on 24 December 1776, to be followed by a 9-mile march to reach Trenton. As the result of the successful attack, two of the best Hessian regiments (the Regiment *von Rall* and the Regiment *von Lossberg*) surrendered, but the Regiment *von Knyphausen* escaped to try to warn the British about the Americans. Between the two captured regiments, Washington and his troops had 948 prisoners,[10(pp166–169),11(pp118–119)] but they had to reach Princeton before the escaping Hessians did. The third Hessian regiment was subsequently located and driven to a creek, and gave up shortly thereafter.[12(pp303–304)] The Americans defeated Howe's troops left at Princeton before Cornwallis could intervene with his forces. The Trenton victory has been regarded as the first meaningful Continental victory of the war. Washington gained 40 horses, six artillery pieces, and 1,000 muskets, along with valuable supplies. The material gains were great, but the morale lift was even greater.[1(p87)]

The victory over the Hessian regiments at Trenton added luster to the Continental cause.[4(pp51–61,69–70)] One Hessian officer said that he and his troops had not slept one night in peace. Colonel von Rahl, one of the Hessian commanders, had been mortally wounded in the fighting at Trenton. Certainly these factors added to Washington's chances of success.

Many Hessians were captured and taken to Philadelphia where there was British criticism of their treatment.[13(p355)] One effect of the 10-day Colonial victory celebration at Princeton and Trenton was that militia volunteers became numerous. In fact, there were so many volunteers that Washington couldn't handle the numbers, despite gaining all of the Hessian supplies. The victory at Trenton was a turning point for Washington's reputation, which had been threatened by the popularity of American General Charles Lee.[13(p274)]

Washington decided to move his troops some 20 miles away from the British at Philadelphia to Valley Forge. His 6-month encampment there in the winter of 1777 tested the young Continental Army in the extreme. Washington designed the 14 x 16 foot log cabins himself. The cabins housed the majority of soldiers, but some tents were needed. Supplies became very scarce there, with shortages of food, clothing, and feed for the animals.[12(p356)] Typhus was common. The polluted water led to cases of typhoid and dysentery. Food shortages were such that "fire cake" was the main staple. It was a mixture of flour and water cooked on heated firestones. It has been estimated that of the approximately 10,000 troops who went to Valley Forge, 2,500 died during the period, and another 2,000 deserted.[12(p357)] It was at this point in the war that a group of officers, including Horatio Gates and Thomas Conway, worked against Washington, suggesting to Congress that he was a weak leader who should be replaced by Gates. The support of Marquis de Lafayette, with his connections at the French court, greatly helped Washington's cause during this difficult winter period.[12(pp365-368)] (While encamped at Valley Forge, there was also an issue with the poor discipline of doctors, especially in regard to their frequently taking leaves and furloughs. Washington had to order that only leaves signed by Director General John Cochran would be honored.[3(pp86-87)] Cochran was the physician in charge of the Valley Forge "flying hospital," which consisted of two huts per brigade. General Washington requested that the soldiers be hospitalized as close as possible to camp.[3(pp85-87)])

THE WAR CONTINUES

Other Major Battles of the Revolutionary War

British General John Burgoyne provided a victory for the British with the capture of Fort Ticonderoga, on 6 July 1777, which caused morale issues among the Continental forces in the north. The American defenders included many inexperienced militia members under the command of the American General Arthur St Clair.[12(pp324-325)] Ethan Allen and Benedict Arnold had captured the fort originally in 1775. Ticonderoga was located on Lake Champlain between New York and Quebec Province. At that time, the New Englanders won control of the lake, which could be viewed as a way to the heart of Canada.[10(p107)]

However, at the Battle of Bennington, on 16 August 1777, a Tory/German mercenary force was defeated by the Americans. The American Northern Army (a part of the Continental Army but designated as a specific command) was first commanded by Phillip Schuyler and later Horatio Gates. Burgoyne was later defeated at Saratoga by the same Northern Continental Army. British forces under Burgoyne's command included British Regulars, Hessian and Brunswick German troops, Canadians, and Indians.[14(p245)] The

American Northern Army relied on volunteers entirely.[14(p9)] Logusz makes the case that there was varied ethnic makeup of the American forces.[14] He describes some 30 languages and dialects used within the Northern Army.[14(p10)] He also addresses minorities and women in the conflict. He even mentions that a group of "400 armed women rallied to defend Pittsfield, Vermont."[14(p13)]

The Americans suffered another defeat on 11 September 1777 at the Battle of Brandywine as part of the Philadelphia Campaign. The American casualties were significant with the loss of 1,100 men.[1pp115–120] Lafayette received a leg wound at Brandywine, and was taken to Bethlehem, where Moravian sisters cared for him. Lafayette wrote to his wife that the wound healed quickly due to his excellent care at the orders of General Washington.[12(p347)] After his wounding, Lafayette, who was a major general, was given his own command by Congress upon Washington's recommendation.[12(p348)]

The British defeat at Saratoga on 19 September 1777 had far-reaching consequences, in that an entire British Army had been subdued. Among the British officers taken captive were six members of Parliament. The British and Hessian prisoners were sent to Boston, while the captured Canadians were returned to Canada.[15(p256)] Ketchum views Saratoga as the watershed event in the fight for American independence. He points out that because of the American win at Saratoga, France entered the war as a Colonial ally.[13(p1)] The famous Jonathan Trumbull painting of the surrender at Saratoga, titled "The Turning Point," shows British General Burgoyne offering his sword to General Gates, who subsequently returned it. Not only did Gates return the sword, he also invited Burgoyne to dine with him in his tent.[10(pp197–198)] However, Corbett, in his book, *No Turning Point: The Saratoga Campaign in Perspective*,[16] written after examining archival sources, describes Saratoga as a stage in a civil conflict that continued and that little changed for people in the region. Corbett describes civil discord going back at least 15 years, with animosity between the local inhabitants of New York and surrounding states. Furthermore, there were residents loyal to England as well as those favoring independence. The larger group just wanted to be left alone. He did not see Saratoga as a "turning point." Corbett feels, instead, that British General Burgoyne's plans were altered by the civil war in the region.[16(p5)]

After the events at Saratoga, the wounded of both sides were numerous. It is noteworthy that the Indian allies of the British inflicted cruel wounds.[15(pp257–258)] Indeed, the wounded that fell into the Indian allies' hands after Saratoga were often tortured before being scalped and killed. Duncan cited a case of a Captain Gregg, who survived scalping and other wounds despite being left for dead.[15(p258)]

Logusz also points to one factor contributing to the British defeat: General Howe decided to move his troops, normally based in New York, to Philadelphia rather than north to join Burgoyne.[14] Saratoga, a village west of the Hudson River, provided natural positions of strength for the Americans. Burgoyne's forces were defeated at the battles of Bemis Heights and Freeman's Farm. The Americans encircled the British, leading to their surrender on 17 October 1777.[14(pp14–16)]

The French were awaiting such a triumph as that of Saratoga to provide a basis for assistance. The French were more concerned with causing problems for England after their losses in the French and Indian Wars. After signing a treaty with America on 6 February 1778, the French formally recognized America's independence on 4 May 1778.[1(plxiii)]

The Spanish also provided financial and material support for America, starting in 1776. In 1779, the Spanish attacked the British in Louisiana, Mississippi, and west Florida. Spanish naval forces supported land forces in the capture of Pensacola and the Spanish naval presence allowed the French to participate in the Yorktown campaign.[1(pplxvi–lxvii)] The siege of Pensacola, from 9 March 1781 to 10 May 1781, was a factor in Great Britain's defeat that is often overlooked. Spanish Governor Galvez won victories that secured Pensacola, navigation on the Mississippi River, and the Caribbean. As Savas and Dameron point out, "the multi-national effort at Pensacola was eerily similar to what General Cornwallis was about to face in Virginia at Yorktown."[1(pp302–303)] As these authors also note, in both campaigns, a siege on land was coupled with control of the seas to bring about the surrender of the British.[1(pp302–303)]

Naval Battles

Although the majority of writings about the Revolutionary War focus on the battles on land, the conflict also involved naval engagements. However, the Continental Congress had few naval assets of its own available. To remedy this deficiency, the Continental Congress issued commissions for privateers (private shipowners granted license to wage war). The privateers had limited successes against British warships and merchant vessels, but they did provide transport for French and Dutch supplies.[2(p487)] All matters improved when the French signed the Treaty of Amity and Commerce in 1778 with the colonies. This signing happened after the American successes on the Great Lakes with vessels under the command of Benedict Arnold.[2(p487)] After the Americans' naval victory on the Great Lakes, General Howe returned to England, turning over the command to General Clinton. Hearing of a rumored French fleet coming, Howe ordered the evacuation of his troops from Philadelphia and a return to New York.[2(p487)]

Other Battles to Consider

The tactical draw that resulted from the Battle of Monmouth Court House (in Monmouth, New Jersey) on 28 June 1778 was the last major battle in the Northern colonies for the rest of the war. Monmouth was the longest continuous battle of the war (lasting from 10:00 AM until 6:00 PM) with the largest artillery exchange of the war. Even if the Battle of Monmouth Court House was not a resounding victory, the ability of an American Army to meet a British Army as an equal had come.[1(p177)] For this battle, the British and the Americans each had approximately 15,000 troops. The British reported 65 killed, 170 wounded, and 70 missing, while the Americans had 70 killed, 161 wounded, and 131 missing. Several churches and the courthouse of Monmouth were used as makeshift hospitals.[15(p268)]

Because there was promise of a strong loyalist contingent in the South, the British turned their attention there. North Carolina had a varied population but many were loyal to England. Tory forces and British Army recruits were organized in the state.[15(p310)] The Siege of Savannah, Georgia, from 16 September 1779 to 19 October 1779, ended in disaster for the French and Americans. The French Admiral d'Estaing was wounded and his French Marines sustained significant losses. Admiral d'Estaing was unhappy with the performance of the American troops, led by Major General Benjamin Lincoln. The loss of

French confidence led d'Estaing to withdraw and to sail his ships and men back to France after the defeat.[1(pp227-232)] In a repeat loss, the Siege of Charleston, South Carolina, of 18 April 1780 to 12 May 1780 was a serious loss for French and American forces. It brought a worldwide loss of confidence in the American cause. As an example of the fallout from the loss, the Spanish had declared war against England in June 1779, but delayed a formal alignment with the Americans.[1(pp233-237)]

The British and the Americans both suffered significant illness in the Southern climate. Indeed, both armies in the Carolinas were ill with "[m]alarial fevers and diarrhoeas not usually fatal."[15(p311)] In fact, it was reported that the British General Cornwallis was himself ill at one point. It was speculated that he had malaria.[15(p312)] In a letter to General Henry Clinton, Cornwallis wrote that the climate in South Carolina was so bad within 100 miles of the coast from June until the middle of October that British troops could not be stationed there during that time without being rendered useless due to illness.[15(p312)] It was not just on land that the troops were ill. American prisoners (after the defeat of General Gates in 1780) were held on prison ships where illness prevailed, especially smallpox and dysentery.[15(p319)]

The Battle of Cowpens, South Carolina, on 17 January 1781 represented a victory for the American General Daniel Morgan, which raised morale in all parts of the country. Clark describes it as "the most brilliant single victory of the Revolutionary War."[12(p495)] Morgan defeated the forces of General Banastre Tarleton, one of the more notorious British commanders, while escaping with his forces into North Carolina to join General Nathaniel Greene and his American troops. Cornwallis tried to catch Morgan, but Morgan's successful exit into North Carolina precluded Cornwallis's catching up.[1(pp281-282)] The Battle of Guilford Courthouse, North Carolina, on 15 March 1781 resulted from the pursuit. The British held the field but lost 25% of their force. General Greene's forces survived with presumably fewer casualties. A large number of the American missing were said to be militia that left when the fighting ended.[1(p291)]

The Yorktown, Virginia, campaign was a major victory for the French-American forces.[4(pp262-263,268-269)] At Yorktown, the French fleet caught the English on one side, gaining control over the Chesapeake Bay, and blockading Cornwallis from British naval support. The Continental Army caught the English on the other side, coming down from New York City. This forced Cornwallis to surrender.[1(p488)] The Siege of Yorktown lasted from 28 September 1781 until 18 October 1781. On 19 October, the British and Hessian troops defending Yorktown surrendered. Although it showcased Washington at his best, the French contribution was critical to his success. This victory meant the end of fighting in the North and Middle States (aside from minor skirmishes), although the British remained in New York until 25 November 1783.[1(p336)] The French thereafter withdrew any financial support because they became financially stretched with the major costs involved in a conflict with the British. The Dutch stepped in to offer loans, with the American John Adams pushing the concept.[12(p552)] After Yorktown, the fighting was limited to local fighting and two battles. In present day Kentucky, the Battle of Blue Licks took place on 19 August 1782. The other major battle, the Battle of Arkansas Post, transpired on 17 April 1783 in Spanish Territory (Louisiana and West Florida).[1(pp337-343)]

Revolutionary War Casualties

In the period 1775 to 1783, approximately 184,000 to 250,000 men were estimated to serve in the various American forces, including the militias. Of the recorded casualties, the Defense Casualty Analysis System lists 4,435 died and 6,188 as wounded within the Regular forces.[17] As Savas and Dameron point out, however, these numbers do not include militias, which had significant casualties.[1(ppxxvii–xxviii)] Reliable numbers for British, German, and Indian forces are not available. Peckham, in his 1974 *The Toll of Independence: Engagements and Battle Casualties of the Revolution*,[18] reported 7,000 Americans died in battle and 10,000 died of disease.[18(p130)]

The Continental Army's Medical Department

The Continental Army's Medical Department was created by the Continental Congress in July 1775. The inexperienced staff had to contend with no existing infrastructure, little funding for medicines and supplies, and a poorly defined organizational structure. The Continental Congress did not deal with the expansion of the department beyond Massachusetts, so as to define the reporting relationships of the heads of hospitals to the Director General and Chief Physician (who was appointed as the nominal head in July 1775). Congress established the "Hospital for the Army," which was, in fact, to be the Army Medical Department.[19(p25)] Massachusetts' surgeons and facilities were being used for the Continental Army that General George Washington took command of on 3 July 1775. As Gillet points out, only legislation passed by Congress in April 1777 and later in March 1781 gave the Director General authority to supervise all medical services.[3(p23)]

In September 1775, the Continental Congress created the Medical Committee to deal with medicine shortages. Its role expanded with the participation of Dr Benjamin Rush, until he lost his bid for reelection to Congress in 1777. A Medical Committee in various iterations remained until its functions were taken over by the Board of War in May 1781.[3(p23)]

The terms used for the highest authority in the Medical Department varied over the course of the Revolutionary War. The office of "Director General and Chief Physician" was established in July 1775. In September 1775, in addition to the office of Director General, another Director General and a Chief Physician in the North were added. In June 1776, a Director General and a Chief Physician in the South were added to the Medical Department. The relationship of these offices to the main Director General was unclear.[3(p23)] In August 1777, in addition to the Director General, a Director of the Hospitals in the South was appointed. In September 1780, a Deputy Director General for areas south of Virginia was named. The reporting schemes for these various medical officers were unclear for much of the time. The distinction between physicians and surgeon generals was to remain until 1780.[3(p37)] Finally in March 1781, a Director General was named along with a Deputy Director in the South.[3(p23)]

THE BRITISH MEDICAL SYSTEM—TO BE EMULATED

By 1660, the English King, Charles II, had created a standing Army and a standing surgeon staff. The British surgeons purchased their positions and could also serve in combat. Of interest, the British soldier had to pay for his own medicines. Later, Winston Churchill's ancestor, John Churchill, the Duke of Marlborough, developed regimental aid stations.[20(p4)]

The British had an enviable number of medical leaders to provide tradition for the provision of medical services to their military. The relationship of American and British medicine was further enhanced by the fact that many of the Colonial medical leaders had studied at London, England, or at Edinburgh, Scotland. The Hunter brothers were an example of this. Dr John Hunter was renowned for his pioneering and controversial operations. He achieved some notoriety for his methods of securing anatomical parts for which he was said to pay above the norm for materials.[21(p5)] Among his accomplishments, he had removed a massive tumor from the neck of a coachman.[4(p3)] John Hunter had also removed a popliteal aneurysm,[21(p7)] devising the technique with input from his brother, William Hunter. The Hunters used a dog to research the procedure.[21(p8)] It is rumored that they also completed a successful appendectomy in 1789.[22(p13)]

A number of important Revolutionary War physicians spent time in London with John and William Hunter. William Shippen,[3(p38)] appointed the Director General (charged with leading the department) of the Continental Hospital Department on 11 April 1777, studied with the Hunters after gaining his MD degree from Edinburgh.[23(p40)] John Morgan, an earlier Director General, studied with the Hunters after receiving his MD from Edinburgh.[23(p11)] John Cullen of Edinburgh was another European medical luminary who was sought out for training by many students.[3(p19)]

The colonies had only the British medical system as a role model. To that end, it is of interest that a number of the influential doctors in the Continental Hospital Department had prior service with British and Colonial troops in the French and Indian War. This experience helped prepare them, to some extent, for the events ahead. They also gained familiarity with the British system, which had not changed appreciably by the time of the Revolutionary War. John Morgan, a Director General, was a surgeon in the war. John Cochran, also a Director General, was a surgeon's mate in the French and Indian War. Cochran was apprentice trained in England.[23(p41)] Ammi R Cutter, later a Physician General, served with the British forces at Louisburg in the French and Indian War and on the Indian frontier with the rangers.[23(p41)] Samuel Stringer, a Director of Hospitals in the North, served in the British Army in the regular forces. James Craik, a Chief Physician and Surgeon General of the Army, had trained in Edinburgh and served in the French and Indian War. Dr Philip Turner, later in charge of the Eastern Department, served as an assistant surgeon with General Jeffrey Amherst at Ticonderoga in the French and Indian War.[23(p43)]

There were some deficiencies in the British system. For instance, at the time of the Revolutionary War, the British had no regular bearer troops to carry the wounded; furthermore, the British were always short of wagons.[16(p8)] The British soldier had a portion of his pay deducted to pay for the surgeon. Each regiment (approximately 550 men) had one surgeon and 12 assistants.[20(p4)]

In many areas the Continental Army Hospital Department attempted to emulate the British system. One of the earliest handbooks consulted by the British and the Americans, detailing the treatment of wounded soldiers, was published in 1758 by Baron Gerhard Von Swieten, titled *Swieten's Diseases Incident to Armies*. Reiss points out that it filled the same need as the *Merck Manual* in modern times. Treatments were outlined in the manual. It was thought to be most useful when a surgeon was not available and the care of the sick was left to whomever was there to minister aid.[3(p4)]

Of note, in contrast to the American Army, a British physician had to be a graduate of one of the great European medical colleges or of the College of Physicians of London. However, the requirement to be a surgeon was less rigorous.[15(p18)] For example, regimental surgeon commissions were purchased as were other Army commissions. The purchase funds were paid to the retiring officer, which served for him as an annuity or retirement fund. Duncan quoted cash payments for regimental surgeon positions—one example was £150. Positions were purchased for rates as high as £500 to £600.[15(p18)] At this time, the practice of medicine was sharply distinguished from that of surgery. The physicians were presumed to treat the sick in general hospitals, while the regimental surgeon treated the wounded soldiers in regimental hospitals. In practice, there was less distinction.

John Hunter reformed the purchase system in 1790 (but the old system returned after his death in 1793[15(p18)]). The regimental surgeons were not eligible for promotion, which made the required purchase less desirable. Hunter mandated that the highest positions could be filled only by men who had seen prior service. Hunter also removed restrictions on promotions for regimental and higher surgeons (but that also ended with his death[15(p18)]).

The leadership of the British Medical Service was in the form of a council, consisting of a physician general, a surgeon general, and an inspector general. These men were chosen from the famous or favored London professionals, and were not necessarily experienced Army medical officers.[3(p20),15(p18)] The council members were actually civilians, which would be unexpected for a military system.[3(p20)]

A typical British army as fielded would consist of 20,000 to 30,000 men who would be divided into divisions of 4,000 to 5,000 soldiers. The fielded army would have an inspector general, while the divisions would each have an inspector. The regimental surgeons had no real rank, although they had commissions. They were ranked with the chaplain and listed after the lowest-ranking ensign.[15(p19)] The British intended that each regiment would have its own surgeon. In wartime, the regimental surgeon would have two assistants, along with a tent or house for a hospital. In the French and Indian War, the British found that a sergeant and two orderlies were needed to maintain order in the larger hospitals.[3(p20)] Most surgeons preferred the small regimental hospital instead of a large general facility due to the presence of many sick in the latter. It was noted that disease mortality and morbidity were actually increased in the larger facilities.[15(p20)]

A general hospital was set up in existing facilities for the army, while the regiment would have a small hospital in a building such as a church. Tents were the choice of last resort. The typical general British hospital would have 400 beds, with six medical officers and 48 assistants, clerks, and nurses. The officer group would be composed of a physician (with two assistants) and a surgeon (with two assistants), as well as an apothecary to provide the medicines. Apparently the assistants were hired because there were no enlisted medical troops in the British Army.[15(p19)] No special areas were designated for surgical operations generally. A room in a house or a designated tent in a field might be used for surgery.

The British provided wine as a part of the daily ration for all troops. Duncan comments that the free-flowing liquor in the hospital cost more than the bread ration. Aside from bread rations, the patients ate much the same fare as the regular troops. Often the rations were obtained locally by foraging sweeps and could include chickens, pigs, cattle, and available fruits and vegetables in season. Generally, the menu was not varied or nutritious.[15(p20)]

THE AMERICAN MEDICAL SYSTEM

The American medical experience is difficult to evaluate because, as Gillet points out, there were few surviving official records until 1814. She speculates that the few records kept were lost by fire in 1800 or in the 1814 British burning of Washington, DC. Much of the records extant were kept in state archives or in private records and correspondence. Gillet's book, *The Army Medical Department 1778–1818*,[3] provides an excellent coverage of the Revolutionary War medical issues.[3(pxi)]

In America at the beginning of the Revolutionary War, there were only two medical colleges—one in New York City and the other in Philadelphia, Pennsylvania. They were closed during the war because both New York and Philadelphia were under British occupation at various times in the war. However, they had only had 50 graduates total prior to the onset of hostilities. Apprenticeships of varying lengths with practicing physicians were the norm for most.[15(p7)] As already noted, some of the prominent medical men, such as Rush, Shippen, and Church, studied in European medical colleges such as at Edinburgh in Scotland.[15(p8)]

Most surgeons/physicians did not have the benefit of a European course of study leading to a formal medical degree. Indeed, most were either apprentices (studying 3 to 7 years with a mentor) or self-trained.[3(p1)] The majority of the surgeons entering Colonial military service had no prior experience, unlike the British, with the exception of some surgeons who had served with British or Colonial forces in the French and Indian War.[3(pp19–20)] Gillet points out that during this time the traditional humoral explanation of disease was beginning to lose its appeal. The humoral medicine approach had been given great prestige by Galen, to the extent that it lasted until the 18th century. The humoral approach posited that health and disease were determined by the presence of the four body humors—blood, yellow and black bile, and phlegm—and their relationship with the four elemental humors—fire, air, earth, and water.[24(p10)] In its place, conflicting ideas for competing systems attempted to use fact rather than theory to explain disease. While diagnosis was gaining momentum, the treatments all were still reduced to bleeding, blistering, and purging.[3(p1)]

The Dutch system devised by Hermann Boerhaave placed emphasis on chemical and physical qualities to explain disease. He used qualities such as acid and base, or tension versus relaxation, instead of the humors. Boerhaave felt that nature should be used to aid in any cure. However, William Cullen, of the University of Edinburgh and the mentor to many Revolutionary War surgeons, challenged that view, instead favoring the approach of nervous tension underlying disease.[3(pp1–2)] Cullen felt that an excess or debit of nervous tension would cause a disease. A fever meant an excess of nervous tension, which would be dealt with by bleeding, purges, restricted diets, and sedation. A chill would mean a lack of nervous tension, which called for restorative methods.[3(p2)] Specific diseases were not singled out, but Cullen called for their study. In time, Benjamin Rush would somewhat modify Cullen's approach and advocate limited study of each disease as an entity. In general, however, Rush applied Cullen's principles in a rigid fashion.[3(pp2–3)]

Hospitals in America and Organization of Continental Medicine

As previously noted, only two civilian hospitals existed in America in the colonial period. One was in New York City (hospital founded in 1711) and the other was in Philadelphia (hospital founded in 1755). As with many other philanthropic efforts, Benjamin Franklin was involved in the Philadelphia effort.[15(p8)] Nonetheless, hospitals in the colonies and in Europe had high death rates, which is not surprising given the lack of antibiotics and the dearth of knowledge about human physiology and disease processes.[15(p9)]

The history of the hospital department of the Army started with the siege of Boston in 1775. After the Battle of Breed's Hill in Boston, a hospital was established in Cambridge within private homes. Director (Doctor [Dr]) John Warren was placed in charge of the hospital.[23(p4)] [Note that these physicians were referred to both as a Director and a doctor, hence Director (Dr) in the text that follows.] The Second Provincial Congress ordered "that the President pro tempore, Doctor Church, Doctor Taylor, Doctor Holten and Doctor Dunsmore be a committee to examine such persons as are, or may be recommended for Surgeons for the Army."[23(p4)] In a screening of 16 applicant surgeons, six were rejected.[23(p4)]

A letter, or warrant of appointment, was issued by the Provincial Congress of Massachusetts Bay recognizing the status of the military surgeons. In 1775, General Washington had accepted appointment as Commander-in-Chief. The Colonial Provincial Congress provided for the appointment of general officers and officers of the general staff, but made no provision for the creation of a hospital department.[23(p6)] General Washington wrote a letter about the lack of a hospital litter and Congress passed a resolution after a committee provided in a bill that they would approve the appointment of one Director General and Chief Physician (pay of four dollars per day). Four surgeons were to be appointed (at one-and-a-third dollars pay per day). Furthermore, one apothecary would be employed at the same rate of pay per day. Twenty surgeon's mates were to be selected with pay of two-thirds of a dollar per day. The bill also provided for the appointment of one clerk, two storekeepers, one nurse, and laborers as needed.[23(pp6–7)]

The necessity for a reorganization of the Hospital Department was increasingly apparent by 1780. The inefficiencies of separate departments with their own hierarchies were finally dealt with in the reorganization plan put to Congress. The resolution to accomplish this renovation before Congress was presumably the work of Director (Dr) John Cochran. The most important piece of the plan was that the Medical Director was to have centralized authority and would have three assistants. The separate departments and their staff were abolished. A "flying hospital" (a field hospital) was to go with the Army and the Medical Director was to remain in the field. This was a response (and a rebuke) to Director (Dr) Shippen, who was always seeking comfortable lodgings.[15(pp329–330)]

Congress appointed surgeons to the battalions in New Jersey and Pennsylvania at a monthly pay of $25. They later added that each regiment should have a surgeon's mate, paid $18 a month. Congress did this because most regiments were raised by various states without regard to the provision for medical attendance. In the winter of 1775 to 1776, very severe weather was experienced. At the time, there was the appearance of smallpox in the north. The troops of the middle and southern states presented with typhus, typhoid fever, and dysentery.[23(p14)]

As troops were being assembled in the late summer and early fall of 1775 for an invasion of Canada,[3(p57)] a new and separate department was considered necessary—the Northern Department. General Philip Schuyler was given command.[3(p57)] However, a smallpox epidemic had struck the Northern Department troops in Quebec in the spring and summer of 1776, with particular severity.[3(p59)] An attempt was made to start an inoculation program, which was not successful. The American men at Sorel and Montreal numbered 3,200, of which 1,900 were ill with smallpox. Smallpox threatened to destroy the Northern Army before the invasion plans were cancelled because the force required evacuation. In fact, the epidemic was so widespread that Major General (MG) John Thomas, who commanded at Quebec, died of smallpox.[3(p60)] The surgeons were unable to obtain medical supplies and medications (including opiates), which would have been of little use in dealing with the epidemic.[3(p62)] The only treatment for the pox was isolation.[3(p74)] Interestingly, the British Army did not have smallpox, but it reportedly had significant dysentery.[3p63]

The colonies varied in their responses to smallpox. Maryland, for instance, advocated inoculation and offered to pay for it. On the other hand, The Council of Massachusetts asked that the practice be stopped after hearing that MG Ward was allowing inoculation of troops outside Boston. Inoculations were banned in Boston because it was feared that those inoculated would spread smallpox. The official Continental Army order to inoculate all troops came in February 1777, although Virginia would not allow its troops to be inoculated. Washington ordered segregation of recently inoculated troops, and was thus able to reverse the Virginia policy after he wrote personally to the Virginia Governor, Patrick Henry.[3(p75)] The mortality rate from this inoculation effort was reported as four of every 500 Continental soldiers inoculated. The rates of infection for noninoculated troops were quite variable but could involve the majority of the contingent. Washington ordered the inoculations repeated at Valley Forge in 1778.[3(p75)]

As discussed in John Morgan's *A Recommendation of Inoculation According to the Baron Dimsdale Method*,[24] the inoculation method used in America was styled after the Dimsdale or Sutton methods of the English, which required an arduous 2-week period of preparation, consisting of purges, bleeding, and the use of mercury. The inoculation involved taking a piece of tissue from a pox lesion of an active human case and placing it in a puncture wound, thereby introducing the foreign tissue.[25] Arnold Klebs wrote an involved history of the evolution of variolation, which showed much experience leading up to the procedure as practiced in the Revolutionary War.[25] The use of mercury in the preparation period involved its own toxicities, as Cochran pointed out in 1772.[3(p14)] (It is now known that complications include mercury-induced cognitive impairments such as inattention, excitement, and hallucinations. In addition, there also can be neuronal damage and cerebral infarctions.[26] Vaccination would come after Jenner's work in 1798, with the American Army finally ordering vaccination for all of its soldiers in May 1812.[3(p14)])

Several categories of hospitals existed in the Continental system. The "Regimental Hospitals" were built and run by regimental surgeons for their own regiment. The "Flying Hospitals" were temporary and perhaps more mobile facilities, often located in a hut or a tent with a few beds and a surgeon's table. They were run by Continental Army personnel. The "General Hospitals" were run by Continental personnel located in more stable (less combat) locations. These were not dedicated facilities in the modern sense, but rather were conducted in homes, churches, government buildings, or college buildings.[23(pp25,26)]

Surgeons/Physicians of Note

JOHN JONES

Rogers, in an article published in 1972 in the *Plastic and Reconstructive Surgery—Journal of the American Society of Plastic Surgeons,* clearly felt strongly about the Revolutionary War contributions of Dr John Jones. He states in his article that, "Our knowledge of Revolutionary War surgery comes to us exclusively from one man, John Jones . . . a New Yorker by birth, [who] was and should be rightfully called [the] 'Father of American Surgery.'"[27(p1)]

Jones studied medicine under his father and later studied in England (under John Harvey's direction), Scotland (Edinburgh), and France (Paris).[15(p23)] Jones received his degree in medicine from Rheims (in France) in 1751.[15(p18)] Jones was a founder and the first full Professor of Surgery of the Medical School of King's College in New York City. For a surgeon, such a position was not possible in European medical schools or in Philadelphia (the other American medical center). Distinct chairs of surgery did not exist because of the subservient role of "surgeons" to "physicians" of the times.[3(p1)] Jones' manual of surgery, *Plain Concise Practical Remarks on the Treatment of Wounds and Fractures,* was the first surgical text published by an American in what would become the United States. The treatise was published in 1775; two editions were later printed in 1776 and, posthumously, in 1795.[27(pp1–2)]

Jones made a number of recommendations. For example, most compound fractures called for amputation as the prevailing standard of practice. In gunshot wounds, he suggested removal of the ball; to deal with bleeding he suggested a ligature. The British used a smooth bore musket that had a ball about ¾ inches in diameter.[15(p13)] The musket could cause significant damage within its 100-yard range. As in later conflicts, the bayonet was used infrequently and there were few artillery wounds. Due to the use of Indian fighters by the British, there were reported a number of knife, hatchet, and club wounds.[15(p12)] Jones recommended expanding the opening of many wounds. For chest or abdominal wounds, however, bleeding was often excessive and the prognosis was grim.[15(p12)]

BENJAMIN CHURCH

Director (Dr) Benjamin Church was selected as the first head (the Director General and Chief Physician) of the Hospital Department of the Army.[3(p26)] Church was appointed through an act of Congress dated 17 July 1775.[15(p60)] In addition to being a prominent physician, he was a member of the "Sons of Liberty." Church was also described as a poet who wrote "liberty songs."[3(p26)] He had graduated from Harvard College in 1754 and studied medicine with Dr Joseph Pynchon, a prominent Boston physician. Church then went on to study medicine in London. He later practiced in Boston. Church became a member of the Continental Congress in 1775, and a member of the Committee on Public Safety.[15(pp61-62)]

The wounded and sick were being cared for in 30 or more hospitals. Massachusetts' surgeons were generally the only ones to work with Church because he was from the state. Church felt that general hospitals were more efficient; he did not trust the care provided in the small regimental hospitals. The regimental surgeons would complain to their Army commanders whenever the general hospitals would not give them medicines. Church got Washington to support the general hospital concept but the controversy continued.[3(p27)] Washington said that a soldier who was too ill to stay in camp should be sent to the general hospital.[15(p62)] Washington established a Court of Inquiry within each brigade to call on the regimental surgeons and the Director General to testify as to their views. However, the inquiries did not proceed because of Director Church's arrest (as detailed in the following paragraphs).[3(pp27-28),15(pp62-63)]

Church's term was also beset with controversy as to the reporting structure for the newly appointed Chief Physician and Surgeon for the Army in the Northern Department. Dr Samuel Stringer had been so appointed by the Congress, although his exact status vis-a-vis Church was not spelled out by the Congress.[3(p27)] Church had so many complaints filed against him that General Washington had to seek an investigation; inquiries were conducted at the brigade level. Church felt the regimental hospitals were too expensive to operate (as well as inefficient), and that their supplies should largely be sent to larger hospitals, which added to the political rumblings.[3(p28)] Before the various disputes could be resolved, Church was arrested on charges of treason because he was trying to pass correspondence to the British in Boston.[3(p11)] Church had written a letter in cipher to a British major and given the letter to a young woman to transmit. The letter was taken from her and indirectly given to General Washington.[15(p63)] A Reverend Ward was able to decode the letter, which described disposition of American forces, but its total reading was not viewed as rising to the level of treason.[15(pp63-64)] Still, Church was removed from office and placed in confinement for a period. When he was released, he set sail from Boston, but the vessel apparently sank. Church's wife applied to King George III for a pension, stating that Dr Church was, in fact, a loyalist.[3(p28)] Congress replaced him with Director (Dr) John Morgan of Philadelphia. A noteworthy suggestion of Church's was his urging that special units for convalescents be set up because there was a very high relapse rate after soldiers were released from the hospital.[15(p62)]

JOHN MORGAN

Director (Dr) John Morgan (Figure 1-2), from Pennsylvania, had graduated from the College of Philadelphia in 1757.[15(p65)] He then studied in Europe in 1760 with John Hunter, and later spent time in France and Italy. Morgan obtained a Doctor of Medicine degree in Edinburgh in 1764. When he returned to America, he was elected the first Chair of the Theory and Practice of Medicine in the newly formed medical school in Philadelphia. He held the position until he died in 1789.[3(pp28-29)]

Morgan was selected by the Congress on 17 October 1775 to be the next Director despite General Washington's preference for Dr William Shippen. Morgan took more than a month before he reported for duty, even though Washington implored him to promptly report for duty because the medical situation required urgent attention.[3(p29)] Morgan also experienced the same conflicts between the general hospital and the regimental hospitals as did Church. Morgan saw his role to be that of increasing the efficiency and organization of hospital medical care. However, it was felt by some that Morgan was stockpiling medicines and supplies rather than releasing them to the regimental units.[3(pp30-31)] Like Church, Morgan ran into problems with Dr Stringer, who was attempting to carve his own independent niche.[3(pp32-33)] The intrigues and charges came from a number of sources, but especially from Shippen. Morgan had prepared his rebuttal of charges.[28(p826)] Congress did not resolve the controversy, but instead created another Physician and Director General for a system based in Virginia as a way of avoiding more controversy.[3(pp32-33)] Congress dismissed Morgan on 9 January 1777.[3(p35)] Although he was eventually cleared of any charges of wrongdoing in 1779, Morgan was not reinstated.[3(p35)] While he did receive vindication from Congress, he failed to resume his prior leadership role in Philadelphia by not resuming his professorship and subsequently resigning from the staff of the Pennsylvania Hospital.[28(p826)]

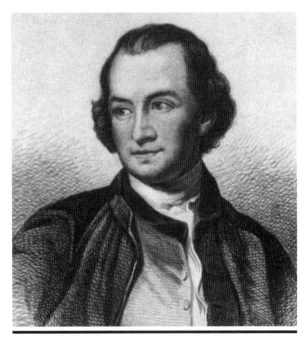

FIGURE 1-2. John Morgan. Despite the fact that General George Washington preferred another candidate, Congress appointed Dr John Morgan as the Director in the fall of 1775; he left his post in early 1777, amid accusations of misconduct. Although he was exonerated in 1779, Morgan did not regain his post. Artwork courtesy of the National Library of Medicine, Image #B019169.

BENJAMIN RUSH

Director (Dr) Benjamin Rush (Figure 1-3) is perhaps the most famous of the physicians/surgeons of the Revolutionary War period, in part because of his overall impact medically and politically. Rush was one of the 56 signers of the Declaration of Independence, for which he is today remembered.[29(p8)] Although he was not the head of

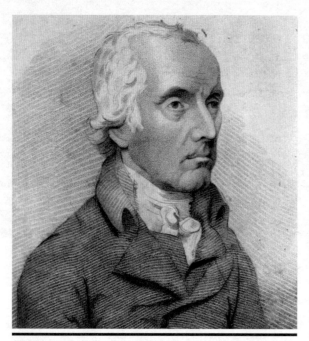

FIGURE 1-3. Benjamin Rush. Dr Rush remains the most famous of the physicians/surgeons of the Revolutionary War period because of his overall impact both medically and politically. Rush was a member of the Continental Congress and served on its Medical Committee. Artwork courtesy of the National Library of Medicine, Image #B022631.

the Medical Department (but was appointed to head the Middle Department), Rush had great influence due to his professional reputation and his position as a member of the Continental Congress, as well as being one of the physicians on the Medical Committee of the Congress.[29(pp8–9)]

When Benjamin Rush was just 6 years old, his father died. Rush then studied at the school run by his maternal uncle. He graduated at age 14 from Princeton, from which he received a bachelor's degree in 1760.[29(p11),30(p24)] After an apprenticeship with Dr John Redman (a leading physician and apothecary) of Philadelphia, which ran between 1760 and 1766, Rush attended medical courses at the University of Pennsylvania, during his last 2 years as an apprentice. Dr Redman advised him to study further in Europe. Hence, Rush went to the University of Edinburgh,[30(p46)] where Director William Cullen was his mentor. Of interest, Benjamin Franklin, who had been in London representing the Colonies since 1764, provided a reference for Rush to the Edinburgh faculty.[30(p43)]

Rush returned to Philadelphia in July 1769 and joined the Philadelphia militia in 1775. He took care of the militia sick and wounded in various encounters around the Philadelphia area. There are no totals on the numbers involved or of the sick and wounded.[30(p59)] Rush offered his services to Washington's forces after the Continental Congress adjourned in 1776. Rush and John Cochran took care of the wounded at Trenton, New Jersey, before Washington moved to Princeton, New Jersey.[3(p72)] The wounded were moved by Rush and Cochran to Bordentown, New Jersey, and later Princeton, after they obtained wagons. (In contrast to Rush, Cochran had a more rudimentary training, first as an apprentice trained in England and later service as a surgeon's mate in the French and Indian Wars.[15(p333),23(p42)])

Rush was appointed to the Congressional Medical Committee in August 1776. The committee was set up "to devise ways and means for supplying the Continental Army with Medicines,"[3(p23)] but became involved with hiring and firing of medical personnel and other details of operation. Rush was not reelected to Congress in February 1777 and therefore left the committee.[3(p23)]

As part of Rush's plan to reorganize the Army medical services (in his role as a Congressional Medical Committee member), Director (Dr) John Morgan was removed and Director (Dr) William Shippen was named the new Director General of the medical department. Dr Benjamin Rush was then named the Director General of the Middle Department of the Army on 1 July 1777. The Middle Department's jurisdiction extended from the Hudson River in New York to the Potomac River, south of Maryland. Rush held the position for over a year.

Rush then became a chief medical officer of the area that was under the personal command of George Washington, although he was not the overall director.[31(p177)] Rush was officially appointed as Physician General of the Middle Department of the Continental Army.[30(p200)] Rush reported to Director Shippen and to his deputy, Director Thomas Bond Jr. Rush reported to Morristown, New Jersey, where the winter quarters of George Washington's troops were located.[30(p181)] Rush was stationed at Princeton but he moved constantly around military hospitals scattered throughout New Jersey to supervise the attending surgeons and their staffs.

After the Battle of Brandywine, Pennsylvania, Rush had to deal with over 900 soldiers killed and 600 wounded. Rush led a group of surgeons into the British camp under a flag of truce granted by General Howe of the British forces to "dress the American wounded."[30(p187)] Rush was quite impressed by the way the British tended to the men, both the British and American wounded, in marked contrast to the way the Americans treated their own.[30(p187)] Rush stated that British officers went out of their way to make sure their surgeons treated the Americans and their own wounded well. He attributed this to the standards of their medical establishment.[30(p188)]

Rush became involved in the controversy over the poor administration of the Army hospital, which was but one of many controversies in which he was involved. Rush reported on Shippen's many failures[30(p189)]; the controversy ultimately led to Rush's 1778 resignation. Much of the controversy involving Army medicine was due to infighting within the Continental Congress.[30(p177)] However, Rush's involvement in controversy in many areas really did not help the Continental Army's cause. In that regard, Rush was also said to have engaged in criticism of General Washington.[30(p209)]

After the war, Rush was named in October 1789 to succeed Morgan as the Professor of Theory and Practice of Medicine in the College of Philadelphia. He continued to make contributions in many areas of medicine. Rush initially endorsed William Cullen's view of disease as involving disordered nervous tension,[30(p49)] but later modified it somewhat, although it remained essentially Cullen's. In fact, Rush was said to think of himself as Cullen's chief disciple.[30(p49)] Rush called for treatment to include purges with calomel (mercury chloride) and jalap (a purgative), and bleeding until the patient fainted.[3(pp2-3),30(pp254,341)] He recommended purges to begin the cure of all "febrile diseases."[30(p91)] Rush discussed the cause of yellow fever epidemic in Philadelphia in 1793 and spoke to fact that yellow fever and malaria were avoidable through proper hygiene and appropriate environment.[3(p3),30(pxvii)] To his great credit, Rush purged the Army formulary of many medications that he recognized as ineffective. He did so also for the civilian sector, purging the material medical of many remedies that simply didn't work or could cause serious side effects.

The fact that Rush advocated more progressive treatment of the mentally ill has been an often cited accomplishment that seems forward looking in scope as opposed to some of his other practices.[30(pxvii)] During his tenure, Rush was said to have trained more than 2,500 students who made their own contributions.[30(pxvii)] (In 1804, Rush learned that letters he had written critical of Washington had been received by John Marshall, who planned to use it in his written life of Washington. Rush protested to Marshall, who used the letters without Rush's name.[30(p375)])

WILLIAM SHIPPEN

The controversy and charges surrounding John Morgan led to his replacement by Director (Dr) William Shippen (Figure 1-4).[3(p40)] As with other privileged elites, Shippen graduated from Princeton, then studied medicine in his father's office for 3 years. At the recommendation of his father, he went to Europe to study medicine, where he lived in the home of Director (Dr) John Hunter, with whom he studied anatomy. He studied midwifery with his brother, William Hunter. He then studied at Edinburgh under Director (Dr) Cullen and graduated in 1761, after which he studied in France for a year. He ultimately became the professor of anatomy at a medical college in Philadelphia. Shippen became the head of a "flying camp," which was considered a more mobile field facility, at Trenton and later the head of all hospitals on the west bank of the Hudson River.[3(p40)]

Shippen came into his own criticisms, especially from Benjamin Rush, who was one of his more energetic critics.[30(p189)] Supplies were short and personal rivalries were prevalent. Shippen was especially under fire for continuing to teach anatomy and not devoting his time and energies fully to his military job.[3(p38)] Rush accused Shippen of selling hospital supplies for his own profit. In 1779, Shippen asked for courts-martial for himself to provide a forum to rebut the charges. The protracted proceeding was finally

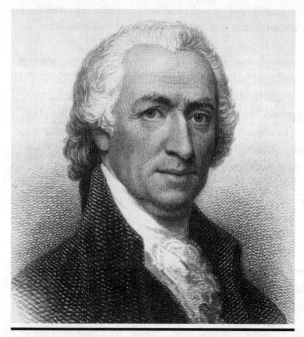

FIGURE 1-4. William Shippen. Prior to becoming the Director, Dr Shippen had been the head of a "flying camp" in New Jersey. Dr Benjamin Rush was an ardent critic and supported charges against Shippen, who requested a courts-martial in 1779. The lengthy proceedings were not finally settled until August 1780, resulting in no conviction. After the decision, Shippen was reinstated but resigned shortly thereafter.
Artwork courtesy of the National Library of Medicine, Image #B023782.

settled on 18 August 1780, with no conviction. Subsequently, Shippen was reinstated as Medical Director in 1780, but resigned on 3 January 1781.[3(pp42–43)]

JOHN COCHRAN

Director (Dr) John Cochran (Figure 1-5), appointed Director General of the Hospital Department in 1781, was the last of the medical directors during the Revolutionary War.[3(p44)] Cochran had been surgeon's mate in the French and Indian War, which gave him some military experience.[3(p44),15(pp333–334)] He had studied medicine as an apprentice with Director John Thompson of Lancaster, Pennsylvania. He was practicing in New Jersey when the war started. Cochran was an Assistant Director of a flying camp hospital in 1776, and in 1777 became the Surgeon General of the Middle Department. Cochran became the Chief Physician and Surgeon of the Army in 1780 before becoming the Director General in 1781 (after Director Shippen resigned).[3(p44)]

In the 1780 to 1781 period, severe shortages of supplies were experienced.[3(p45)] Robert Morris, appointed as the Superintendent of Finance, restored some order to Congressional finances, but it took the French supplement to alleviate the crisis.[3(p46)] Further help was on its way from France, which in 1782 sent supplies and gold,

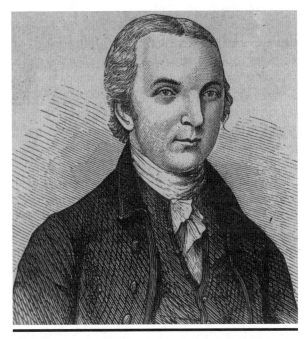

FIGURE 1-5. John Cochran. Cochran was the last of the medical directors during the Revolutionary War. Before the war had ended, he was ordered to start closing hospitals to save money. Cochran remained the Medical Director until Congress dissolved the Army in late 1783. Artwork courtesy of the National Library of Medicine, Image #B04815.

even though the war was winding down.[3(p46)] Pay was 2 years behind for both officers and enlisted. Financial difficulties had reached the point that Director Cochran could not afford to get to Philadelphia in performance of his oversight duties.[3(p47)] In an effort to resolve the situation, Congress issued some warrants for pay, which were devalued due to inflation. Attempts to deal with the inflation loss of income for medical officers led to warrants being issued to be filled by the states. New York refused to participate.[3(pp46,47)]

Cochran was ordered to start closing hospitals for financial reasons by the Board of War even before the British surrendered at Yorktown. He tried to delay the closure of the Boston and the Albany hospitals. Cochran remained until after the signing of the Treaty of Paris on 3 September 1783; Congress dissolved the Army on 3 November 1783. The Hospital Department existing during the war was replaced by an institution to aid the veterans.[3(p48)]

The American Soldier

For the Colonial Army, the recruits had to meet certain standards. Traditionally, men from the countryside were preferred because they were considered better able to handle the stresses of soldiering. The rural men were thought to benefit from the healthy country life with its hard work, availability of a more varied diet than the city dweller, and less exposure to the contagions of close living. The recruit was to be healthy and without obvious skin sores. Venereal disease, hernias, epilepsy, and alcoholism were to be avoided in the recruit.[23(p6)]

Benjamin Rush observed the British, Hessian, and American forces and concluded that men under 20 were more likely to experience "camp diseases,"[20(p6)] under which he included all diseases with fever as a common symptom (malaria, dysentery, various gastrointestinal illnesses, and typhoid, among others). During the war, Rush described many of his views regarding cleanliness and the proper environment for troops. Rush opined that Southern troops were more sickly than Northern troops, and that Native Americans were more sickly in the Army than foreign born. Rush concluded that the healthiest soldiers were above age 30. He dismissed the Southern troops for being ill due to "lack of salted provisions."[20(pp6–7)] In all armies, standards depend upon supply and demand. In the 18th century, infantry soldiers were to be at least 5 feet 4 inches tall while cavalry were to be 5 feet 3 inches to 5 feet 6 inches in height. The age range was to be from 18 to 40 years.[20(p8)] There was generally agreement that an army on the march was healthier than one in camp.[20(p11)] The problems that the permanent camps had in common were poor sanitation, animal and human waste, and contaminated water.[20(p11)]

At the start of the Revolutionary War, the men from Connecticut had the most liberal ration allowance. The weekly ration called for 1 pound pork or beef, 1 pound bread/flour, and 3 pints of beer. Weekly, the Connecticut soldier would also get rice, butter, peas, or other vegetables. Calorie counts were not available for the Continental soldier because the diet varied according to local availability.[20(p8)] The Continental Congress set out specifics for a daily ration. Feeding an Army on the march was a difficult problem. Rations, including meat, generally were salted for preservation. However, because most salt was obtained from Britain, the meat to be eaten had instead to be "driven on the hoof."[20(p7)] Rations could be supplemented with flour, which could be added to water and cooked on rocks in a fire (a concoction called "fire cakes" by the soldiers). Purchasing vegetables and fruits was difficult for the Colonial troops because farmers preferred the hard currency of the British rather than the Continental currency. In places like Valley Forge and during the first winter at Morristown, New Jersey, scurvy was common.[20(p9)] Food was seasoned only with vinegar and salt. Vinegar was used especially during the summer because it was believed that it kept away disease. Spruce beer (one of America's oldest beer styles, which utilized the distilled oils from local spruce trees, molasses, and dates, when available) was added to the diet to prevent scurvy.[20(p7)]

The Army's clothing was always an issue. For the Continental Army, standardized uniforms were late in coming to the war. Militias and the troops often wore whatever clothing they had on hand. Director Benjamin Rush recommended "that officers wear flannel shirts next to their skin rather than linen to protect them from fever and disease."[20(p10)] Director John Jones called for lighter clothes during the excessive heat of colonial summers.[20(p10)] Indeed, the ever-present threat of the heat was always a concern for the troops and the consequences could be dire. For example, at the Battle of Monmouth, New Jersey, 59 Hessians, wearing all-wool uniforms, died of heat exhaustion and sunstroke before meeting the Colonials.[20(p10)]

Van Swieten's *Diseases Incident to Armies* (originally published in 1758) was a useful guide to common diseases and their treatments. The book was published in 1762 in England, where it became available to Colonial outlets. The book was then published in Philadelphia and later Boston (1776 and 1777, respectively).[20] Specifics for the disposition of a camp were discussed. The camp was to be on dry land with a low water table and located away from the forest where animals of the forest could be a problem. Van Swieten described illnesses in early spring including sore throat, cough, pleurisy, pneumonia, and rheumatism. Bleeding and purges were featured in the treatments. He discussed jaundice, especially after prolonged or intermittent fevers.[20(pp12–14)]

Diseases of the day included dysentery, "camp fever," smallpox, and the most feared, putrid fever. Putrid fever included typhoid fever and typhus. (There is controversy concerning whether the doctors of the day could distinguish between them.[31(p232)]) Cures included mercury,[32] "Peruvian bark" (containing quinine) mixed with wine,[33] and salts.[15(p14)] Venereal diseases were common.[34(p59)] Dr John Hunter felt that gonorrhea and syphilis were both a form of the same disease.[34(p117),35(p450)]

In the Revolutionary War, diseases were the main nemesis for the military surgeon/physician. There really was no signature wound of the conflict other than an abundance of disease. There were certainly some wounds to be treated, but disease was the main issue. Musket wounds, bayonet and knife wounds, the assorted Indian arrow and tomahawk wounds, and attempted scalpings would otherwise occupy the surgeon.

Vaccination for smallpox wasn't available until 1798. (Vaccination involves the introduction of a vaccine functioning as an antigenic stimulus. The individual's immune system is prompted to form an adaptive immunity to a pathogen—bacterial or viral.) Inoculation (or variolation) involved the direct introduction of material from the pustule of a smallpox victim into another person. A milder form of smallpox would result with consequent immunity to the disease. Morgan didn't favor inoculation but his successor, Shippen, did recommend its use. As previously discussed, George Washington was apparently himself inoculated.[15(p16)]

The most common disease in the Colonies was termed "fever," thought by Boyd, writing in the *American Journal of Tropical Medicine and Hygiene,* to be malaria. It was endemic from New England to Florida.[33(p229)] The incidence of malaria was said to be increased during the Revolutionary War, perhaps related to the large numbers of people traveling in endemic areas. Malaria was an issue for the British, the Loyalists, and the Colonial regular and irregular forces without discrimination. Yellow fever had a terrible reputation for severity. Fortunately, yellow fever was endemic largely in the deep South, although outbreaks in port cities such as Charleston, South Carolina, also occurred.[23(p4)]

Fresh air was advocated for health; Benjamin Franklin was one of the major proponents.[3(p7)] Good air supply was central to planning for hospitals; it could be helped by high ceilings in buildings and by avoiding overcrowding. Use was made of the Hales ventilators (manually operated large bellows) to remove poor air. Eighteenth-century hospitals also used incense or burned berries or sulfur. Placing hospitals in forests was to be avoided because the air could not circulate as well under a canopy of trees.[3(p9)] Sanitation in hospitals meant scrubbing of floors, walls, ceilings, and bedframes. Straw was easier to change in pillows/mattresses than feathers, and felt to be cleaner and less expensive.[3(p9)] The British were also interested in avoiding overcrowding, providing good sanitation, and having sufficient air circulation and ventilation.[3(p20)] Mercury was often prescribed for pleurisy, inflammatory diseases, pneumonia, and rheumatism, but was increasingly given for an expanded list. Opium was also increasingly used, usually in the form of laudanum.[3(pp7–8)] Scurvy was the only recognized deficiency disease. James Lind had shown that oranges, lemons, and limes cured even the most severe cases of scurvy.[3(p11)] There may have been a recognition of cases attributable to scurvy as evidenced by large orders for lime juice in 1778.[3(p84)]

THE WAR COMES TO AN END

In the period 1778 to 1781, the majority of the operations of the Continental Army were in the South,[3(p101)] where malaria severely affected the Army. There were rumors that the British had used infected slaves to spread smallpox to the Colonials, but this was not confirmed.[3(p125)] A Corps of Invalids was established at this point (1782–1783) to deal with the convalescents. The fact that there was a general improvement of health in the period 1780 to 1783 spoke to inoculation for smallpox, and improved sanitation and discipline of the troops to follow health guidance.[3(p102)]

The wounded in the North were largely replaced with soldiers afflicted with diseases, which were not abated due to shortages of medicines and medical supplies. For example, in the period of 1777 to 1778, there were extreme shortages of lint (used for dressings) and bandages.[3(p83)] Moravian women in the North were tasked with making more lint to help with the diminished supplies. The shortage of medicine bottles was helped when the glass works at Manheim, Pennsylvania, was reopened to make glass bottles.[3(p87)] The shortage of surgeons' chests was also an issue. These chests, made from wood with felt linings, were to hold instruments such as scalpels and saws, and medicines. There was a controversy in the Medical Department as to the optimal size: large or small. The smaller chests won out because they were less costly to procure.[3(p84)] There were also shortages of surgeons because they were often prisoners of war. However, Washington reached an agreement with British General Frederick Howard, the Earl of Carlisle, that surgeons, surgeons' mates, and chaplains would not be treated as prisoners of war when captured. They would instead be returned to their respective lines when possible, otherwise they were not to be incarcerated if return could not be readily accomplished.[3(p47)]

In the waning days of the war, the British were largely quartered in New York City proper. The British had set up their fortress in New York because Washington had not stopped the British withdrawal to New York at the 1778 Battle of Monmouth. However, from November 1781 going forward, there was an unofficial truce in the area.[3(p123)]

At the close of the war, on 23 October 1783, the Hospital Department was replaced by an organization to aid the "invalids of the Army and Navy."[3(p48)] In 1783, after lobbying efforts, Congress agreed to provide the same pensions for physicians and surgeons as other officers.[3(p6)] As early as 1636, Plymouth Colony had passed a law to care for its soldiers injured in various wars with the Indians in the region. In 1776, Congress made provisions for pensions to invalid soldiers and officers. Officers were to receive half pay for total disability, and a proportionate amount for less, while enlisted received about $5 per month. Incomplete records and the ever-present lack of funds prevented payments to an estimated 6,000 wounded.[3(pp127–128)]

The success of the Revolutionary War was in question for much of the conflict. Lockhart highlights the importance of a number of men in the early pivotal times.[36(pp2–6)] Dr Joseph Warren was the principal organizer of the Massachusetts forces, but he was killed at Bunker Hill. General Artemas Ward was the field commander of those forces, but had to resign his commission due to illness. His deputy, Dr John Thomas, died of smallpox. All of these men were connected with the identification and resolution of numerous medical issues. One can only speculate about their impact had they not died prematurely.[36(pp2–6),37]

ADVANCES RESULTING FROM THE REVOLUTIONARY WAR

While there were no revolutionary medical/surgical advances that resulted from the war, there were, in fact, some advances. One advance that is not often appreciated was the use of various types of tourniquets. The crude tourniquet was replaced in 1718 with a screw type of tourniquet devised by the French surgeon Jean Louis Petit. Various types of ligatures and sutures were tried. The famed English surgeon John Hunter preferred "dry sutures" (the use of "sticking plaster"), except for penetrating injuries.[1(p16)] Amputations exposed the injured to more blood loss. The higher up on the extremity the amputation, the greater the risk of blood loss. Ligatures provided improved blood loss control over the previous use of cauterization.[37(pp101–103)]

Eichner, in a 2003 paper, noted positive effects coming from the Revolutionary War that included: (*a*) beginning principles of sanitation and hygiene were recognized; (*b*) steps in disease control were initiated; (*c*) importance of smallpox inoculation was established; (*d*) policy for battlefield treatment of the wounded, and the importance of the evacuation of those injured was recognized; and (*e*) initial efforts to structure a military medical department were made.[19(p32)]

AFTER THE REVOLUTIONARY WAR

The first Treaty of Paris, in 1763, ended the Seven Years War (the French and Indian War) and allowed the English to receive control of North America, and to neutralize French bases in India. The second Treaty of Paris, in 1783, ended the Revolutionary War, which also had global dimensions involving England, Spain, and France, as well as the financial involvement of the Dutch. The newly independent nation was now on its own.[38(p12)]

The American citizenry had an aversion to standing armies after the war. This aversion and suspiciousness was also fueled by a strong dislike of taxes.[23(p70)] The English aversion to standing armies can be traced to the English Civil War. The populace felt that standing armies could lead to loss of independence and more taxes because they would need to pay for the armies. Congress and the populace seemed to prefer militias to stand up when needed on the frontier. Thus the standing army of the war period would soon be gone, to be replaced by militias and volunteer units. By June 1784, only eight soldiers were left in the Continental Army. Seven hundred men were called up from state militias to form an active regiment for a 1-year period of service.[3(p130)] These troops were to secure the Northwestern frontier and to take possession of Western forts vacated by British forces. These were militia troops of the states and any surgeons were provided by the involved states.[23(p70)] There was no formal medical department during this period.[3(p130)] From 1785 until 1789, there was one surgeon and four surgeon mates to care for the next 700-man regiment.

After the Constitutional Convention was concluded in 1787, the first Congress (meeting in New York) created three executive departments while setting up the organization of the government. The War Department, the Treasury Department, and the Department of Foreign Affairs were the three departments. A formal Department of War was created in 1789.[3(p129)] The newly created Department of War was to be guided by MG Henry Knox as the Secretary of War in 1789. Knox had a small number of clerks to help him in the newly created organization. He first directed his attention to increasing the number of soldiers serving in the military.[15(p71)] The Indians were an issue in the West where British agents were stirring up trouble. A federal force of 700 troops was organized to serve there.[23(p71)]

Of interest, the three Secretaries of War that served between the Revolutionary War and the War of 1812 were all physicians (Henry Dearborn, William Eustis, and James McHenry).[3(p129)] In December of 1792, the Army was reorganized into a legion, with four sublegions (1,280 soldiers each). (By comparison, a regiment prior to 1812 had 1,000 soldiers.) There was one appointed surgeon general for the legion. Each sublegion had one surgeon and three surgeons' mates. The legion configuration lasted until May of 1796, when the Army was organized into four regiments. The Medical Department was created by Congress in 1799 to care for the troops.[3(p130),15(p74)]

War threats arose again in 1794 concerning issues of failure to indemnify for lost slaves, British occupation of Western forts, and the activities of British agents with the Indians. John Jay settled the issues by diplomatic work in London.[11(p74)] The reorganization of the Army in 1796 was brought about by concerns of war with Revolutionary France.[11(p75)] The France that had been an American ally in the Revolutionary War was the Royalist France. The Revolutionary France that replaced the monarchy seemed to back away from its prior friends, including America. France tried to prevent all trade with England, which remained a major trading partner with America.

The military had it first postwar engagement in 1791 against the Indians in the Northwest Territory. No specifics of medical care available are extant, although contemporary commentaries note a high rate of illness. The first incursion resulted in an Indian victory. In 1792, Arthur St Clair, Governor of the Northwest Territory and later designated a major general in the Army, launched a second campaign against the Indians. St Clair had a force of 1,500 militia and 600 Regulars; he also had prior medical training of note. Unfortunately, St Clair suffered from severe gout, which hampered his leadership. The Miami Indians defeated the force, inflicting many casualties.[3(pp133–135)] St Clair lost 632 killed and 264 wounded. Not all the wounded were taken with the retreating force, but those that were taken were left at Fort Jefferson for care.[3(p134–135)]

With the appointment of MG Anthony Wayne, the young nation had a victory over the Indians at the Battle of Fallen Timbers, Ohio, in 1794. Wayne likewise suffered from gout, which flared even before the Fallen Timbers campaign. Malaria also became a major health issue for his command. Medicine and supply shortage issues plagued the command through 1796. The last Indian campaign in the Northwest came in October to November of 1811. Three hundred Regular troops and 600 or so militia were deployed against an unknown number of Indians. William Henry Harrison was the general engaging Tecumseh at Vincennes. Harrison had also trained as a physician.[2(pp136–137)]

Harrison won a victory against the Indians at the Tippecanoe River near Lafayette, Indiana. Harrison had 900 to 1,000 men in his command and had been commissioned as a brigadier general. The Indians launched the attack on 7 November 1811. (This victory became part of a slogan for Harrison's later presidential campaign.) He received 200 casualties, of which 137 were wounded. In the evacuation by boat, an additional 25 of the wounded died before reaching the fort.[3(pp138–139)]

James Wilkinson had also trained as a physician but left the practice of medicine to become a soldier. He was appointed a brigadier general for service in 1808 in the Louisiana Territory.[3(p142)] In 1813, Wilkinson became the Army Commanding General. He was ordered to the Canadian border to lead troops, but was dismissed from the Army in 1814 for his incompetence in battle. (Wilkinson was also involved in many scandals, most notably his involvement with Aaron Burr. The Burr scandal resulted in a famous trial and acquittal for Burr. He and his colleagues, including Wilkinson, were charged with attempting to make Spanish territory and Louisiana a separate country. Wilkinson was also alleged to have been a paid informant for the Spanish.[3(p141),39(p230)])

The provision of healthcare for the soldiers was the sole responsibility of the individual surgeons and surgeon mates because there was little organization or support for a nonexistent medical department. Because the British had been impressing American seamen and giving aid to the western Indians for some years, the coming of the War of 1812 was anticipated. Despite this, the preparations were inadequate. The actual declaration of war did not come until 18 June 1812, but America was ill prepared for another war so soon after the Revolutionary War and the various skirmishes with the Indians in the West.[1(p148)]

REFERENCES

1. Savas TP, Dameron JD. *A Guide to the Battles of the American Revolution*. El Dorado Hills, Calif: Savas Beatie LLC; 2013.
2. Paine L. *The Sea and Civilization*. New York, NY: Alfred A. Knopf; 2003.
3. Gillet MC. *The Army Medical Department 1775–1818*. Washington, DC: US Government Printing Office; 1981.
4. Wood WJ. *Battles of the Revolutionary War. 1775–1781: Major Battles and Campaigns*. Chapel Hill, NC: Algonquin Books of Chapel Hill; 1990.
5. Allen D. *Our Declaration: A Reading of the Declaration of Independence in Defense of Equality*. New York, NY: Liveright Publishing Corporation; 2014.
6. Hall JW. An irregular reconsideration of George Washington and the American military tradition. *J Mil Hist*. 2014;78(3):961–993.
7. Desjardin TA. *Through a Howling Wilderness: Benedict Arnold's March to Quebec, 1775*. New York, NY: St Martin's Griffin; 2006.
8. Lefkowitz AS. *Benedict Arnold's Army: The 1775 Invasion of Canada During the Revolutionary War*. El Dorado Hills, Calif: Savas Beatie LLC; 2014.
9. Anderson MR. *The Battle for the Fourteenth Colony: America's War of Liberation in Canada, 1774–1776*. Lebanon, NH: University Press of New England; 2013.
10. Lancaster B. *The American Revolution*. New York, NY: Houghton Mifflin Harcourt; 2001.
11. Randall WS. *Alexander Hamilton: A Life*. New York, NY: Harper Collins Publishers; 2003.
12. Clark H. *All Cloudless Glory: The Life of George Washington From Youth to Yorktown*. Washington, DC: Regnery Publishing, Inc.; 1996.
13. Ketchum RM. *The Winter Soldiers: The Battles for Trenton and Princeton*. New York, NY: Henry Holt and Company; 1973.
14. Logusz MO. *With Musket and Tomahawk: The Saratoga Campaign and the Wilderness War of 1777*. Havertown, Penn: Casemate Publishers; 2012.
15. Duncan LC. *Medical Men in the American Revolution 1775–1783*. Carlisle Barracks, Penn: Medical Field Service School; 1931.
16. Corbett T. *No Turning Point: The Saratoga Campaign in Perspective*. Norman, Okla.: University of Oklahoma Press; 2012.
17. Defense Casualty Analysis System. *Principal Wars in Which the United States Participated: US Military Personnel Serving and Casualties*. https://www.dmdc.osd.mil/dcas/pages/report_principal_wars.xhtml. Accessed 19 March 2015.
18. Peckham HH. *The Toll of Independence: Engagements and Battle Casualties of the Revolution*. Chicago, Ill: University of Chicago Press; 1974.
19. Eichner LG. The military practice of medicine during the Revolutionary War. http://www.tehistory.org/hqda/pdf/v41/Volume41_N1_025.pdf. Accessed 19 March 2015.
20. Reiss O. *Medicine and the American Revolution: How Diseases and Their Treatment Affected the Colonial Army*. Jefferson, NC: McFarland and Co.; 2004.
21. Moore W. *The Knife Man: Blood, Body Snatching and the Birth of Modern Surgery*. New York, NY: Broadway Books; 2005.
22. Hunter J. *Treatise on the Blood, Inflammation and Gunshot Wounds*. (Originally published London, England, 1794). Bethesda, MD: Classics of Medicine Library (Gryplon Edition); 1982.
23. Brown HE. *The Medical Department of the United States Army from 1775 to 1783*. Washington, DC: Surgeon General's Office; 1873.
24. Morgan J. *A Recommendation of Inoculation According to the Baron Dimsdale Method*. Boston, Mass: J Gill; 1776.

25. Klebs AC. The historic evolution of variolation. *Bull Johns Hopkins Hosp.* 1913;(24):69–83.
26. Bynum W. *The History of Medicine: A Very Short Introduction.* Oxford, England: Oxford University Press; 2008.
27. Rogers BO. Surgery in the Revolutionary War: contributions of John Jones, MD (1729–1791). *Plastic Reconstr Surg.* 1972;49(1):1–13.
28. Editor. John Morgan (1735–1789) Founder of American medical education. *JAMA.* 1965;194(7):826.
29. Barton D. *Benjamin Rush: Signer of the Declaration of Independence.* Aledo, Tex: Wall Builders; 1999.
30. Brodsky A. *Benjamin Rush: Patriot and Physician.* New York, NY: St Martin's Press; 2005.
31. Duffy J. *Epidemics in Colonial America.* Baton Rouge, La: Louisiana State University Press; 1953.
32. Olson DA. Mercury toxicity. http://emedicine.medscape.com/article/1175560-overview#aw2aab6b2b2aa. Accessed 19 March 2015.
33. Boyd MF. An historical sketch of the prevalence of malaria in North America. *Am J Trop Med Hyg.* 1941;(21):223–244.
34. Hunter J. *A Treatise on the Venereal Disease.* [Reprinted by Nabu Press (book in common domain originally published 1789)] Charleston, SC: Nabu Press; 2011.
35. Applegate HL. Remedial medicine in the American Revolutionary Army. *Mil Med.* 1961;(126):450–453.
36. Lockhart P. *The Whites of Their Eyes: Bunker Hill, the First American Army and the Emergence of George Washington.* New York, NY: Harper Collins; 2011.
37. Wangensteen OH, Smith J, Wangensteen SD. Some highlights in the history of amputation reflecting lessons in wound healing. *Bull Hist Med.* 1967;(41):97–131.
38. Miranda J. When lions sailed: naval strategy and the rise of Europe. *Strategy & Tactics.* 2011;268:6–12.
39. Melton BF. *Aaron Burr: Conspiracy to Treason.* New York, NY: John Wiley and Sons; 2002.

"In the War of 1812, there had been little change in the art of surgery since the Revolutionary War. As in the previous conflict, field surgery was a very crude attempt to extract a bullet or a piece of shell fragment. The wound would be cleaned and dressed. Extremity wounds often resulted in amputation, particularly if the fracture was complicated, although simple fractures could be splinted. Mortality rates were 9% for simple fractures, 42% for compound or complicated fractures, and 50% for gunshot wounds."

Chapter Two

Surgery and Medicine in the War of 1812: A New Nation Challenged

LANCE P. STEAHLY, MD

THE WAR OF 1812

Contemporary Views of the War

A NUMBER OF CONTEMPORARY AUTHORS have written about the War of 1812. Yet, the war has not enjoyed very much fame or even notoriety among America's conflicts. Hickey, in his book *The War of 1812: A Forgotten Conflict*,[1] attributes this, in part, to a lack of a defined "war leader." President Madison was not a war president such as Lincoln, Wilson, or Roosevelt would be in later years. Nor was Madison a skilled orator or a leader who inspired confidence. Hickey points out that Madison was unable to impose his will on Congress or indeed the country.[1(p34)] Furthermore, Hickey feels that the best generals (by his choice Andrew Jackson, Winfield Scott, and Jacob Brown) were confined to secondary theaters. He also cites the complex issues that motivated the war and the fact that the Treaty of Ghent ending the War of 1812 brought only the benefit that America didn't have to make significant concessions or reparations.[1(pp1–2)] In fact, the outcome was a treaty that returned both countries to the status quo that existed at the beginning of the war. Hickey also points out that prior to 1812, the incompetence in the American officer corps had reached such a level that the enlisted detested most of the officers.[1(p8)] There was little professionalism because most of the leaders had no formal military training. Most, in fact, owed their appointments to political connections. The state of the forces was due to Republican fiscal economies and the intent to rely on militias and privateers (privately owned ships with government licenses to wage war) in the maritime arena.[1(p9)]

Taylor, in his book *The Civil War of 1812: American Citizens, British Subjects, Irish Rebels, & Indian Allies*,[2] saw the war as a civil war "between competing visions of America: one still loyal to the [British] empire and the other defined by its republican revolution against that empire."[2(p12)] Sheads, in his book *The Chesapeake Campaigns 1813–15: Middle Ground of the War of 1812*,[3] saw the war as a "culmination of the struggle for the North American continent"[3(p5)] that involved the French and Indian War, the Revolutionary

War, and the War of 1812.[3(p5)] And Vogel, in his book *Through the Perilous Fight: From the Burning of Washington to the Star Spangled Banner: The Six Weeks That Saved the Nation*,[4] points out that the British during the Napoleonic Wars were fighting in their view for their very survival and that Britain would not hesitate to impinge on American rights to survive.[4(p6)] And, finally, Latimer in his book, *1812: War With America*,[5] has an excellent discussion about the war, but from a British perspective. Latimer points out that the "strain of war and threat of invasion loomed large in British minds."[5(p19)]

Background

In 1796, George Washington decided not to run for a third term as president. Washington's party, called the Federalist Party, represented the commercial interests of New England and the mid-Atlantic states. The opposition party, the Democratic Republicans, represented largely southern agricultural interests. John Adams, the Federalist candidate, succeeded Washington as president.[5(p14)] The Federalists expanded the military gradually until 1798, enlarging the almost nonexistent Army and restarting the Navy, which had been retired after the Revolutionary War. The Federalists clearly were pro-British in their policies and attitudes, as evidenced in 1794 by their signing the Jay Treaty with England, which brought continued peace with England and allowed American commerce to flourish. One aspect of the treaty allowed the British most favored nation trading status. The French (who were at war with England at the time) did not like the Jay Treaty, viewing it as a unilateral break with the French nation despite its help in the Revolutionary War. The French Revolution, however, had changed the attitude of the French because America had previously dealt with the French monarchy. The radical Republican French government resulting from the French Revolution seized more than 300 American ships carrying British goods as part of France's war with England.[5(pp14–15)] The United States subsequently had a limited, undeclared naval war, the "Quasi-War," with the French, lasting from 1798 until 1801. The Quasi-War involved real conflict despite its undeclared status. In response to these ship seizures, the American Navy was created in 1798 under the Federalists' direction. In a series of individual ship actions, they took control of 80 French privateers and put out of action three French warships.[5(p15)] The French privateers, fortunately, were more interested in prize money than fighting and thus would often decline battle.[1(p7)] The Quasi-War was ended by the strong Federalist naval campaign. In 1801, the Republicans gained power at the end of the undeclared war, reversing course because they viewed the policies under the Federalist Party as being too pro-British, the taxes too burdensome, and the attempts to control immigration too restrictive to continue.[1(p7)]

James Madison was hostile to the British, in part to counter the pro-British leanings of Alexander Hamilton and the Federalists. Madison had been Jefferson's Secretary of State during the near war with Britain after the 1807 *Chesapeake-Leopard* affair in which a British ship, looking for English deserters, stopped an American ship and involuntarily impressed Americans into the British Navy. The *Chesapeake-Leopard* affair revived the hope of the Indians for a new conflict that they could join with the British against the Americans.[6(p38)] Indeed, the British Indian Department began to enlist Indian help in the event of another American invasion of Canada.[5(p25)] The British were aware that an invasion of Canada was being advocated in America, especially by those in the southern states. The taking of Canada had been a feature of the Revolutionary War, with continued interest in the years following. The Americans reasoned that the French Canadians could not be happy with their lot in an English colony. The British started negotiations with Indian leaders such as Tecumseh and his brother, Tenskwatawa, to enlist their help in the event of an American invasion.[5(p25)] Latimer points out that there were as many reasons for America to go to war with France as England. However, there was no interest in the quarters of Jefferson and Madison for such a war because Jefferson's Republicans were more in tune with the revolutionary sentiment of the French.[1(p7)] Latimer also points out that America could have enjoyed unhindered trade and protection for its ships had it allied itself with England.[5(pp25–26)]

Strategies and Goals

President Madison outlined five grievances against the British (representing the ideas of those favoring war with the British) in a secret message to Congress. Four of the five areas that he outlined dealt with maritime issues relating to blockade, search and seizure, and impressment of seamen (presumed to be British). The British recognized as American those who lived in the United States before 1783 or were born in the United States subsequently.[5(p17)] The fifth area concerned British support for Indian warfare on the frontier. The maritime states were busily evading the British rules and were engaged in smuggling. The states of New York and those to the north were in favor of peace. The states of Pennsylvania and those to its south were for war. War against Great Britain was finally declared on 18 June 1812, barely passing Congress, with the votes for or against reflecting regional differences.[5(p34)] The Americans were unaware that the British had suspended the 1807 "Orders" (Orders-in-Council—regulations issued by the British that hindered American trade with the European Continent, specifically France) with the plan that envisioned that the Americans would repeal their Non-Importation Act of 1811 (in essence an embargo or restrictive system that cut trade with belligerents in the Napoleonic Wars).[3(p6)] It is certain that the war bill would not have passed at this juncture had the Congress known about these recent British moves. As it unfolded, the bill received the least amount of Congressional support of any declaration of war in America's history. The senators and congressmen from New York to Maine voted for peace, while the senators and congressmen south of Pennsylvania voted for war.[5(p34)] This stark geographical difference in voting was explained by the different economies of the North and South, and the impact of British actions on these respective economies, as described below.

It was policy that the British would seize any ship sailing for France. The British had already seized approximately 400 American ships by 1812, which necessarily caused problems for American commerce. An economic depression in the South resulted from an inability to successfully export cotton and tobacco, and further explained why the senators and congressmen in the region voted for war. Furthermore, British agents were suspected of stirring up Indian tribes to attack. In addition, many Americans believed that some Canadians really wanted to be Americans. As noted by Berton in his book, *The Invasion of Canada: 1812–1813*,[6] aside from the old Loyalists and the British in residence, most Canadians were "at best apathetic or at worst disaffected."[6(p24)] He points out that some 500 Canadians were identified as supporting the "enemy" (the United States). Berton notes there were probably more as witnessed by the reluctance of the Canadian militia to do battle.[6(pp24–25)] As in the Revolutionary War, Americans attempted to lure the French Canadians of Quebec Province into the American camp and, as in the Revolutionary War with Arnold's and Montgomery's attempt to take Quebec, pursuing this same idea on the battlefield some four decades later would also end in failure.[6(pp24–25)]

Lieutenant General (LTG) Sir George Prevost was appointed Governor-in-Chief of Upper and Lower Canada in September 1811. Prevost's defensive strategy was to hold on to the territory until help could come from England. He was aware that to take Quebec City, the Americans would need to first take Montreal, where he decided to concentrate his troops. Prevost could not expect much help from Britain because the war with the French was of paramount importance on the European continent, and thus consumed both manpower and resources.[5(pp43–44)] When war was finally declared in June of 1812, Prevost cancelled the planned return to England of the 41st and 49th Regiments, and the relocation of the 100th Regiment to Halifax.[5(p49)] Local volunteers, known as "fencibles" (who could only serve in Canada), and commanded by Regular Army officers, were established to augment the regulars. Prevost and General Sir Issac Brock also had 13,000 militia and variable Indian adjunct forces.

American troop strength consisted of 17 infantry regiments, four artillery regiments, two regiments of dragoons (cavalry), one regiment of riflemen, and a Corps of Engineers.[7(p131)] On 26 June 1812, a few weeks after war was declared, the regiment size was standardized at 900 soldiers and the authorized regiment number was increased to 25. By January of 1813, 20 more regiments had been authorized.[7(p131)] In addition, the American states in 1811 had over 700,000 troops on the militia rolls. In practice, the Federalist governors in Massachusetts, Rhode Island, and Connecticut refused a request by General Henry Dearborn, the regional commander, to call out militia companies that would have allowed Regulars to serve at the front. American planning and operations were complicated by such domestic opposition.[5(pp57–58)]

The early American campaigns included the infamous invasion of Canada in July 1812 that failed. In the envisioned three-prong invasion, General William Hull was to attack Canada from the village of Detroit in one phase, with General Henry Dearborn attacking in the east, and General Stephen Van Rensselaer attacking in the Niagara region.[3(pp6,157)] All three incursions would be unsuccessful by the end of 1812.[3(p157)]

It appears that the US military leadership initially was not adequately briefed on political war plans. For instance, Secretary of War William Eustis had sent orders to Brigadier General (BG) Hull only hours before war was declared, but he did not tell Hull of this war declaration. He ordered Major General (MG) Henry Dearborn to command the North forces, but did not specifically assign Detroit to his command. Dearborn assumed Detroit wasn't his responsibility due to this failure of communication. This lack of preparedness and leadership resulted in John Armstrong Jr replacing William Eustis on 13 January 1813 as the Secretary of War.[7(p148)] Armstrong served from 1813 to 1814 and supervised the Canadian campaigns.

At the start of the Canadian invasion, the three American armies were poised to take the border strongpoints of Montreal, Kingston, Queenston, and Amherstburg. It appeared that Upper Canada would fall, to be followed by the collapse of Quebec. Berton points out that three out of every five settlers in Upper Canada were actually Americans who had come in response to the lure of cheap land. Some of these may have had familial loyalist sympathies for the Crown dating back to the Revolutionary War. Berton spoke of three factors leading to American failure in the invasion of Canada: (1) the British troops were better disciplined, although fewer in number; (2) America's lack of military aptitude; and (3) the military alliance between the British and the Indians.[6(pp26-27)]

Dr James Mann was placed in charge of the upstate New York medical services, and later the forces under MG Henry Dearborn assembled at Greenburgh (in the Albany area), New York. The forces were largely militia, which returned home after being repulsed in their Canadian invasion attempt. Mann attended the sick there; in addition, he was required to distribute supplies to Niagara and Plattsburgh. Mann observed the diseases that soldiers suffered and opined that rheumatism impacted men over 40 years of age the most.[7(pp157-159)] Dr William Beaumont, of later international fame for his work in digestion, served under Dr Mann as a surgeon's mate in New York. Dr Beaumont saw respiratory diseases as his soldiers' main health problem. He favored bleeding as a treatment for respiratory issues, to be followed by "raising of blisters" in more extreme cases.[7(pp159-160)] Dr Mann toured the hospitals at Plattsburgh and Burlington, Vermont, where he was pleased with the work of Dr James Lovell (later Surgeon General of the Army). Lovell was in charge of the hospital at Burlington. Drs Mann and Lovell were both Regular Army surgeons.[7(p160)]

Many of the American forces along the frontier were in poor health.[5(pp81-83)] Indeed, in 1812, the situation in Buffalo was not good; the 100 wounded held by the British at Queenston had died. The prisoners had fought in the Buffalo, Lewiston, and Erie areas.[7(pp161-162)] Mann found that measles and dysentery were the most common illnesses suffered by the men.[7(p161)]

When Secretary of War John Armstrong took office in January 1813, he found the logistical supply infrastructure in dire shape, chronic shortages of Regular troops with training, and a major financial shortfall.[5(p115)] To address this, Congress doubled import tariffs in 1813, but otherwise taxes were not raised, due to Republican opposition.[5(pp120-121)]

Albert Gallatin, Secretary of the Treasury, encouraged Congress to authorize a war loan to be raised by nonconventional means to stave off insolvency. Subsequently, Congress authorized a war loan with the help of three wealthy merchants. The merchants included John Jacob Astor (of fur trading fame), Stephen Girard, and the financier David Parish. Their collective experience as financiers helped Congress arrange a $16 million war loan, with higher interest rates than normal (highlighting the need for increased taxes). Thirteen million dollars of the loan proceeds were given to the War Department. Gallatin directed Armstrong to use no more than $1,480,000 each month, which necessarily meant that there would be shortfalls in supplies and manpower.[5(p121)] Armstrong used some of the funds to appoint a number of Regular brigadier and major generals and to reorganize the Army into nine military districts.[5(p121)]

The shortages of supplies and trained personnel were evident in the medical arena as well. For example, Dr William Beaumont described 300 casualties from an ammunition dump explosion in Toronto.[8(p16)] Because of the shortage of Army doctors, he operated on 50 of those injured over a 2-day period. He also described working for 48 hours straight in the spring of 1813. Some of the surgeons with Beaumont later worked on ships of the American Great Lakes Squadron.[7(p170)] Beaumont continued as a surgeon's mate and participated

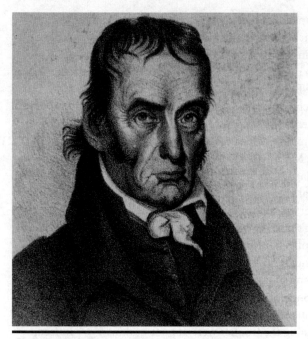

FIGURE 2-1. Surgeon James Tilton was appointed to the newly created office of Physician and Surgeon General in June of 1813. Tilton's appointment allowed him to manage medical personnel as needed, which had not been the case up until that time. Artwork courtesy of the National Library of Medicine, Image #B08882.

in the September 1814 Battle of Plattsburgh. He drew the praise of Surgeon Mann and Surgeon General Tilton for his work there.[8(pxiii)] Interestingly, Beaumont had only obtained his license to practice medicine in June 1812.

From June 1812, when war was declared, until June 1813 and the appointment of Surgeon James Tilton (Figure 2-1) to the newly created office of Physician and Surgeon General, the Army's medical care was relegated to the individual physician/surgeon. Changes were over a year in coming. Tilton's appointment as the Physician and Surgeon General allowed him to assign and then move surgeons, surgeon mates, and hospital steward personnel as needed.[7(pp169–170)]

In the 13 October 1812 Battle of Queenston Heights (across the Niagara River from Lewiston, New York), Sir Isaac Brock was killed. The British prevailed in the battle, with General Sir Roger Sheaffe assuming command after Brock's death. American MG Van Rensselaer negotiated a ceasefire with the British, which was extended several times. It was reported that it took three attempts to find someone in authority to bring about a truce.[5(p82)] The British listed 20 killed, 85 wounded, and 22 taken prisoner; the American casualties were not officially recorded. MG Van Rensselaer, however, stated in correspondence that 60 Americans were killed and 170 wounded. The British reported taking 925 American prisoners.[5(pp82–83)]

In 1813 in the South, Andrew Jackson had success in actions against the Creek Indians in Mississippi Territory. Jackson later became aware that the British were planning to attack Mobile and New Orleans in 1813 from their location at Pensacola, Florida. Jackson sent 160 Regulars and a few artillery pieces under the command of Major William Lawrence to garrison at Fort Bowyer at the beginning of Mobile Bay.[5(p370)]

In the North, Navy Master Commandant Oliver Hazard Perry won a seminal victory on Lake Erie. This brought that entire region around Lake Erie under American control.[7(p164)] The Battle of Lake Erie also made Perry a national hero.[5(p184)] The Battle of the Thames near present-day Chatham, Ontario, in October 1813 resulted in the death of Tecumseh and the end of the Indian Confederacy, an alliance between the Indian tribes and the British, and thus the threat from the British Native American allies was alleviated.[5(p191)]

The American campaign's move toward Montreal ultimately failed when the British were victorious at the Battle of Crysler's Farm (11 November 1813)[5(p210)] in Ontario and the Battle of Chateauguay (26 October 1813)[5(p202)] in Quebec province.[4(p21)] The Battle of Lundy's Lane at Niagara Falls on 25 July 1814 was one of the war's bloodiest encounters. The Americans lost 173 killed, 571 wounded, and 117 missing in action. The British losses were stated to be 84 killed, 559 wounded, and 193 missing. The missing could include deserters and casualties not recovered. The American casualties amounted to 45% of troops engaged and 30% for the British.[5(pp296–297)]

Winfield Scott, as a brigade commander, received great praise for his command at Lundy's Lane. General Brown sent for Scott, who arrived in the afternoon of 25 July 1814. When he saw the number of British facing him, Scott considered withdrawal, but instead attacked. Scott was credited with being one of the few aggressive and decisive American young generals in the war.[5(p289)] The American wounded were sent to a hospital made up of tents at Williamsville, near Buffalo, New York. The British wounded were taken to Fort George, the westernmost of the British fortified posts on Lake Ontario, Upper Canada, where only a single surgeon and a sergeant attended 320 of the wounded. The Americans were transferred to an inadequate hospital at York (the provincial capital of Upper Canada)—the general hospital was so small that other buildings, including a church, were utilized. The wounded were typically carried on litters made from blankets slung between two poles as opposed to being transported on an available wagon. The dead were so numerous after the engagement that burning of the dead had to be used instead of burial.[5(p298)]

The British perfected their version of power projection by sea landings, such as the raid on Essex, Connecticut, in 1814, which only lasted 24 hours. This tale of the raid was recast in Roberts' *The British Raid on Essex: The Forgotten Battle*.[9(p1)] The British sent 136 Royal marines and sailors (rowing 6 miles), launched from two warships in the Long Island Sound, to attack the American privateers of the village of Pettipaug, Connecticut. The British burned 27 American vessels, which was the most American vessels lost in a single event in the war.[9(pp1–5)] The British also used these sea-borne raids, raised to an art form, in the Chesapeake. Vogel presents as a theme of his book, *Through the Perilous Fight*,[4] that in the context of the larger war as a whole, the Chesapeake operations were an intended British diversion from American operations in the North, where the land armies were mainly concentrated.[4(p20)] British Admiral George Cockburn told the communities in the region that they would be spared if no resistance was offered but that severe retribution would come if they did resist. Some communities, such as Havre de Grace,[5(p160)] offered no resistance, while Georgetown and Fredericktown (on the Sassafras River) resisted and suffered destruction of the towns. No more resistance ensued for the next 12 days of Cockburn's incursions.[5(pp161–162)] In a continuation of the landings from the sea, the British threatened Washington, DC, in 1813.[4(p21)] Cockburn came within 25 miles of the city in mid-March 1813, but he felt that his strength was not sufficient at the time to attack the American capitol.[5(p156)] In May 1813, the British attacked Havre de Grace in Maryland.[4(p25)]

Although the Americans knew that the British had threatened Washington in 1813, they took no serious actions to defend the capital from attack.[5(p303)] Howard, in his *Mr and Mrs Madison's War; America's First Couple and the Second War of Independence*,[10] stated that Madison failed to exercise his role as Commander-in-Chief when Washington was threatened. There were many clues as to the threat to the city.[10(p196)] Indeed, British prisoners had already told the military and Secretary John Armstrong Jr of coming plans for the invasion.[5(p303)] Unfortunately, Armstrong believed that Baltimore was actually the intended British target, and Madison did not want to overrule his Secretary of War. Furthermore, both Armstrong and Madison overlooked the psychological and morale benefits that would accrue to the British from an attack on Washington. Cockburn, the British admiral who led the coming attack, was thus certain that Washington would not resist an attack. Cockburn was an experienced commander who had amassed 1 year of coastal operations. Due to the lack of resistance to date and his awareness of the state of things in Washington, he felt resistance would not amount to much.[5(p311)]

By 1814, Washington, DC, had been the country's capital for 14 years. The city was becoming increasingly important to the United States as the seat of power, making it more attractive as a symbolic target. The population of the city and neighboring Georgetown was listed as 13,156 (including 2,559 slaves).[5(p316)]

The British attack resulting in the destruction of Washington on 24 August 1814 caused outrage among Americans; even some British considered it to be excessive. The British used a force of only 4,000, which advanced 50 miles, to defeat an American force three times larger, before burning the public buildings, including the White House, with property loss given as $1.5 million.[5(p322)] The defenders of the city were defeated soundly by the British outside the city.[9(p196)] The Americans set fire to the Washington Naval Yard on the night of the attack, under the orders of the Yard Commandant, Captain Thomas Tingey of the US Navy. The Commandant ordered the fire to deny the Naval Yard's stores from falling into British hands. The fire spared only the Marine Corps Commandant's house.[5(pp316-317)] Howard suggests that Madison was able to survive politically only by the popularity of his wife Dolly, who early on had become the leader of Washington's social scene.[10(p223)]

The subsequent defiance of Baltimore, Maryland (September 1814), and the victory at Plattsburgh, New York (11 September 1814), offered some solace for the Americans. After the ruin of Washington, there was some resolve to move the capital. However, influential lawmakers and businessmen interested in the status quo resisted the move.[11(p1)]

In September 1814, the British had taken the eastern part of Maine with 100 miles of coast.[5(p347)] By the end of the war, the British had captured or destroyed 55% of America's naval forces. The Battle of Plattsburgh on 11 September 1814 was won by the Americans, as was the naval action on adjacent Lake Champlain, which helped precipitate the British loss on land. British General Sir George Prevost blamed the loss by his troops on land to the success of the American naval action. Latimer makes the point that it is possible a more confident commander could have prevailed against the smaller American force.[5(p359)] Prevost led 11,000 troops against an American force of 1,500 Regulars and 500 militia.[5(p359)] The losses of the battle reported for the Americans were 38 killed, 64 wounded, and 20 missing. The British reported 37 killed, 150 wounded, and 55 missing, although more may have deserted to the Americans, attracted by the American offer of higher pay than they received from the British side. Indeed, BG Alexander Macomb, the American ground commander, reported that over 300 British troops came over to the American side in part because they were upset at the British retreat and in part because of the American offer of higher pay for their services.[5(p358)]

As mentioned previously, the British also had Indian allies in the War of 1812. The conflict with the Creek Indians ended with General Andrew Jackson's assault against a Creek group at Tohopeka (Horseshoe Bend) on the Tallapossa River in Alabama. Eight hundred Indians were killed, compared to the loss of only 45 Americans. The Creek power was broken, ending the war with the Indians.[5(pp220–221)] Andrew Jackson's victories over the Creek Indians resulted in the Treaty of Fort Jackson, which was signed at Fort Jackson, near Wetumpka, Alabama, on 9 August 1814. The Creeks were required to give up claim to 23 million acres and to move west beyond the Mississippi River. (The British later maintained that the treaty was a violation of the Treaty of Ghent [ending the war], which had a clause protecting the Indians.[5(pp369–370)]) Jackson then recruited a militia force, a small force of several hundred, and proceeded to Mobile, Alabama. Jackson was promoted to the regular rank of major general and took command of Military District No. 7 based at Mobile.[5(p221)] He had received reports that the British were set to invade New Orleans or Mobile because they were interested in securing control of the Mississippi River.[5(p370)]

Later, on 16 September 1814, the British attacked Fort Bowyer with two English ships and two sloops. The naval craft carried 60 Royal Marines, 12 Royal Artillerymen, and 130 Indians. The forces were defeated with the British suffering 32 killed and 37 wounded, in contrast to the Americans' 4 killed and 5 wounded.[5(p372)] Meanwhile, the British were trying to enlist the help of the pirates under Jean Lafitte at Barataria, some 60 miles away from New Orleans. The Lafitte pirate group eventually sided with the Americans at New Orleans.[5(p371)]

In preparation for the British advance at New Orleans, Jackson held a fortified line with 3,500 men and 100 more in reserve. The Battle of New Orleans extended from 24 December 1814 until 8 January 1815. The battle took place some 10 miles south of New Orleans on the east bank of the Mississippi on the Plains of Chalmette. The 8,000-man strong British Army had a plan to take New Orleans and to meet up with troops from Canada coming down the Mississippi River. The opposing Army of Americans, by then numbering around 4,000, was made up of militia, Regulars, Indians, and pirates.[12(pp5–6)] Many of the British troops came directly from the battles of Europe with the defeat of the French.[5(p383)] The end result was that the British sustained a humiliating defeat at the hands of a ragtag American force, which proved to be unnecessary given that the peace treaty (the Treaty of Ghent) had been concluded on Christmas Eve, 24 December 1814.[5(p388)] Total American casualties at New Orleans were reported as 13 killed, 39 wounded, and 19 missing,[5(p387)] as opposed to the greater British losses of 289 killed, 1,262 wounded, and 484 missing (some of which are presumed to have deserted).[5(p386)]

The Treaty of Ghent was concluded to insure no further cause for war by either side. America was not able to take Canada[5(p402)]; the war ended in a stalemate. The two countries were to take their argument of which side owned the islands in Passamaquoddy Bay, the northeast boundary between the United States and Canada, to the commissioners appointed from each country. The clause inserted by the British to protect native Indian lands from encroachment became inoperable due to the pressure of growing American populations anxious for new farmlands. Nationalism of the Canadians was increased as a result of the War of 1812.[5(pp401–408)]

State of Medicine and Surgery in the War of 1812

By the War of 1812, there had been little change in the art of surgery since the Revolutionary War. As in the previous conflict, field surgery was a very crude attempt to extract a bullet or a piece of shell fragment. The wound would be cleaned and dressed. Extremity wounds often resulted in amputation, particularly if the fracture was complicated, although simple fractures could be splinted. Mortality rates were 9% for simple fractures, 42% for compound or complicated fractures, and 50% for gunshot wounds.[13(p1071)] As in the Revolutionary War, most of the surgeon's attention was directed to the many diseases, although smallpox played a lesser role in this conflict due to vaccination (available since 1798 with Jenner's work).[13(pp1071–1073)]

Howard, in *Wellington's Doctors*,[14] provides a view of contemporary war surgery from a British perspective. Amputation was deemed to be required to save the life of the soldier in certain circumstances, such as compound fractures and uncontrolled bleeding.[14(p130)] They cautioned, however, to let the soldier first recover from the shock of the wounding before proceeding to amputation.[14(p136)]

The French impact on America's Army, both tactically and medically, began years before the War of 1812. In the period preceding the war, General Winfield Scott bought French textbooks on war, which he studied carefully. Scott's use of French techniques allowed him to win the only land war victories of the War of 1812.[15(p8)] Hence it would be appropriate for significant regard to also be given to French military surgery greats such as Napoleon's surgeon, Dominique Jean Larrey, Surgeon-in-Chief of the forces. In the Napoleonic Wars, Larrey spoke to the need to recover from the initial wounding before carrying out definitive surgery, such as amputation.[7(p130)]

The need for a professional Army, including the medical component, was recognized by leaders following the end of the War of 1812. It would be several years later before a permanent Medical Department was established in 1818. However, before that happened, a Congressional legislative move in 1815 reduced the size of the military to 10,000 men and eliminated the position of Physician and Surgeon General.[7(p186)] Curiously, the Apothecary General position, with two assistants, was left. In 1816, further legislation attempted to deal with medical support to the military and made the position of Apothecary General permanent.[7(p187)] The Apothecary General was tasked with a number of functions, such as purchasing and handling all medicines, surgical equipment, and dressings. He was to handle the pay of stewards, ward masters, and nurses of the hospitals. The Apothecary General was also charged with preparing medicines under the direction of physicians.[7(Appendix J)]

STATUS OF DISEASE AND MEDICATIONS AT THE END OF THE WAR OF 1812

Following the War of 1812, much of the attention of the surgeons was directed to patients with illnesses/wounds resulting from the conflict, although some new patients came from existing forces. The surgeon had to sign a certificate for a soldier to receive a pension.[7(p190)] Nevertheless, most of the practice of military surgeons in this time frame was directed at disease, rather than surgery. Vaccination was not practiced as hoped within the Army. The Apothecary General appointed a team of six surgeon mates to act as a "vaccinating team." However, he had no command authority to require immunization. Materials for vaccination were sent to the commanding officers, who did have the authority but often neglected the use of it. Despite this inability to insure that the commanders or the "vaccinating team" did meet success, there were no recorded smallpox epidemics in the War of 1812.[7(pp191–192)]

Dysentery and other related disorders caused the so-called "camp diseases" of the War of 1812. Purges and emetics, baths, and medicines such as "Dover's powder" (a combination of opium and ipecac) were used. Many physicians held that diseases of "diarrhea and dysentery" were to be treated by increasing perspiration, often by using Dover's powder.[7(p192)] Some confusion was caused by physicians such as Dr John Warren of Revolutionary War service, who in 1813 opined that typhus and yellow fever were the same disease.[7(p193)] There were some reservations about bleeding as a therapy and the use of certain medicines such as mercurials, arsenicals, and opiates, but these practices were slow to die.[7(pp193–194)]

Purges and emetics were standard fare for the physician in the first quarter of the 19th century. Purges containing mercury were favored. Calomel (also known as mercurous chloride) was another purgative that had its advocates. As time passed, the side effects of the mercurial purge were recognized and it was slowly discontinued.[16(pp6,13)] Mercury toxicity can cause many side effects that can be appreciated today in retrospect. However, even in the early 19th century, toxicities such as these were noticed. Long-term exposure may cause numbness, pain, tremor, memory problems, seizures, and death. Mercury can also cause vomiting, diarrhea, and kidney failure.[17] Purges and emetics remained popular in the war period. However, despite the fall from use of purges, emetics were seen effective to treat fever and inflammatory issues.[16(p8)]

There were only a few apothecary shops at the turn of the century. Most medications were dispensed by the physician after his apprentice put the medication together. Some physicians did cross between being a doctor and an apothecary. Apothecaries and druggists in the early 19th century often branched into chemical manufacturing. The War of 1812, with the loss of English medicines, spurred the domestic development of drug preparations. After the war, the quinine alkaloid was isolated in 1820 by Pierre Pelletier and Joseph Caventou.[18(p10)] They started work on the bark of the cinchona tree from which they isolated a yellow gum, which the two termed quinine. By 1821, a treatment guide for the use of quinine was set. The listing of medicines took a significant step forward with the publication of James Thacher's 1810 *The American New Dispensary* and with the more definitive 1820 *Pharmacopoeia of the United States of America (USP)*.[18(pp10–11)] In England, the Society of Apothecaries was founded in 1790, but its educational mandate was not established until the Apothecaries Act of 1815.[19(p6)] Poor quality medicines were a problem in the War of 1812. However, in the 1840s, as European standards increased, poor quality drugs became an increasing problem in America. There were no universal standards in America; most drug preparation was simply left to the apothecaries. (Quality started to improve with the formation of the American Pharmaceutical Association in 1852 and the creation of pharmaceutical industries.[18(pp12–13)])

Quinine had previously been used in the form of bark of the cinchona tree in the treatment of fevers. After 1820, quinine sulfate was extracted from the bark with greater dosage accuracy and predictability due to the work of Pelletier and Caventou.[18(p10),20] Surgeons were using higher doses (20–30 gms at a time) than previously, with good result. They found that the quinine sulfate was better tolerated from a gastrointestinal standpoint than the bark of the cinchona tree. Physician/surgeons often used it for other fevers than malaria, including typhus, typhoid fever, cholera, and pneumonia, among the many diseases causing fever.[16(pp6–8)] (A survey of Army surgeons in 1843 found that the majority of them were using a few larger doses rather than numerous smaller doses. The survey also found that the majority of physicians did not relate the gastrointestinal symptoms due to the higher doses and confirmed that physicians were indeed using quinine for all types of fevers in addition to malaria.[16(p7)])

Opium had been used for dysentery or severe pain, but its constipation side effects were undesirable. Morphine and codeine were refined from opium products in the first part of the 19th century. The newly refined drugs were popular and their use was increased. The addictive properties were often overlooked and not condemned. Gillet points out that even active Army officers might indulge without censure. The opiates were usually taken by mouth. However, some physicians applied the drugs directly to exposed skin that had been scraped or abraded.[16(p7)]

Malaria became less common in the East but was nonetheless a nationwide problem. Interestingly, malaria was prominent in the Midwest. Malaria was thought to be spread by evil vapors and was felt to be largely a disease of the rural areas. In the writings of the time, malaria was called many names, such as intermittent fever, marsh fever, and ague, to name a few.[16(p8)] Relapses with malaria were common in the day. A combination of tuberculosis with malaria was often fatal. Malaria could be also fatal in men already debilitated with wounds, other diseases, or poor diet. Prior to the refinement of quinine sulfate, bleeding still remained the treatment for malaria in addition to emetics, purges, and cinchona bark.[16(pp9–10)]

Venesection for bleeding became less prevalent during this time period. However, some physicians still used leeches or vacuum cups to extract blood. (Even in the Civil War some bleeding was practiced for the appropriate "relaxation" of the body, which would imply weakening of the patient secondary to blood loss.[16(p8)]) Bleeding had been the treatment of choice for malaria before quinine's use.[16(p9)]

Typhoid fever was a widespread problem. The etiology was not clear and the treatment even less so. Quinine was used to deal with the fever. Dengue fever, yellow fever, and cholera were additional diseases for the surgeon to contend with. These diseases were also not understood and no effective treatment was entertained. Because there were no methods of rehydration available to the cholera patient, death from that disease was cruel.[16(pp10–12)] Cholera was endemic in India, the Near East, Russia, and Asia in 1814 to 1815. It became periodically present in America after 1832.[16(pp10–11)] The rapid mortality and the therapies, such as bleeding, which didn't work, brought panic.[21(p1)]

Scurvy was still a problem for the troops despite the British Navy's use of fruits to prevent the disease. Indeed, the understanding of the role of fruits and vegetables to prevent scurvy and to treat the disease was limited. Vinegar was thought, incorrectly, to help, although doctors of the period found potatoes worked. The isolated posts often had potatoes available, which helped somewhat. Army surgeons came to learn that native plants such as maguey, wild onions, prickly pears, and poke weed seemed to work as antiscorbutics.[16(p14)]

POST-WAR OF 1812: THE MEDICAL DEPARTMENT GOING FORWARD

The Medical Department had been created after the War of 1812 started, and its organization was ended with the end of the war. The office of the Physician and Surgeon General was no longer in existence after the legislation of 3 March 1815. The Army was reduced to 10,000 effectives at the time by this legislation. While the office of the Physician and Surgeon General was eliminated, Congress did retain the office of Apothecary General, along with two assistants. These positions were created by a Congressional order on 17 May 1815. The Apothecary General and his assistants were retained to ensure some economy and efficiency in the procurements of medicines.[7(pp186–187)] Only one surgeon and two surgeon mates per regiment were allowed, which caused many otherwise experienced surgeons and mates to be dropped from the roles as the overall numbers were reduced.[7(p186)]

In April 1816, the War Department established regulations for the Army that actually delineated the duties of medical officers in detail. The position of Apothecary General (and his assistants) was made permanent. The regulations discussed roles of the hospital surgeon and surgeon mates, as well as allowances for food and quarters. The Army was organized into a Northern and a Southern Division. A ratio of four surgeons and eight mates for each division was established. There was still no single medical superior to coordinate the surgeons and to provide medicine needs to the Apothecary General.[7(pp186–187)]

On 14 May 1818, the new regulations were approved, establishing the post of Surgeon General as well as slots for two Assistant Surgeons. The Surgeon General reported directly to the Secretary of War.[16(p27)] The Apothecary General reported to the Surgeon General now.[16(p27)] The Apothecary General post was also approved, along with two Assistant Apothecary Generals. Forty post surgeons were mentioned. One regimental surgeon and two mates were to be assigned to each regiment specifically.[22(p107)] There were four regiments of artillery, seven regiments of infantry, a Corps of Engineers, and topographical engineers.[22(pp126–127)]

From the establishment of the Army Medical Department in 1818, Wintermute points out that those medical officers faced many challenges, including that of their exercising authority. Doctors struggled to get legitimacy and social status. Wintermute uses the term "marginalized subordinates" to describe their status.[23(p22)] He points out that the Regular line officer often saw the doctors as interlopers, not deserving of recognition.[23(p21)] He notes that some Regular officers did not always implement the surgeon's recommendations, instead seeing the surgeon as a "contractor." The Regular officer could say that command was his sole concern.[23(p6)] (As late as 1840, Surgeon General Lawson still had to fight for the privilege of wearing epaulettes on the surgeon's uniform.[16(p79)])

Congress again reduced the size of the Army in legislation dated March 1821. The Apothecary General position was removed. The Surgeon General appointed a physician to be the purchasing officer, but he had the authority to appoint any qualified person to the position.[22(p126)] The surgeons were all now to be classified as surgeons or assistant surgeons.[16(p28)]

In 1832, four more surgeon positions were added to the active roster, along with 10 more assistant surgeons. At this time, Secretary of War John Eaton proposed abolishing the Surgeon General's office, but Surgeon General Lovell fought the proposal, and was successful.[16(p30)] However, in 1834, Congress raised the pay levels for all physicians, except for the Surgeon General. The Surgeon General received $2,500 per year, which was lower than comparable salaries paid to other Army branch chiefs. Although the record is silent on the failure to increase Lovell's pay, some "pay back" may have been in play. The senior surgeon received pay of a major, that is, $50 per month. The assistant surgeon would receive the pay of a captain. The lowest assistant surgeon would receive the pay of a first lieutenant. The surgeons still had no actual military rank. The assistant surgeon who had more than 10 years of service would get double rations.[16(pp30–31)]

THE MEDICAL DEPARTMENT IN THE INDIAN WARS

First Seminole War (1814–1819)

The Seminoles were an aggregate of Indians (mostly Creeks) and runaway slaves. The Indians had sided with the British in the War of 1812. Andrew Jackson was sent with 3,000 troops to deal with the Seminoles. Jackson was successful in defeating the Seminoles and captured several forts in Florida. The Adams-Onis Treaty of 1819 with Spain gave America possession of Florida in exchange for cancelling Spain's $5 million debt.[24] The treaty was signed by the US Secretary of State John Quincy Adams and Spain's Minister Luis de Onis. Florida was subsequently divided into two counties and an infrastructure was established. Florida became an official territory 3 years later in 1822. Settlers from the North "invaded" Seminole territory. The result was that the Indians and former runaway slaves were pushed farther into the Everglades.[24]

Black Hawk War (1832–1833)

Andrew Jackson became President in 1829; the Indian Removal Act was passed in 1830. The Black Hawk War of 1832 to 1833 evolved because the Sac and Fox Indian tribes (led by Black Hawk) were attempting to return from Iowa (where they had been sent by the Indian Removal Act) to their former lands, east of the Mississippi River in Illinois. General Winfield Scott was the commander of the forces opposing the Indian move.[16(p50)] Scott had 1,000 men that came from the east and 200 men at Jefferson Barracks in Saint Louis. Surgeon General Lovell appointed Josiah Everett as the Medical Director for the campaign. Other surgeons from other posts were ordered to join Everett. Two additional battles were fought successfully against the Indians, with minor American casualties.[16(pp50–51)] The Black Hawk War was known at the time as the "Cholera Campaign," reflecting the high incidence of the disease among the troops in the Army. Cholera spread to many forts despite the attempts by Lovell and his surgeons to limit its extent.[16(p52),22(pp149–150)]

Second Seminole War 1835–1842

The exploits of the Indian chief Osceola, who led his people to a number of victories, were historic as recorded in Hatch's *Osceola and the Great Seminole War: A Struggle for Justice and Freedom*.[25] In a December 1835 attack on the troops of Major Francis Dade, who was on his way to Fort King with his detachment (in the area of Tampa Bay, Florida), over 100 troops were killed in an event known later as "Dade's Massacre." Three soldiers survived but two of them died later of their wounds.[25(pp321–323)] Such a complete massacre had not previously been known in Indian warfare.[25(p324)] BG Duncan Clinch had been in charge until General Winfield Scott took over as the Commanding General. Scott was called away to wage another campaign against the Creeks.[24(p350)] Osceola came to negotiate a treaty, but was instead captured and imprisoned in September 1837. He became ill with fever and died a few months later in 1838 in prison at Fort Moultrie in Charleston, South Carolina.[25(p452)] The conflict, however, didn't end with Osceola's death.[25(p453)]

The Second Seminole War was the only major conflict during the period starting in 1835 but extending to 1842. The conflict centered on the removal of the "Five Civilized Tribes"—the Creeks, Cherokees, Chickasaws, Choctaws, and Seminoles—to lands west of the Mississippi River. Attempts to remove the Creeks, and especially the Seminoles, brought troops into territories where malaria was endemic, complicating the work of the Army Medical Department.[16(p53)]

Malaria and cholera were the major diseases in this period. Cholera was a major problem on the *Henry Clay*, a steamer transport chartered to move the tribes. It was thought that rats infected the steamer before its charter.[22(pp150–152)] Even Surgeon Josiah Everett, who had played an important role as Winfield Scott's Medical Director in the Black Hawk War, died of cholera in 1832. At the time, Everett and the ill troops had just been landed from the transport *Henry Clay*. After Everett died, Assistant Surgeon Robert E Kerr was the remaining medical officer.[22(p150)] Kerr took care of the survivors unassisted.[22(p151)] Of a force of 400 soldiers, approximately 250 soldiers were lost (27 died and the rest as desertions); 150 effective soldiers remained.[16(pp50–51)]

The 7-year Seminole conflict alone accounted for 1,200 of 1,500 deaths in the Army in the 1835 to 1842 period. Over 75% of the Army deaths in Florida were due to disease. The small-unit type warfare was best geared to the Army due to its reduced troop size. However, the smaller size could mean no medical support on deployment.[16(p58)]

Third Seminole War (1855–1858)

There was a Third Seminole War from 1855 to 1858. The third conflict was between the few remaining Seminoles in Florida (who had withdrawn to the Everglades) and the white settler population. The Seminole population was reduced to 200 by the end of the conflict in 1858.[26]

SURGEONS GENERAL DURING THE INTERWAR PERIOD

Joseph Lovell (1818–1836)

Before 1818, there was no position of Surgeon General in the US Army. In May 1818, Congress established the post of Surgeon General, appointing Dr Joseph Lovell to the position (Figure 2-2). He had graduated from Harvard College and Harvard Medical School, and then studied medicine with Dr William Ingalls of Boston.[22(pp107–108)] Lovell had previously served as the surgeon of the 9th Infantry and served as a hospital surgeon on the Northern frontier.[16(p28)] He was the head of the hospital at Burlington, Vermont, with the forces of General Winfield Scott and General Jacob J Brown.[22(pp108–109)] Lovell had occupied progressively superior positions despite his youthful 30 years of age. Lovell was concerned about physician quality and the level of care provided by them. He had to hire civilian physicians at various times and locations, with varying quality. Lovell was able to modify the regulations to allow for competitive examinations both for appointment and promotion. Only two attempts were allowed to pass the test. An assistant surgeon had to take an examination within 5 years of initiating military service to remain in the Army. However, Lovell allowed the medical officer to refuse a promotion because it usually brought with it a transfer. Apparently refusals of promotion for this reason were not that uncommon. Lovell tried to accommodate requests for postings. As a result, surgeons and assistant surgeons were known to have stayed at one post as long as 20 years. However, because some surgeons were quick to request a new post if they were not happy with their lot, Lovell required they stay at least 2 years in one post before moving to another post.[16(pp31–33)]

Surgeon General Lovell died on 17 October 1836; the cause of his death was not specified. After Lovell's death, Assistant Surgeon Benjamin King was appointed the interim replacement.[22(p157)] King continued in the office while President Jackson considered suggested successors. Thomas Lawson was the favored candidate from the Army medical staff.[22(p159)] There was a movement to appoint a civilian Surgeon General, but this was successfully resisted by the military doctors.[27]

Thomas Lawson (1836–1861)

Lawson (Figure 2-3) began his medical career in the US Navy as a surgeon's mate, but became an Army garrison surgeon in 1811. There is little information about Lawson's early education or even of his medical training; although it is assumed he had been trained through a preceptor arrangement. He participated in the War of 1812 and was commended for his work at Plattsburgh, New York.[27] Prior to his medical appointment as Surgeon General, Lawson served as a volunteer Army line officer at the rank of lieutenant colonel. He was second in command of a Louisiana volunteer infantry regiment during the Second Seminole War, from February 1836 to May 1836. Lawson served later as the medical director of troops engaged in the Second Seminole War.[16(p53)]

Lawson became the Surgeon General in May 1836. He delayed taking over the duties of the office while he accompanied the retiring President Jackson to Tennessee. Upon his return to Washington, Lawson left again to assume command of a volunteer unit in late

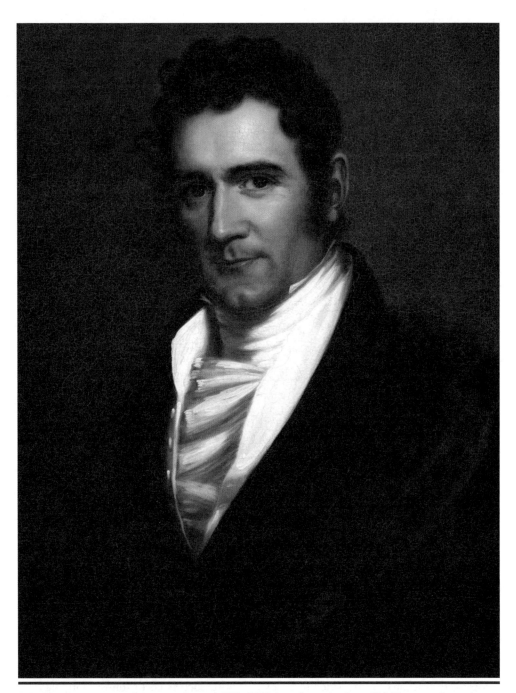

FIGURE 2-2. James Lovell, Surgeon General (1818–1836). Lovell was the first official Surgeon General, appointed to the post in May 1818. He was concerned about the provision of medical care during the Mexican-American War. Of the more than 100,000 troops that went into Mexico for the war, about one in nine died, the majority of diseases of the time. Artwork courtesy of the National Library of Medicine, Image #B18125.

1837.[16(p53)] He was the serving Surgeon General during most of the Second Seminole War (1835–1842). Lawson had to deal with severe doctor shortages, particularly in Florida where many soldiers became ill. A number of the surgeons themselves came down with diseases. Lawson had few resources with which to remedy the shortages, but he had little tolerance for surgeons who did not do their duty.[16(pp58–60)] Lawson faced innumerable challenges in supporting the Second Seminole War as well as the other scattered Army posts nationally, due to an inadequate staff and supply/transportation issues.[16(p94)] Lawson had to supply medical support for many temporary forts—indeed, there were 31 forts in the 1838 to 1839 period alone.[16(p66)] In 1838, Lawson had 15 surgeons and 60 assistant surgeons but only one clerk in his office. In 1842, a few more surgeon positions were added by Congress.

The medical examinations for recruits were a problem for Surgeon General Lawson because many potential soldiers failed the basic standards.[16(p74)] Standards for recruits had evolved slowly since the Revolutionary War. In that war, Congress spoke only of men ages 16 to 50. The first specific standards were set in 1814 and spoke of able-bodied men ages 18 to 35, whose healthiness had to be demonstrated. Examination went to showing use of joints and limbs and the absence of tumors, sore legs, and rupture and disease enlargement of bones or joints. Admission of physically unqualified men was recognized as leading to discharges for preexisting problems. Examination practices for newly recruited soldiers up to and including the Civil War were very lax.[28(p148)]

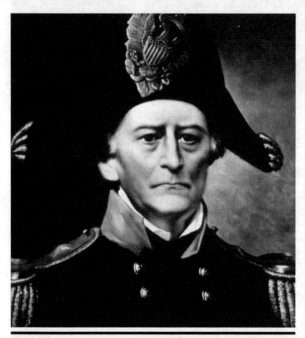

FIGURE 2-3. Thomas Lawson, Surgeon General (1836–1861). Lawson was the second physician appointed to the post of Surgeon General. Like some other physicians of the era, he had previously served as a volunteer Army line officer at the rank of lieutenant colonel. Lawson served later as the medical director of troops engaged in the Second Seminole War, where he faced many challenges in supporting the action in Florida, as well as the other scattered Army posts nationally, due to staffing and supply issues. Artwork courtesy of the National Library of Medicine, Image #B16886.

During Lawson's tenure, sick troops were evacuated from Florida to East Coast posts such as Fort Monroe (Virginia) and Fort Hamilton (New York City Harbor), with the idea that in these locations the climate would be healthier. In fall 1840, an additional evacuation point was added, with Fort Columbus becoming the second New York City Harbor evacuation point.[16(p64)]

WILLIAM BEAUMONT, PROMINENT ARMY PHYSICIAN

The international fame of William Beaumont (Figure 2-4) was in recognition of his pioneering work in gastric physiology due to a fortuitous encounter with a wounded 18-year-old French Canadian. This fame brought great credit to Army medicine. While Beaumont's career started out in a traditional manner, the move to a basic research topic was not typical.

Beaumont's Army career spanned the period from 1812 until his resignation in 1839. He served well in the War of 1812, but his star began to rise with his assignment in 1820 to Fort Mackinac at the northern point of Michigan. Fort Mackinac, with its island location overlooking the Great Lakes, was one of the healthiest posts from the standpoint of absence of disease.[16(p42)] When he arrived in 1820 at the fort, Beaumont had responsibilities for a garrison of 50 to 100 soldiers. Because his duties were not that rigorous, he had permission to also treat civilians, as long as the private patients did not take away from his official duties.[16(p42)]

Beaumont's path became famously intertwined with that of Alexis St Martin, an 18-year-old Canadian who experienced an accidental wounding on 6 June 1822 with a musket loaded with "duck shot." He developed a wound on the left side, which healed as an opening 7 inches in circumference. The gastric contents could be viewed through the fistula. Beaumont initially had to keep a bandage over the wound to keep the gastric contents inside the fistula. However, a fold of the stomach eventually created a type of valve.[22(p161)] Beaumont used this eventful accident as an opportunity to study gastric digestion. He placed scraps of various foods into the stomach attached to a silk string through the fistula hole directly. He established that digestion was due to a chemical process rather than mechanical process.[16(pp23–25)] Beaumont encouraged St Martin to stay with him so that these studies could continue. At one point, he enrolled St Martin as an Army orderly to help defray St Martin's personal expenses.[16(p25)] In 1834, St Martin left for Canada for a proposed short family visit, but he never returned. Beaumont was unable to entice his return after that point.[16(p25)]

Beaumont published a book in 1833 titled *Experiments and Observations on the Gastric Flora and Physiology of Digestion*,[27] which recorded his unique observations. The book was translated into French and German, which helped facilitate the dissemination of his work.[22(p162)] He was displeased that he could not get chemists to provide analysis of the gastric contents to an acceptable level.[22(p161)]

Brown provided an interesting report on Beaumont's 1825 participation in a courts-martial. A lieutenant at Fort Niagara saw Surgeon Beaumont for a sore arm. Beaumont thought he was malingering and gave him a compound of calomel and a tartar emetic. Beaumont also reported him to his commanding officer, who pressed charges and the lieutenant was dismissed from the service. The lieutenant appealed his dismissal and the details came to the President's attention because he was the final authority in such actions. The President disapproved the verdict, and was critical of Beaumont's testimony and conduct. Beaumont applied for a Court of Inquiry, which was refused. Beaumont wrote a pamphlet to be circulated in the Army in which he set out the facts of the case. Apparently the matter rested after the pamphlet's publication.[22(pp131–132)]

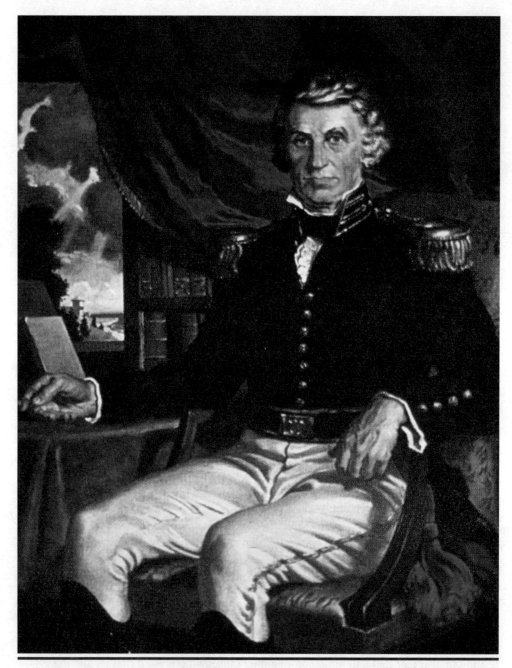

FIGURE 2-4. William Beaumont, Army Surgeon (1812–1839). While Beaumont's career started out in a traditional manner, the move to a basic research topic was unusual. Beaumont's Army career spanned the period from 1812 until his resignation in 1839. Artwork courtesy of the National Library of Medicine, Image #B29606.

Beaumont had issues with Surgeon General Lawson, who had succeeded Lovell. Lawson did not like the attention that the prior Surgeon General gave to Beaumont, who by this time was internationally famous. In particular, the two of them had a conflict over leave. Beaumont applied for leave in 1839, with the request that his replacement be supplied by the Army at its own cost. (At the time, the officer seeking leave had to make arrangements for a replacement and defer some of the costs.) Beaumont gave "personal reasons" as the rationale for the leave. Lawson denied the leave. Furthermore, Lawson planned to transfer Beaumont to Florida to serve on a medical examining board. Because the St Martin experiments were over, Beaumont didn't have as strong a case to remain in Michigan. Beaumont offered his resignation in an attempt to pressure Lawson to rescind his actions. Beaumont was not expecting Lawson to accept the resignation because he felt he would not be replaceable, given his celebrity. The acceptance of his resignation by the Surgeon General effectively ended Beaumont's Army career, which spanned the period of the War of 1812 until 1839.[16(p80)]

STATUS OF MEDICAL CARE PRIOR TO THE MEXICAN-AMERICAN WAR

Diseases and Treatment

A number of diseases, such as cholera and scurvy, continued to be a problem in the lead up to the Mexican-American War. Cholera was epidemic in 1832 and again in 1849. Scurvy continued to be a problem because authorities were slow to recognize the value of fruits and vegetables as prevention aids, despite Lind's work in the prior century. Slowly, the destructive effects of mercury used to treat scurvy were acknowledged.[16(pp12–13)]

Lead poisoning was also a significant medical problem. For example, a lead-covered roof could contaminate the cistern water running off the roof. Lead was also often found in utensils associated with cooking and eating—pots, pans, and drinking cups. A form of lead was used to clean boots. Paint usually contained lead constituents as well.[16(p15)]

Alcohol abuse continued to be a problem for both officers and enlisted, in garrison and in the field. The Army supplied whiskey, brandy, and/or rum until 1838 as a ration to its troops. Additional alcohol was available for purchase. In 1838, the Army substituted a ration of coffee and sugar for the alcohol ration. Temperance societies certainly played a role in reducing alcohol use, at least officially.[16(pp15,84)]

Poor diet was a problem that Surgeon General Lovell tried to alleviate. He issued instructions calling for less meat and more diverse foods, including grains, vegetables, and fruits as available. He discussed beer and the use of molasses and water to make whiskey. He liked pickles for the diet because Lovell felt they worked to prevent too much bile production.[16(p16)]

Anesthesia and Surgery

In surgery, ether had been demonstrated in 1846 in Boston. However, ether was not popular among medical personnel due to its explosive nature. Ether was used only for a short time in the Mexican-American War (1846–1848) but was discontinued because of its flammability. Indeed, often no anesthesia, other than alcohol spirits, was used. Ether was first sanctioned for use by the Army in 1849. Chloroform, which had enjoyed more popularity in the South, was also approved for Army use in 1849. Sulfuric ether (a more stable form) and chloroform, or a combination of the two, was the anesthetic of choice before 1861. Army surgeons used anesthetics routinely during operations after 1852.[16(pp17–19)]

Surgery would typically be necessary for compound fractures, as well as in the cases of extensive damage to joints or blood vessels.[16(p20)] Typical instruments that were standard issue for the surgeon's case would include the following: tourniquets, saws, bone cutters, silver catheters, artery forceps, tenaculum (a type of forceps), and a stomach pump (used as now for removing stomach contents in overdoses and for operations).

Transportation

Transportation of the wounded had been largely an *ad hoc* arrangement up to the Mexican-American War. Typically wagons, carts, or horses were used to move the wounded. In the Seminole and Black Hawk wars, there was no organized method of transport. The Mexican-American War featured a two-horse litter system or a nondedicated wheeled wagon. The two-horse litter system consisted of two poles with a blanket carried between two horses. The wagon was any available wheeled vehicle that could be utilized.[16(p22)] It was not until 1859 that an organized Army Board considered an approved wagon of conveyance. They evaluated both a two- and a four-wheeled vehicle. The idea of a dedicated ambulance was finally established in 1860. A four-wheeled ambulance was first tried out at Fort Leavenworth, Kansas, in 1861 prior to the Civil War onset because troopers there would be close to Indian hostilities. The two-wheeled ambulance was also evaluated at the fort for the same reason.[16(pp132–133)]

Medical Education

The state of medical education was not impressive in the years prior to the Mexican-American War and, for that matter, up to the Civil War. Many medical students who could afford to travel continued to go to the major medical training schools in Europe. English, Scottish, and German schools were most popular, with French and Italian schools following. In America, there was a proliferation of for-profit schools of varying quality. Preceptor training was still common, especially in the first half of the 19th century, and could be the whole or part of the training. As in the late 18th century and early 19th century, most apprenticeships in the trades lasted 7 years, as was the case for medicine. Often the for-profit medical schools required a 3-year apprenticeship in addition to attending several sessions of medical lectures.[16(p22)] Unfortunately, many people just put out signs without any real training. During this period, licensing by the states also declined. After the Army instituted competitive examinations in 1832, only 50% of candidates qualified.[16(pp31–31)] The examinations were required even for former Army surgeons who were trying to return to active duty. The examining boards consisted of three surgeons or assistant surgeons who conducted 3-day examinations and traveled to locations near the examinees.[16(p32)]

THE MEXICAN-AMERICAN WAR (1846–1848)

Contemporary Views of the War

A number of current books provide a good understanding of the Mexican-American War, which was a complex conflict. A sense of the times can be gathered from these books. Greenberg's book, *A Wicked War: Polk, Clay, Lincoln and the 1846 Invasion of Mexico*,[29] tells the story of the Mexican War from the perspective of five men—John Hardin, Nicholas Trist, James K Polk, Henry Clay, and Abraham Lincoln. Hardin was an Illinois congressman who was the first to volunteer for the war from Illinois. Trist successfully negotiated peace in a manner against the desires of his party and the president. President Polk was so identified with the war that it has been called "Mr Polk's War." Clay was the most famous politician of his time but he did not become president. His role in the prosecution of the war was central to the war effort. Lincoln was noted for his opposition to the Mexican conflict during his term in Congress.[29(pviii)]

Merry's book, *Country of Vast Designs: James K Polk, the Mexican War and the Conquest of the American Continent*,[30] provides a view of the war from the perspective of President Polk's actions. It is worthy of note that future presidents Lincoln and Grant did not favor the Mexican War, Lincoln serving in his only term in Congress and Grant serving as a first lieutenant in the war.[30(p474)]

Henderson's book, *A Glorious Defeat: Mexico and Its War With the United States*,[31] seeks to provide the Mexican perspective as to why it went to war with the United States in 1846. Mexico had only gained its independence from Spain in 1821. Mexico had many internal problems to deal with, given its recent independence. Finances were always a problem for a poor country and the political instability as to control of the country added to the problems. The relative instability helps explain some of the Mexican decisions in the conflict. The book explores the complex societal and hierarchical structure defining the Mexican state at the time.[31(pp6–8)] Henderson points out that Mexico made halting attempts to overcome obstacles such as the many different races, regions, cultures, and classes that made up the nation. He identified these obstacles as preventing a common identity and cause.[31(ppxviii-xix)]

Background

As noted, Mexico had gained independence from Spain in 1821. BG Antonio Lopez de Santa Anna proclaimed a republican regime in 1822.[32(p14)] The presence of American settlers (called Texians) in Texas caused instability for the Mexicans because the Americans did not follow Mexican rules and, furthermore, were independent in nature. The fall of the Alamo (6 March 1836) and the Battle of San Jacinto (a signal victory for Texas on 21 April 1836) were all part of the history of Texas.[32(p12)] In the ensuing years, new migrants to Texas established their own independent Lone Star Republic in 1836. The Mexicans were displeased with the outcome but did not move against the new republic due to their own internal issues.

The Texans were largely in favor of annexation by the United States, which happened in February 1845. War with Mexico seemed very certain with the annexation.[16(p95)] War on

Mexico was declared 15 months later by the United States on 13 May 1846.[22(p177)] Mexican forces had crossed the Rio Grande River while attacking an American patrol. Taylor had stationed an army of 3,500 in preparation at Corpus Christi in late 1845.[33(p150)] The many factors leading to war made it controversial even then. President Polk personified the energy of the country that created a political need for expansion. Henry Clay and Martin Van Buren (among others) opposed this idea, but the populace of America chose to go along with Polk.[30(p476)] In essence, the war caused conflict between those favoring growth and those satisfied with the status quo.

President Polk, a Democrat, was a driving force in the war. His two main generals were Winfield Scott and Zachary Taylor, who were both Whig Party members with political aspirations. President Polk liked the idea of volunteer soldiers, while General Scott favored Regular Army troops.[33(p78)] General Taylor's Army was not typical; it was a regular organization with disciplined troops, as opposed to the more typical militia troops of past military ventures. Over one-half of Taylor's Army was made up of recent immigrants, largely from Germany, Poland, and Ireland.[22(p60)]

Goals and Strategies

Polk held that the Rio Grande was the border with Mexico, while the Mexicans held that the Nueces River was the southern Texan border.[33(p149)] Polk hoped to secure his idea of a border with Mexico and to encourage Mexico to sell the territories of New Mexico and California. As the war progressed, the purchase approach was not pursued due to Mexican opposition.[34(p57)] Polk's military strategy was to have the Navy enforce a blockade of Mexico's ports (in the Gulf of Mexico) and Taylor's Army to proceed from Corpus Christi in a southwestern direction into Mexico to occupy it. A second force, composed of Missouri volunteers and commanded by Colonel (COL) Alexander Doniphan, was to take New Mexico and California.[22(p78)] Taylor's forces would occupy northeastern Mexico.[22(p88)] General Stephen Kearney conquered New Mexico before proceeding to California.[34(p111),35(p196)] COL Doniphan's Missouri volunteers then captured Chihuahua.[34(p142)] General Scott was to take half of Taylor's forces and proceed against Mexico City. Polk decided that Scott, if victorious, would be less of a political threat than Taylor. Taylor was mentioned in political circles as the favored Whig candidate for president in 1848.[33(p160)] Hence, using this political calculus, Winfield Scott was selected for the attack on Mexico City.[34(p141)]

Taylor's Forces

BG Zachary Taylor was ordered to move his troops from Louisiana to Texas in summer 1845. In August 1845, he had set up near Corpus Christi, Texas. General Taylor's forces, including his medical assets, landed at Corpus Christi where President Polk wanted his force in the area where he could react to Mexican provocations. Regimental hospitals were quickly set up in tents, while general hospitals were incorporated into existing buildings. Taylor's troops soon became ill, with 90 officers and 118 enlisted out of every 1,000 soldiers sick with various diseases.[16(pp98–99)]

Taylor was then ordered to move south to Point Isabel (where he set up Fort Texas). Taylor's surgeons received casualties from the Mexican bombardment of Fort Texas (and subsequent battles of Palo Alto and Resaca de la Palma). Point Isabel and Fort Texas were located directly opposite from Matamoros, Mexico.[16(p99)] Taylor's forces consisted of 3,000 troops, who had marched the several hundred miles from Corpus Christi to Fort Texas.[34(p58)] The first wounded were received from hostilities in May 1846, with 50 killed and 130 wounded. The Mexican wounded were turned over to Mexican surgeons by Taylor's forces.[16(p99)]

Taylor established general hospitals as his troops moved further into Mexico. Hospitals were set up at Mier, Camargo, Cerralvo, and at Matamoros (this one for smallpox isolation patients). These hospitals were set up in tents or existing buildings, when available. Some of these hospitals stayed open until the time when Americans started to leave Mexico in late spring 1848.[16(pp101–102)]

Matamoros was evacuated by the Mexicans; the Americans then occupied the city, but malaria increased due to heavy rains. In June 1846, as Taylor moved his Army further into Mexico, malaria and scurvy were problems.[16(pp100–101)] Taylor made it to Monterrey in September 1846. Surgeon General Lawson did not increase the ranks of the 20 surgeons with Taylor's Army, resulting in the surgeons working tirelessly. Monterrey capitulated after a 5-day battle. The Americans lost 120 killed and 368 wounded; the Mexican losses were not known.[16(p102)] The wounded were transported by litter or wagon to one of three Army hospitals set up in existing buildings in the city of Monterrey.[16(p102)] Wound infections were common. Malaria afflicted the wounded as well as complicating any recovery. At Saltillo, which the American forces took next, shortage of medicines required their local purchase. Malaria and a measles epidemic plagued the troops.[16(p104)] The Battle of Buena Vista was the end of Taylor's active campaign.[16(p105)]

Doniphan and his Missouri Volunteers

Although much attention has been directed to the Regular forces, the success of COL Doniphan and his Missouri Volunteers reflect the contribution of the citizen-soldier and of the natural citizen leader. Doniphan was a small town Missouri lawyer who enlisted as a private in 1846, but in a month was elected the colonel of the 1st Regiment of Missouri Mounted Volunteers (consisting of 800 soldiers). The volunteers were formed to protect Texas, a newly admitted state of the United States.[35(p1)] President Polk had selected COL Kearny, a regular officer, to lead a force consisting of 300 Regulars, 400 other volunteers, and Doniphan's regiment to invade the area that is now New Mexico (but was then part of Mexico). Doniphan's regiment played a key role in the capitulation of New Mexico. Doniphan led his regiment in the Battles of Buena Vista (a General Taylor victory) and Chihuahua.[35(pp193–194)] Doniphan placed emphasis on the contribution that the Regular Army troops made to the volunteers. After the war, Doniphan gave credit for his military success to the 3-month time his troops served with Kearny (who was later promoted to general).[35(p202)]

Kearny's forces in the "Army of the West" continued to California with a difficult journey from Fort Leavenworth, Kansas, to Santa Fe, New Mexico. Doniphan's volunteer forces were split off to remain in Santa Fe. None of Doniphan's physicians were from the Army Medical Department. His volunteer physicians included a civilian contractor that Doniphan hired. Doniphan's troops had a high sick rate, approaching one-third of the force at times, while showing a high death rate from disease (not specified). Measles, fevers, and diarrhea were all mentioned as involving the command. In their Chihuahua fight, Doniphan lost one killed and five wounded. His surgeons also cared for wounded and ill Mexicans.[16(p106)]

Scott's Move toward Mexico City

Johnson, in his book *Winfield Scott: The Quest for Military Glory*,[33] felt that General Scott was very well qualified to lead the American Army to Mexico City. He developed what Johnson terms "an astute strategy" and had become in this time of his life "the consummate field commander."[33(p208)] Scott was a student of history who had studied the French experience in the Iberian Peninsula during the Napoleonic Wars. The French, due to their poor treatment of the Spanish peasants and soldiers, had a guerilla action on their hands.[33(pp166–167)] Scott had firsthand experience with guerilla action in the Florida Seminole Wars during his inability to cancel out an 1836 Indian guerilla action.[33(p169)] Scott was able to use politics and diplomacy in support of his military action.[33(p170)]

Scott's 9 March 1847 assault upon Veracruz was the largest American amphibious operation until World War II. Scott landed 8,600 men in 5 hours without any losses.[33(p174)] The Veracruz operations were completed by 29 March 1847. Casualties included 13 Americans killed and 55 wounded. The Mexican casualties were unknown but estimated to be about 200 killed.[33(p178)] After Scott took Veracruz, he imposed martial law. He paroled enemy prisoners, distributed food to the city, and provided clean-up funds for the streets. Scott's measures led the people of Veracruz to accept the occupation by his troops.[33(p179)]

Veracruz was Scott's valued supply base (especially for medical supplies) as the troops moved into Mexico.[33(p180)] Veracruz became an important general hospital site due to its location. The fear of yellow fever was, however, a reality at Veracruz; at least two surgeons died of yellow fever.[16(p117)] Yellow fever treatments at Veracruz included quinine (for fever), mustard plasters (to even the temperature and circulation), mercurials (to promote bowel movements), and cupping to draw off blood.[16(p117)]

Surgeon General Lawson traveled with General Scott's army, joining him at Veracruz in December 1846 and remaining until early spring 1848. He did not exercise direct control of Scott's medical staff, but rather acted as the senior surgeon on the field. The duties of the Surgeon General in Washington, DC, were assumed by the very competent Surgeon Henry Heiskell.[16(p111)] One consequence of Lawson being in Mexico dealt with supplies, in that the New York supply officer did not receive reports from Lawson in the field and incorrect quantities were shipped.[16(p114)]

Scott sent BG David E Twiggs with his division to capture Jalapa (60 miles away) while MG William Worth was ordered to stay in Veracruz.[33(p181)] As the troops moved inland from Veracruz in March 1847, they were plagued with intestinal disturbances (diarrhea) from "bad water."[16(p118)] Along the march route, the Battle of Cerro Gordo was an American victory. The subsequent battle for Cerro Gordo Pass resulted in 64 Americans killed and 353 wounded. (Mexican figures are not available).[16(p118)] Jalapa fell to the Americans and, again, Scott's civil pacification strategy kept the citizens quiet.[33(p188)] At Jalapa, Scott had to send home several regiments whose terms of enlistment were soon to expire.[33(p189)] The hospital at Jalapa was located in a church. The facility had few amenities and sustained a 20% mortality of the 1,000 estimated patients to pass through it.[16(p119)] A hospital was set up San Augustin and later at Mixcoac within 10 miles of Mexico City. On 8 September 1847, the Americans battled the Mexicans at Molino del Ray. One surgeon was killed leading troops after their officers were killed.[16(p120)] The surrender of Mexico City ended the active prosecution of the war. (As an interesting side note, Robert E Lee had been assigned to the US Engineers starting in 1831. He was assigned to the staff of General Scott. Lee's engineering background helped in locating an unused trail at Chapultepec, Mexico that allowed the American troops to come behind the defending Mexican forces.)[36(p41)]

Disease continued to be a health problem in Mexico City. Diarrhea was the major problem for troops there.[16(pp121–122)] Evacuation of the ill and wounded took 18 days in a wagon to reach Veracruz. The evacuated were then taken to New Orleans and Baton Rouge. Overcrowding led the Army to send patients as far north as Jefferson Barracks near St Louis, Missouri.[16(p123)] Fort Monroe, Virginia, was the stopping point for other evacuees.[16(p124)]

Medical Care During the Mexican-American War

As the war progressed, some changes were made to the medical side of the Army. In 1846, the volunteer surgeons were accorded the same professional status as Regulars. In February 1847, ranks were accorded to medical officers, although they were not to command outside of medical channels. The Surgeon General was to be a colonel, surgeons were to be majors, and assistant surgeons were to be captains.[16(pp97–98)] The Medical Department leaders serving on site in Mexico included a medical director and the director of a general hospital. There was also an office of purveyor. The purveyor was a surgeon who served as a purchasing officer as well.[16(p97)]

As noted above, an act of Congress had instructed that medical officers would have official rank. Congress ruled that medical officers would have equal remuneration to that of other officers for allowances and housing. However, the US Army Adjutant General mandated that the old rules would remain in effect because in his view the new law was deemed to be inconclusive. In effect, medical officers would still be expected to obey orders from the most junior officer. Indeed, medical officers could be brought before courts-martial for refusing orders, as was the case with Major (Surgeon) Clement Finley, who would later become Surgeon General. Finley refused an order from Brevet Lieutenant Colonel (LTC) Braxton Bragg (of later Confederate Civil War fame). LTC Bragg had a Regular rank of Captain, which Finley held to be Bragg's true rank, and Finley, as a major, therefore refused his order. Finley was convicted by courts-martial. President Millard Fillmore upheld the conviction, but remitted Finley's dismissal from the Army.[16(p129)] (A senior medical officer could lead a Court of Inquiry if he were the most senior in rank, but even such a role was not applied consistently.) Thus, the exact status of the medical officer remained to be clarified in the future.[16(p129)]

The volunteer surgeons and the contract surgeons did not have to pass examinations, as did the Regular Army surgeons. The volunteer surgeons, in particular, were not familiar with military discipline and the need to adhere to accepted medical standards of sanitation planning in the military environment. The surgeon was required to advise the line command as to the placement of latrines and water supplies and to pick a "healthy" site for the camp (if possible, not in an area known for yellow fever or malaria). In the Mexican-American War, Surgeon General Lawson did not make the most in all situations of the surgeons and staff that he had on hand, because he did not plan to staff both regimental and general hospitals at the same time.[16(p97)] At the start of the conflict, Congress allowed only three surgeons per regiment. In 1846, Congress authorized the call-up of two surgeons per volunteer regiment. In February 1847, Congress increased the size of the medical staffs. One surgeon and two assistant surgeons could be appointed for new regular regiments. However, the difficult examination for Regular surgeons still remained. Hence, the hiring of civilian surgeons was necessary to staff Army posts and to provide care in Mexico.[16(p96)]

As part of the logistical planning for the Mexican-American War, Surgeon General Lawson favored procuring supplies from New York City, where he wished to set up a medical supply depot. He believed that better prices could be obtained in a larger city. Supplies were to then be stockpiled in New Orleans because this would be a large port closer to the points of conflict. Not surprisingly, there were losses of materials and supplies due to pilfering along the supply chain, as well as shipwrecks at sea.[16(p98)]

Although disease seemed to be the major focus of medical care, there were wounds to deal with in the war. The Mexicans used old musket smoothbore pieces, which fired round projectiles. They could be superficial and could be more easily removed than the Minié ball, which would be used extensively in the Civil War. Artillery fire from cannons was more lethal but, due to the relative lack of Mexican field pieces, was used infrequently. Wounds could be more serious, especially if shot or metallic pieces were fired into massed troops.[16(p118)]

During the time of the Mexican-American War, the deaths from disease were 10 times greater in the Army than at home in the civilian communities.[16(p124)] Out of 100,000 soldiers who served in Mexico, Gillet reports 1,500 killed and 10,000 dying of disease. (Nevertheless, the ratio of battle deaths to disease deaths for the Mexican-American War was improved from the approximate figures for the Revolutionary War.[16(pp124–125),35,37]) Total battle deaths for the Mexican-American War (as listed on the Congressional Research Service site) are reported as 1,733, with total deaths largely due to disease of 11,550. Woundings not leading to death were listed as 4,152.[37]

The Treaty of Guadalupe Hidalgo ended the war after it was signed on 2 February 1848. The treaty was ratified by the US Congress on 30 May 1848 and by the Mexican Congress on 15 July 1848. The treaty provided for the use of the Rio Grande River as the boundary between Texas and Mexico. The United States paid $15 million to Mexico and would settle the claims of United States citizens against Mexico. Mexicans could be United States citizens if they lived within the new boundaries. In bringing about this settlement, Nicholas Trist represented the United States in negotiations with a special commission.[31(ppxv,172–178)] The treaty also specified that the Indians residing in the newly acquired territories would be restrained by the United States from entering Mexico.[34(p221)]

The successful prosecution of the war launched several political careers. General Taylor, a hero of the Mexican-American War, and a slaveholder, became the Whig candidate opposing President Polk, a Democrat. General Scott had previously been a candidate for the Whig nomination. Scott in a later election became the Whig candidate for president but he lost to Franklin Pierce. Taylor won easily due to his wartime prestige.[34(p222)] President Taylor died on 4 July 1850 of a gastrointestinal ailment. (The symptoms suggest to the modern physician reader a recurrence of amebic dysentery or cholera.) His death illustrated how diseases of the time could afflict even the most powerful person.[16(p143),34(p222)]

The Mexican-American War outcome promoted the need for a professional military. The graduates of West Point brought their engineering and military strategy education to the conflict. Their professionalism and the need for a standing army to deal with the country's expanded territory retired the notion of an all-volunteer force.[34(p222)]

MEDICAL DEPARTMENT INVOLVEMENT OUTSIDE MEDICINE

In the same tradition of Generals Ainsworth and Wood, who would later move to areas outside medicine in the Army, Assistant Surgeon Albert Meyer became very interested in new signal techniques. He would later become the head of the newly created Signal Corps in 1863.[16(p148)] In 1852, Surgeon General Lawson asked for the Army surgeons to collect meteorological data for scientific completeness and to report statistics for sickness and wounds. (It was later in the 1870s that Dr John Shaw Billings pushed for the collection of mortality statistics. He, too, asked for meteorological statistics. He also collected examples of unique medical anatomical specimens.[22(p210)])

THE APPROACH OF THE CIVIL WAR

Army surgeons had generally dealt with the health issues of small and often isolated posts. The scale of casualties to be had in the coming Civil War would not be even imagined by veteran surgeons of the War of 1812 (1812–1814) or the Mexican-American War (1846–1848).

Surgeon General Lawson died on 15 May 1861. Clement Finley would become the next Surgeon General. It was said that only his 40 years of service would be a qualification for office because he was not felt to be otherwise qualified by his subordinates.[16(pp153–154)]

In peacetime prior to the Civil War, the Army Medical Department had to contend with limited budgets, isolated posts, and bureaucratic rules. Army medicine and its practice were largely as it was prior to the Mexican-American War. Medical practice remained more art than science. There were no central plans in the Army for medical supply and evacuation so needed in the coming large conflict.[16(p149)]

REFERENCES
1. Hickey DR. *The War of 1812: A Forgotten Conflict*. Urbana, Ill: University of Illinois Press; 2012.
2. Taylor A. *The Civil War of 1812: American Citizens, British Subjects, Irish Rebels, & Indian Allies*. New York, NY: Alfred A Knopf; 2010.
3. Sheads SS. *The Chesapeake Campaigns 1813–15; Middle Ground of the War of 1812*. London, England: Osprey Publishing Company; 2014.
4. Vogel S. *Through the Perilous Fight: From the Burning of Washington to the Star Spangled Banner: The Six Weeks That Saved the Nation*. New York, NY: Random House; 2013.
5. Latimer J. *1812: War With America*. Cambridge, Mass: The Belknap Press of Harvard University Press; 2007.
6. Berton P. *The Invasion of Canada: 1812–1813*. Toronto, Canada: Anchor Canada (Division of Random House of Canada Ltd); 1980.
7. Gillet MC. *The Army Medical Department: 1775–1818*. Washington, DC: US Government Printing Office; 1981.
8. Beaumont W, Miller G, eds. *William Beaumont's Formative Years: Two Early Notebooks 1811–1821*. Whitefish, Mont: Kessinger Publishing Company; 2007.
9. Roberts J. *The British Raid on Essex: The Forgotten Battle of the War of 1812*. Middleton, Conn: Wesleyan University Press; 2014.
10. Howard H. *Mr and Mrs Madison's War. America's First Couple and the Second War of Independence*. New York, NY: Bloomsbury Press; 2012.
11. Pitch AS. *The Burning of Washington: The British Invasion of 1814*. Annapolis, Md: The Naval Institute Press; 1998.
12. Remini RV. *The Battle of New Orleans: Andrew Jackson and America's First Military Victory*. New York, NY: Penguin Books; 2001.
13. Phalen J. Landmarks in surgery: Surgeon James Mann, US Army: observations on battlefield amputations. *Surgery*. 1938;(66):1071–1073.
14. Howard M. *Wellington's Doctors: The British Army Medical Services in the Napoleonic Wars*. New York, NY: History Press; 2008.
15. Bonura MA. *Under the Shadow of Napoleon: French Influence on the American Way of Warfare From the War of 1812 to the Outbreak of WWII*. New York, NY: NYU Press; 2012.
16. Gillet MC. *The Army Medical Department 1818–1865*. Washington, DC: Center for Military History United States Army; 1987.
17. Medline Plus. Mercury. http://www.nlm.nih.gov/medlineplus/ency/article/002476.htm. Accessed 19 March 2015.
18. Higby GJ. Chemistry and the 19th century American pharmacist. *Bull Hist Chem*. 2003;(28):10.
19. Bynum WF. *Science and the Practice of Medicine in the 19th Century*. Cambridge, England: Cambridge University Press; 1994.
20. Royal Society of Chemistry. Quinine. http://www.rsc.org/chemistryworld/podcast/CIIEcompounds/transcripts/Quinine.asp?playpodcastlinkuri=%2Fchemistryworld%2Fpodcast%2FCIIEcompound%2Easp%3Fcompound%3DQuinine. Accessed 19 March 2015.
21. Whooley O. *Knowledge in the Time of Cholera: The Struggle Over American Medicine in the Nineteenth Century*. Chicago, Ill: University of Chicago Press; 2013.
22. Brown HE. *The Medical Department of the United States Army From 1775 to 1873*. Washington, DC: Surgeon General's Office; 1873.
23. Wintermute BA. *Public Health and the US Military: A History of the Army Medical Department, 1818–1917*. New York, NY: Routledge (Taylor and Francis Group); 2011.

24. Exploring Florida. The Seminole Wars. http://fcit.usf.edu/florida/lessons/sem_war/sem_war1.htm. Accessed 19 March 2015.
25. Hatch T. *Osceola and the Great Seminole War: A Struggle for Justice and Freedom*. New York, NY; St Martin's Press; 2012.
26. US Army Medical Department. Office of Medical History. *Surgeons General. Thomas Lawson*. http://history.amedd.army.mil/surgeongenerals/T_Lawson.html. Accessed 19 March 2015.
27. Beaumont W. *Experiments and Observations on the Gastric Juice and the Physiology of Digestion*. Plattsburgh, NY: Maclachlan and Stewart; 1833.
28. Mahmoud RA, Clark KL, May L. *Military Preventive Medicine: Mobilization and Deployment*. Vol 1. Chapter 7. Evolution of military recruit accession standards. https://ke.army.mil/bordeninstitute/published_volumes/mpmVol1/PM1ch7.pdf. Accessed 19 March 2015.
29. Greenberg AS. *A Wicked War: Polk, Clay, Lincoln, and the 1846 US Invasion of Mexico*. New York, NY: Alfred A Knopf; 2012.
30. Merry RW. *A Country of Vast Designs: James K. Polk, the Mexican War and the Conquest of the American Continent*. New York, NY: Simon and Schuster; 2009.
31. Henderson JJ. *A Glorious Defeat: Mexico and Its War With the United States*. New York, NY: Hill and Wang (Division of Farrar, Strauss, and Giroux); 2007.
32. Nofi AA. *The Alamo and the Texas War for Independence; Heroes, Myths and History*. San Antonio, Tex: De Capo Press; 1992.
33. Johnson TD. *Winfield Scott: The Quest for Military Glory*. Lawrence, Kans: University Press of Kansas; 1998.
34. Christensen C, Christensen T. *The US-Mexican War*. San Francisco, Calif: Bay Books; 1998.
35. Dawson JC. *Doniphan's Epic March: The 1st Missouri Volunteers in the Mexican War*. Lawrence, Kans: University Press of Kansas; 1999.
36. Lee F. *General Lee: A Biography of Robert E Lee*. Wilmington, NC: Broadfoot Publishing, Inc; 1989. (Original publication 1894 by D Appleton and Company, New York, NY.)
37. Congressional Research Service. *American War and Military Operations Casualties: Lists and Statistics*. http://fas.org/sgp/crs/natsec/RL32492.pdf. Accessed 19 March 2015.

" The Civil War was an epic conflict involving forces engaged in large-scale battles. The military's medical resources were stretched almost to the breaking in the early phases of the fighting. The Confederacy was limited in its medical response by lack of resources due to the blockade of many of its ports. Because the statistics and records of the Confederate Medical Department are limited, most of the discussion in this chapter will be focused on the Union Army. It was a time of 'forward surgery' in its simplest form."

Chapter Three

The Civil War: Military Medical Care in the War Between the States

LANCE P. STEAHLY, MD

INTRODUCTION

THE CIVIL WAR WAS AN EPIC CONFLICT involving forces engaged in large-scale battles. The military's medical resources were stretched almost to the breaking in the early phases of the fighting. The skills of men such as William Hammond, Jonathan Letterman, and John Shaw Billings helped the Union meet the challenge. The Confederacy was limited in its medical response by lack of resources due to the blockade of many of its ports. Because the statistics and records of the Confederate Medical Department are limited, most of the discussion in this chapter will be focused on the Union Army. Prior to the Civil War, the "action" in Army medicine was centered in the military outposts in the West. It was a time of "forward surgery" in its simplest form. In the West, the Army surgeon treated broken bones, the occasional arrow wound, and the many illnesses of the time. The postwar transition to peace signaled a return to many features of prewar medicine. The late-1860s to the mid-1890s were characterized by small-unit Indian conflicts with just the bare essentials of "forward surgery." The Spanish-American War in 1898 showed the inadequacies of preparation for large-scale conflicts. However, the brevity of the conflict meant that the inadequacies of supplies and personnel did not affect the outcome. After the Spanish-American War, new national responsibilities in Cuba, Puerto Rico, Panama, and the Philippines highlighted the importance of public health advances (control of yellow fever, malaria, immunization programs, and sanitary reforms) for Army medicine.

THE COMING OF WAR

In the decade before the onset of the Civil War, there were fundamental changes that had impact on the coming conflict. In the 1850s, most people in the North and the South were living in rural areas. A large influx of immigrants in that decade brought many Irish and Germans to the United States. (Many of these same immigrants would enlist in the Union Army in the conflict ahead.) Most of these new immigrants settled in urban areas. The North, especially, developed a large manufacturing infrastructure; the South had some manufacturing gains, but it remained largely focused on agriculture. Cotton was the main economic engine in the South.

The slavery question was heavily tied to the agrarian economy of the South. Over the years, the US Congress had taken up the issue of slavery. The Northwest Ordnance of 1787 originally stipulated that states north of the Ohio River were to be free, while those states to the south were to be slave. The states were balanced until 1819, when Missouri sought admission as a slave state. Maine came in as a free state to balance the number again, which was codified in the Missouri Compromise of 1820. Further accommodation had to be made in the Compromise of 1850. In the Congress, Henry Clay of Kentucky was the central manager of the agreement, with aid from Daniel Webster of Massachusetts. The Compromise admitted California as a free state and prohibited slavery in the District of Columbia. However, it allowed new states that were to be admitted henceforth to decide the slavery issue for themselves.[1(p6)] At issue here, as a common thread, was the concern about "state's rights."[1(pp5–6)]

The election of Lincoln in 1860 added weight to the South's perception that the federal government would seek to abolish slavery. The secession of the Southern states, starting with South Carolina, was a point of no return. The 12 April 1861 4:30 AM firing upon Fort Sumter, South Carolina, was the opening volley in a civil war that would last several years and affect almost every family in both the North and the South. Major Robert Anderson, the commander of Fort Sumter, surrendered on 13 April 1861 because the fort lacked adequate supplies and manpower to withstand the ongoing attack.[2(p166),3(p5)]

Lieutenant General (LTG) Winfield Scott, the aging Army Chief of Staff who played such a prominent role in the War of 1812, the Indian Wars, and the Mexican-American War of 1848, devised the Anaconda Plan of 1861 to deal with the insurrection. The plan envisioned blockade of the entire 3,000 mile southern coastal line (both Atlantic and Gulf ports) and the capture of the Mississippi River, which bisected the Confederacy. The plan required an expedition of 84,000 troops, supported by gunboats, to go down the Mississippi and capture New Orleans, Louisiana.[2(pp168–169)] LTG Scott was replaced as the Army Commander because of his health, obesity, and advanced age (74 years old) by Major General (MG) George McClellan on the orders of President Lincoln (Figure 3-1). Nonetheless, the Anaconda Plan devised by General Scott was basically the strategy for the military and economic offense that was followed going forward.[1(p41),3(p5)]

OVERVIEW OF THE MAIN BATTLES OF THE CIVIL WAR

To set the stage for this discussion of the Civil War, a brief review of the timelines involved and the subsequent important battles follows:
- An Ordinance of Secession was passed by South Carolina on 20 December 1860,

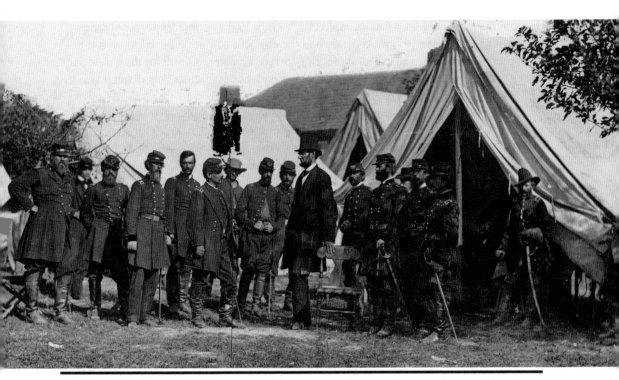

FIGURE 3-1. President Abraham Lincoln, in his familiar top hat, with his commander, Major General George B McClellan and other officers, Antietam, Maryland, October 1862. Photograph courtesy of the Library of Congress, Image #04352.

making it the first state to secede. Over a 6-month period, it was followed by 11 other states, with Tennessee joining the last of the states on 8 June 1861.[1(p31)]
- The Confederate attack on Fort Sumter (Charleston Harbor, South Carolina) was carried out on 12–13 April 1861. On 15 April 1861, President Lincoln proclaimed a state of insurrection. He issued a call for 75,000 Union volunteers.[1(pp85–87)]
- The First Battle of Bull Run was fought; both the North and the South were hoping for a quick victory and to rapidly occupy their respective opposing capitals. The battle began on 21 July 1861. The Confederates gained victory while the Union had a disaster as their forces retreated in a chaotic manner. The Union fielded some 35,000 troops in the Army of the Potomac, of which 2,896 were killed. The Confederates had 1,982 killed, out of a force of 21,000 Confederate troops.[1(pp87–90)]
- The Battle of Shiloh, fought at Pittsburg Landing on the Tennessee River in Tennessee during the period of 6–7 April 1861, was considered a Union victory, although much criticism was leveled at Grant for his losses. The Union lost approximately 13,000 wounded and killed (of the 30,000 troops in the Army of the Potomac) compared with the Confederacy's 10,694 casualties (out of 21,000 troops).[1(pp91–93)]
- The Battle of Antietam was preceded by the Confederate victory at the Second Battle of Bull Run. The Antietam Battle on 17 September 1862 was a signal Union victory

and the premiere McClellan triumph.[1(pp95–96)] Only 40,000 Confederates faced more than 75,000 Union troops. Antietam had the distinction of being the battle with the most casualties in a single day, amounting to approximately 12,400 for the Union and 10,300 for the Confederates.[1(p94)] (Gettysburg had more casualties overall but it was a 3-day engagement.) The Army of the Potomac (Union) tried to keep Lee's Army of Northern Virginia from entering Maryland at Frederick, Maryland.

- Chancellorsville was one of General Lee's greatest victories. Union MG Joseph Hooker had replaced MG Ambrose Burnside as the Commander of the Army of the Potomac. General Lee and his forces were able to severely defeat Hooker's Union forces. The battle lasted from 1–3 May 1862. The Union sustained 17,000 casualties, while the South had 13,000 casualties. The South had some 60,000 troops involved under the command of General Robert E Lee. The Union had 134,000 troops under the command of MG Hooker.[1(pp97–98)]

- The Battle of Gettysburg lasted from 1–3 July 1863. It was the Confederate's last major incursion (Frederick, Maryland, at Antietam was the first) into the North. It was a costly encounter for both sides but the Confederates withdrew, without pursuit, to safety. In a 3-day battle, the losses were so great that 50,000 combined casualties were noted. MG Hooker's Army of the Potomac fielded over 90,000 men to oppose Lee's 75,000 men.[1(pp99–100)]

- The Battle of Chickamauga was from 19–20 September 1863. The battle, named for a Georgia creek, provided a victory for the Confederacy.[1(pp102–103)] The Union Army of the Cumberland, commanded by MG William Rosecrans, had taken areas in Tennessee including Chattanooga, an important transportation and supply hub. The Confederate Army of Tennessee was commanded by the Confederate General Braxton Bragg. Union MG George Thomas' performance was credited with keeping the Union losses controlled. Fortunately for the North, Bragg did not provide decisive leadership that could have resulted in a crippling blow to the Union.[1(pp101–103)]

- Chattanooga, Tennessee, was a victory for the North in October and November 1863. Chattanooga was the South's important regional supply and communication center. The loss of such a center was impossible to mitigate.[1(pp105–106)] The Union forces had seized Chattanooga in November 1863 and had fended off attempts to retake the center. MG Braxton Bragg and his Confederate forces besieged the city. MG (later LTG) Ulysses S Grant came to the rescue, using MG William T Sherman's and MG Hooker's troops.[1(pp104–106)]

- The Battle of the Wilderness transpired from 5–7 May 1864, but was indecisive for either side. It was followed by the 8–21 May 1864 Battle of Spotsylvania, which had Lee and Grant in play. The losses were great: 17,500 Union casualties and 10,000 Confederate casualties. The Union fielded approximately 119,000 troops, poised against the undermanned Confederates (64,000 strong) of Lee's Army of Northern Virginia.[1(pp110–112)]

- Atlanta, an important Southern manufacturing and communication center, fell to Sherman's troops after a 4-month long campaign from 1 May to 2 September 1864.[1(pp112–113)]

- The Battle of Nashville, 15–16 December 1864, brought about the defeat of Confederate General John Bell Hood and the Army of Tennessee. It would be the last major battle in the West.
- The Battle of Petersburg, Virginia, ran from 15 June 1864 until 3 April 1865. The 10-month siege of Petersburg ended in a Confederate defeat, despite their victory earlier at the Battle of Cold Harbor, Virginia, on 3 June 1864.
- General Lee surrendered his Army to General Grant at Appomattox Court House on 9 April 1865, which is usually perceived as the war's end. However, other Confederate commands continued the war for another 10 weeks.[1(p217)] LTG Kirby Smith fought on 12–13 May 1865 in Texas. LTG Simon Buckner surrendered in New Orleans, Louisiana, on 25 May 1865. The last to surrender was the Cherokee force headed by Confederate Brigadier General (BG) Stand Watie, which quit fighting on 23 June 1865.[1(p218)]

BATTLEFIELD SURGERY: THE RUN-UP TO THE CIVIL WAR

French Influence on Western Medicine

During the Napoleonic Wars, the French Surgeon Dominique Jean Larrey described "temporary hospital establishments, organized near the divisions of an army."[4(p1)] Larrey started out as a young surgeon from Beaudeau in the Pyrenees Mountains,[4(p13)] and later became the medical chief of the French Army of the Rhine. Larrey was appointed to his position in the Army of the Rhine only 13 months after the start of the Reign of Terror during the French Revolution.[1(p14)] He developed two- and four-wheeled light wagons, which he organized as a "flying ambulance," that carried surgeons and their assistants to the front and then brought the wounded to the surgeons.[4(p14)] The surgeons could then do amputations, remove bullets, and dress wounds. There was some tradition for regimental surgeons treating soldiers on the line already in England and with multiple Continental armies at Fontenoy, Belgium, in the mid-18th century.[4(pp14–15)] Yet another French surgeon, Pierre Francois Percy, organized a trained corps of ambulance litter-bearers to gather the wounded and to carry them to a surgical support station.[4(p15)] He created the Percy surgical wagon, similar in concept to that devised by Larrey.

In the Crimean War (1854–1856), the French, unlike the English and Russians, were prepared with a complete system of army hospitals, including the "flying ambulances" (and the ordinary ambulance).[4(p17)] The flying ambulance consisted of a light cart with one officer, two surgeons, and two attendants. The ambulance was posted near the battle to treat and evacuate the wounded. The ordinary ambulance consisted of five wagons carrying more extensive dressings and material. Five officers, six surgeons, 25 attendants, several apothecaries, and an instrument maker made up the ambulance staff.[4(p17)] Most surgeons followed the wisdom of Pare and Larrey that immediate amputation was desirable. Chloroform became popular in the Crimean conflict as the anesthetic of choice.

The Beginnings of the Nursing Profession

In the Crimea, Florence Nightingale was appointed the superintendent of the Female Nursing Establishment of the Eighth General Hospital in Turkey. She set up for business with 38 women trained as nurses just 4 days after the "Charge of the Light Brigade" at Balaclava in October 1854. The British (unlike the French) were not able to care for their wounded and had a poorly organized evacuation system.[4(pp19-20)] The advances to come from the Crimean conflict included improved amputation techniques, the use of prefabricated wooden buildings along the pavilion system lines, and the care brought forth by Nightingale.[4(p17)] Florence Nightingale and her recruited nurses were not initially appreciated by the medical establishment and many of the surgeons, despite the fact that the nurses were appreciated by the wounded troops. However, their hard work and dedication won the belated respect of the surgeons and more so of the international community.[4(p21)]

Contributions of the Prussians

The Prussians first introduced a system of dedicated litter bearers to bring the wounded off the field in 1855. The Prussians learned much from Larrey (and later Letterman) in setting up specialized and dedicated wartime surgical treatment.[4(p69)] The Prussians made a significant advance in their armaments with the advent of the breech-loading Dreyse needle-fire rifle. The rifle's cartridge was set off by a steel pin pushed by the hammer into the base of the cartridge. This firearms advance resulted in more casualties to be treated for the opponents of the Prussians. On the field of battle the dedicated litter carriers helped to evacuate the enemy casualties, in addition to their own troops.[4(p96)]

It was with this introduction that the medical and surgical needs of the US Civil War were to be met.[4(p21)] In the Civil War, the medical establishments were as unprepared as was the military for the soon-to-erupt carnage. Years of fighting in small engagements, or quickly won small wars, would soon be replaced by the need to field massive armies. The medical support necessary to tend to the needs of the casualties would overwhelm the initially inadequate medical establishment.

WAR FOR AMATEURS—LINE AND MEDICAL

For both the North and the South, despite the small cadre of military academy graduates (West Point, the Citadel, Virginia Military Institute, and the Military College of Vermont), the armies were populated by amateurs. In the same way, the small number of professional military surgeons would be joined by a majority of military medical "amateurs." These inadequacies were soon tested in the First Battle of Bull Run, which failed to be the easy victory that many in the Union sought. They had hoped it would bring an early end to the rebellion, but instead the South was the victor. The Confederate victory led to the South's expectations that the rest of the war could be prosecuted just as efficiently and successfully. It was unfortunate that the South's expectations were unrealistically elevated so early. In their enthusiasm, it led to the perspective that the South could be victorious, while ignoring their inadequate resources necessary for victory in the long term.[1(p88)]

Just before the start of the Civil War, the US Army Medical Corps had only 30 surgeons and 83 assistant surgeons. Of these, three surgeons and 21 assistant surgeons resigned to join the Confederate States of America (CSA). Another three assistant surgeons were dismissed because they would not sign loyalty oaths.[4(p23)] The 80-year-old and dying Surgeon General, Thomas Lawson, a veteran of the War of 1812, cut budgets because he was frugal; furthermore, he denied his surgeons leave. He also cut the medical supply inventory to a minimum.[5(p2)] Additionally, only 62 new surgeons were appointed out of 116 applicants.[6(p9)] Surgeon General Lawson's 1860 budget request for appropriations was a mere $90,000 ($27,000 of the total would be paid for contract surgeons). Lawson's frugal obsession was aided by Congress, which appropriated only $115,000 in March 1861.[6(p5)] Lawson had become the Surgeon General only because of seniority at the time of the administration of John Quincy Adams. He stayed in office for the period up to the Civil War because there was no retirement law.[6(p4)] Thus, the US Army Medical Corps was woefully unprepared for the massive casualties it would soon be called on to care for in the war. The coming of the Sanitary Commission would put additional pressure on the Medical Department and Congress to spend at more appropriate levels.[6(p5)]

THE CIVIL WAR: ITS IMPORTANCE TO MILITARY MEDICINE

The number of Civil War deaths had been believed to be 360,000 Union dead (and 281,000 wounded) and 285,000 Confederate dead (and 194,000 wounded) ever since an 1889 report, based on imprecise after-action reports for the South compiled by William F Fox, who served as a lieutenant colonel of USA Volunteers, and had served at Antietam, Chancellorsville, and Gettysburg.[7] Fox wrote that of 2.3 million enrolled Union troops, an additional 199,970 died of disease. Confederate figures are not as accurate, but are in the range of 150,000 died of disease.[7] In a recent book, Young explores the murky Confederate casualty numbers in the Overland Campaign, a series of battles fought in Virginia during May and June 1864. He studied letters, diaries, and, best of all, Confederate newspapers, which were often the most accurate sources for reliable statistics.[8(ppix–x)] Young found that Lee's numbers at the start of the campaign were larger than reported. Furthermore, Confederate losses were greater than previously held to be the case.[8(px)] In a 2011 article, Hacker revised the number of deaths upward by 20%, based upon recently digitalized 19th-century census data. He noted that the data are not final because the number of civilian dead can only be estimated.[9] Blaisdell points out that these casualties exceeded the total of all preceding or subsequent US wars. He further notes that the losses affected, directly or indirectly, nearly every family in the North and the South.[10] These casualties occurred at the more than 10,000 battles and combat encounters that took place during the 4 years of the Civil War.

The history of Civil War medicine for Union forces has been thoroughly reported in several volumes, including *The Army Medical Department 1818–1865*[11] and *Medical Recollections of the Army of the Potomac*.[12] There was no comparable reporting of Civil War medicine for the Confederate forces. Yet there are glimpses of Confederate military medicine. As one example, the second CSA Surgeon General, Dr Samuel Preston Moore (replacing the inept David C Deleon), had been a US Army surgeon until 1861. He is credited with reform of Southern hospitals and creation of an ambulance corps. His work included efforts to find substitutes from the Southern flora for pharmaceuticals (which were affected by the Northern blockade). Interestingly, he was the editor of the *Confederate State Medical and Surgical Journal*, which is available (in DVD [digital video diskette] format) from the Francis A Countway Library of Medicine at Harvard University in Boston.[13]

The enormous battlefield carnage, infection, and disease sorely tested the US Army Medical Department in the Civil War. Viewing it from a 21st-century perspective, the medicine practiced in the 1860s seems primitive. However, as Schroeder-Lein commented, a sense of context and humility is needed to evaluate the medicine and surgery of the time. Schroeder-Lein wrote that surgeons were trying to do their best generally, with the equipment and techniques available, and trying to learn from their experience.[14(p2)]

The Sanitary Commission

The Sanitary Commission was formed to assist in the massive undertaking of caring for the wounded and sick of the North. The Sanitary Commission could be thought of as a combination of today's American Red Cross and the United Service Organizations (USO). It was actually more in practice, assuming many of the roles that the military/government would have today. The Sanitary Commission was to play a unique role in relation to the Army Medical Department, acting as a "'gadfly' in 'stinging' the moribund department into more effective activity."[6(p5)]

The Sanitary Commission was established in New York in 1861 by a combination of physicians, ministers, and women interested in improving the life of the soldier.[6(p5)] It was said to have resulted from a happenstance New York City curbside meeting of the Reverend Henry W Bellows and Doctor (Dr) Elisha Harris. Hoping to avoid the medical disaster of the Crimea, the two, supported by a number of prominent New York women, formed the Women's Central Association of Relief. The society's organization was carried out at a meeting at the Cooper Union.[6(p5)] This organization asked the Army Medical Department about its needs, to which the Surgeon General responded that they didn't need help.[6(p6),15(p42)]

A delegation representing these groups then went to Washington with a view that a sanitary commission like the one formed in the Crimea should be created.[6(p7)] The original document sent to the War Department (with a supporting letter from Army Surgeon General Lawson's office) on 18 May 1861 outlining the mission and intent of the Sanitary Commission was signed by Henry W Bellows, DD; WH Van Buren, MD; J Hansen, MD; and Elisha Harris, MD. The document listed three organizations from New York that would participate in the proposed commission.[15(pp63–64)] These were the Women's Central Association of Relief for the Sick and Wounded of the Army, the New York Medical

Association for Furnishing Hospital Supplies in Aid of the Army, and the Advisory Committee of the Boards of Physicians and Surgeons of the Hospitals of New York. The letter also pointed out that commissions in the Crimean War followed the war. The signers proposed that this commission should be established immediately because the war had already begun.[15(pp45–47,53)]

A delegation met with General Winfield Scott, the Army Chief of Staff, which resulted in the order being given for series of "preventive measures," such as increased attention to sanitary matters in the layout of troop camps. The delegation met next with the Army Acting Surgeon General Robert C Wood.[15(pp47–48)] Wood, although very polite, was not inclined to have interference from an outside agency.[15(p49)]

The official 9 June 1861 order for the establishment of the Sanitary Commission came from the War Department and was signed 4 days later by President Abraham Lincoln (13 June 1861).[15(pp63–65)] The Women's Central Association of Relief offered to train and provide cooks. The association also offered the use of several hundred women who had registered as nurses with the group.[6(p7)] In addition, the proposal called for the association to select 100 female volunteers. The document further proposed that a group of "volunteer dressers [male volunteer nurses who would apply and change bandages among other duties], composed of young medical men, drilled for this purpose by the hospital physicians and surgeons of New York . . . [would be made available to come] to the aid of the regular medical forces."[15(p65)] While awaiting the final approval, Surgeon General Lawson died and was succeeded by Clement A Finley, who had been an Army surgeon since 1818. Finley was skeptical of the Sanitary Commission, but yielded to public pressure and signed off on the proposal. He added a stipulation that the commission concern itself only with volunteer troops rather than Regular Army soldiers.[16(p8)]

Frederick Law Olmsted, who would later design Central Park in New York City, was the organization's General Secretary.[15(p106)] Olmsted was one of the original members of the US Sanitary Commission appointed on 20 June 1861.[15(p64)] Olmsted, assisted by Dr Harris representing the Sanitary Commission, wrote a report in 1861 on the conditions of 20 Army camps in the Washington area that found many deficiencies. Olmsted put the root of the problems to the lack of experience on the part of the officers and the consequent poor discipline of the soldiers.[15(p86)] When General George McClellan assumed command of the Army of the Potomac, he was receptive to the Sanitary Commission's recommendations.[15(p93)] The commission pushed to build a model hospital system based on the "pavilion system." The system envisioned separate wards in the form of detached buildings.[15(p84)] The Sanitary Commission had searched among the medical officers for someone to recommend for Surgeon General. They identified Dr William A Hammond, who had a career as an Army officer and had been Professor of Physiology and Anatomy at the University of Maryland.[15(p130)] The commission's members put their considerable weight behind his ultimately successful candidacy.[15(p134)]

The Sanitary Commission provided inspections, supplies, hospitals, and transportation for the wounded. Commission members inspected Army hospitals and camps to make sure they were as healthy as possible. Clean Army facilities were shown to have less disease than dirty ones, even though the role of bacteria was not yet known. In many facilities, the Army officers were unhappy with the commission finding that they failed to adhere to Army regulations, especially concerning sanitation. The Sanitary Commission also transported supplies and maintained its own organic transportation systems, including river steamboats, wagons, and ambulances. Although chartered by Congress, its operation and finances were solely from private sources.

Among the Sanitary Commission volunteers was Walt Whitman, best known for his poetic works.[17(pp85,87)] Whitman was also a war correspondent who wrote about war from behind the lines. He came to Washington seeking his brother who had been wounded in the Battle of Fredericksburg in Virginia. He finally found him recovering near Fredericksburg. Whitman stayed in Washington until the end of the war. He made over 600 hospital visits while speaking to an estimated 100,000 wounded soldiers.[18(pp52,59)] His humanitarian work brought much comfort to the wounded and ill soldiers, as well as to their families.[6(p89),18(pp52,59)]

Women were significantly involved in the 7,000 regional and local offices of the Sanitary Commission. Although the top leaders of the commission were men, women assumed public roles that were uncommon before the time by becoming involved with providing local and regional leadership.[19(p62)] The commission established Soldiers Homes to provide housing while soldiers were on furlough.[16(pp291,292)] It also provided long-term care convalescent centers.[19(p62)]

The local chapters (branches) raised $15 million in supplies and $5 million in cash for the Sanitary Commission.[19(p62)] Much of the fundraising came from special events. Contributions large and small came from people anxious to help relieve the suffering of the wounded and ill troops. The commission's fundraising received especially large contributions from "Sanitary Fair" events. Indeed, the fairs in New York and Philadelphia were compared to international expositions on the order of the Great Crystal Palace exposition in England. Various celebrities also donated items for sale. At one Sanitary Fair, for example, President Lincoln provided a handwritten copy of the Emancipation Proclamation, which brought a $3,000 bid.[19(p63)] The actual contributions and disbursements for supplies and expenses are listed in detail in the 1864 *The United States Sanitary Commission*, which has been digitally reproduced by the Cornell University Library in Ithaca, New York.[20(pp539–549)]

The Sanitary Commission was vitally important to the Army Medical Department. For instance, after the Battle of Antietam, the commission delivered to the area hospitals, independently of the Army, a variety of items in quantity including dry goods, condensed milk, beef stock and beef, farina (a cereal), bottles of wine, and various beverages such as tea and coffee along with sugar.[21(pp120–121)] The commission also set up an overall hospital directory that allowed family members to find where their soldiers were situated. Surprisingly, the War Department did not keep such records on an official basis.[19(p62)] After the Civil War, the Sanitary Commission also helped veterans file claims for pensions.[19(p62)] Other charitable organizations, like the US Christian Association, sent personal items to soldiers such as socks, stamps, paper for letters, soap, and canned foods. It was associated with the Young Men's Christian Association.[22(p78)]

Surgeons and Their Training

Many surgeons of the era learned their profession as apprentices, although there were formal medical schools in operation. As an example, William Henry Corbusier, who served as an acting assistant surgeon for the 6th Illinois Cavalry, didn't receive his Medicinae Doctor degree from the Bellevue Hospital Medical College in New York until 1867 after "having attended lectures and clinics. I had also received instruction in a special class under Dr Stephen Smith . . . . and a course in auscultation and percussion and diseases of the heart and lungs, under Dr Austin Flint."[23(p62)] The sparse nature of the curriculum can be seen as Corbusier found it necessary to supplement his training with "special" classes (requiring fees) under the direction of New York specialists. His path in medicine was typical of many of his Civil War colleagues. Corbusier started to study medicine and surgery with a Dr JJ Braman of Gilroy, who "wanted a helper who could speak Spanish."[23(p36)] He studied "[p]harmacy and made all of the tinctures, syrups, mixtures, powders, pills, etc."[23(p39)] He later met an English surgeon in the area who "was well educated and had had much experience, some of which he imparted to me."[23(p39)] In 1864, with this limited training, Corbusier gained his position as an acting assistant surgeon with the 6th Illinois Cavalry. "The Army needed surgeons and I had no difficulty in getting a position."[23(p47)]

The quality of the surgeons certainly varied from the very good to the poorest excuse for a surgeon. The Army surgeons that were initially recruited were young, inexperienced, and frequently not of good quality. The best medical recruits were said to take the Surgeon General's Office examination for "surgeons of volunteers" and, if successful, were generally assigned to staff positions in general hospitals rather than field duty.[6(p46)] Many of these newly acquired surgeons refused assignment to Washington hospitals, preferring to ply their trade in the field.[6(p73)] The lack of the "best" surgeons on the battlefield had consequences for the Army. At the Second Battle of Bull Run, for example, the medical situation was worse than at the first battle. Letterman had worked in July and August 1862 on the preliminary start to what would be an effective medical plan, but the confusion and disarray of troops during the battle precluded its effectiveness. The Union alone sustained 10,000 casualties (killed and wounded) out of 62,000 Union troops, while the victorious Confederates had 8,300 casualties (killed and wounded) out of 50,000 troops.[6(p73)] The medical side had poor coordination with other departments in the matters of transportation and supply. Furthermore, the volunteer surgeons were said to have displayed ignorance of military order and procedure and showed no teamwork.[6(p63)] It was reported that the Surgeon General dismissed 2,000 volunteer surgeons, paying their way home, believing that they would not obey orders and would be more trouble than their value.[6(p57)]

The extremes of care are illustrated in the following case. As a Private Chase was quoted after his wounding in the Overland Campaign and transport to Fredericksburg: "The worst treatment I received in all my Army service was from the brute that called himself an Army surgeon. He appeared to be void of all feeling for humanity, and seemed to delight in torturing the wounded men as much [as] a savage."[24(p188)] Yet the next day, the same private was attended by a Dr William Sawin of the 2nd Vermont. Chase said, "It was his kind hands that fixed me up, gave me a quieting powder, and spoke cheerful words to me . . . . He said to me . . . . 'I am very tired. I have amputated 100 limbs today.'"[24(p188)]

How did it come to be that there was such a range of skills among Army surgeons? Many of the medical schools in the United States were little more than "diploma mills."[6(p50)] (It would take the Flexner Report of 1906 to close down many of these schools.) Even Harvard Medical School, one of the leading schools of the time, had no stethoscope until 1868, which was 30 years after its invention. Corbusier, in his memoirs, said that in 1864 his unit had "a wooden tube about four inches long with a trumpet shaped piece at one end and a flat disk at the other, as a stethoscope to listen to the sounds of the heart and lungs."[23(p47)] Harvard had no microscope until 1869, even though the microscope had been devised by Anton van Leeuwenhoek in 1674.[6(p50)] By contrast, the achromatic microscope (no distortion), developed in the early 1860s, did find its way to the headquarters of the Army Medical Department in a matter of a few years (1863).[6(p51)]

Many medical schools started to appear in the late 18th and early 19th centuries. However, many surgeons still gained their training by working with a preceptor. The preceptor was a surgeon who took on an assistant to learn the trade, usually over a 7-year period. The preceptorship could be augmented by medical courses or even attendance at a traditional school of medicine. It was the medical equivalent of "reading the law" at the side of a practicing lawyer, rather than attending a law school.

At first, most medical schools were in the North and the southern students trained there. Transylvania University (1799) in Kentucky and the University of Maryland (1807) were early schools. Transylvania University was the first university west of the Allegheny Mountains. The medical department was formed by the trustees in 1799. Harvard, in Massachusetts, and the University of Pennsylvania were very highly regarded. The Jefferson Medical College in Philadelphia, Pennsylvania, opened its doors in 1825. This tendency toward a Northern education is reflected in the fact that the membership of an 1830 North Carolina medical society had a majority graduating from three Northern schools.[25(p10)]

The South was soon to follow with medical schools. The Medical College of South Carolina in Charleston (1824) became a leading center. The University of Virginia had a medical department in 1828. In the next decade medical schools were established in Richmond, Virginia; New Orleans, Louisiana; and Augusta, Georgia.[25(p10)] However, most physicians studied at these Northern and Southern institutions for a period of only 4 to 5 months of lectures. Virginia expanded its lecture schedule to 9 months in 1837, allowing more anatomical instruction. The Medical College of Georgia in 1837 proposed the extension of its 6-month course, started in 1832.[25(p11)] The numbers of faculty employed by the medical schools were limited; eight was a typical number.

Some surgical advances were made in the first part of the 19th century. For instance, a Danville, Kentucky, surgeon (Dr Ephraim McDowell, from Virginia originally) in 1809 performed a successful ovariotomy that he later repeated a number of times (with no patient deaths). In 1849, Dr James Marion Sims completed a successful repair of a vesico-vaginal fistula. Of course, Dr Crawford Long of Georgia, a rural surgeon, first used ether in 1837 as an anesthetic prior to the Boston use in 1848.[25(p18)] Dr Benjamin W Dudley, who was a professor at Transylvania University (Kentucky) from 1817 until 1850, did impart in his teachings to medical students from the South the value of boiled water and cleansing of the surgical field. He felt that dirt and impure water could somehow lead to disease.[25(p19)]

The Contributions of Jonathan Letterman

Jonathan Letterman became the medical director of the Army of the Potomac (Figure 3-2) following the failure of Charles Tripler to deal with the disastrous Peninsula Campaign casualties. During this campaign (March–June 1862), the Union suffered defeat and many casualties received delayed and substandard care, attributed to Tripler's lack of planning and direction. As detailed in his memoirs, on 1 July 1862, Letterman reported to MG George McClellan, Commanding General, for duty as the Medical Director of the Army of the Potomac. McClellan was then at Harrison's Landing on the James River in Virginia, following the Peninsula Campaign.

Letterman then received orders on the 23rd of July to report to the White House, but didn't get there until the 28th where he met with Frederick Law Olmsted and other members of the Sanitary Commission.[12(pp6–10)] Letterman recorded in his memoirs that the greatest need of the troops then was for proper food. Slowly the situation improved but not without much suffering of the troops. At the instigation of Letterman, McClellan issued orders for the organization of an Ambulance Corps (Special Orders No. 147, dated 2 August 1862).[12(p24)] He later issued an order discussing the use of the Ambulance Corps and that of Ambulance Trains (General Order No. 85, dated 24 August 1862). Congress passed an "Ambulance Corps Act of 1864," enacted on 11 March 1864, that codified its operation.[12]

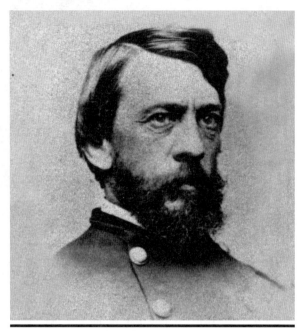

FIGURE 3-2A. Jonathan Letterman. Letterman became the medical director of the Army of the Potomac in 1862 following the failure of Dr Charles Tripler to deal with the disastrous Peninsula Campaign casualties. His ambulance evacuation system revolutionized Army medical care. He served in his post until 1864, at which time he resigned from the US Army. Photograph courtesy of the National Library of Medicine, Image #B011098

Letterman was born in Washington County, Pennsylvania, on 11 December 1824. His father was a well-regarded physician and surgeon in western Pennsylvania in his own right. He engaged a private tutor to educate his son. Jonathan Letterman graduated from the Jefferson Medical College in Philadelphia, in March 1849. He passed a comprehensive medical examination after which he was appointed as an Army assistant surgeon. Letterman served in Florida where he took part in the Seminole Indian campaigns until March 1853. He then was assigned to Fort Defiance in New Mexico. As a young Army assistant surgeon, Letterman participated in campaigns against the Indians, treating disease

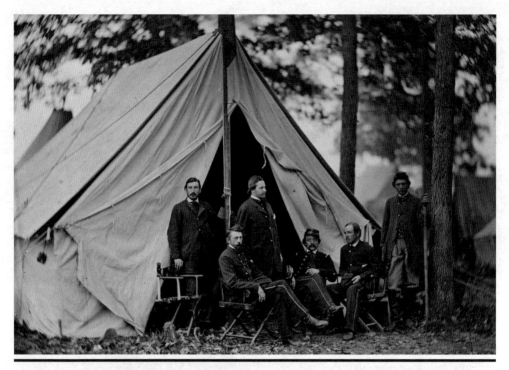

FIGURE 3-2B. Dr Jonathan Letterman (seated, left) with his medical staff. Warrenton, Virginia, 1863. Photograph courtesy of the Library of Congress, Image #03769v.

and inflicted arrow wounds that might later become infected. By 1859, he was assigned to Fort Monroe, Virginia. In 1860, he was posted to California where he participated in a campaign against the Pah Ute Indians. In 1861, Letterman was assigned to the Army of the Potomac. In May 1862, he was appointed as the Medical Director of the Department of West Virginia.[12(p1)] Letterman was then ordered to the position as Medical Director of the Army of the Potomac. He was later promoted to the rank of surgeon on 2 July 1862 (effective date 16 April 1862). William Hammond, the Army Surgeon General, requested in July 1862 that the position as Medical Director further be enhanced by appointing the Director as an aide-de-camp to the Commanding General and be afforded the rank of colonel. Secretary of War Edwin Stanton denied the request. It finally took an act of Congress in February 1865 to provide the extra rank.[26(pp227–228)]

In the position of Medical Director of the Army of the Potomac, Letterman followed Charles Tripler, who was faulted for the poor handling of the casualties of the Peninsula Campaign. Tripler was then offered other posts and he selected the position as chief surgeon of the Department of the Lakes in Detroit. The office later moved to Columbus, Ohio, and then to Cincinnati, Ohio. Tripler received brevet promotions to colonel (1864) and to brigadier general (1865). While still on duty at Cincinnati in 1865 Tripler died, secondary to neck cancer. Tripler's past accomplishments are worth noting. He was born in 1806 and graduated from the College of Physicians and Surgeons in New York in 1827. Tripler worked for several months in New York's Bellevue Hospital. He spent time in Florida in the Seminole War and later in the Mexican-American War, where he served under General Twiggs. He organized and supervised a variety of hospitals. In those days, disease put more troops out of action than wounding. He later spent time in Michigan, New York, and California. On 12 August 1861, he was assigned as the first Medical Director of the Army of the Potomac. Paradoxically, Tripler had been chosen for this position to bring order after the poor showing by the medical assets after the Second Battle of Bull Run.[6(pp60,73,245)] He probably performed better than he was credited in the Peninsula Campaign fiasco. Tripler's own assessment in his final report of the campaign was that he neither was "a complete success nor a very decided failure."[6(p73)] He listed many mitigating issues (described below) that he was not able to affect.[6(p73–74)]

The Peninsula Campaign, which was Tripler's downfall, was designated such as fighting took place on the York Peninsula on the Virginia coast near Richmond.[6(p61)] McClellan's Peninsula Campaign was designed to capture Richmond; however, it had ultimately failed by July 1863. McClellan had envisioned an offensive strategy featuring the largest US Army fielded thus far in the war. The Army of the Potomac made an amphibious landing at Fort Monroe, Virginia. A temporary camp was established there with many supplies and a temporary tent city housing 100,000 Union troops.[21(p69)] The Union ultimately had some 105,000 troops, while the Confederates fielded only 60,000. The Union sustained 5,031 casualties including 790 killed, 3,594 wounded, and 647 missing. The Confederates, on the other hand, had 6,134 casualties including 980 killed, 4,749 wounded, and 405 missing.[27(p147)]

The Confederates had established three lines of defense from the York River to the James River. The first line of defense at Yorktown stalled McClellan's Army in a siege that lasted a month.[21(p70)] The Confederates later attacked the Union troops at Seven Pines. After only 2 days' fighting, the Union had 3,600 wounded.[21(p71)] The wounded number had expanded to 8,000 by the end of the engagement.[21(p72)] McClellan halted his offensive. General Robert E Lee attacked the forces on 25 June 1862, at the start of the Seven Days Battle. McClellan withdrew then to the James River.[21(p70)]

The Peninsula Campaign's medical efforts were characterized by lack of supplies (which became exhausted), medical tents missing or in need of repair, and the lack of surgeons. The extensive outbreak of dysentery in the Union Army has been cited as one of the reasons for McClellan's withdrawal from the peninsula. The soldiers called the dysentery the "Tennessee trots" or the "Virginia quick-step."[2(p232)] The Sanitary Commission provided significant criticism of the medical operations. Although Tripler did not receive the logistical support requested, the outrage at the extent of the casualties and their poor management doomed any chance that he could have remained at his post.[21(p72)]

A unique perspective of the scale of the Peninsula Campaign medical disaster comes from several eyewitnesses as recalled 68 years later.[29(p27)] In May 1862, Union troops were advancing through Virginia's lower peninsula as part of the campaign. The Confederate rear guard action, as part of a delaying tactic, resulted in the Battle of Williamsburg, which took place east of the historic town. In 1930, the Reverend Dr WAR Goodwin shared on "recording discs" the oral history of what transpired as recalled by two then-teenagers. One said:

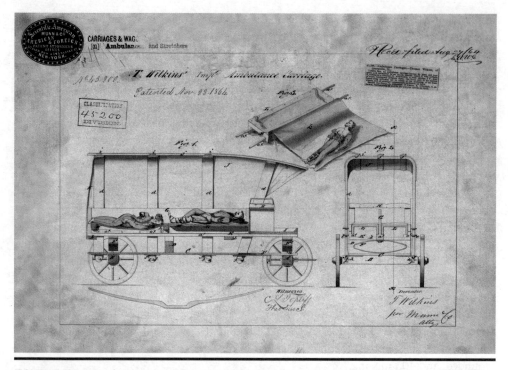

FIGURE 3-3. Design of an improved ambulance to upgrade the basic Letterman Ambulance, November 1864. The Letterman ambulance made possible the rapid and potentially life-saving evacuation of the Civil War wounded. Letterman's ambulance system greatly improved the treatment of the Civil War soldier. At the instigation of Letterman, McClellan issued orders for the organization of an Ambulance Corps. Photograph courtesy of the National Archives and Records Administration, Image #16652.

I went on the battlefield the next day . . . . and there wasn't a hospital or anything of the kind to take care of the wounded. And the Confederates and the Yankees, the Federals were all in a barn . . . My father . . . heard the suffering . . . he went down [and brought] . . . up some of the Confederate soldiers [to his home.] The Federals . . . . took care of their men as well as they could. They took care in fact of both sides. But there was nothing, no hospitals, or anything of that kind.[29(p28)]

The people of Williamsburg nursed soldiers in their own homes and turned the town church into a basic hospital. "A Baptist church visitor chanced upon a pile of limbs amputated by Yankee surgeons operating there."[29(p30)]

Letterman provided his views of the eastern campaigns through 1864 in his *Medical Recollections of the Army of the Potomac*, published in 1866.[12] Letterman resources also include for review here Clements' *Memoir of Letterman*[30] and Tripler's brief biography (regarding the Peninsula Campaign).[31] Letterman began his book[12] with the "Aftermath of Seven Days" in the wake of the peninsula disaster when Letterman became the Medical Director for the Army of the Potomac. He details how he tried to improve the diet and provide sanitary disposition of the encampment. Letterman reported that he examined the hospitals (under the Army of the Potomac) at Point Lookout, Fortress Monroe,

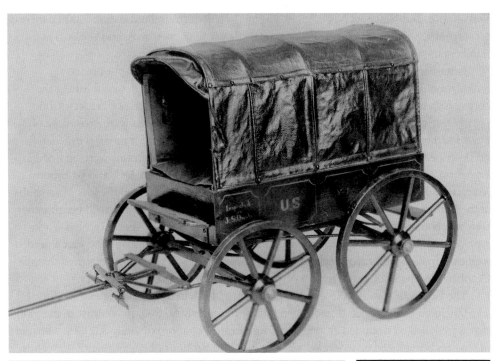

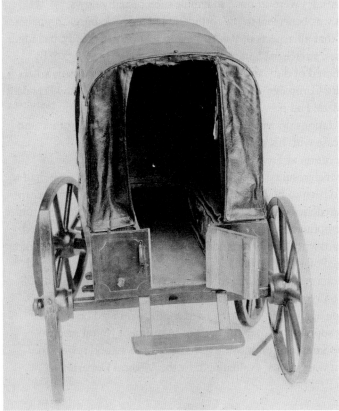

FIGURE 3-4. Views of the Letterman ambulance. The ambulance formed the centerpiece of the Ambulance Corps organized by Jonathan Letterman. The ambulances featured springs in their suspension that were much more comfortable for the occupants than a regular wagon. They were drawn by horse or mule with canvas roofs and sides of canvas. Two-wheel ambulances were followed by the four-wheel ambulance pictured here. Photograph courtesy of the National Library of Medicine, Image #19999137-2.

Portsmouth, and Newport News, all in Virginia. There he found more than 7,000 patients, 66 surgeons, 500 nurses, and miscellaneous medical cadets, stewards, and cooks. The numbers found there highlight the scale of care that was needed.[12(p33)]

Letterman organized the Ambulance Corps with two-horse and four-horse ambulances[12(p27)] (Figures 3-3 and 3-4). McClellan had issued an order establishing the corps on 2 August 1862.[11(pp190–191)] The system was tested at the Battle of Fredericksburg on 13 December 1862, with good results. The Maryland campaigns were even more of a test for the Medical Director because the trains were a problem for medical evacuation (as described in the section in this chapter on transportation). The trains were boarded at Frederick, Maryland, for transport of the wounded to Washington, DC, and Baltimore, Maryland. There were other problems facing Letterman. He described the loss of surgeons at the Battle of Antietam. Some contract surgeons just deserted the battlefield because they were not bound by Army regulations. He also described a Dr CR Agnew of New York, representing the Sanitary Commission, coming to Maryland and distributing much needed medical supplies. Letterman, seeking to avoid supply issues in the future, reported that in October 1862 he instituted a system of "brigade supplies" with accountability.[12(pp50–53)]

The battles of Antietam Creek and Sharpsburg, both in Maryland, accounted for 11,600 Union troops killed or wounded (of approximately 50,000) in contrast to the 9,000 that were killed or wounded among the Confederates (of approximately 33,000). The rate of soldiers being killed or wounded was put at 2,000 per hour of engagement.[21(p114)] Thus, the medical resources of both sides were strained to handle such casualty flows.[21(pp114–115)]

Letterman's preparation was beneficial to the forthcoming Fredericksburg Campaign. Specifically, he made certain that all aspects of the Ambulance Corps were ready, including inspection of horses, harnesses, stretchers, lanterns, and related equipment.[12(pp65–66)] By then McClellan had been relieved of duty and it was to be MG Ambrose Burnside who would lead the Fredericksburg Campaign in Virginia. (McClellan was relieved by President Lincoln who felt that the general had been too slow to pursue Lee after Antietam.[2(pp242,262)]) Letterman had had a good relationship with McClellan, who gave him wide latitude and support, which was not the case with his successor.

The Union's plan of execution at Fredericksburg was complicated by a delay in erecting a pontoon bridge, which resulted in high casualty lists, to which Letterman had to respond. The Union plan had been to build a bridge to cross the Rappahannock River to engage the Confederates in Fredericksburg. However, Confederate sharpshooters continued to pick off Union troops attempting to complete the bridge. The approximate combined casualties included 2,000 dead, with 13,000 wounded and 2,500 missing.[21(p146)] The Union casualties (total forces engaged of 114,000) included 1,284 killed, 9,605 wounded, and 1,769 missing. The Confederate casualties (total forces engaged of 72,500) included 608 killed, 4,116 wounded, and 653 missing.[32(p405)]

The Sanitary Commission again supplied many needs of the wounded because the Army did not have sufficient supplies. Despite the need to supplement Union medical supplies due to shortages, the Sanitary Commission gave Letterman a good review for preparation. The commission was, in fact, evaluating how the Medical Department functioned in various battles.[21(pp147–148)]

MEDICAL CARE AT THE TIME OF THE BATTLE OF GETTYSBURG

In the lead up to the Battle of Gettysburg (in Pennsylvania), the extreme carnage of the Civil War was exemplified by the Antietam casualties for both the North and the South.[4(p94)] The surgical performances of both sides at Antietam had been criticized in public talk of "butcher surgery."[6(p115)] During the Chancellorsville fighting, despite the South's victory, Letterman was proud of the Union medical response and, in particular, cited a successful amputation at the hip joint of a private who was struck in the upper thigh by a conical ball, creating a comminuted fracture. The surgery was done in a field hospital without loss of much blood. The private survived despite being captured (while he was recuperating) and being moved to Richmond.[12(pp117–119)]

As pointed out in the book *Doctors in Blue: The Medical History of the Union Army in the Civil War*,[6] there was a great deal of controversy regarding the issue of when and how to amputate. One faction advocated "conservative" measures that might preserve the injured extremity. The other faction favored prompt, speedy surgery/amputation.[6(pp131–132)] The latter faction favored speed due to the enormous workloads in battle. They termed the amputation as "primary" in this situation[6(p134)] (Figures 3-5A and 3-5B). The risk of infection after amputation was ever present. Civil War surgeons, such as John Shaw Billings, considered that the surgeon's hands might spread infection, which had already been demonstrated in obstetrical circles in the case of puerperal fever.[6(p140)]

In his memoirs, Letterman described the actions and medical care in the Union Army in significant detail in the period leading up to the battle at Gettysburg. As an example, in describing the Battle of Chancellorsville, Virginia, Letterman noted that 1,200 of the Union wounded fell into Confederate control. Letterman organized a relief column of 26 medical officers and five wagons loaded with supplies. Nineteen Union surgeons had remained with the wounded and were augmented by the 26 medical officers in the column. Also of interest is that General Lee offered free passage to the Union ambulance trains to Chancellorsville and, as Letterman put it, "to avoid the suffering that would be endured if our wounded were carried in the enemy's transportation, and transferred to our ambulances."[12(pp139–140)]

The 1863 Gettysburg Campaign was the second attempt by the Confederates under Lee to invade the North. The first was the 1862 push into Antietam. After Antietam resulted in a Union victory, Lee viewed an invasion of the North as a way of forcing a political settlement. Gettysburg was a 3-day battle that resulted in huge casualties for both sides (a combined total of 46,386 killed, wounded, or missing out of a total force of approximately 160,000 men). The Union (94,000 total troops) had casualties of 23,055 (3,151 killed, 14,531 wounded, and 5,369 missing). The Confederates (66,000 total troops) had casualties of 23,231 (4,708 killed, 12,693 wounded, and 5,830 missing).[21(pp186-187)] The last day of the engagement ended with the Confederate charge (led by MG George Pickett) at Cemetery Ridge that netted only a small part of the Union line that could not be secured.[4(pp99–100)] It would take until 14 July 1863 for the Confederates to be across the Potomac marking the end of the Gettysburg Campaign. Lee remarked to the officer escorting the wounded: "Too bad! Too bad!" in reference to the battle.[32(p25)]

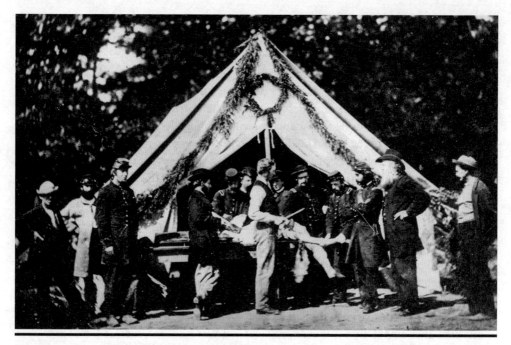

FIGURE 3-5A. Amputation, Gettysburg, July 1863. Civil War surgeon in a posed scene preparing to amputate a wounded soldier's leg. Amputation was the method of choice for compound fractures and vascular injuries of the extremities. The speed of the surgeon was judged to be a point of pride. The Minié ball wound was responsible for many amputations because the bone was often shattered. A flap method of amputation left more tissue to cover the stump (the preferred Union method). Chloroform and ether were readily available anesthetics, with chloroform being the preferred agent. Ether's explosive nature made its use dangerous. Photograph courtesy of the National Archives and Records Administration, Image #520203.

During the Gettysburg Campaign, Letterman remarked that the Ambulance Corps performed well and that he was able to remove the wounded from the battlefield within 6 hours.[12(pp158–159)] Letterman requested that the Surgeon General send 20 more surgeons. The surgeons that came included some that worked well, but the majority were poorly trained and of little use. Letterman used the occasion to remark to Surgeon General Hammond that three surgeons per regiment must accompany the Army into the field.[12(p159)]

The Union medical organization under Letterman during the Gettysburg Campaign consisted of 650 medical officers, 1,000 ambulances, and 3,000 ambulance drivers and litter carriers to service the 94,000 Union troops.[6(p91)] Many Northern women came to Gettysburg after the fighting ended to serve as nurses and attendants. The Union forces even allowed Southern women to come to Gettysburg to perform the same functions for wounded Confederate forces.[6(p70)] Letterman used hospital tents and "nearly every house formed a hospital ward"[6(p92)] in the small town. Letterman moved the wounded from the houses and other points to Camp Letterman, a central medical facility composed of 400 tents of varying size and capacity.[6(p214)] The wounded at Gettysburg were then sent to hospitals outside the area as soon as possible. The main tent hospital in Gettysburg closed more than 4

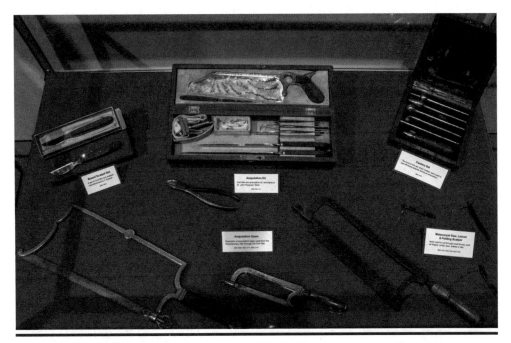

FIGURE 3-5B. Civil War era amputation kits and implements. Photograph courtesy of Army Medical Department Center of History and Heritage.

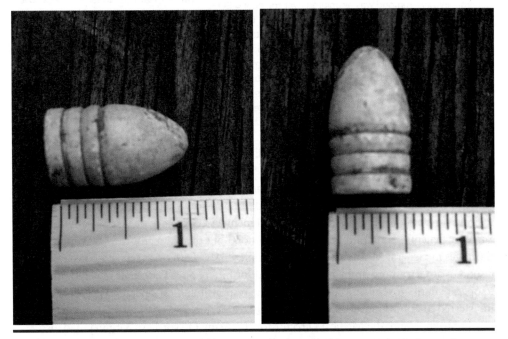

FIGURE 3-5C. Minié ball, .58 caliber. From the Battle of Fredericksburg, Virginia. Minié ball wounds were responsible for the majority of the amputations. Photographs courtesy of Ronald Sparacino.

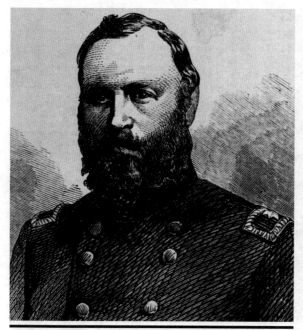

FIGURE 3-6. Surgeon General William A. Hammond (1862–1864). Surgeon Hammond came to the attention of the Sanitary Commission members as a replacement for Surgeon General Finley. Hammond was appointed over the acting Surgeon General (Colonel Wood) and over a candidate backed by Secretary of War Stanton. Hammond was the catalyst for Letterman's reforms and ambulance organization. Hammond's courts-martial for alleged irregular procurement of medical supplies resulted in his dismissal in 1864. He subsequently went on to academic success in New York. Congress restored his brigadier general rank in 1878. Photograph courtesy of the National Library of Medicine, Image #B08356.

months after the battle ended, on 20 November 1863, the day following Lincoln's Gettysburg Address dedicating the new military cemetery.[22(p79)]

The Sanitary Commission came to Gettysburg on 4 July 1863, the day after Pickett's Charge. The Commission raised large amounts of money to respond to the needs of the wounded, bringing in over 40 tons of food and supplies.[22(p78)] The Sanitary Commission and the US Christian Commission (an outgrowth of the Young Men's Christian Association) supply wagons that came from Frederick to Gettysburg had avoided most of the fighting in the region and brought much needed materials to the various Union hospitals.[6(p184)] The US Christian Commission sent along soap, towels, paper, stamps, and food as well.[22(p78)]

The Confederate Medical Director at Gettysburg, Lafayette Guild, said that the Confederates left behind 6,000 wounded and 100 surgeons to provide care for them in 24 hospitals within a 12-mile radius of Gettysburg.[21(p188)] Letterman's medical troops already were dealing with their own 15,000 wounded at Gettysburg.[21(pp188–189)] Regardless of the tremendous burden resulting from such horrific casualties, Letterman received criticism for the care of the wounded, despite how well he performed. In response to criticism from the press and Congressional members, Secretary of War Stanton sent Surgeon General Hammond to inspect. Hammond put the blame for medical supply shortages in General Meade's line of responsibility.[21(p196)] Letterman left surgeons and resources at Gettysburg and a hospital named for him (Camp Letterman), which continued to operate until November 1863, although the responsibility for operations had been transferred to another surgeon.[21(pp196–197),33(p15)]

Lafayette Guild, the Medical Director for the Army of Northern Virginia, had also graduated from the Jefferson Medical College 1 year before Letterman. He had served in the Union Army in western posts, including California. Guild and Letterman met in person at Gettysburg to deal with the wounded.[21(pp290–291)]

There was also combat activity, and thus medical activity, in the "western" part of the theater of operations during this time. To Letterman's credit, the "Letterman system" was more integrated in the West, in the Army of Tennessee for the 1863 to 1865 campaigns.[6(p106)] In contrast, the South had a confused and disorganized medical activity in the West. The hospitals were makeshift at Magnolia, Mississippi, and Ringgold, Georgia.[25(p49)] Also in the West during the Civil War, some of the Indian tribes saw an opportunity to cause trouble while the armies were otherwise engaged. For instance, the Dakota War of 1862 left several hundred settlers dead. BG Henry Sibley brought revenge for these killings in the summer of 1863 in the present North Dakota when he located a large encampment of Sioux. The later Sand Creek Massacre had further repercussions.[34(pp241–242)] BG Alfred Sully's own punitive expedition in 1864 followed, with further loss of life for all involved.[34(p177)] It is important to note that the Dakota War brought much more destruction to the people of Minnesota than did the Civil War.[34(pxi)] These campaigns took place during the time of the Civil War, although their campaigns and medical/surgical response were more typical of the Plains wars to follow in the upcoming decades.

Surgeon General William Hammond (Figure 3-6) was the catalyst for Letterman's reforms. The tier-hospital system and the effective Ambulance Corps were the highlights of the advances. When Hammond became the Union Army Surgeon General, he worked with Letterman to implement pavilion-style hospital design, which featured open ventilation and efficient operation.[11(pp66,67)] Unfortunately, Hammond ran into political difficulties with Secretary of War Stanton. Hammond was arrested on 17 January 1864 and charged with malfeasance and fraud. The core of the charges was that he allowed medical supply purchases without going through the standard channels. There were also allegations of substandard supply quality. His trial lasted 4 months and ended with Hammond's dismissal from the Army on 18 August 1864.[21(pp216–220),28(p234)] Hammond campaigned to seek vindication of his courts-martial in 1878. An Act of Congress in 1878 restored him to the Army (retired) with a rank of brigadier general, but with no back pay.[35]

By the second year of the Civil War, the two-wheeled ambulances were replaced by the four-wheeled model. The four-wheeled model came in two variations: one was drawn by a two-horse team and the other by a four-horse team. Most came with springs, which was a blessing for the injured. The larger ambulances could carry four to six stretcher cases.[14(p8)] Until Letterman's implementation of his Ambulance Corps, the Army Quartermaster had control of hospital and ambulance procurement and disposition. Ambulances were often diverted to other purposes before Medical Department control.[6(p34)]

Letterman was subsequently appointed as the Medical Inspector of the hospitals in the Department of the Susquehanna, where he stayed until 1864. This appointment was important because the Department of the Susquehanna was responsible for the entirety of the Virginia operations. Although he could not truly be replaced, Letterman was succeeded as Medical Director of the Army of the Potomac by Surgeon Thomas A McParlin.[4(p57)]

In his new position, Letterman inspected the Department of the Susquehanna's 18 hospitals, which accounted for 10% of the Union hospitals at the time.[21(pp217–219)] He also involved himself in the Congressional proposals to create an Army-wide Ambulance Corps, which passed and became law on 11 March 1864. It was noted that it was largely the same as McClellan's General Order No. 147 of 1862.[21(p218)] One of the provisions of the Ambulance Corps creation was that only Corps personnel could help the wounded from the field, rather than random troops.[6(p97)]

When Letterman learned that he was slated to receive new orders assigning him to the Department of the Missouri, he declined the position; he submitted his resignation from the Army on 22 December 1864. After 15 years in the Army, Letterman departed to take up private business opportunities in California. He had been married for only a year when he made this decision. Thus, despite his significant contributions to the war effort, Letterman left the Army before the end of the war because of increasing frustrations in his position and continued problems in procurement and supply. Unfortunately, the promising opportunities in California didn't work out; Letterman then started a medical practice and later became the coroner in San Francisco, California.[21(pp224,238,247-258)] The coroner's job provided a steady source of income and a prestigious position. Letterman retired from his coroner's position in 1871; he died on 15 March 1872 of what may have been chronic dysentery.[21(pp260-261)]

SURGEONS GENERAL DURING THE CIVIL WAR

Thomas Lawson (30 November 1836–15 May 1861)

Thomas Lawson served for almost 25 years as the Surgeon General. His period in office was during conflicts such as the Seminole Wars, the Mexican-American War, the pre-Civil War Indian conflicts, and finally the start of the Civil War. His signal accomplishment while in his long tenure was his fight for rank and recognition of his surgeons. His tenure was marked by conflicts with superiors and subordinates. He doggedly pursued medical officers who he felt were not a credit to the Army. However, he was unable to respond to the fall of Fort Sumter because he was quite ill. Lawson died on 15 May 1861.[36]

Clement Finley (15 May 1861–14 April 1862)

The next Surgeon General was Clement Finley, who was 64 at the time of his appointment. He had also served in the Seminole Wars and the Mexican-American War. The rank of the Surgeon General had been that of colonel. An act was passed by Congress on 16 April 1862 that made the Surgeon General a brigadier general and provided for an assistant surgeon general and a medical inspector, who were to be colonels. Finley was not promoted to the rank of brigadier general because he retired on 14 April 1862, 2 days before the act was passed. Assistant Surgeon General Robert C Wood was the interim office holder until the appointment of William Hammond, who took over on 25 April 1862.[37] Finley received praise for his dedication to the care of his patients. General Winfield Scott praised him for his care of cholera patients in the Black Hawk War. His tenure in office was characterized by efficient operation, although his assistant garnered some of the credit there.[37]

William Hammond (25 April 1862–18 August 1864)

William Hammond and Jonathan Letterman were both classmates at the Jefferson Medical College.[21(p285)] William Hammond was appointed an assistant surgeon in 1849, just missing the Mexican-American War. He served in a variety of posts and participated in a campaign against the Sioux Indians. Hammond was interested in physiology and botanical studies, which he pursued in his off-duty time. In fact, he won an 1857 award from the American Medical Association for his essay dealing with the nutritional and physiologic effects of albumin and gum used as a food.[35] In 1860, he resigned from the Army to accept a teaching position in Baltimore, Maryland. On 28 May 1861, Hammond reentered the US Army as an assistant surgeon. He served in a number of positions after the start of the Civil War but came to the favorable attention of the Sanitary Commission members, who were not happy with Surgeon General Finley. Hammond was appointed over the acting Surgeon General (Colonel Wood) and over a candidate backed by Secretary of War Stanton.[35]

Hammond's courts-martial for conduct unbecoming to an officer and alleged irregular procurement of medical supplies resulted in his dismissal in 1864.[21(p285)] He subsequently went on to academic success in New York as a neurologist (a newly evolving specialty). He held a series of academic appointments subsequently.[21(p285)] Although he did not return to active duty, Congress restored his brigadier general rank in 1878 and placed him on the retired list as surgeon general. He published extensively and established a sanatorium.[21(p285),35]

Joseph Barnes (22 August 1864–30 June 1882)

Joseph Barnes followed Hammond in 1864 as the next Surgeon General. He had also served in the Seminole conflict and later in the Mexican-American War. He was serving in the West at the onset of the Civil War. He was ordered back to the Surgeon General's Office where he was designated the surgeon for Washington. While in this position, he made a favorable impression upon Secretary of War Stanton. Indeed, Stanton was influential in Barnes being chosen to replace Hammond. Barnes became the Surgeon General in August 1864 and remained in office for almost 18 years.[38] Barnes assigned officers to compile the *Medical and Surgical History of the War of the Rebellion*, which was an exhaustive record of the conflict and the main achievement of his long tenure as Surgeon General.[21(p264)]

CONFEDERATE MEDICAL SERVICES

The primary focus in this chapter is on the Union Army as a continuation of the US Army. The book entitled *Doctors in Gray: The Confederate Medical Service*,[25] authored by Horace H Cunningham, was first published in 1958. It is one of the best descriptions of the Confederate Medical Service organization.[25] The Confederates' problems in 1861 included lack of medical personnel, food, and supplies. These problems increased as the war endured, in part due to the effective blockade of all Confederate ports.

Many of the South's physicians had received training in the North before the war began. Cunningham states that in 1860 the majority of the members of the North Carolina Medical Society received their training in the North. As time went by, more schools developed in the South, including the Medical College of South Carolina (1824) and the University of Virginia (1828); other institutions were established in the 1830s.[25(pp10,12)]

Dr Joseph Jones is quoted as saying that he believed there were 600,000 Confederate troops mobilized and 200,000 of these died as a result of action, wounding, or disease during the conflict.[25(p3)] Only 50,000 deaths were directly attributable to battle as described by Jones.[25(p5)] (Cunningham, quoting other authorities, concluded that deaths from disease may be understated for the South.[25(pp5-6)]) Dr Jones was a graduate of the University of Pennsylvania School of Medicine and taught at the Savannah Medical College, the University of Georgia, and the Medical College of Georgia before the war. He became a Confederate surgeon of note.[25(p3)] Disease was very prevalent in both armies. Even General Robert E Lee was afflicted with an unspecific illness in May 1864 during the Battle of the Wilderness. Indeed, illness affected outcomes for both the North and the South.[25(p8)]

The Confederate medical system also had to contend with the prisoner-of-war sick and wounded at Southern prisons. Andersonville, Libby, Belle Isle, and Salisbury Prison were the most famous of the Confederate prisons.[25(p7)] The prison hospital at Andersonville recorded 15,987 cases of illness, of which 11,086 died, which would confirm a frightful mortality rate.[25(pp7-8)] Cunningham reported 42,686 deaths from disease or wounds in the prisons for 6 months in 1864 alone.[25(p7)] Records for the Danville, Virginia, prison hospital for the period November 1864 to March 1865 reflected a 30% mortality for sickness. However, records were incomplete in the Confederacy; even the number of overall prisoners of war is vague.[25(p8)]

At the start in 1861, the Surgeon General of the Confederacy was to have a rank of colonel, while surgeons and assistant surgeons would rank as majors and captains, respectively.[25(p21)] The Confederate Medical Department had on its rolls one Surgeon General, 1,242 surgeons, and 1,994 assistant surgeons.[25(p37)] The Confederate Surgeon General received pay of 3,000 Confederate dollars per year. The pay rates listed were 162 to 200 Confederate dollars per month for a surgeon, while an assistant surgeon received 110 to 150 Confederate dollars per month[25(p21)] (the Confederate dollar declined in value as the war proceeded). (By comparison, the Union surgeon was paid only $80 to $100 per month until the rates were raised in 1864.[6(p175)])

The first CSA Surgeon General was Dr David C Deleon, who lasted only a few months. He was named the Acting Surgeon General on 6 May 1861. His tenure was ended on 12 July 1861 due to perceived incompetence. Dr Charles H Smith served for a few weeks as an interim Surgeon General. He was followed by Dr Samuel Preston Moore, who served until the end of the war.[25(p28)] Dr Moore prevailed upon the CSA Secretary of the Treasury, who controlled office assignment, that his office could not operate out of the one room assigned to the Surgeon General's Office. He received a larger space.[25(p28)]

Moore was an 1834 graduate of the Medical College of South Carolina. In 1835, he became an assistant surgeon in the US Army. He served at many posts and his service included the Mexican-American War, after which he became a full surgeon. Moore was the medical purveyor in New Orleans (managing the purchase and distribution of medicines and supplies), but left for private practice when the Civil War broke out. He was then selected to become the Confederate Surgeon General.[25(p28)]

The arrival of German immigrants who were trained as pharmacists enhanced possibilities of formulating medicines from indigenous sources to offset the effects of the North's blockade.[25(p16)] In the South, almost all of the surgeons were allopathic physicians who had graduated from a medical school. However, because the type of school was not specifically stated, technically a homeopathic physician could be appointed.[14(p5)] Moore implemented medical examining boards, which generally provided thorough examinations. Some criticisms were inevitable, but the results were usually fair.[25(pp34–35)] The Medical College of Virginia was the only Southern medical school to keep its doors open during the Civil War. Hence, the supply of new surgeons was affected.[25(p35)] Some 3,000 medical officers served in the Confederate Army and Navy.[25(p36)]

Confederate surgeons made great efforts to prevent surgical fevers in the hospitals. They separated infected patients and called for disinfection and whitewashing of hospital walls to slow the spread of disease.[25(p242)] Surgeon General Moore spoke of the value of surgical records, in which many surgeons were remiss.[25(p242)] Indeed, Moore was quite critical of hospitals and surgeons that did not keep accurate records. In fact, many of his facilities kept such minimal records that they were of no value.[25(p257)] Moore had his critics, but Jefferson Davis in a speech recognized the value of his hospital organization in 1863.[25(p251)] Moore is credited with the concept of a one-story hospital pavilion, which became the preferred model even after the war.[25(p267)] Moore had good relations with the Confederate Congress, which paid close attention to his estimates of medical needs. The Confederate Congress increased the amounts for medical services as needed, eventually reaching 74 million Confederate dollars.[25(p43)]

Confederate hospitals came to have good ventilation and light for their patients with infectious disease and "surgical fever." Because the blockade precluded the use of many medications, the new use of natural remedies, including no medications, had a beneficial effect. Without the ingredients of many "quack" medications, perhaps the public was better off also.[25(p268)]

Richmond, Virginia, became the hub of medical care for the sick and wounded in the region, with 11 hospitals situated there. Chimborazo, named after a Mexican War battle site, was the most recognized and the largest of the purpose-built hospitals. (Both the North and the South found that purpose-built hospitals meant better recovery rates.[19(p60)]) It could serve as many as 8,000 patients with its more than 150 buildings. The hospital bakery produced approximately 10,000 loaves of bread per day. It also had five ice houses and 200 cows on the nearby grounds to provide milk and butter.[19(p60)] Other Richmond Confederate hospitals included Camp Lee and Howard Grove.[25(p286)] Twenty hospitals were ultimately located in the Richmond area.[25(p53)]

Another of the hospitals in Richmond was the Winder Hospital; it was similar in design to the Chimborazo Hospital. The Winder Hospital had grounds of 125 acres and had a capacity of 5,000 patients.[25(p52)] The Jackson Hospital, another main Richmond hospital, had wooden barracks, which housed approximately 2,500 patients. It had two water closets, two icehouses, a bakery, a garden, and 60 cows.[25(p52)] Gardens were attended by recovering patients. Canal boats brought food from Lexington and Lynchburg for the patients. The Confederates had ambulances, although (aside from captured Union ambulances) they were difficult to acquire. Regular wagons generally had to suffice. The Richmond Ambulance Committee was formed from volunteers in 1862 and provided service to the Army of Northern Virginia. The regular Confederate Ambulance Corps, in theory, had two ambulances per regiment.[14(p6)]

The Confederate Medical Department recognized the value of professional dentists and ensured the availability of dentists to the troops. (The Union was not as proactive.[25(p273)]) The skills developed by CSA surgeons provided for advances when Lister's concepts and improved anesthesia were available. It was the lancet for blood letting that was not used further as the popularity of that therapy declined.[25(p268)] Confederate surgeons used the Smith anterior splint (as did the North) for fractures of the lower extremity, unless the fracture was more complicated, thus requiring pulley and weight. The Smith anterior splint had been designed by a University of Maryland surgeon before the war. The South used maggots to clean wounds. The North, with its copious medical supplies, did not utilize this technique, while the South had to improvise often. The practice had been forgotten after the Napoleonic Wars. It was again forgotten after the Civil War.[25(pp268–269)]

CIVIL WAR DIET, VACCINATIONS AND MEDICATIONS, AND TRANSPORTATION

Diet

By the time Letterman left the service in 1864, the Army's diet and hygiene had improved greatly over the previous 3 years, due in large part to his efforts. It was apparent that dietary additions, such as fresh vegetables and fruits, reduced the risk/rate of scurvy. In the Civil War, the Union soldier used considerable hardtack, which was a form of a cracker that had to be soaked or broken up to eat. A soldier was said to consume up to 10 crackers a day. Bakeries cut the dough into 3-inch squares and perforated them with 16 holes. Typically, soldiers of both sides would carry 3 days' rations before going into combat.[39(pp45,47)] The Southern soldier used ground corn as his staple because corn was plentiful in the South. Pork was more commonly available than would be beef or chicken. Fresh meats, vegetables, and fruits were only periodically available.[19(pp20–22)]

Vaccinations and Medications

Smallpox vaccinations (used first in the Revolutionary War) were required for Confederate soldiers.[40] Corbusier commented that smallpox was "very fatal to the Negroes,"[23(p60)] while the whites and the soldiers were protected by "vaccination from scabs."[23(p59)] However, the source of the smallpox material was "not always well selected when there was so great a demand for them at the beginning of war [resulting in] very sore arms [and that the] persons were not always rendered immune."[23(pp59–60)]

Most of the medications then used by physicians were not particularly useful, with the exception of quinine for the treatment and prevention of malaria. Opium had its use as a pain medication; it could also help in some diarrhea cases by slowing the digestive system.[19(p57)] Many drugs that were used included harmful contents such as mercury, lead, and strychnine. Thus, the South's inability to get many of these medicines due to the blockade may have been beneficial to the Confederate troops.[19(p56)]

Quinine was the closest thing to a "miracle drug" in the Civil War because it provided an effective treatment for malaria. Quinine was obtained from the bark of the Peruvian cinchona tree and was bitter in taste; indeed, whiskey was often used as an inducement to take the medicine. Whiskey didn't always work, as noted by Dr Corbusier in his *Memoirs*,[23] who said that his first time on tour with his regiment, "I took several barrels of whiskey along to issue with quinine for malarial fevers."[23(p50)] Corbusier found that the whiskey was unnecessary for the drug to work and that the alcohol tended to "evaporate." Alcohol was a key feature of medicines in both the North and the South. Alcohol was used in whatever form to help with surgery and its aftermath. It was a key ingredient in medicines such as quinine and opium. It was also used to preserve specimens of tissue.

Alcohol was always in short supply, especially in the South. Theft for recreational use was a significant problem.[14(p3)] Quinine was used as a "stimulant drug," along with dilute sulphuric acid.[6(p140)] Ipecac (a plant) and calomel had been used for diarrhea. Ipecac, generally used as an emetic, had become more popular again in the Civil War following British experience with it in India. (Ipecac has some bactericidal action in bacterial dysentery cases.) It was noted to be useful in amebic dysentery (apparently having amoebicidal components) but no one knew why it worked.[19(p57)] Quinine was used by some surgeons for diarrhea because they believed the diarrhea might be due to malaria.[6(p218)] Alcohol was used in the war as an antiseptic and as a remedy (alcohol was a main ingredient in many remedies in the Civil War and continuing into the 20th century). Alcohol was appreciated by soldiers for its obvious benefit.[6(pp128,140,144)]

In the context of medications in the Civil War, there was a conflict between the allopathic or "regular physicians" and the homeopathic physician. The homeopathic view was begun by Dr Hahnemann, who advised against bloodletting and use of "heroic" medications. The allopathic physicians stemmed from the teachings of Dr Benjamin Rush of Revolutionary War fame. The allopathic physicians formed the American Medical Association and controlled the medical boards appointing surgeons in the North. The surgeons in the South had a more lenient attitude toward the use of botanical drugs.[14(p5)] Dr Oliver Wendell Holmes said in an 1860 talk before the Massachusetts Medical Society that the populace was "overdosed" with medications. While he gave the medical profession part of the blame, he also said that the public "insisted on being poisoned."[25(p16)]

Trains and Ambulances: Medical Evacuation

Letterman's ambulance system greatly speeded treatment for the Civil War soldier. The ambulance system and the use of trains improved the care of the Union soldier, although transportation remained a problem in the West. The ambulances featured springs in their suspension; they were so much more comfortable than a regular wagon that they were often requisitioned for the use of officers and their wives. They were horse or mule drawn with canvas roofs and sides of canvas that could be raised or lowered depending on the weather.[6] Letterman's organization of the Ambulance Corps via General Order No. 85, issued on 24 August 1863, initially detailed the use of two-wheeled ambulances (to be followed later by four-wheeled vehicles) and described the details of ambulance organization, parking, and order of march. For instance, medicine wagons were to follow the ambulances. Letterman's organization prohibited the ambulances to be used for other purposes as they had in the past.[26(pp162–178)]

The "travelling general hospitals" were an interesting use of the railroads utilized by the Army of the Cumberland to follow its march when rail lines were in proximity.

Transportation to a convenient rail head would be the alternative. The railroads were used to move the wounded to larger hospitals in a safer and more expedient manner. Corbusier describes being in charge of a "railroad train of sick and wounded in freight cars."[23(p57)] The wounded had to travel on the "bare floor, having only one or two blankets as bedding."[23(p57)] Dedicated ambulance trains that were purpose designed would come in much later conflicts.

The Civil War was the first American conflict in which the military made great use of railroads to transport troops, move supplies, and transport the wounded.[19(pp50-54)] Getting the wounded onto a train, however, did not always mean a convenient or comfortable trip to a hospital. For instance, railroads were generally local or regional in operation, although a few larger operations existed, such as the Pennsylvania Railroad. There were often no through trains, as in the case of Baltimore, where travelers would come in at one station and have to go to another station to continue. Even when lines were linked, the companies might unload and reload their cargo as the route changed to a different company. At the start of the war, the North had a transportation advantage with 21,000 miles of track, compared to the South's 9,000 miles. In addition, the South had not spent money in the decade before to improve its infrastructure. Furthermore, the locomotives were largely built in the North. The Richmond-based Tredegar Iron Works built some engines, but not enough to meet the demands of the war.[19(p50)] Also, due to the poor state of the tracks in the South, most trains were limited to 15 to 20 mph. The engines burned wood largely and required significant supplies of water along the rails for steam.

The railroad hospital transportation of the Medical Department in the East "continued to be crude down to the end of the war."[6(p105)] The trains (Union Army) running from Nashville to the front were painted a "glaring scarlet while at night three red lanterns were hung beneath the headlight"[6(p108)] to distinguish them from regular trains. Often the rail routes were threatened by enemy troops. In the Overland Campaign, for example, General Grant had planned to move the wounded across the Rapidan River for evacuation by train to Washington. However, the threat of raiders caused the plan to be modified, eventually transporting the wounded by boat from various points along the Potomac River.[24(p186)] The wounded had first been transported to Fredericksburg in "spring less wagons."

CSA evacuation trains also had problems. Confederate surgeon Frank M Dennis, in charge of Confederate ambulance trains in 1863, described the day train, in which the worst cases were placed in bunks, while another 200 sat in the seats. The night mail train had no bunks. Only the wounded were to be on the evacuation train, whose schedules were irregular due to equipment failures and poor scheduling. The train surgeons were described as a disciplined group whose main problem was getting the wounded off to the hospitals. Many of the wounded were reported to have travelled 20 to 25 miles to get to the railhead. Fortunately, the destination hospitals were generally located close to the transportation railheads.[25(p282)] The North and the South both had some designated ambulance trains. Union General John Fremont was credited with setting up such a train in 1861.

Union hospital ships were used along the Western rivers. The medical evacuation in the first part of the war was irregular and confused at times. Oftentimes civilian captains of the vessels would not set off until the ship was filled. Early in the war, riverboats were dedicated to the sick and the wounded, with the leased *City of Memphis* being the first in 1862. The Western Sanitary Commission, operating on the Mississippi River and west of it, arranged to outfit the captured *Red Rover* as a hospital ship that same year.[41(p62)] (The Western Sanitary Commission was independent from the main Sanitary Commission.) The USS *Red Rover* became the first US Navy hospital ship and transported 1,697 wounded in its first two and a half years. Both sanitary commissions ran hospital ships, with the Army supplying the doctors, while the nurses were employed by the Sanitary Commission.[41(p64)] The main Sanitary Commission controlled all hospital vessels in the East.[41(p70)]

ADVANCES IN MEDICAL CARE

Writing in the *Archives of Surgery*,[10] Dr William Blaisdell described a number of medical advances that he viewed as important during the Civil War. He identified recordkeeping; management of mass casualties in a timely fashion (including Letterman's ambulances); and the improved design of hospitals, sanitation/hygiene, and use of female nurses. The pavilion-style hospital construction (Figure 3-7), featuring open ventilation and clean details, was championed by Surgeon General Hammond, Letterman, and John Shaw Billings. Blaisdell viewed as most important the physician lessons learned in management, surgery, and anesthesia.[10(p1045)] The Civil War surgeon also acquired invaluable experience in the management of infectious disease and the rapid treatment of fractures and wounds.[10(pp1045–1050)]

An interesting addition to the Union Army Medical Service was the attempted introduction of the Autenrieth Wagon to carry surgical instruments and supplies into the field. An earlier 1862 attempt was directed at building a light wagon to carry medications, which would travel with ambulances. The wagon proved impracticable.[42(p244)] It was to be a dedicated special supply source that could be targeted in the direction or area needed. The wagon would go to wherever surgery was being done, whether in makeshift hospitals in the field or in homes or churches. The idea was to get surgical needs to the surgeons quickly. It had one storage case specifically for major operations, such as amputations, readily available. Unfortunately, the Autenrieth Wagon was not of interest to the Union medical authorities during the war because it was too complex and costly to manufacture.[42(pp244–245)]

Wounds and Diseases

In addition to the wounds from bullets and artillery, the Civil War is notable in that more soldiers died of camp diseases, such as pneumonia, typhus, and dysentery, than from battle wounds. In the era before germ theory, deaths could come from outbreaks of typhoid fever, yellow fever, smallpox, dysentery, and cholera. Typhoid, typhus, and the so-called "continued fevers" were common in both armies. Various fevers that could not be diagnosed seemed to be placed into the "continued fevers" category.[25(p194)] Unsanitary camp conditions certainly didn't help limit diseases. It was not uncommon to locate latrines near water sources. Childhood diseases, such as measles, also took their toll, especially in the crowded camps. Soldiers from rural areas, who had often lived in relative isolation,

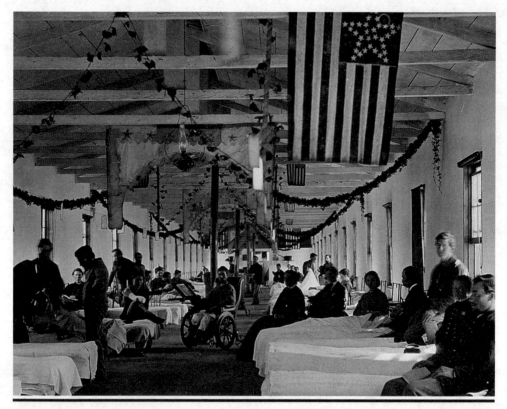

FIGURE 3-7. Convalescing soldiers at Carver Hospital, 1865, one of the Washington area's hospitals. The pavilion-style hospital construction was utilized. Walt Whitman, a Sanitary Commission volunteer, made over 600 visits to military hospitals in the Washington area for the purpose of visiting the wounded. The pavilion style of hospital construction featured open ventilation and light. Photograph courtesy of the National Archives and Records Administration, Image #524592a.

suffered more than those from urban centers. Population dislocations had their impact as well. Jim Downs, writing in the *Lancet*, points out the dire effect of disease upon freed slave populations of the Civil War era.[43(pp1640–1641)]

Pneumonia had been treated in the period before the war with antimony and the lancet for bleeding. During the war, opium, rest, and "snakeroot" (a low-growing perennial found in central and southern climates) were utilized. Snakeroot was considered a remedy to produce "expectoration." Snakeroot was also used as a cure for snakebites. It had been used since colonial times for fevers and malaria.[25(p203)] For both the North and the South, scurvy was undoubtedly underreported or was misdiagnosed. Scurvy was reported as early as 1862 in the Army of the Potomac. Scurvy was likely unreported in Southern hospital records. As an example, only 110 cases of scurvy were reported in records at Chimborazo Hospital in Richmond, Virginia, among Confederate patients.[25(pp206–208)]

Smallpox was both endemic and epidemic despite attempted vaccinations, which featured often ineffective vaccines and failure to vaccinate enough of the nonvaccinated troops in both the North and the South.[25(p199)] As an example, The Smallpox Hospital in Richmond had 250 cases resulting in 110 deaths in 1 week in December 1862.[25(p196)] Smallpox patients at Army camps were isolated in remote buildings.[25(p198)] Smallpox was a problem for prisoner of war camps in both the North and the South. It was medical policy for both the North and the South to vaccinate all prisoners who did not have vaccination scars. However, there were ineffective vaccines that did not prevent the disease.[42(p294)] Smallpox also was an issue among Freedmen (freed slaves) who had not been vaccinated, and caused the majority of deaths in this group.[42(p291)] The attempts by physicians on both sides to treat smallpox once it developed were largely ineffective.[42(p296)]

Meier wrote an interesting book, published in 2013, that presents a unique thesis that the healthy soldier was distanced from the infirm by what she terms as "self-care."[44] Healthy soldiers bathed more often, washed their clothes, sought out good footwear as available, and sought better shelter. They would seek to supplement their camp diets with fruits and vegetables. To meet these ends, these soldiers might "straggle" behind their formations to forage for what they could along the route of the march.[44(pp1–7)]

Anesthesia

In the period leading up to the Civil War, anesthesia was not universally employed in the United States in either civilian or military settings. Of note, ether was utilized in a few cases in the Mexican-American War (1846–1848).[45(pxii)] Anesthetic agents had been available since the 1840s after the early use (1842) by Crawford Long, a surgeon.[45(pp2–5)] Several men were involved in the introduction of ether as an anesthetic: Horace Wells, a Boston dentist; Charles Jackson, a Boston surgeon (who fought with Morton over claims for its use); and William Morton, a dentist (1846). An Edinburgh physician discovered chloroform's use as an anesthetic in 1847. Indeed, Queen Victoria had used chloroform in 1853 for the birth of one of her children.[45(pxii)] However, in the aftermath of the Crimean War, the British Surgeon General believed general anesthetics were dangerous in serious cases.[6(p120)] Even some medical journals in 1861 enunciated the belief that the patient's excitement might carry them through and that anesthetics should be avoided.[6(p120)] Nevertheless, the surgical use of anesthesia accelerated during the Civil War in response to the sheer numbers of wounded. Chloroform and ether were both available as anesthetics, but chloroform was the preferred agent when available, due to ether's explosive nature. Alcohol (ie, liquor) was used to supplement these agents or to substitute for them when supplies were exhausted.

During the Civil War, Union forces had no difficulty obtaining anesthetic agents. ER Squibb and other companies made both ether and chloroform. Squibb had been a Navy surgeon who later became a pharmaceutical manufacturer.[46(p46)] In fact, more than 1 million ounces of each agent were purchased by the North during the conflict.[46(p46)] The South attempted to obtain adequate supplies of anesthetics through various methods. For example, some supplies were obtained by blockade running and the use of supplies captured from Northern troops.[14(p9)] Also, small amounts of ether and chloroform were manufactured in the South during the Civil War.[46(p46)] The South generally used chloroform anesthesia, which had been discovered in 1847 by Dr Simpson and used almost exclusively by the British in the Crimean War.[25(pp225–226)] WTG Morton, who had given one of the first anesthetics in Boston (1846), later gave many anesthetics during the Battles of Spotsylvania and the Wilderness, both in Virginia.[46(p46),47(pp1068–1078)]

Surgery

Surgeons had antiseptics and disinfectants available, but they often didn't use them effectively. For example, antiseptics might not be used until a wound was infected. Disinfectants were often used to get rid of odors associated with infections, but instruments and dressings were not routinely disinfected. Carbolic acid as an antiseptic had use in the Civil War, but it would not be used as a standard agent until Lister published his work with carbolic acid in 1867.

Antiseptics included potassium iodide; potassium permanganate; carbolic acid; bromine; chloride; turpentine; and the nitric, sulfuric, and hydrochloric acids. The US Sanitary Commission published a pamphlet in 1863 on the use of disinfectants.[6(p128)] The Commission favored quicklime, chloride, bromine, and sulfate of lime.[6(pp126–127)] Some surgeons even washed their hands in chlorinated soda, which was shown in the 1840s to reduce childbirth fever.[14(p9)]

Dressings and bandages were a priority in medical supply. Bandages were often rolled. Dressings were termed wet or dry. Dry dressings, without added ointments or liquids, often resulted in improved healing. Wet dressings might involve placing a beeswax ointment (cerate). There was a further distinction between the cold and the warm dressing. The cold version might involve applying water continuously to the wound.[14(p34)] The warm version was associated with obtaining suppuration as a result of infection.[6(p233)]

The most common surgery involved bullet removal and wound cleaning, although amputations, with the images of piles of limbs, seem more common. The Minié ball wound was the responsible agent for many amputations. The Confederates preferred the circular method of amputation, while the North preferred a flap approach. The South considered the circular approach more efficient; in this method the skin and tissues were rolled over the stump and then closed. The flap method involved two strips of skin and tissue that were tied together and closed. The flap method left more tissue to cover the stump, in the view of those favoring the technique.

Surgeons used scalpels, hemostats, and saws that would be familiar today. Instruments were kept in lined cases and were usually just washed off with stream or well water, or just wiped off before replacing in the case. Some instruments passed into history, such as the "Nelaton's probe," which had a ceramic knob that would show scratches when it was passed close to a bullet.[19(p57)]

Introduction of Female Nurses and Physicians

During the Civil War, the use of female nurses was a signal event. As Keegan pointed out in his article, "Reinventing the Battlefield," combat of the Civil War period involved heavy and extensive rifle fire with entrenched soldiers, leading to more casualties, which made the role of nurses immediate.[49] In 1862, the Secretary of War, upon the recommendation of Surgeon General Hammond, authorized a squad of 11 nurses to take care of 100 patients. The use of female nurses followed the precedent set in the Crimean

War. Dorothea Dix was appointed Superintendent of Female Nurses for the Union.[50(p40)] The Catholic religious orders supplied many well-trained nurses, although Dix was not in favor because she (like many of her time) was suspicious of Catholic institutions.[6(pp176–179)] In the nursing heritage, the name of Florence Nightingale stands out. She established a nursing training program at St Thomas' Hospital in London during 1862. In America, nurses were often referred to as "Nightingales" because of her work.[51(p408)] Nurses during the Civil War performed many duties, including dispensing medications, changing dressings and bandages, and washing the wounded. They often cooked food for the wounded or ill. The role of the friend, the confidante, the letter writer, and the purveyor of hope were all extremely valuable.[51(p424)]

Clara Barton was one of the most famous of women involved in the Civil War. Barton started as a teacher but gained a position as a clerk in the US Patent Office (in Washington, DC). She worked there from 1854 to 1857 and then again from 1860 to 1865, which provided support for her Civil War pursuits. She obtained influential backers, which allowed her to operate independently of The Sanitary Commission and Dorothea Dix and her nurses.[14(p37)]

Barton provided care in 1861 for wounded soldiers injured by Baltimore mobs. She gathered donated supplies and took them to Culpeper and Fairfax Station, Virginia. Barton attended the wounded at Fredericksburg in 1864. She set up an office in Annapolis, Maryland, that would help families find their soldier relatives. She went to the infamous Confederate prison at Andersonville, Georgia. She made a list of all that had died the past year and where they were buried. She continued her important work running her missing person office, receiving only a small amount of government aid in 1866.[14(p39)]

Dr Elizabeth Blackwell, the first female American graduate in medicine, established a nurses' training program to provide skilled individuals.[43(p424)] There were always issues about the nurses, including concerns about the baggage accompanying them. There was criticism that the nurses were too interested in carrying clothes, and personal items such as brushes and combs.[6(p183)]

Dorothea Dix's organization supplied nurses to Army field hospitals. The exasperated reaction of the medical director, Dr John Brinton, of the large facility at Cairo, Illinois, was not unusual for the time. The doctors were most upset with the fact that the nurses did not understand military order. Dr Brinton was quoted as saying of the nurses: "They defied all military law."[41(p54)] Mary A Bickerdyke (known as Mother Bickerdyke) openly challenged the authorities in Union Hospitals. She told them she received her authority from the Creator.[41(p57)] The attitudes of both the physicians and the nurses softened as the war progressed.

In the Confederate hospitals, good nursing was recognized early and the best nurses were deemed by the patients to be women. A number of women were employed in military hospitals, although the role was not generally supported in public thought.[25(pp267–268)] In the South, local women's organizations provided assistance. Mrs Opie Hopkins, for instance, was sent to Richmond with food and clothing for the wounded by the Ladies Aid Society of Montgomery (and later the Ladies Aid Society of Alabama). They continued their growing assistance until they aided the Alabama section of the noted Chimborazo Hospital in Richmond.[41(p54)]

Another interesting personage is that of Dr Mary Walker, who graduated in 1855 from Geneva Medical College. Dr Walker worked to become an official assistant surgeon, even to the point of showing up for duty in a uniform she had created herself. She was first allowed to work only as a nurse; then in late 1861 to work as a volunteer field surgeon. In 1863, she was hired as a civilian contract assistant surgeon, finally quietly being integrated into the ranks of medical professionals.[41(p60)] In the Confederacy, Jefferson Davis gave a commission (as a captain) in the Confederate States of America to nurse Sally Tompkins so she could continue her work after all Confederate hospitals were placed under military control.[41(p58)]

WEAPONS AND WOUNDS OF THE CIVIL WAR

Rifles

Captains Claude-Etienne Minié and Henri-Gustave Delvigne of the French Army devised a rifle, the Minié rifle, in 1849 that would fire a conical hollow-base projectile with three ring bands that would deform when fired and create a good seal in the chamber to prevent the loss of gases. The bands expanded into the rifling of the barrel after firing. The ball could be easily and quickly inserted down the muzzle loader's barrel.[39(p8)] By 1851 the British had equipped their forces with the Minié rifle, firing the feared Minié ball projectile.

By contrast, smooth-bore muskets required actively ramming the ball down the muzzle with a rod, which took extra time and effort. Interestingly, Jefferson Davis (later the President of the Confederate States of America), while serving as the US Secretary of War, held tests of the rifle in 1854 that led to the direct production of the 1861 Springfield rifle. The Springfield, using the Minié ball ammunition, was accurate out to 1,000 yards.[17(p191)] Davis standardized the .58mm caliber Minié ball as the Federal ammunition. The shorter-length barrel of the Harpers Ferry .58 caliber rifle was a limiting factor in terms of range, but the Confederates came into possession of many of these weapons when they took the Federal Armory at Harpers Ferry, West Virginia, in October 1859.[39(p6)] The English-manufactured Enfield was respected and used by both sides for its quality of manufacture. It was held almost to the standard of the 1861 Springfield rifle. Other foreign weapons were used, especially by the Confederates, including the .54 caliber Austrian Lorenz rifle musket and a .71 caliber Belgian rifle musket.[39(p6)] The Confederates manufactured copies of the Springfield rifle for their troops, such as the "Richmond" rifle.

By 1860, percussion cap and Minié ball rifles were the standard infantry weapon of the Union forces. The Spencer and Henry breech-loading repeating rifles were introduced soon thereafter, although not widely used until later in the war. Breech-loading and relatively rapid-firing percussion weapons such as the Henry (featuring an elegant brass receiver) were expensive because they required critical machining. The Henry rifle was the forerunner of the 1873 Winchester repeating rifle. All of the small arms used black powder, which added to the haze over a battlefield, hindering accuracy.[50(pp94–95),51(pp56–62)]

Bilby calls 1863 the "year of the rifle-musket"[50(p95)] because both sides were finally equipped with the standard weapon for the conflict, which was a single-shot rifled weapon such as the weapons produced at the Springfield Armory.[2] However, he terms 1864 the "year of the repeating rifle"[52(p95)] because increasing numbers of Spencer rifles, and to a lesser extent the Henry rifle, started to be seen more.[50(pp94–95)] These breech-loading rifles used copper rim-fire cartridges that contained the powder and the primer.[50(p95)]

Corbusier explained that his 6th Illinois Cavalry of 1,000 men were armed with "sabres and Spencer carbines, having one shot in the chamber and six in the breech."[23(p50)] He further describes the carbines having "cartridges [that] were metallic . . . unlike the paper cartridges used in standard weapons . . . which required good teeth to tear"[23(p50)] the packets open to load the weapon. Corbusier speculated that the use of the Spencer carbine with its metallic cartridges allowed men with few or no teeth to be recruited. The carbines had issues that he described in his writings of a soldier using a carbine that had mechanical loading problems or, as Corbusier described, "the cartridges soon gave out on the advanced line"[23(p50)] and he came back carrying his "hat full of cartridges."[23(p50)] Despite glitches in the weapon as noted by Corbusier, the Spencer used .56-.56 caliber cartridges; the rifle could be very effective in combat.

The Union in 1864 contracted with the Spencer factory to buy every Spencer rifle it could manufacture. Many units clamored to be equipped with the new rifle. The Henry rifle (the 16-shot rifle) was usually obtained as a private purchase item; however, the Ordnance Department provided the ammunition for the Henry. The South came into possession of some captured repeating rifles, but ammunition was always a problem, unless it was also captured.[50(p116)] Union units used the Henry repeating rifle as an enlistment inducement.[51(p62)] The Spencer repeating rifle made a considerable contribution to Union firepower, especially the cavalry. The rifle was not manufactured beyond 1865 because the Army had a need for a large-caliber round, which could be accommodated only with a single-shot rifle at that stage of technology.[51(p62)]

Handguns

Handguns were the favorite of cavalry troops. The Union purchased over 370,000 pistols in the war. The weapons of choice included the .44 caliber Army Colt and the .36 caliber Navy Colt pistols. The Union purchased approximately 12,000 Lefaucheux French pistols, which fired a unique .41 caliber pin-fired self-exploding cartridge.[1(pp136–137)] Revolvers were issued to cavalry and officers, but not to the enlisted men. However, the enlisted men managed to equip themselves. Oftentimes, infantry troops found the revolvers were not as useful as they thought they would be and frequently sold or simply disposed of them. The Confederates, when faced with a shortage of handguns for the cavalry, confiscated such guns from the infantry. Handguns used in the South came from captured stocks and imported weapons. The British-made Adams and Deane, and the Kerr revolvers, were imported in quantity. The Colt revolvers of the Army and Navy versions were also sought-after weapons.[1(p137)]

Projectiles

The infamous Minié ball, a low-velocity projectile, caused severe wounds. The bullet could shatter bone and tear soft tissue, while bringing fragments of clothing and other forms of contamination into the wound. Infection would often follow. The fractures resulting from the ball were complex enough to challenge surgeons today.[11(p282)] The Minié ball was said to have caused 108,000 wounds (where the type of projectile could be determined), as opposed to only 16,000 for the older round ball.[6(p114)] Most of the Confederate rifle wounds were caused by the Minié ball.[25(p220)] There were some explosive Minié balls that embedded copper, lead, and pewter into the wound.[11(p282)]

Artillery

Artillery weapons were common on the battlefield. The "Napoleon" was used most commonly by both the North and the South. It was a smooth-bore muzzle-loading cannon that used a 12-pound ball projectile. It was developed in France during the Napoleonic years, but it was only introduced into the United States in 1856. The rifled artillery pieces were used somewhat less frequently and included the Parrot and the 3-inch ordnance. The rifled weapons had longer range but were best against fortifications because the accuracy depended on line-of-sight visualization. These weapons were all muzzle loading. Breech-loading weapons were starting to be used, but were troublesome. The early breech-loading artillery had problems with the breech seal (to prevent escaping gases) and the seating of the shell.[1(pp140–141)]

John Keegan noted that "[u]ltimately, Civil War battles came to be characterized by heavy rifle fire, by the [relative] absence of artillery, and the prevalence of earthworks."[49(p87)] Keegan felt that artillery and the cavalry were comparatively insignificant in Civil War encounters. He went on to note that heavy casualties were typical of Civil War battles, which he attributed to local terrain making it difficult to maneuver or escape. He would include such a situation as those at Antietam and parts of Gettysburg's battlefield.[48(p87)] Of special note, there were few bayonet or edge weapon (sword) wounds, despite the popular image of forces charging each other with fixed bayonets and drawn swords.[6(pp113–114)]

THE WAR CONTINUES

In September 1863, the Battle of Chickamauga (named for a creek in northern Georgia) proved to be a bloody affair. Despite being a Confederate victory, General Braxton Bragg failed to deliver a decisive defeat to the Union. However, the South did get a morale lift in Chickamauga after its defeats at Vicksburg and Gettysburg.[52(pp101–102)] By the midpoint in the war, both sides had shortages of physicians, treatment facilities, and medical supplies.[52(p106)] Rubenstein points out that the Medical Directors for the North (the Army of the Cumberland) and the South (the Army of Tennessee) had treatment schemes in place at the Battle of Chickamauga that proved to be inadequate, which resulted in needless deaths.[52(p110)] For example, the Union hospitals were not placed well. The location of the hospitals was said to have been poor as they were exposed to artillery and assault. The main hospital was located at Crawfish Springs, which at least did offer water for the Union. (The entire area had sustained a drought.[52(p74)]) The wounded were evacuated by the Union by scheduled day and mail trains to the general hospitals, while an equal number were sent by troop transport trains on the backhaul route (trains returned empty after off-loading cargo, hence they were available for carrying wounded).[52(p109)]

The Confederates, led by General Bragg, assaulted Union forces at Chattanooga, Tennessee. Ulysses Grant had recently been appointed commander of the Military Division of the Mississippi. The Confederates in the end were defeated in their combat attempts; more importantly, their defeat opened the way for Sherman's advances into the South.[1(pp105–106)]

Lee and Grant faced each other as adversaries for the first time at the Battle of the Wilderness in Virginia. It is of note that in 1864 the Confederate Surgeon General directed that a Reserve Surgical Corps be set up so that the reserve could be used in emergencies. However, Lafayette Guild, the Confederate Medical head at the Battle of the Wilderness, was unable to get as many of the reserve members as needed.[25(pp116–117)] Despite heavy losses for both sides, the Wilderness Campaign ended in a stalemate, which was followed by the May 1864 Battle of Spotsylvania, also in Virginia. This latter battle also resulted in huge losses for both sides, but the casualties could be better absorbed by the North with its greater overall population.[1(pp11–12)]

At the start of the war, captured medical officers were held as prisoners of war in the same manner as regular line officers. Generally, surgeons would be left to attend the wounded when the forces of either side retreated. However, an agreement of 31 May 1862 between medical officers of both sides was followed by a General Order from McClellan's headquarters and copied to General Lee that medical officers would be exchanged.[25(pp130–131)] The ready exchange worked well, despite an 1863 issue concerning a Union surgeon who was sought for civil charges by the Richmond authorities.[25(p132)]

THE WAR ENDS

As the Confederate defeats continued, Lee was given overall command of the Confederate armies in 1864. However, the South continued to experience shortages of almost everything. A string of defeats at Petersburg, the fall of Richmond, Sherman's wins (Atlanta, Georgia; the Carolinas; and Savannah, Georgia), and Sheridan's victories in the Shenandoah region in Virginia all led up to the final events. The end was signaled by Lee's surrender to Grant at the Appomattox Court House. America's greatest battle carnage was finally over.

MEDICAL OUTCOMES

The implementation of an effective ambulance evacuation scheme was perhaps the signal advance of the Civil War. Limb immobilization, using splints such as the Hodgen Splint, provided improvement in the handling of orthopedic injuries. The beginnings of specialty division care started in the war, with reconstructive surgery and neurological surgery being first. Dr S Weir Mitchell was a neurologist to whom Surgeon General

Hammond dedicated a hospital for Mitchell to study neurological disease. Mitchell and his associates looked at the relief of phantom limb problems and various nerve injuries (among many areas of interest).[11(p283)]

Considerable progress was made in the creation of artificial limbs for those soldiers with lost extremities. Mobility in the ankle of the prosthesis was a new advance. Surgeon General Hammond appointed a committee of physicians to approve the dispensation of an artificial limb. The soldier could then choose a prosthesis from a number of manufacturers that cost $50 or less.[11(p287)]

Many surgeons gained improvement in their skill set, which would benefit future patients. The following surgeons are examples of the later successes of the many surgeons who served during the Civil War. Dr William W Kean, a veteran of Gettysburg and other campaigns, went to Europe for additional training after the war and became one of the first American surgeons to adopt Lister's antiseptic techniques. John Shaw Billings helped establish the Army Medical Museum and went on to design the new Johns Hopkins Hospital.[21(pp289–290)] Dr William Corbusier continued to serve in the Army and served through World War I. Many other less famous surgeons were to serve their country in myriad ways after this terrible war.

REFERENCES

1. Turner TR. *101 Things You Didn't Know About the Civil War: Places, Battles, Generals—Essential Facts About the War That Divided America.* Avon, Mass: Adams Media; 2007.
2. Davis KC. *Don't Know Much About the Civil War: Everything You Need to Know About America's Greatest Conflict But Never Learned.* New York, NY: William Morrow and Company, Inc; 1996.
3. Jensen LD. *Johnny Reb: The Uniform of the Confederate Army, 1861–1865.* Mechanicsburg, Penn: Stackpole Books; 1996.
4. Haller JS. *Battlefield Medicine: A History of the Military Ambulance From the Napoleonic Wars Through World War I.* Carbondale and Edwardsville, Ill: Southern Illinois University Press; 2011.
5. Straubing HE. *In Hospital and Camp: The Civil War Through the Eyes of Its Doctors and Nurses.* Harrisburg, Penn: Stackpole Books; 1993.
6. Adams GW. *Doctors in Blue: The Medical History of the Union Army in the Civil War.* Shreveport, La: Louisiana State University Press; 1996.
7. Fox WF. *Regimental Losses in the American Civil War, 1861–1865.* Albany, NY: Albany Publishing Company; 1869. Available online as an e-book at https://archive.org/stream/regimentallosses00foxw#page/n9/mode/2up. Accessed 23 March 2015.
8. Young AC III. *Lee's Army During the Overland Campaign.* Baton Rouge, La: Louisiana State University Press; 2013.
9. Hacker JD. A Census-based count of the Civil War dead. *Civil War Hist.* 2011;57(4):307–348.
10. Blaisdell FW. Medical advances during the Civil War: presidential address. *Arch Surg.* 1988;123(9):1045–1050.
11. Gillet M. *The Army Medical Department 1818–1865.* Washington, DC: Center of Military History, United States Army; 1987.
12. Letterman J. *Medical Recollections of the Army of the Potomac.* New York, NY: D Appleton and Company; 1866.
13. Medical Heritage Library. Internet Archive. *Confederate States Medical and Surgical Journal.* https://archive.org/details/confederatestate12conf. Accessed 23 March 2015.

14. Schroeder-Lein G. *The Encyclopedia of Civil War Medicine*. Armonk, NY: ME Sharpe, Inc; 2008: Introduction.
15. Stille CJ. *History of the United States Sanitary Commission Being the General Report of Its Work During the War of the Rebellion*. Philadelphia, Penn: JB Lippincott and Company; 1866.
16. *The Sanitary Commission of the United States: A Succinct Narrative of Its Works and Purposes*. Ithaca, NY: Cornell University Library; 1864.
17. Naythons M. *The Face of Mercy: A Photographic History of Medicine at War*. New York, NY: Random House; 1993.
18. Morris R. The soldier's missionary. *Civil War Q*. 2014;Spring:52, 59.
19. Norris DA. Life during the Civil War. *History Magazine* (Toronto, Can: Moorshead Magazine, Ltd.); 2009.
20. Howe SG. *The United States Sanitary Commission*. Ithaca, NY: Cornell University Library; 1864.
21. McGaugh S. *Surgeon in Blue*. New York, NY: Arcade Publishing Company; 2013.
22. Schultz D. A strange and blighted land. *MHQ: Q J Mil Hist*. 2013;25(4):78.
23. Corbusier WH, Wooster R (ed). *Soldier, Surgeon, Scholar: The Memoirs of William Henry Corbusier 1844–1930*. Norman, Okla: University of Oklahoma Press; 2003.
24. Coffin H. *The Battered Stars: One State's Civil War Ordeal During Grant's Overland Campaign*. Montpelier, Ver: Country Man Press; 2002.
25. Cunningham HH. *Doctors in Gray: The Confederate Medical Service*. Shreveport, La: Louisiana State University Press; 1958.
26. Garrison FH. *John Shaw Billings: A Memoir*. New York, NY: GP Putnam's; 1915.
27. Sears SS. *To the Gates of Richmond: The Peninsula Campaign*. New York, NY: Ticknor and Fields; 1992.
28. Brown HE. *The Medical Department of the United States Army From 1775 to 1873*. Washington, DC: Surgeon General's Office; 1873.
29. Barbour JH. And now a few words on the battle of Williamsburg. *Colonial Williamsburg*. 2014;Spring:27–30.
30. Clements BA. *Memoir of Jonathan Letterman, MD, Surgeon United States Army and Medical Director of the Army of the Potomac*. In Medical Recollections. http://history.amedd.army.mil/booksdocs/civil/lettermanmemoirs/Bennett_Master.html. Accessed 23 March 2015.
31. Office of Medical History. US Army Medical Department. *Biographies. Charles Stuart Tripler*. http://history.amedd.army.mil/biographies/tripler.html. Accessed 23 March 2015.
32. Eicher D. *The Longest Night: A Military History of the Civil War*. New York, NY: Simon and Schuster; 2001.
33. Trudeau NA. Did Lee doom himself at Gettysburg? *Q J Mil Hist*. Summer2009;21(4):14–25.
34. Beck PN. *Columns of Vengeance: Soldiers, Sioux, and the Punitive Expedition, 1863–1864*. Norman, Okla: University of Oklahoma Press; 2013.
35. Office of Medical History. US Army Medical Department. *Surgeons General. William Hammond*. http://history.amedd.army.mil/surgeongenerals/W_Hammond.html. Accessed 23 March 2015.
36. Office of Medical History. US Army Medical Department. *Surgeons General. Thomas Lawson*. http://history.amedd.army.mil/surgeongenerals/T_Lawson.html. Accessed 23 March 2015.
37. Office of Medical History. US Army Medical Department. *Surgeons General. Clement A Finley*. http://history.amedd.army.mil/surgeongenerals/C_Finley.html. Accessed 23 March 2015.
38. Office of Medical History. US Army Medical Department. *Surgeons General. Joseph K Barnes*. http://history.amedd.army.mil/surgeongenerals/J_Barnes.html. Accessed 23 March 2015.
39. Field R. *Eastern Theater 1861–1865: Union Infantryman Versus Confederate Infantryman*. Botley, Oxford, United Kingdom: Osprey Publishing Ltd; 2013.

40. Army Heritage Center. *A Deadly Scourge: Smallpox During the Revolutionary War.* https://www.armyheritage.org/education-and-programs/educational-resources/education-materials-index/50-information/soldier-stories/282-smallpoxver. Accessed 23 March 2015.
41. Freemont F. *Gangrene and Glory: Medical Care During the Civil War.* Carbondale, Ill: University of Illinois Press; 2001.
42. Bollet AJ. *Civil War Medicine: Challenges and Triumphs.* Tucson, Ariz: Galen Press; 2002.
43. Downs J. Emancipation, sickness, and death in the American Civil War. *Lancet.* 2012;380(9854):1640–1641.
44. Meier KS. *Nature's Civil War: Common Soldiers and the Environment in 1862 Virginia.* Chapel Hill, NC: University of North Carolina Press; 2013.
45. Snow SJ. *Blessed Days of Anaesthesia: How Anaesthetics Changed the World.* Oxford, England: Oxford University Press; 2008.
46. Wright AJ. The merciful magic of ether-anesthetics in the Civil War. *Anaesth News.* 2013;393. http://www.anesthesiologynews.com/ViewArticle.aspx?d=Ad+Lib&d_id=384&i=March+2013&i_id=937&a_id=22708. Accessed 23 March 2015.
47. Morton WTG. The first use of ether as an anesthetic at the Battle of the Wilderness in the Civil War. *JAMA.* 1904;42(18):1153.
48. Keegan J. Reinventing the battlefield. *Q J Mil Hist.* 2009;22(1):80–87.
49. Beller SP. *Medical Practices in the Civil War.* Cincinnati, Oh: Betterway Books; 1992.
50. Bilby JG. The guns of 1864. *Am Rifleman.* 2014;162(5):94–95.
51. Bilby JG. The guns of 1865. *Am Rifleman.* 2015;163(3):56–62.
52. Rubenstein DA. *Thesis: A Study of the Medical Support to the Union and Confederate Armies During the Battle of Chickamauga: Lessons and Implications for Today's US Army Medical Department Leaders.* Submitted to the Faculty of the US Army Command and General Staff College. Fort Leavenworth, Kans: US Army; 1990. http://history.amedd.army.mil/booksdocs/civil/ThesisRubenstein/rubenstein.html. Accessed 23 March 2015.

Chapter Four

Transitions: Army Medicine in the Post-Civil War Period to the Start of World War I

LANCE P. STEAHLY, MD

INTRODUCTION

AT THE END OF THE CIVIL WAR, the size of the US Army was reduced to prewar levels and its missions were redirected. The Army reverted to its prewar model of dealing with Indian irregular warfare, with a limited role as an occupation force in the reconstruction of the South. Years later, the Army had to quickly gear up for a more modern conflict in the Spanish-American War. The Army also saw action in China (the Boxer Rebellion), the Philippines (the Philippine Insurrection), and in Mexico, all in the prelude to World War I.

In the Civil War, the Regular Army became less attractive as a destination for recruits as the war progressed due to the popularity of the volunteer units. This was because the volunteer units of the states had more favorable terms of service and bounties than did the Regulars.[1(p381)] The whole issue became more of an academic topic once peace came and the separate militaries of the North and the South melted away.

The Civil War resulted in casualties of a magnitude not seen in warfare up to that time. However, largely due to medical innovations introduced during the Civil War, the mortality rate was reduced significantly as the war went on. As an example, the mortality rate sustained by soldiers at Gettysburg was only one-third of the mortality experienced during the Peninsula Campaign just one year earlier.[2(p214)] However, as the war ended, the lessons learned about mass casualty management were not applied because monies became scarce and the once great Army was reduced to a fraction of its previous size.

As a detractor from the aftermath of the Civil War, the Army's attention was focused again on the international stage with potential changes for both the North and the newly defeated South. The French intervention in Mexico was guided by Napoleon III; the French government also established the Austrian Maximillian as Emperor of Mexico. This incursion of a European power literally in the backyard of both the North and the South represented an additional threat as the Civil War ended. One of the agendas of the

Confederacy at the 1865 Hampton Roads Conference dealt with this Mexican/French issue. Prior to the end of the Civil War, on 3 February 1865, President Abraham Lincoln and Secretary of State William Seward met with representatives of the Confederacy aboard a steamboat in the James River at Hampton Roads, Virginia. The Confederate delegates included the Confederate Vice President Alexander Hamilton Stephens and two others. The Confederates hoped that the Union could be persuaded to work with the South in dealing with the French incursion.[3(pp210–211)] However, the Mexicans dealt with Maximillian after the French abandoned the venture. After the end of the French adventure in 1867, the Army did not plan for any larger conflicts.

IMMEDIATE POST-CIVIL WAR PERIOD

A monumental effort by the Army Surgeon General's Office, under the guidance of Surgeon General Joseph Barnes, resulted in the publishing of six volumes between 1870 and 1888. The *Medical and Surgical History of the War of the Rebellion, 1861–1865* was the result of that effort using much data from the Provost Marshal General's Bureau.[4] This compilation of the statistics and experience of the US Army Medical Department should have been an aid to planning for conflicts of the future. Unfortunately, as in many wars, the lessons learned were forgotten and had to be relearned for future conflicts.

The volunteers were rapidly and completely released from duty while Congress reduced the number of Regular troops from 54,000 in 1867 to 26,000 in the 1870s.[5(p218)] Immediately following the Civil War, the Medical Department, like the Army as a whole, spent much of its energy reducing personnel and hospitals. Contract surgeons were reduced to 187 by 1870 from the many thousands used in wartime.[6(pp4,7,8)] A peacetime Medical Corps was established in 1866 by Congress. It featured a Surgeon General at the rank of brigadier general and an Assistant Surgeon General as a colonel. Field surgeons were continued as a surgeon (ranked as a major) and an assistant surgeon (ranked as either a lieutenant or a captain).[4(p901)] The Regular surgeons and assistant surgeons who remained in the Army had to meet high standards. While these positions might look good to a young physician without prospects, the slow promotions and low pay that characterized the peacetime Army had a negative effect on recruiting the best physicians for these positions.[7(p106)] It was not until 1876 that Congress increased the number of colonels to three and doubled the number of lieutenant colonels, potentially benefiting recruitment by freeing up more spaces at the top of the pyramid. Otherwise, Congress did not address the recruitment issue.[8(pp250–251)]

As mentioned above, the post-Civil War Army reverted to its prewar Indian fighting model but gained a role as a limited occupation force enforcing Reconstruction in the South. The many physicians, the large general hospitals, and the hospital trains and ships were no longer needed. The medical service in the South involved dealing with the inevitable diseases and with the health of troops and Freedman's Bureau clients. The Indian war fighting role involved frontier post medicine and surgery, punctuated by various campaigns to deal with irregular warfare.

Dr William Henry Corbusier actually experienced both roles in his career. In 1864, Dr Corbusier accepted a contract offer as an Acting Assistant Surgeon in the US Army for 1 year. He was ordered to Amite, Louisiana, where he was stationed with the 1st US Infantry under Brevet Major Offley. His book, titled *Soldier, Surgeon, Scholar: The Memoirs of William Henry Corbusier*,[9] provides a uniquely personal experience of that time in Louisiana.[9(pp62–63)] He requested that his contract end early on 14 June 1865 because he wished to earn a medical degree. Although he was a surgeon in the war, he didn't receive his medical degree until 1867 from the Bellevue Medical College, after attending lectures and clinics.

As in the case of Corbusier's commanding officer, brevet ranks were used in several ways. Brevet rank could be conferred when a position called for a higher rank, much as services may "frock" someone with a command requiring a higher rank. Brevet ranks were conferred, as were substantive regular ranks, by a nominating process requiring Senate confirmation. Eicher and Eicher note that in the period of rapid demobilization and military occupation of the South during Reconstruction, brevet ranks conferred during the Civil War were all given the "omnibus" date of rank of 13 March 1865.[10(p34)] However, for medical officers the rank situation remained murky. The formal ranks granted in 1847 were not clarified so the rank equivalents in the form of the titles of "surgeon" and "assistant surgeon" continued. However, the Surgeon General did have an official brigadier general rank and prevailed as one of the all-powerful bureau chiefs. These Army bureau chiefs ran their own departments and had direct access to the Secretary of War.[11(p4)]

Army duty in the period of Reconstruction in the South presented its own medical challenges. Disease remained the Army's major problem in the immediate post-Civil War era. Preventive medicine remained the only real defense against disease available to the Army surgeon. Unfortunately, the surgeon's recommendations to the line officer concerning preventive medicine measures were often disregarded. However, in 1874, the Army did require the surgeon to make sanitary and public health recommendations that had to be approved or disapproved by the commander. The commander had to forward his reasons for his actions to the territorial/regional commanding general.[11(pp39–40)]

There were areas in which medical care was inadequate for a variety of reasons. For example, smallpox vaccinations were required for Army soldiers, but local communities were frequently not protected due to antivaccination movements. Sometimes lax enforcement of the vaccination requirement was the problem. For instance, approximately 600 Black soldiers died of smallpox in 1866, which the authorities attributed to a postwar letdown in precautions.[11(pp39–40)] Other diseases were also prevalent. Yellow fever was always a peril in the South. Yellow fever epidemics were reported in Florida in 1867, causing the death of one soldier at Key West and 27 at Fort Jefferson. Dr Samuel Mudd, of Lincoln conspiracy fame and a prisoner there, was given permission to work at Fort Jefferson to deal with the illness. Cholera was also a real threat, although the death rate from cholera declined after 1867 due to the implementation of better medical practices, while yellow fever rates climbed. In 1869, yellow fever caused 12 soldier deaths in Pensacola, Florida. Captain George Sternberg, the future Army Surgeon General, was a surgeon at Fort Barrancas (Pensacola). Sternberg came down with yellow fever but survived, after which he gained a special interest in the disease. After 1869, the death rates fell as yellow fever and cholera cases decreased in part due to the isolation of the troops from other populations.[11(pp40–41)] As Gillet notes, the Army moved troops away from involved areas, which helped, but the mortality rate with yellow fever cases could nonetheless exceed one-third of the total number of cases.[11(p41)]

A major postwar development for the Army Medical Department was the creation of the Hospital Corps in 1886. The Corps would be composed of hospital stewards, acting stewards, and privates. Hospital corpsmen still had to be trained for their wartime roles as soldiers because they might be called upon for defense, especially in the West. Schools of instruction were set up to teach horse care, first aid, anatomy, physiology, nursing, and pharmacy. More than 400 hospital corpsmen were trained from 1891 to 1896, but many were lost to attrition due to lack of interest or academic failure. Because they were also soldiers, those dropping out would serve in the ranks.[11(pp100–101)] However, random soldiers could not be picked to work as nurses in the hospitals—only stewards of the Hospital Corps with appropriate training could work there. Especially in the West, stewards were dispersed among the posts and did not have the ability to work and train together beyond their initial steward course. In the late 1880s, the reduced Indian threat brought some attention to the prospect of medical readiness for other threats. In 1883, the Surgeon General recommended that the Medical Department's enlisted soldiers train together.[5(p396)]

Despite the number of posts declining after the Civil War, the individual medical officer had more responsibilities. By the 1890 to 1891 year, the Army had closed more than one-fourth of these posts[5(p80)]; the surgeon had little staff and almost no respite. The posts were often in remote areas with little to offer in terms of diversions or amenities for a family. Families had difficulty obtaining clothing and household goods, which often had to be ordered from cities or sent by relatives. The medical officer had to care for the soldiers and their families. The doctor trained his stewards and litter carriers to his specific requirements beyond any initial school training. There was a professional need to pay more attention to antiseptic principles and the consequent need for more skilled surgical interventions, as improved techniques became known.

SURGEONS GENERAL CONTRIBUTIONS IN THE PERIOD 1865 TO 1917

The period from the end of the Civil War to the start of World War I can be viewed through the accomplishments of the respective Army Surgeons General. The Surgeons General all faced challenges to provide care at the many widely separated posts with limited resources. The expected budget cutting following a major war persisted as a political feature up to the Spanish-American War. The Surgeons General from 1865 to 1893 were all Civil War veterans; six of the number had served prior to the war.

Joseph K Barnes (22 August 1864–30 June 1882)

The first of these men was Brigadier General (BG) Joseph K Barnes, who entered office in 1864. Barnes attended, but did not graduate from, Harvard College. He received his medical degree from the University of Pennsylvania in 1838. He served at various Army posts and was a participant in the Mexican-American War. After serving in many posts, he served in various Civil War commands in Missouri and Kansas. He was then assigned to Washington, DC, where he became the attending military surgeon in that city. The duties included caring for the ranking military and civilian office holders. Barnes made a favorable impression upon Secretary of War Edwin Stanton.[12]

Barnes' appointment as the Surgeon General was the result of the court-martial conviction of the prior Surgeon General, William Hammond. Barnes was officially appointed as a brigadier general, but was given a brevet appointment as a major general due to his Civil War service. Stanton was instrumental in Barnes' appointment. Barnes developed the Army Medical School and Medical Museum. He was one of the attending physicians for President Garfield during his illness. He left office in mid-1882 due to nephritis, which ultimately caused his death in April 1883.[13(pp233,247)]

Charles H Crane (3 July 1882–10 October 1883)

Barnes was followed by his Assistant Surgeon General, BG Charles Crane, who held the position until he died of a hemorrhage from an oral tumor a little over a year after becoming Surgeon General. Both Barnes and Crane were involved in the dramatic drawdown of forces.[14(p52)] Crane graduated from Yale College and then Harvard Medical School in 1847. He served at Veracruz during the Mexican-American War, and also participated in the Seminole Wars for 3 years (1849–1852). Crane went on to serve in California and Oregon, and later in Florida. He served in the Civil War as the primary assistant to Surgeon General Barnes. Barnes had retired in 1882 because Congress had passed legislation in June 1882 mandating retirement for age, and he was a year beyond the maximum age. Crane followed Barnes to the Surgeon General post in July 1882.[15]

Robert Murray (28 November 1883–6 August 1886)

Crane was followed by another Assistant Surgeon General, BG Robert Murray, in November 1883. Murray had served in the Army Medical Department since 1846, hence providing a long historical perspective ranging to the Mexican-American War.[14(pp74–76)] Murray received an MD degree from the University of Pennsylvania in 1843. He became an assistant surgeon in 1846. Murray spent the Mexican-American War years in California until 1850, when he returned to the East. In 1854, he was again posted to California and he remained there until the start of the Civil War. He served with what became the Army of the Cumberland and was its medical director until 1862. Murray was then posted to Philadelphia, Pennsylvania, as the medical purveyor commanding a depot from which he was the principal purchasing agent for medical supplies and medicines. In 1866, he became the medical purveyor at San Francisco and remained there until 1876. In 1880, he became the medical director of the Division of the Atlantic. As the ranking medical officer, he became the Assistant Surgeon General to the newly appointed Surgeon General Crane. When Crane died in 1883, President Arthur advanced the senior man, namely Murray, to the Surgeon General's office. Murray recognized advances in surgery and advocated antisepsis and antiseptic surgery in reports. He was responsible for a report citing contaminated water at posts as a disease source. Murray retired due to age in 1886.[16]

John Moore (18 November 1886–6 August 1890)

After much political maneuvering by the various eligible senior officers, President Grover Cleveland appointed BG John Moore, who had been Major General (MG) William Sherman's medical director near the end of the Civil War, to be the next Surgeon General. Moore received a medical degree in 1850 from the University of the City of New York. He did an internship at Bellevue Hospital and then worked for several years at the New York Dispensary. He passed the examination for assistant surgeon in the Army in 1853, receiving an appointment in June. Moore was posted at various assignments, including duty at the Marine Hospital at Cincinnati, Ohio, where he remained until 1862. In 1862, he was assigned to the Army of the Potomac as medical director of the Central Grand Division. In 1863, he became the medical director for the Department of Tennessee. Murray then became the medical director for the Army of Georgia and Tennessee (the designation for a larger command) and later the medical director at Vicksburg, Mississippi. He remained in Mississippi until 1866, when he relocated to New York. After 2 years in New York, he spent the period from 1868 until 1880 as an attending surgeon at area hospitals (private practice) and served on various boards while based in New York City. He became the medical purveyor at San Francisco until appointed Surgeon General in 1886.

Moore was instrumental in having first aid taught throughout the Army. Various teaching and training manuals were produced. Under his guidance, Army regulations were issued for the conduct and training of the Hospital Corps, which Congress established in 1887. He encouraged sanitary reports, adding awareness to the sanitation efforts of posts. Moore retired in 1890 for reasons of age.[17]

Jedidiah Baxter, MD (16 August 1890–4 December 1890)

BG Jedidiah Baxter, the chief medical officer in the Provost Marshal's office,[13(p76)] became the next Surgeon General after being involved in political infighting for most of his career. Baxter received his medical degree from the University of Vermont in 1860. He spent some time providing care at Bellevue and Blackwell's Island hospitals in New York. Following the start of the Civil War, Baxter received an appointment as a surgeon to the 12th Massachusetts Volunteers in 1861. Following this and a later stint with the Army of the Potomac, he was moved to Washington where he became chief medical officer for the Provost Marshal General's Bureau until the end of the war. He served as a medical purveyor during some of the time in Washington and he was credited with getting the medical supply chain running smoothly.

Baxter apparently developed a busy medical practice at the White House during the Garfield term, treating numerous members of Congress and various influential leaders. Baxter even earned a law degree from Columbia during this period while on active duty as a military surgeon. After much infighting (which had been building over the years), he secured the office of Surgeon General but died 4 months into the term after a severe stroke.[18] Even with only 4 months in office, Baxter made a contribution inasmuch as he was responsible for sending Walter Reed to study bacteriology and pathology with Dr Henry Welch at Johns Hopkins School of Medicine in Baltimore, Maryland.[13(pp75–78)]

Charles Sutherland (10 May 1831–10 October 1895)

Sutherland graduated from Jefferson Medical College in Philadelphia, Pennsylvania, in 1849, and gained his commission in 1852. He served at the following locations: Jefferson Barracks, Missouri; Fort Riley, Kansas; and New Mexico. Sutherland was serving in Texas on the border when the Civil War started. He was sent to Florida for a year. In 1862, he became the medical purveyor for MG Henry Halleck's command, centered in Mississippi. He was credited with setting up and supplying numerous hospitals in the command. He later became the medical director for the Department of Virginia and medical purveyor for the Army of the Potomac.

After the Civil War, Sutherland became the medical purveyor for Washington and New York. From 1879 until 1884, he was the medical director of the Division of the Pacific and from 1884 until 1893 he was the medical director for the Division of the Atlantic.[19] In May 1893, Sutherland became the next Surgeon General. By all accounts, he was a capable administrator with an amiable disposition. Due to his age, he retired in 1893 on a mandatory basis. As was the case with all of the Surgeons General in the post-Civil War period, much of his work revolved around the continued drawdown after the Civil War (closing facilities, reducing physician staff, and always watching the limited budget).[5(p218)]

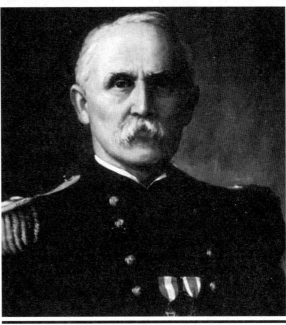

FIGURE 4-1. George Sternberg. Sternberg was a prominent scientist in addition to being the Army Surgeon General. He was responsible for setting up the Army Medical School (1893–1894) and oversaw its evolution into the Army Institute of Research. Sternberg encouraged his doctors to seek more training. Among his achievements, he obtained early radiograph machines for some post hospitals. He retired in 1902 and was the recipient of many honors. Photograph courtesy of the National Library of Medicine, Image #B03026.

George M Sternberg (30 May 1893–8 June 1902)

George M Sternberg followed Sutherland in the Surgeon General's Office in 1893. In view of his relative junior standing and his lack of administrative experience, Sternberg (Figure 4-1) would seem an unlikely choice. However, he was a scientist rivaling the best European scientists. He had studied with Koch in Germany. Sternberg became skilled with the microscope and the camera while establishing himself as a serious researcher. He published and developed a prominence in scientific circles and he had a serious quest for recognition.[20(pp178–179)] Sternberg was responsible for the establishment of the Army Medical School, which functioned in conjunction with the established Medical Museum.[15(p153)] The first class of the Army Medical School was held from November 1893 to March 1894. The success of that group ensured the school's continuation and its evolution into the Army Institute of Research. The School had four instructors, including Major (MAJ) John Shaw Billings (associated with the founding of the Army Medical Museum) and MAJ Walter Reed.[11(pp97–100)]

Sternberg was instrumental in getting the new radiograph machines for several post hospitals. To his credit, he assigned physicians to posts near medical schools and encouraged them to become involved in more training. Sternberg also concerned himself with the training and organization of the Hospital Corps. He looked at the hospital corpsman as having an important role in the future. He worked to improve post sanitation, the quality of the water supply, and to implement preventive medicine procedures. Under his guidance, Army rations were evaluated and a new emergency 4,100-calorie ration was devised for use in the field and in action. Sternberg called for the creation of operating rooms to reduce infection and laboratories to help with diagnosis.[11(pp100–108)]

Surgeon General Sternberg's 9-year tenure witnessed the entrance of Army medicine into an era of modern medicine. However, the department was still geared to medicine on the frontier and at posts, rather than to major wartime needs. The department did not incorporate any lessons that could have been learned from the casualty management of the Franco-Prussian War. For example, the Prussians insured that every German soldier carried emergency bandages that a treating medic would use. The Germans started using identification cards for the wounded that stated what treatment had been given. Furthermore, the Prussians had dedicated litter carriers at all times. The medical casualties of the coming Spanish-American War and the invasions of Cuba and the Philippines would suffer because of that neglect to incorporate the latest innovations pioneered in Europe.[11(p112)]

Surgeon General Sternberg retired in 1902 due to mandatory age requirements. He received many honors and was at one time the President of the American Medical Association, the American Public Health Association, the Military Surgeons of the United States, and the Washington Biological Association.[21(pp70–74)]

William H Forwood (8 June 1902–7 September 1902)

William Henry Forwood served as the Surgeon General from June 1902 until September 1902. Of special interest, when he was appointed to the office he had only 3 months before his age-mandated retirement date.[21(pp75–78)] Forwood graduated from the University of Pennsylvania in 1861. In August 1861, he became an Army assistant surgeon. He served in many battles and survived a chest gunshot wound at the Brandy Station Battle in Virginia. Forwood served at various stations in the West (Kansas, Texas, and Nebraska), as well as in Georgia. He participated in several expeditions, including an exploring expedition in the summer of 1883 with Robert Lincoln, the son of the slain president, and President Chester A Arthur. Forwood became the Professor of Military Surgery at the Army Medical School when it was opened in 1893. He held various positions there until 1898 when he was appointed the chief medical officer for a hospital and convalescent center in Georgia. He was posted to California but returned to the Washington Army

Medical School in 1901. Although a colonel at this point, he was appointed to the rank of brigadier general and to the post of Surgeon General (replacing the retiring Sternberg) with only 3 months remaining until his own mandatory retirement date. His 41 years of service culminated in his being considered one of the great military surgeons of his day.[22]

Robert M O'Reilly (7 September 1902–14 January 1909)

O'Reilly was Surgeon General from September 1902 until January 1909. Interestingly, he served in the Civil War as a medical cadet. The medical cadets were formally recognized by the Union Army as medical students who had not graduated but could offer more advanced care than a layman. Resuming his studies after the end of the war, he received a medical degree from the University of Pennsylvania in 1866. He served at various posts until 1870, when he became involved in numerous actions against the Indians. He later became the personal physician to President Grover Cleveland. He served in various spots including Havana, Cuba, during the Spanish-American War. He was sent to Jamaica to study British methods in the tropics. He became the Surgeon General by virtue of a new rule that required the candidate to be able to serve 4 years before the mandatory retirement age. The three colonels ahead of him were not eligible. His greatest accomplishment was the enlargement of the Medical Corps and of the Hospital Corps.[23] He was also able to create the Medical Reserve Corps. O'Reilly maintained good political relations in Washington after his appointment as Surgeon General. Funding for the Walter Reed Hospital in Washington was passed during his tenure.[23]

George H Torney (14 January 1909–27 December 1913)

Torney graduated from the University of Virginia School of Medicine in 1870. He started his military career with the Navy in 1871 but resigned in 1875 due to severe seasickness. He accepted an Army commission the following day. He served in a variety of assignments including field duty in New Mexico and Colorado until 1895, when he was posted to Virginia for 4 more years with the start of the Spanish-American War. During the years of the Spanish-American War, he was assigned to Hot Springs, Arkansas, until 1902. He was then sent to Manila, in the Philippines, where he commanded the 1st Reserve Hospital. He was the commander of the Presidio Hospital, in San Francisco, California, from 1904 to 1908. He was involved in directing and supervising emergency care during the 1906 earthquake and fire in San Francisco. His good work there helped the momentum for his selection as Surgeon General in 1909. During Tourney's time as Surgeon General, the newly built Walter Reed Army Hospital was opened in 1909. The Dental Corps was established in 1911. Laboratories were added to the Army Medical School and typhoid immunizations were standardized for the Army.[24]

William C Gorgas (16 January 1914–3 October 1918)

Gorgas was appointed Surgeon General in January 1914 and served almost to the end of World War I (October 1918). Gorgas (Figure 4-2) was the son of a West Point graduate and later brigadier general in the Confederate Army. The young Gorgas was interested in a military career but could not get admitted to West Point. He decided to gain a military

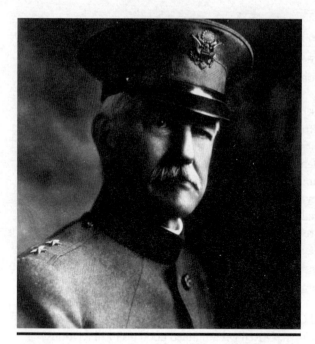

FIGURE 4-2. William C Gorgas. Gorgas was an 1879 graduate of New York's Bellevue Medical College. He began his Army career as an assistant surgeon in 1880, serving at posts in the West and in Florida. General Leonard Wood later appointed him to be the chief sanitary officer in Havana, Cuba. Gorgas was credited with all but eliminating malaria and yellow fever (by mosquito control) during the building and operation of the Panama Canal. Photograph courtesy of the National Library of Medicine, Image #B13204.

career by entering the Army through medicine. He graduated from Bellevue Medical College in New York in 1879. He served a year of internship in New York and received an Army commission in 1880.[25]

Gorgas started in the Army as an assistant surgeon. Like Leonard Wood, Gorgas was stationed in the West, where he had a number of tours, and also in Florida. He survived yellow fever while in Florida; he also survived typhoid fever. After being appointed the military governor of Cuba in 1899, BG Leonard Wood appointed him as the chief sanitary officer in Havana. Gorgas, as a colonel, worked on the health aspects of the Panama Canal project until 1913. Gorgas is credited with removing the mosquitoes, all but eliminating malaria and yellow fever from the Canal Zone. He was appointed the Surgeon General in 1914 and was later promoted to the rank of major general in 1915. Although he had planned to retire in 1917, the onset of World War I and all of the needed mobilization planning kept him on until his mandatory age retirement just short of the armistice.[25]

Gorgas is best known for his sanitary efforts in Cuba and the Panama Canal Zone. His work in eradicating yellow fever brought major acclaim. The canal could not have been built had diseases not been curtailed. During his Surgeon General tenure, Fitzsimons Army Hospital in Colorado opened in 1918 under his direction and the Army School of Nursing in Washington, DC. Gorgas was involved in the many facets of World War I care and the early phases of the influenza pandemic, which became more pronounced in late 1918 and 1919.[25]

Meritte Ireland (5 October 1918–31 May 1931)

Ireland succeeded Gorgas as the next Surgeon General in October 1918.[11(pp88–93)] Ireland became an assistant Army surgeon in 1901 by examination after graduating from the Detroit College of Medicine and then the Jefferson Medical College. He served in Cuba and later in the Philippines. In the immediate lead up to World War I, General Pershing selected him as the American Expeditionary Forces (AEF) Medical Director. However,

Surgeon General Gorgas appointed another colonel for whom Ireland served as deputy. He deployed to France with General Pershing as the deputy to the AEF Medical Director, Colonel Bradley. He was quickly promoted to colonel, then brigadier general, and finally major general, Assistant Surgeon General, AEF, in 1918. He was recommended for Surgeon General following Gorgas' retirement. He was to remain in this office until 1931.[11(pp94–100)] MG Ireland will be discussed further in the chapter on forward surgery in World War I.

THE DOCTOR BECOMES A SOLDIER: THE ROLE OF LEONARD WOOD IN THE INTERWAR YEARS

The study of the career of Dr Leonard Wood (Figure 4-3) is an effective vehicle to illustrate the life and times of a physician in the Indian Wars, the Spanish-American War, the Philippine Insurrection, and the lead up to World War I. Although other physicians had many similar medical experiences (Exhibit 4-1), Wood was unique in his combination of medical and nonmedical assignments. While Leonard Wood reached the military pinnacle of becoming the Army's Chief of Staff, and later became a near-run candidate for president, it should be remembered that he started as an Army contract surgeon. Even though he later switched roles and became a line officer, he always paid attention to the medical needs of his commands. As his career progressed, the role of Army medicine is highlighted through his actions.

His medical training arguably enhanced his future commands by increasing his awareness of public health, preventive medicine, and the handling and disposition of casualties. In his governing roles in Cuba and the Philippines, his attention to public health and disease control greatly enhanced his role as commander.[26(p30)] Wood's experience nicely highlights the events leading to a transition of the Army from an Indian fighting force to an Army preparing for overseas conflicts.

EXHIBIT 4-1. WILLIAM CORBUSIER, ARMY SURGEON SPANNING MANY ERAS

In addition to Leonard Wood, another interesting figure from the era was Dr William Corbusier. His career was different from Wood's in that he stayed with Army medicine. His career ran from 1877 to World War I. Dr Corbusier and his wife both wrote separate books detailing their frontier and later experiences. Fanny Corbusier wrote from the perspective of an Army officer's wife raising her children in often rather primitive posts.[1] William Corbusier described being in the field in 1885 in pursuit of Geronimo. Corbusier was unique in that he took a leave of absence to study advances in surgery from November 1881 until March 1882. In the Spanish-American War, Dr Corbusier was sent to the Philippines for the first of two tours. He described being in charge of the wounded sent by rail from the front at Caloocan, which was the main railroad terminus in central Luzon located north of Manila.[2(p130)] Corbusier was involved in evacuation of the wounded by boat following an attack on Malolos by General Arthur MacArthur.[2(pp130,202)]

References: (1) Corbusier FD. *Fanny Dunbar Corbusier: Recollections of Her Army Life, 1869–1908*. Norman, Okla: University of Oklahoma Press; 2003; (2) Wooster R, ed. Corbusier WH. *Soldier, Surgeon, Scholar: The Memoirs of William Henry Corbusier 1844–1930*. Norman, Okla: University of Oklahoma Press; 2003.

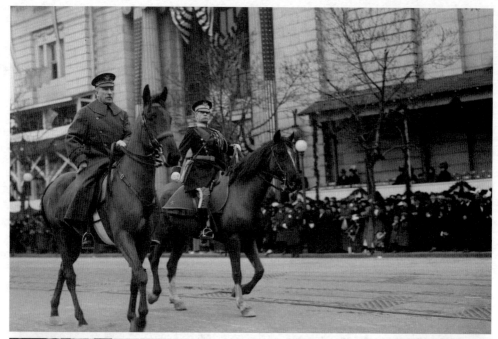

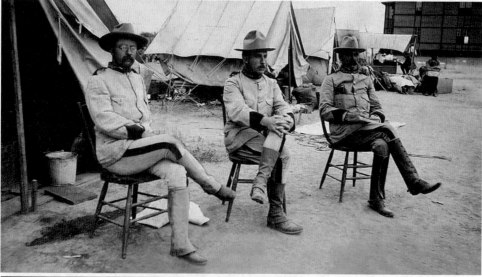

FIGURE 4-3. Leonard Wood. Wood began his Army career as an Army assistant contract surgeon after graduating from Harvard Medical School. His career was aided by Generals Miles and Crook. Wood belatedly received the Medal of Honor for his efforts in the capture of Geronimo. He made a transition to become a line Army officer and also served as the physician to the White House and particularly to President McKinley's wife, Ida Sexton McKinley. He commanded the Rough Riders in the Spanish-American War with Theodore Roosevelt. Wood became the Army Chief of Staff before the start of World War I. (A). General Leonard Wood as Chief of Staff (Wood is in uniform). Photograph courtesy of the Library of Congress, Image #11338V. (B) Theodore Roosevelt, Leonard Wood, and Alexander Brodie in 1898, in San Antonio, Texas. Photograph courtesy of the Library of Congress, Image #37599V.

Leonard Wood's father had attended the Massachusetts Medical School (a precursor of Harvard Medical School) and Dartmouth Medical School, but exhausted his funds before he could complete his studies. He obtained a diploma from the Eclectic Medical College of Pennsylvania (a version of a homeopathic school), but was unable to earn a satisfactory living from his practice.[27(p11)] Due to his incomplete training, Wood's father could not get an appointment as a physician in the Union Army. Instead, he became a hospital steward and was an enlisted soldier, rather than an officer, for an 11-month tour in Louisiana.[27(p12)]

Leonard Wood's Medical Training

Leonard Wood was able to enroll at the Harvard Medical School in 1880. His enrollment was made possible by the loan of money by HH Hunnewell, a prominent Wellesley businessman. At the start of his second year, he received a scholarship. The Harvard course at that time was 3 years in length. As part of his training, he received an appointment as an intern at Boston City Hospital. In the hospital setting, the interns were largely to be observers while senior staff surgeons carried out procedures. Wood, however, did not adhere to the requirement that he only observe surgery. He was placed on probation for operating without supervision. One month later, he was released from his internship for continuing to operate without supervision (the episode didn't surface until much later in Wood's life [during his quest for promotion to major general] when the mayor of Boston got access to the records of the Boston City Hospital and used this information against Wood). There was little recourse for him but to find a type of limited practice opportunity that did not require some type of hospital connection.[26(p30)]

Wood took over the practice of a classmate who had not done well with it. He had patients but most could not afford to pay, so he mentored medical students to supplement his income. Wood decided to take the examinations for an Army medical appointment; he wasn't sure he wanted to be an Army medical doctor but he needed the security and the money of the position. Wood placed second in the examination out of a field of 59 applicants.[27(p12)] Because there was only one commission available at the time, he was offered a 1-year stint as an assistant contract surgeon with pay of $100 per month.[28(p20)] The $1,200 to $1,500 per year paid to assistant and contract surgeons (contract surgeons were paid slightly more money than the assistant) equaled or exceeded the average civilian doctor's income at the time. The contract surgeons wore officer's uniforms, were treated as officers, and were included in officer functions and entertainment as a courtesy. The two ranks at the time were an assistant contract surgeon and the (full) contract surgeon.[26(pp30,31),29] The contract surgeon and the assistant surgeon were required to reapply each year for a renewal of the appointment; the contract was subject to cancellation at any time by the Surgeon General (often related to budget problems). There is still some confusion among historians as to the status of the contract surgeon. For instance, in a recent book about Dr Henry Porter, who was a contract surgeon with Custer's 7th Cavalry, the author uses the term "non-commissioned contract surgeons,"[29(p11)] which creates the false impression that they were noncommissioned officers (enlisted sergeants).

Wood took the job of assistant contract surgeon and reported to Fort Whipple in Arizona. Interestingly, he met Fred Ainsworth, another fellow contract surgeon, at Fort Whipple; both Wood and Ainsworth would ultimately decide to leave the Medical Corps after they had later become commissioned Medical Department officers. Ainsworth, an industrious bureaucrat, rose to become the Adjutant General of the Army, while Wood picked a route that led him to become the Army Chief of Staff. Ainsworth was to become a nemesis to Wood when they both achieved high positions. It is an interesting note of history that these two men, who both started as contract surgeons at the same time, should end up in conflict when they had both reached a high point in their respective careers.[28(p252)] Wood, with the help of Secretary of War Stimson, ultimately won the bureaucratic battle between the two of them when Stimson sided with Leonard Wood.[28(p252)] Ainsworth essentially wanted to continue acting independently of the Chief of Staff's direction as a bureau chief. Ainsworth, despite his position, power, and ability to block many actions, was forced to retire. As McCallum points out, Ainsworth and Wood shared the same beginnings and demonstrated many of the same assets and flaws that would cause them to become bitter antagonists. They both were very intelligent, motivated, hard working, and believed in their own vision. Neither man could really bring himself to readily compromise, but saw conflicts as power and control issues.[28(pp250–251),30(p178)]

Wood's Early Military Career: The Frontier Indian Wars

Two generals, George Crook and Nelson Miles, played an important role in Wood's early military career and in the frontier Indian wars. General Crook was an 1852 graduate from West Point. Assigned to frontier duty before the Civil War, Crook survived being shot with a poisoned arrow during the Oregon Rogue River War. Crook later had the dubious distinction of being the highest-ranking Union officer (Major General of Volunteers) captured by the Confederates. His capture occurred while he was staying at a hotel in Cumberland, Maryland. He was imprisoned at Richmond's Libby Prison for 2 weeks before being released in a prisoner exchange.[31(p135)] Secretary of War Stanton wanted to fire Crook for allowing himself to be captured, but General Grant intervened on his behalf.[32(p15)]

In the Civil War, Crook was awarded a brevet major general rank. After the Civil War, he made a mark in the Indian conflicts in the Pacific Northwest. Crook was transferred to command the Department of Arizona in 1871. He fought successfully against the Apaches and was promoted to brigadier general in 1875. He then commanded the Department of the Platte and dealt with the Sioux. He returned to the Arizona command in 1882 and obtained some success using Indian scouts and irregulars to fight and track Geronimo. He had conflicts with his commanding officer, General Philip Sheridan, about the conduct of the Geronimo pursuit. When Crook lost Geronimo (actually on several occasions), his request for transfer was quickly accepted. He was later promoted to major general, but died 2 years afterward in Chicago. Crook thought highly of Wood and used his influence while he held office to promote Wood's career.[28(p25)]

Nelson A Miles was the other general who had a long-term impact on Wood's career. Miles had little formal military training but raised a company of Massachusetts Volunteers after the First Battle of Bull Run in Virginia. Miles emerged from the Civil War as a Major General of Volunteers.[33(pp1,144,195)] Because he was not a West Point graduate, he was selected to serve as the commander of Fort Monroe, which held the former Confederate President Jefferson Davis as a prisoner. The powers-to-be thought he would be less likely to offer

Davis special consideration than a fellow West Pointer.[28(p45)] After the Civil War, he was successful in battle at the Red River War, the Great Sioux War, and the Nez Percé conflict and the Geronimo campaign. Miles was considered by many to be one of the Army's best commanders against the Indians.[9(p200)] Miles became the commanding general of the US Army in 1895 and the mentor of Leonard Wood while advancing his career (and later recommending him for the Medal of Honor[28(pp27–44)]). Miles trusted Wood's medical judgment implicitly, but he also supported Wood's interest in the regular business of being a soldier.

In July 1885, Wood was ordered to Fort Huachuca in Arizona where he established a long-term relationship with Captain Henry Lawton. Lawton was a dedicated soldier who would be Wood's good friend until his death 15 years later.[28(p20)] In Arizona, Wood spent much time outdoors with the troops chasing Apaches. In the difficult pursuit of Geronimo, Wood rode and walked countless miles in the desert and mountains and volunteered to carry dispatches.[28(pp34–40)] Although he was only a contract physician awaiting a commission, he became a functioning officer with Captain Lawton by default. Wood served as a medical officer, and an assistant surgeon with Lawton and under the ultimate command of General Miles.

True to the situation experienced by many Army surgeons, the pursuit of a highly mobile Indian force over nearly impassable terrain allowed for only the minimum in carried supplies. The surgeon would transport all of his instruments and supplies on his own horse and perhaps one or two other animals. As antiseptic surgery was not practiced, only the barest of equipment was needed. Fortunately, the number of wounded was generally limited. Fractures and medical problems were the main stay of the mobile Army surgeon. For transport of the wounded or seriously ill, the surgeon had to rely on a horse or mule litter.[11(pp64,65)] Transportation of supplies always complicated the need to evacuate the wounded. During the Indian campaigns, wagons had to be utilized if other means of transporting the evacuees (rail or boats on waterways) were unavailable.[11(p64)]

Arrow wounds were not all that common after the end of the Civil War, presumably because the Indians were now universally armed with guns. Skilled surgeons devised various techniques to remove the arrows that they did encounter. The sinews used to hold the arrowhead on the arrow shaft would soon break down due to the humidity and enzymes in bodily fluids. Thus an arrowhead could remain behind, embedded, if the shaft were just grasped. Hence, an instrument or a wire placed behind the arrowhead to retract the head, with shaft and all, was preferred.[11(p67)]

Surgeons sometimes had to improvise evacuation techniques. At times a "travois," a litter-like device with one end attached to the horse and the other end dragged on the ground (based on the Indian model), was used to evacuate the wounded. The "travois" could be made with any materials at hand such as tree limbs, teepee poles, or small trees. Some surgeons preferred this device when transporting the wounded over rough country. (While any pack animal could be used, the pack animals tended to weaken if they were on limited rations themselves.[11(pp65–66)]) If the evacuation was in haste, the wounded would have to be slung over a horse or mule if no wagon was available or if a wagon couldn't be used because the terrain would not allow a rapid retreat by that means.

Gillet noted that in the Modoc Wars in the Northwest (Oregon and Northern California) in 1872 to 1873 (also called the Lava Bed Wars) conducted over uneven lava-origin terrain, a chair-like device was fashioned by a carpenter that could be used with a single mule to evacuate the wounded. The wounded of the Indian wars were evacuated to a post hospital or to a field set-up if a post hospital was not possible. Usually tents were used for a field set-up, although other temporary structures could be used.[11(pp65-67)]

Frostbite was always an issue for the military surgeon in cold weather; the surgeon had no effective treatment for such an injury. Amputation of toes and feet were too often the outcome lest gangrene/infection gain a hold.[11(p67)] While in pursuit of hostiles, the surgeon still had to contend with disease, including typhoid, malaria, and scurvy (especially in cold times when rations could not be supplemented with fresh fruits and vegetables).

General Miles and Captain Lawton pushed the recommendation that Leonard Wood be awarded the Medal of Honor, which he finally received in 1898.[28(pp4,45)] The Medal of Honor was essentially the only award for heroism and such an honor would not be justified by today's standards. The award was used rather more commonly then. (General Arthur MacArthur, for example, didn't receive his Medal of Honor for Civil War service until the early 1900s.) General Miles thought highly of Wood's medical experience. Wood was clearly Miles' protégé and his influence in gaining the Medal of Honor and countless later professional opportunities helped the surgeon move toward a nonmedical Army career.[28(p45)] At one point, Miles had suffered a complex compound fracture of his leg in an accident. The attending surgeons wished to amputate but Miles insisted that Wood be summoned. Wood was able to get the fracture to heal, ensuring Miles' lasting gratitude.[28(p47)] Until 1892 (after the Battle of Wounded Knee in 1890), the Army surgeons were also encouraged to help treat the civilians. After that time, the surgeons were to concentrate on their military charges only.

Surgeons like Wood and Ainsworth participated in many diverse Indian conflicts. The Great Sioux War of 1876 to 1877 featured the great effort of the Sioux and Cheyenne at the Little Big Horn. As mentioned earlier, Dr Henry Porter, a contract surgeon also, served with Major Reno, who Custer designated to command a section of his force. Porter handled horrific casualties, as high as 50 injured at one time.[29(p112)] Despite setbacks at the Powder River country of Montana, the Army was the ultimate victor. Hedren, in a book about the Great Sioux War, lists the Army and a contract surgeon involved in the clashes and provides an accurate accounting of the casualties sustained by Army soldiers as well as those of the Indians.[34(Appendices D-F)]

Leading up to the events in which Wood would participate, General Sheridan, who was one of Grant's favorite Civil War commanders, became the commander handling forces in the West and was based in Chicago. Sheridan waged winter campaigns and actively sought out hostiles and their villages with converging troop deployments. In the 1874 to 1875 Red River War, Sheridan's strategy resulted in the defeat of the Comanche and Kiowa. While the Battle of the Little Bighorn was the high point of the Indian's success, their traditional style of war would lead to their ultimate downfall. The Indians did not use cohesive coordinated plans. Each warrior acted on his own, seeking personal combat and triumph. In the end, the constant encroachment of farms, ranches, and towns, coupled with the wholesale decline of the buffalo population, all contributed to the final defeat of the Indian nations.[35(p472)]

Sherman had success in the Indian conflicts of the Southern Plains. The railroads were then able to extend their lines, at which time the conflict shifted to the Northern Plains.[36(p37)] During the 1880s, the Indian expeditions and battles became more rare. The last major engagement of the Indian conflicts occurred at Wounded Knee in South Dakota on 29 December 1890. Army troops were sent to disarm the Lakota Indians. The ensuing events led to the deaths of 150 Indians and 25 soldiers. The events and outcome have been obscured.[37]

In December 1890 during the Battle at Wounded Knee, trains were used to transport medical supplies and men. A 25-bed hospital was expanded to a 60-bed facility. Most of the surgery involved setting fractures and providing homeostasis of wounds. Some triage was done and trained Hospital Corps personnel were first used in this major encounter. Two years later, Captain Charles B Ewing, who was an Assistant Surgeon of the Department of the Platte, gave an address to the Association of Military Surgeons of the National Guard at St Louis on 19 April 1892. He described the various wounds that were attended there. His address was titled: "The Wounded of the Wounded Knee Battlefield, With Remarks on Wounds Produced by Large and Small Caliber Bullets."[37]

After 8 years of frontier medicine, Leonard Wood felt underemployed. He asked General Miles for a line assignment but without success. He sought and received assignment to Washington, which was complicated by political considerations. When he finally arrived in Washington, William McKinley had been elected President. Wood became the attentive doctor for the wife of the President, Ida McKinley. Wood proved a sympathetic ear for Mrs McKinley, who sought his consultation daily. She had a seizure disorder, which may have been a petit mal variant. Because people knew little of epilepsy, the disorder was kept quiet. McKinley was very attentive to her needs and adjusted his schedule and plans to meet her situation.[38(pp267–271)] Mrs McKinley had had a difficult several years. Her first daughter died at age four. Her second daughter died a few months after birth. The death of her mother also added to her precarious mental state. Doctors of the period, including Wood, would have been able to offer only sedatives to alleviate the severity of the seizures. Wood's famous patient provided significant access to the President and other influential people.[39(pp347–361)] During this time, Wood became the strong friend and companion to Theodore Roosevelt, the new Assistant Secretary of the Navy. Roosevelt's influence was to prove to be a definite asset for Wood.[40(p105)]

Coming of the Spanish-American War

The 1898 explosion of the US battleship *Maine* in the harbor in Havana, Cuba, provided the fuse that ignited the Spanish-American War. Surgeon General Sternberg had to change his thinking from that of a scientist to that of a wartime medical leader. Congress provided for the expansion of regular and contract surgeons. Sternberg appointed Colonel (COL) Charles Greenleaf as the chief surgeon in the field.[41] The assigned physicians reported to the line commanders of their units while answering to Greenleaf for their professional work. The states picked the volunteer surgeons with varying success both in

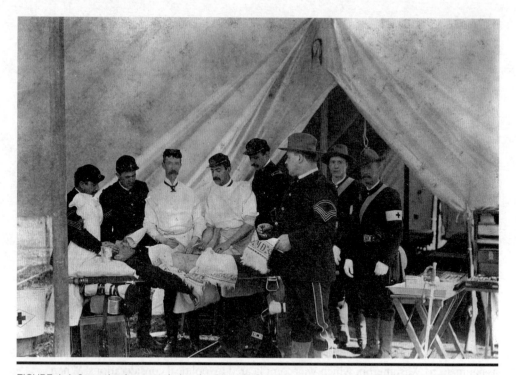

FIGURE 4-4. Operation in a tent during the Spanish-American War. Note absence of surgical gloves even though Halsted had introduced them to Johns Hopkins Hospital in 1871. Photograph courtesy of the National Library of Medicine, Image #A022370.

inducing physicians to serve and to the fact that the physician quality varied greatly. The rapid expansion of the forces required the Medical Department to select contract surgeons largely by references rather than by examination.[11(pp117–120)]

Sternberg pointed out that sufficient supplies were on hand for the 27,000 deployed troops. Despite being allowed to handle bids and to even buy directly on the open market, the need for speedy acquisitions of instruments and medical supplies was frustrated by the bureaucracy. In addition, the Quartermaster Department failed in its responsibility to furnish larger items such as tents.[11(p121)]

Fortunately, Sternberg had the authority to control hospitals and medical trains. He moved to establish hospitals at the division level and away from the previous regimental system. Sternberg established 10 general hospitals specifically for the Spanish-American War within the United States and organized medical trains coming inland from Tampa, Florida. Tampa was a War Department chosen site for deployment due to the proximity to Cuba. Roads and railroads were sparse in the Florida area and the port medical facilities were not developed (Figure 4-4). During his tenure, the Medical Department had continued challenges with the invasions of Cuba and the Philippines. Items such as bandages, medicines, and instruments were always in short supply. (Sternberg came in for major criticism from many quarters for the perceived failures of medical care in the early period of the Spanish-American War in 1898, although the Dodge Commission [appointed to investigate war issues] placed no major blame on the Medical Department.[11(p314)]) The long journey to reach the Philippines added to the dimension of the problems. Because San Francisco was a major supply depot with excellent transportation, the wounded and sick in the Philippines received better care than those in Cuba.[42(p386)] Despite the fact that Cuba and Puerto Rico were closer to the United States, the ports and infrastructure in Florida were not up to the standards and state of infrastructure on the West Coast.

With the Spanish-American War on the horizon, Wood and Roosevelt worked to obtain a volunteer command. Success came finally with the interest in forming "cowboy regiments" and the creation of the United States Volunteer Cavalry. Theodore Roosevelt was offered the command of the First Volunteer Cavalry. Roosevelt agreed to take the second in command slot if Wood would be named the commander.[41,42(pp386–387)] President McKinley was certainly reluctant to have his wife's favorite doctor away from Washington but Wood was able to persuade Ida, and thereby the president, of his strong desire to be a line officer in the war. When Wood's immediate superior became ill with malaria, Wood was promoted to brigadier general (to take over the position) and Roosevelt became the commander of the Rough Riders. (As an aside, Wood and Roosevelt were interested in taking control of Santiago [held by the Spanish] but they needed to get by blockhouses on top of San Juan Hill, Kettle Hill, and El Caney. It appears that the Rough Riders captured Kettle Hill while Lieutenant John Parker's Gatling guns provided excellent covering fire. Lawton and his Second Infantry secured El Carney. Kent held San Juan Hill. However, the hills were contiguous, so it is of little consequence as to who took which hill.[43(pp113,125–129,142–147)])

Tropical Diseases and Sanitation In Cuba

Wood's medical training was to be of assistance to him throughout his career. In Cuba in 1900 to 1902, as military governor, he dealt with a large number of sick and undernourished individuals and a lack of hospitals and medical facilities. Wood created large temporary hospitals in Cuba and supplemented the few Cuban doctors with military surgeons. He built nursing schools and even opened an asylum for the mentally ill in Cuba.[40] In his book *Theodore Rex*,[40] Morris comments that Wood, "A trained surgeon, he . . . transformed Cuba from one of the world's most pestilential countries into one of its healthiest."[40(p105)] During the Spanish-American War, the Cuban hospitals were occupied and utilized fully by the Spanish. The Spanish used the facilities for their troops and civilian dependents, employees, and officials, who used up the limited resources. The work of Leonard Wood and his staff aggressively dealt with the problems of the Havana hospitals and Cuban sanitation.

For decades yellow fever had been a constant problem in Cuba. Army Surgeon General Sternberg, a microbiologist by training, appointed Major (MAJ) Walter Reed to head the Yellow Fever Commission that would investigate infectious diseases in Cuba. The mosquito was identified as the vector of the disease. Wood then ordered mosquito control measures, which his chief medical officer, William Gorgas, successfully applied. By 1901, yellow fever and malaria had been significantly reduced. The famed Johns Hopkins gynecologist Howard A Kelly, in his 1906 book *Walter Reed and Yellow Fever*,[44] spoke of the need to recognize Leonard Wood for "his active and intelligent interest in the work of the Army Commission."[44(p172)] Kelly further credited Wood for his "permission to conduct experiments on non-immune people."[44(p172)] Kelly noted that Wood granted money and authority "to be expended in rewarding volunteers."[44(p172)] Kelly quotes Walter Reed as saying about Wood: "without his approval and assistance their [Yellow Fever Commission] observation could not be counted."[44(p172)] Leonard Wood said of Walter Reed that he knew of no one man "who has done so much for humanity."[44(p232)] Due to the American intervention, "Cuba was free from yellow fever for the first time in two centuries."[40(p105)]

Three medical officers were dispatched by Surgeon General Sternberg to deal with the fevers. They were under the direction of MAJ Walter Reed, who was the microbiologist (officially the professor of bacteriology and clinical microscopy[44(p238)]) of the Army Medical School. The other members of the Yellow Fever Commission included Dr James Carroll, who first met Reed after they were both assigned to the Army Medical School.[44(p255)] Dr Jesse Lazear, another member of the Commission, allowed himself to be bitten by a mosquito, and died of yellow fever at age 34.[44(pp267–268)] Dr Aristides Agramonte, the son of a prominent general in the Cuban insurgency, was a graduate of the Columbia College of Medicine.[44(pp271–272)] Agramonte did the autopsies and pathology work for the Commission.[44(p273)] Wood supplied Reed with $10,000 for his research, with the promise of additional funds as needed.[45(pp2–3)]

In 1902, Harvard University granted Walter Reed an honorary MA degree in recognition of his work in eradicating yellow fever.[44(p242)] In the same year, Reed received a honorary LLD from the University of Michigan.[44(p244)] Reed was also appointed as a professor of pathology and bacteriology at Columbia University in New York at the time he received the Army Medical School appointment.[44(p238)] Sadly, MAJ Walter Reed developed appendicitis, which at operation was found to be infected and perforated. Reed died of peritonitis 6 days after the surgery, on 22 November 1902.[44(p248)]

Wintermute presents the interesting idea that it was during this period that the Army Medical Department sought to reinvent itself as the nation's public health and sanitation resource. The addition of the newly acquired territories of Cuba, Puerto Rico, and the Philippines was a timely catalyst to this reinvention.[46(p4)] However, little progress was noted in combat medicine and surgery until the next great conflict.

Leonard Wood and Army Medicine in the Philippines

During his tenure in the Philippines prior to his becoming the Army Chief of Staff in 1910 (appointed in 1909), Wood preferred to be a line commander, but he applied his medical knowledge in disease prevention for his troops and the local population. Wood was a good administrator who had an interest in efficiency. (Just as Wood had used his medical training to great benefit in Cuba and the Philippines, this skill set was again put to use in World War I while he was sidelined to Fort Riley, Kansas, training divisions for European service. Influenza broke out in October 1918. He recognized that the disease was airborne in its spread. Wood eliminated large assemblies of men, separated dining tables with screens, and dispersed the men in camp. This outbreak quickly subsided in his Kansas station but had worldwide scope.[28(p274)])

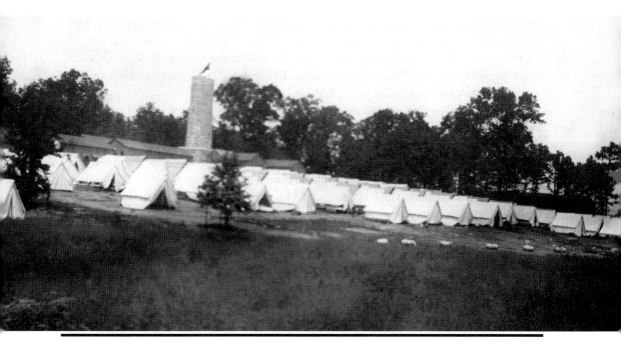

FIGURE 4-5. Sternberg Hospital, Manila, Philippines. In the Philippine campaign, the placement of hospital facilities was very central to the provision of adequate care. Larger facilities, such as the Sternberg Hospital, were designed to receive evacuated wounded and the sick. Photograph courtesy of the National Library of Medicine, Image #19999162.

In 1899, all of the volunteers and one-third of the regular troops returned from the Philippines to the United States. As the conflict escalated against the Filipino rebels, fresh volunteer and regular troops were sent in the autumn of 1899. The Philippine Insurrection was a guerilla war in a tropical environment. The conflict became an insurgent effort, which resulted in dispersion of forces and medical assets. The military medical officers had to deal with dysentery, malaria, and venereal disease among the troops. Medical officers even had to deal with smallpox among the native population. The doctors had to rely on prevention as they had little with which to treat the diseases.[47(p185)] The lack of surgeons and hospital corpsmen was always a challenge.[48(pp202–210)] Placement of facilities was also an important factor in maintaining manpower. Small facilities that were close to the front lines could get soldiers back to duty sooner and lightened the load of the larger facilities. Evacuation to larger cities, such as Manila, could be done by waterways, if needed.[48(p213)] A large facility, the Sternberg Hospital (Figure 4-5), was established in Manila. Initially, as already noted, the Army in the Philippines provided better care for the wounded and ill than provided in Cuba due to the resources available in San Francisco. However, as the Philippine conflict spread to more islands there, the problems mounted. These included more conflict-related casualties and greater requirements for medicines, supplies, and medical personnel.[9(p201),48(pp133–134)] The Army Medical Department maintained a large hospital on each coast of the United States even after the shuttering of the modern hospital at Fort Monroe, Virginia. In 1900, the general hospital in San Francisco (to be named

Letterman General Hospital in 1911) was the receiving point for evacuated Army patients from the Philippine conflict.[48(p337)] In 1901, roughly half of the patients there were from the Philippines. The East Coast facility was initially housed in buildings of the Washington Barracks. When the new hospital, named after MAJ Walter Reed for his contributions in yellow fever research, opened in 1909, it housed only 80 patients.[48(p338)]

The fact that the Filipinos did not accept the American occupation led to a prolonged guerilla war. Medicine had to adjust to a war of small-unit operations in remote isolated areas, often without outside support. The Philippine conflict was controversial in the public view. Linn, in his book about the 1899 to 1902 Philippine War, suggests that US involvement in that country was incremental and accidental.[48(p5)]

The Boxer Rebellion, which occurred in China in 1898 to 1900, was antiforeigner and anti-Christian in its scope. It involved conventional forces and combat. US medical officers had to work with physicians of the other European forces and of Japan. The Boxer Rebellion was like the Philippine conflict in that disease was always a threat to the welfare of the troops.[48(p224)]

The Army Medical Department was also involved in the response to the devastating San Francisco earthquake and fire in 1906. The Army set up hospitals in the Deer Park section of the Golden Gate Park. The Medical Department was instrumental in helping with sanitation, treatment of casualties, and preventive medicine.[49] Dr Henry du R Phelan published an account of his personal experiences as a contract Army surgeon in the earthquake and subsequent fires. It highlighted the good work of the Army and its medical assets in dealing with the tragedy. The Army troops were led by Frederick Funston, who had been promoted to Regular Army brigadier general. Funston declared martial law in San Francisco in the aftermath of the earthquake, fires, and looting.[50(p95)]

ADVANCES IN CIVILIAN MEDICINE

Lister and Germ Theory

A defining event in medicine, which had ramifications for the military, was the English publication in 1867 of Joseph Lister's work titled *On the Antiseptic Principle in the Practice of Surgery*.[51,52(pp326–329)] Lister used carbolic acid in the treatment of a compound fracture in an 11-year-old Scottish boy in 1865. He applied carbolic acid to the wound and found healing later without infection. He gave a lecture describing his techniques before the British Medical Association in London. Lister later published the lecture as an article in the *British Medical Journal*.[53(pp245–260)] Lister's fundamental concept was the germ theory in association with infection. He applied the concepts of Pasteur's 1864 work.[54(pp327–329)]

Lister believed it was important to fill the air with antiseptic, in addition to its use in the wound. He developed a carbolic acid spray apparatus, which he termed a "carbolizer."[46(p17)] It took some time for his principles and practice to become accepted and used, even in Scotland where he was a professor. In fact, physicians in Germany showed more interest in antiseptic surgery than did those in England or Scotland. The United States had resistance to germ theory among some leading surgeons, which persisted until the late 1880s, almost

20 years after Lister published his article. For example, an American Army medical officer, Captain Alfred C Girard, made a visit to observe Lister's techniques in England in 1877. He recommended the techniques highly to Surgeon General Barnes. Barnes then circulated the information to the medical officers, but he did not specifically recommend its adoption. The subsequent Surgeon General Robert Murray (November 1882–August 1886) finally endorsed antiseptic techniques in his 1884 annual report.[55(pp588-591)]

Pasteur and Koch

Louis Pasteur is best known for his work on what came to be known as "pasteurization" and the development of a rabies vaccine (also a military benefit). Pasteur did work that suggested the future use of heat sterilization in surgery, which was given in a paper written in 1878.[56(pp166-167)] Robert Koch, a German physician, did work that correlated disease with disease-causing organisms, resulting in what is known as Koch's postulates. Koch devised four postulates, which briefly were that: (1) the microorganism must be found in the infected host but not in healthy ones, (2) the microorganism must be found in the diseased host and grown in culture, (3) the microorganism will cause disease when introduced into a healthy organism, and (4) the microorganism must be cultured from the original and identified as the organism's causative agent.[57(p19)] Koch presented his findings at the 10th International Congress of Medicine in Berlin in 1890 to formalize the cause and effect of microbes and disease.[57(p20)]

Despite the work of Lister and his followers, the principles of antisepsis were often ignored. For example, after President Garfield was shot by an assassin on 2 July 1885, the wound in his back was repeatedly probed with unsterile instruments and fingers in an attempt to locate the bullet. He died 11 weeks later. (As a side note, Alexander Graham Bell had made available an early "foreign body localizer," which failed due to the overlooked metal in the bedsprings under President Garfield.[11(p50)])

Halsted and Antiseptic Surgery

In the United States a rising star in surgery, William Halsted, had embraced the principles of antiseptic surgery at an early point in his career. He entered the College of Physicians and Surgeons in New York in 1874. It had a 3-year curriculum and was one of the better medical schools at the time. Halsted would become the Professor of Surgery at the newly formed Johns Hopkins School of Medicine.[58(p299)] William Henry Welch, the famed Hopkins pathology professor and Halsted's friend, had spent time with Koch's students and even spent a month with Koch himself in Germany. Hence, Welch provided support for antiseptic techniques.[59(pp72,73)] Halsted (Figure 4-6) became a leader and innovator in American surgery; many of his innovations would also impact Army surgery. For instance, he popularized surgical gloves; the use of surgical shirts and trousers; and rigid attention to surgical detail, homeostasis (prevention of blood loss), and the application of surgical pathology techniques to the operating room. Halsted's clinical interests were in hernia repair (he had perfected a careful and precise herniorrhaphy operation), thyroid surgery (Halsted had performed thyroidectomies regularly), and mastectomy for breast cancer.[59(pp221,222)]

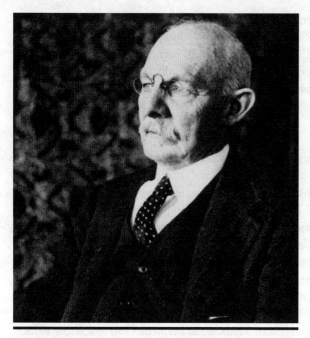

FIGURE 4-6. William Halsted of the Johns Hopkins Hospital, Baltimore, Maryland. Dr Halsted was the first Professor of Surgery at the newly opened Johns Hopkins Hospital. He trained in New York and Europe, and introduced attention to detail in surgery. Halsted also introduced innovations in hernia repair, thyroid surgery, breast surgery, and cholecystectomy. Photograph courtesy of National Library of Medicine, Image #B08313.

Military Adaptation of Civilian Advances

Many of these advances in the civilian world were adopted in the military in an attempt to keep Army medicine current. Medical officers tried an increasing number of operations including abdominal surgery. Dr Halsted's interest in hernia repair was appreciated in the Army because Surgeon General George Sternberg placed emphasis on herniorrhaphy to reduce the numbers of disabled soldiers. In 1895, the Army gave soldiers the option of undergoing hernia surgery or being boarded out on disability. After a successful operation and a "cure" to the hernia disability, they would remain in service. Hernia repair and appendectomy operations were the norm in the later 1890s. Surgeons were even doing hysterectomy, nephrectomy, and cholecystectomy procedures.[59(p111)]

Rubber surgical gloves were originally obtained for the hands of the future Mrs Halsted, who had a severe dermatological reaction to the antiseptic soaps of the time. The use of gloves facilitated her continuing as Dr Halsted's surgical nurse, although the gloves obviously also had a role in infection control. Dr Halsted used gloves that were made finely and withstood frequent heat sterilization.[59(p309)] The Army adopted surgical gloves in 1889.[59(p476)] However, they were not universally adopted by the Army surgeons because their use was not mandated. In addition, many surgeons preferred to have improved "feel" and dexterity without the perceived inconvenience of gloves.

Johns Hopkins was at the forefront of medical advancement, in fact being the only school initially approved by the Flexner Report, which evaluated medical schools in key admissions and curricula areas.[59] The report by Abraham Flexner revolutionized medical education quickly, resulting in the closure of most substandard institutions. Johns Hopkins then became the "gold standard" for the schools going forward.[59(pp199–200)]

President Cleveland: Beneficiary of Medical Advances

The surgery performed on President Cleveland was a marked contrast to that for President Garfield. Cleveland underwent the successful removal of a tumor in the roof of his mouth. The 1893 surgery resulted in no infection, the removal of a portion of his mandible, and the fitting of a prosthetic. Dr Welch, from Johns Hopkins, participated in the evaluation of the mass with indeterminate conclusions as to malignancy. (The pathology was reconsidered as late as 1980 with tissue obtained from the Mutter Museum of the College of Physicians and Surgeons of Philadelphia, Pennsylvania. The study by Brooks and Enterline, published in the *Journal of the American Medical* Association in 1980, was of interest because they reevaluated the Mutter Museum tissue because the fact that the president survived the operation for 15 years spoke to a more benign lesion, rather than the generally suspected sarcoma or oral carcinoma. Brooks and Enterline noted that various more benign diagnoses had been entertained. In their study they concluded that the lesion was a lower-grade malignancy.[60(p2729)])

MEDICAL CHALLENGES AND NEW TECHNOLOGY IN THE SPANISH-AMERICAN WAR AND OTHER MILITARY ACTIONS

Surgeon General Sternberg had ordered supplies in anticipation for war, although the amounts were enough only for a conflict of short duration. Indeed, Congress had not even provided funds sufficient for peacetime stockpiling.[11(p124)] Sternberg took personal charge in many of the details of supply. Despite the Surgeon General's involvement, depots were inadequate to handle the quantities of supplies needed.[11(pp125–126)]

In the mobilization for the Spanish-American War, a great deal of confusion occurred at the embarkation ports for the Army Medical Department, as well as for the troop supplies. At Tampa, for example, medical supplies and ambulances were often left behind in the rush to load troops and munitions. (Similar problems in the shipment of medical supplies were experienced in the invasion of Puerto Rico.[11(pp131,132)])

In the period since the Civil War, the peacetime Army had been centered on post facilities, which ultimately received the wounded and ill from the field in the Indian wars. The size of the Army being formed for the Spanish-American War called for a new approach to care, incorporating Letterman's plans in the Civil War, as opposed to the small-unit Indian wars' approach. The Surgeon General's decision was to base care on a division level with a field hospital following the division in combat.[11(p127)] At the time, the decision to move to a divisional organization was unpopular because most of the regiments reporting had some basic medical facilities organic to their organization. Inasmuch as they were to pool the equipment beyond their needs to the divisional medical facility, parochial concerns were present.[11(p128)]

Fortunately the combat phases of both the Spanish-American War and the invasion of Puerto Rico were short. In the invasion of Cuba in the Spanish-American War, division hospitals could not be landed due to lack of smaller landing craft and the fact that there were problems in unloading from ships, so hospitals were set up on ships. After the Spanish surrender at Santiago, the medical needs switched from dealing with wounds, fractures, and infections (Figures 4-7 through 4-10) to working on public health matters.[11(p142)]

The role of disease in the Spanish-American War follows the military experience as far back as the loss of many men to typhoid fever at Camp Thomas on the site of the Civil War

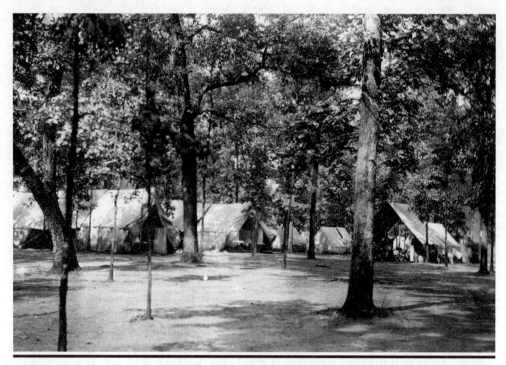

FIGURE 4-7. Sternberg Hospital (distinct from the Sternberg Hospital in the Philippine Islands), 3rd Army Corps, Camp Thomas, August 1898. During the Spanish-American War, many men were lost to typhoid fever at Camp Thomas on the site of the Civil War Chickamauga Battlefield. Diseases such as malaria and yellow fever continued to plague the war effort in the Spanish-American War and were treated at facilities such as the one at Camp Thomas, Georgia. Photograph courtesy of the National Library of Medicine, Image #19999178-2.

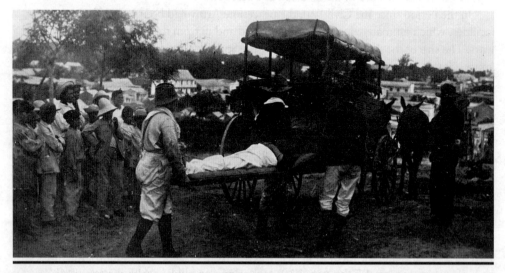

FIGURE 4-8. Soldiers loading a patient into an Army ambulance—little changed since the Letterman ambulance of the Civil War. Photograph courtesy of the National Library of Medicine, Image #9999190.

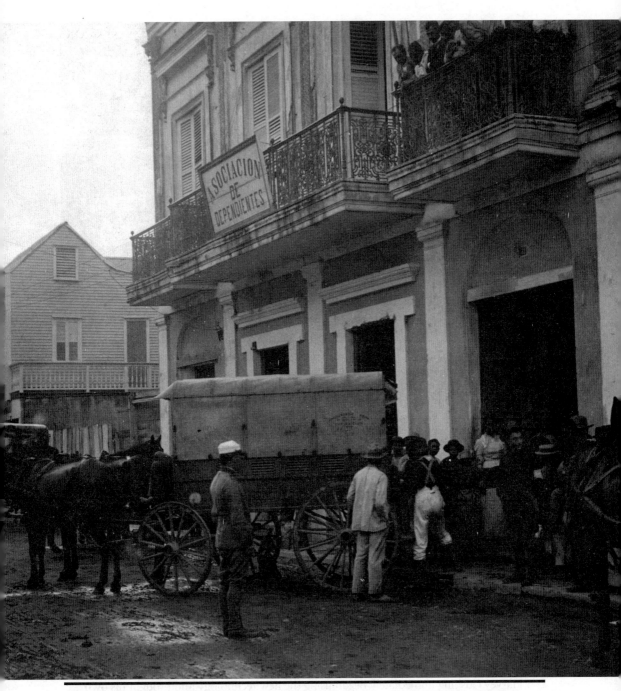

FIGURE 4-9. Casualties of the invasion of Puerto Rico, 1898. The ambulances used in this photograph were rather similar to the Letterman ambulances of the Civil War. In this scene, medics are unloading patients from such an ambulance at a hospital converted from a school. Oftentimes, any shelter available was used as a hospital. Photograph courtesy of the Spanish-American War Photographic Collection, Otis Historical Archives, National Museum of Health and Medicine, Item #8002-28.

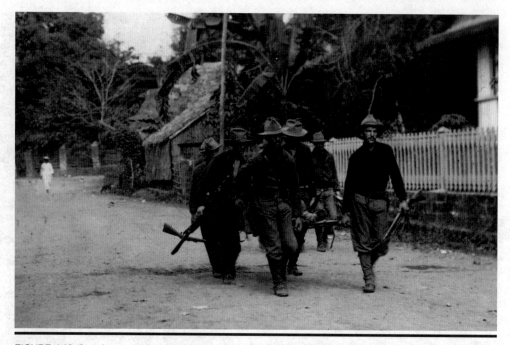

FIGURE 4-10. Carrying wounded to a hospital after action in Santa Mesa, Puerto Rico, 1898. Because dedicated litter bearers were not always available, the scene of armed American soldiers carrying wounded to a field hospital was not uncommon. Photograph courtesy of the Spanish-American War Photographic Collection, Otis Historical Archive, National Museum of Health and Medicine, Item #8002-9.

Chickamauga Battlefield. Diseases such as malaria and yellow fever continued to plague the war effort in the Spanish-American War as in prior conflicts.[61(p283)]

New technology was available to assist the military doctor during this period. Radiographs were developed in 1895. The only radiograph capability in theater was two units on US Army hospital ships and at the general hospitals back in the United States. The use of radiograph technology allowed bullets and shrapnel to be located without manual probing, thus decreasing the likelihood of infection. On the important date of 8 November 1895, Wilhelm Roentgen had taken a radiograph of his wife's hand. The device was shown publicly in Germany during a December 1895 demonstration. Other militaries also took advantage of the new technology. For example, radiographs were used by the British in the medical care of the wounded in the South African War.[62(pp15–20)] Surgeon General Sternberg's Army Medical Museum was the site for early Army experimentation with radiographs. MAJ Walter Reed's initial request to buy a unit was denied, but in 1896 he had obtained a radiograph. He used it to localize a bullet in the thigh of a wounded person.[44(p177)]

Harvey Cushing immediately began using the new technology and brought his own apparatus when he came to Johns Hopkins. Cushing used the radiograph tube energized by a hand-cranked static generator to show a bullet lodged in a woman's spine.[59(pp231,232)] It is noteworthy that the Army embraced this early technology in time for the Spanish-American War.

At the time, the hazards of radiation exposure were yet to be learned, so consequent patient burns due to prolonged exposure were not uncommon. The hazards to the physicians and other personnel were also not recognized, leading to illnesses and loss of digits. For example, at the Johns Hopkins Hospital, Frederick Henry Baetjer had worked with Cushing in the use of the apparatus Cushing brought from Boston. Subsequently, he was selected to take over the work when Cushing finished his residency. In 1902, Baetjer became the radiologist for the hospital. Although he developed the specialty of radiology, he paid a steep price, developing cancer and losing one eye and some of his fingers as a result of radiation exposure.[59(p265)]

In addition to shortages of equipment and supplies, the Army Medical Department also experienced staffing shortfalls. For example, in the Philippines there were shortages of medical personnel. To deal with the shortages and to enhance the skills of the surgeons, the Army opened the new Army Medical School in November 1901 in the Washington Army Medical Museum buildings. Surgeon General William C Gorgas (January 1914–October 1918) encouraged contract and volunteer surgeons to take the examinations for entrance to regular service to expand the core of the Regular Army Medical Department.[11(p319)] In the area of nursing staff, the Secretary of War allowed female nurses to be sent overseas to help with the shortages in combat theaters. While large and small hospitals were established, the medical and surgical care came to resemble that of the Indian wars. The battles seldom were large operations, but rather a series of low-intensity conflicts and counterinsurgencies. The majority of first-line care resembled that of the Indian wars with surgeons embedded with their troops providing most of the care in the field. In general, the Philippine Insurrection and the Boxer Rebellion highlighted the need to deal with tropical diseases, a multiplicity of diseases of vitamin and nutritional disorders, and the problems of long supply lines.

PRELUDE TO THE "WORLD WAR"

There would be many challenges in preparing the healthcare system for the coming large-scale conflict even though there had been many overall technological advances in the provision of care. Army healthcare for troops had been evolving since its inception, but the coming events in Mexico, in the run-up to World War I, further highlighted the need for additional preparation. The incursion into Mexico demonstrated the early use of motor transportation, airplanes, and improved supply methods, but the medical side was not as advanced. The medical equipment that was supplied to regiments was minimal, with the plan being to pass the injured on to dressing stations. The only forward surgery capacity was designed to prepare patients for evacuation.

The Regular Army was organized at the time only on a regimental basis. The regiment consisted of 1,887 men supported by four medical officers and 24 medically trained enlisted men.[11(p400)] Band members and line troops would have to carry litters, if needed. The medical support for the mission had to be organized for the moment and it was felt to be adequate for the smaller number of expected casualties. Although considered forward medicine, the medical support that accompanied the troops was reminiscent of Indian war days. At the peak of manpower, Pershing was backed up by two field hospitals organized as a camp hospital. The field hospitals were described as meagerly equipped shelters. Camp hospitals were 100- to 350-bed sized—smaller than a base hospital but equipped for surgery and related procedures.[11(pp400–401)] They were viewed as semimobile. The National Guard had difficulty with its medical support along the border because it had not been prepared to expand its operations and the Army had not planned adequately for its support.[63(p287)]

Before the US incursion into Mexico, the Germans had been active there since 1910 when the Diaz regime was replaced by that of Francisco Madero in a revolution. Only 3 years later, Victoriano Huerta seized power and killed Madero. Huerta established a military dictatorship, which drew the opposition of President Woodrow Wilson. In 1914, a *Hamburg-Amerika* ship had landed munitions at Veracruz intended for Huerta. Already calling for the restoration of a democratically elected Mexican government and hostile to the Huerta regime, President Wilson dispatched US Marines to Veracruz. The Marines were directed to occupy the Veracruz port to keep the ship from unloading the guns and ammunition, which they did with 19 American and 100 Mexican casualties. Huerta was subsequently overthrown by Venustiano Carranza, one of the leaders of the rival factions. German intelligence transferred its support to Carranza.[64(p254)]

The Army joined forces with the Marines at Veracruz in 1914. Because the military action in Veracruz was quickly over, the Army medical units had time to take on the care of civilians. The Army medical staff provided immunizations, including smallpox, for the local population. The military required mostly routine sick-call duty from the Army and Navy medical units there.[11(pp394–395)]

Because hostilities also threatened the US-Mexico border, the US Army established a post called Camp Furlong at Columbus, New Mexico. Francisco "Pancho" Villa and 500 men attacked the town of Columbus and Camp Furlong on 9 March 1915. The troops at Camp Furlong defended the camp and drove the invaders from Columbus into Mexico. Ten US soldiers and 8 townspeople were killed in the raid.[65(pp26–29)] President Wilson's Administration responded with the formation of a "Punitive Expedition" under the command of Brigadier General John J Pershing (of later fame as the American Expeditionary Forces' commander of World War I). German agents were suspected of encouraging Pancho Villa to raid the United States. (For example, the Germans were mentioned as being the source of munitions supplying Villa in the various ciphers intercepted by British Captain "Blinker" Hall and his "Room 40 operation."[64(p189)])

Pershing moved into Mexico with two cavalry columns; one infantry column and the logistical supply formation followed. Rail transport was only useful to a point due to the lack of rail infrastructure, which then required movement of supplies by wagon and truck. Pershing's troops were all Regular Army troops. He moved 516 miles into Mexico before doing battle with Mexican troops at Parral. The battle did not yield significant results. After the first encounter, the troops then withdrew about 250 miles and at that point set up an occupation line. The troops withdrew from Mexico in February 1917 after engaging some of Villa's forces but without capturing him. The Texas National Guard was then mobilized to protect the border.[11(p400)]

By August 1916, the peak number of National Guard members called to meet the Mexican threat numbered some 128,000 troops, and included 59 field hospitals, along with assorted ambulance companies and sanitary detachments.[11(p400)] Only 60,000 of the 128,000 troops had actual prior military service. These were all federalized but problems of men not reporting, and others resigning once there, added to a poor medical support. The regular troops in the campaign numbered only 42,000.[11(p400)]

A NEW TYPE OF WAR?

As a large-scale conflict for the United States, the Civil War clearly was the closest thing to the coming World War I experience. However, the Europeans had experienced larger scale wars by World War I that included the Crimean War, the Franco-Prussian War, the Boer War, and the Russian-Japanese conflict (among others) in the lead up to World War I.

The US experience in the latter decades of the 19th century was, however, limited in conflicts of any magnitude. Following the Civil War, the Army reverted to small-unit operations conducting a counterinsurgency type of campaign against the Indians. The Army mounted operations from forts that were scattered in the West. Although it had potential for a broader conflict, the Spanish-American War was almost over before it began, so that large-scale mobilizations and a war economy were not required. The Boxer and Philippine insurrections were largely small-unit operations. The Mexican border encounters were small and not particularly successful. The Army did have a chance to use newer technology such as trucks, motorcars, and airplanes on a limited basis. Hence, the learning curve was even greater for the United States as it was on the verge of entering World War I. The Army Medical Department had not been called on to prepare for and treat mass casualties prior to World War I.

Fortunately, visionaries such as Drs Harvey Cushing and George Crile were there to help the country prepare to get into a position to provide emergent medical care in the future conflict.

REFERENCES
1. Newell CR, Shrader CR. *Of Duty Well and Faithfully Done: A History of the Regular Army in the Civil War*. Lincoln, Nebr: University of Nebraska Press; 2011.
2. McGaugh S. *Surgeon in Blue*. New York, NY: Arcade Publishing Company; 2013.
3. Turner TR. *101 Things You Didn't Know About the Civil War: Places, Battles, Generals—Essential Facts About the War That Divided America*. Avon, Mass: Adams Media; 2007.
4. United States, Surgeon General's Office. *The Medical and Surgical History of the War of the Rebellion (1861–1865)*. Washington, DC: Government Printing Office; 1870–1888.
5. Coffman EM. *The Old Army: A Portrait of the American Army in Peacetime 1784–1898*. New York, NY: Oxford University Press; 1968.
6. *Annual Report of the Surgeon General, US Army, to the Secretary of War 1866*. Washington, DC: War Department; 1866.

7. Billings JS. *A Report on the Hygiene of the United States Army*. Washington, DC: War Department, and Surgeon General's Office; 1875. [In paperback, US Government Printing Office; 2012.]
8. Sefton JE. *The United States Army and Reconstruction: 1865–1877*. New York, NY: Greenwood Press; 1980.
9. Wooster R, ed. Corbusier WH. *Soldier, Surgeon, Scholar: The Memoirs of William Henry Corbusier 1844–1930*. Norman, Okla: University of Oklahoma Press; 2003.
10. Eicher J, Eicher D. *Civil War High Command*. Palo Alto, Calif: Stanford University Press; 2002.
11. Gillet MC. *The Army Medical Department 1865–1917*. Washington, DC: Center for Military History, US Army; 1995.
12. Office of Medical History. US Army Medical Department. *Biographies. Joseph K Barnes*. http://history.amedd.army.mil/surgeongenerals/J_Barnes.html. Accessed 15 June 2015.
13. Ingersoll LD. *A History of the War Department of the United States: With Biographical Sketches of the Secretaries*. BiblioBazaar Reproduction Series; 2008. [Originally published Washington, DC: War Department; 1879: Chapter 7, The Bureau of the War Department.]
14. Pilcher JE. *The Surgeon Generals of the Army of the United States of America; A Series of Biographical Sketches of the Senior Officers of the Military Medical Service From the American Revolution to Philippine Pacification*. Washington, DC: Association of Military Surgeons; 1905. [Available as a Google eBook.]
15. Office of Medical History. US Army Medical Department. *Biographies. Charles Crane*. http://history.amedd.army.mil/surgeongenerals/C_Crane.html. Accessed 15 June 2015.
16. Office of Medical History. US Army Medical Department. *Biographies. Robert Murray*. http://history.amedd.army.mil/surgeongenerals/R_Murray.html. Accessed 15 June 2015.
17. Office of Medical History. US Army Medical Department. *Biographies. John Moore*. http://history.amedd.army.mil/surgeongenerals/J_Moore.html. Accessed 15 June 2015.
18. Office of Medical History. US Army Medical Department. *Biographies. Jedidiah Baxter*. http://history.amedd.army.mil/surgeongenerals/J_Baxter.html. Accessed 15 June 2015.
19. Office of Medical History. US Army Medical Department. *Biographies. Charles Sutherland*. http://history.amedd.army.mil/surgeongenerals/C_Sutherland.html. Accessed 15 June 2015.
20. Gibson GM. *Soldier in White: The Life of General George Miller Sternberg*. New York, NY: Literary Licensing LLC; 2011.
21. Phalen JM. Chiefs of the medical department, US Army 1775–1940, biographical sketches. *Army Med Bull*. 1940;52:70–78.
22. Office of Medical History. US Army Medical Department. *Biographies. William Henry Forwood*. http://history.amedd.army.mil/surgeongenerals/W_Forwood.html. Accessed 15 June 2015.
23. Office of Medical History. US Army Medical Department. *Biographies. Robert M O'Reilly*. http://history.amedd.army.mil/surgeongenerals/R_OReilly.html. Accessed 15 June 2015.
24. Office of Medical History. US Army Medical Department. *Biographies. George H Torney*. http://history.amedd.army.mil/surgeongenerals/G_Torney.html. Accessed 15 June 2015.
25. Office of Medical History. US Army Medical Department. *Biographies. William C Gorgas*. http://history.amedd.army.mil/surgeongenerals/W_Gorgas.html. Accessed 15 June 2015.
26. Hagedorn H. *Leonard Wood: A Biography*. New York, NY: Harper and Brothers; 1931.
27. Holmes J. *The Life of Leonard Wood*. New York, NY: Doubleday, Page and Co; 1920.
28. McCallum J. *Leonard Wood: Rough Rider, Surgeon, Architect of American Imperialism*. New York, NY: New York University Press; 2006.

29. Stevenson JN. *Deliverance From the Little Big Horn: Doctor Henry Porter and Custer's Seventh Cavalry.* Norman, Okla: University of Oklahoma Press; 2012.
30. Morison E. *Turmoil and Tradition: A Study of the Life and Times of Henry L Stimson.* Boston, Mass: Houghton Mifflin; 1960.
31. Crook G, Schmitt MF, ed. *General George Crook: His Autobiography.* Norman, Okla: University of Oklahoma Press; 1946, 1966.
32. Magid P. *George Crook: From Redwoods to Appomattox.* Norman, Okla: University of Oklahoma Press; 2011.
33. Wooster R. *Nelson A Miles and the Twilight of the Frontier Army.* Lincoln, Nebr: University of Nebraska Press; 1993.
34. Hedren PL. *Great Sioux War Orders of Battle: How the United States Army Waged War on the Northern Plains, 1876–1877.* Norman, Okla: University of Oklahoma Press; 2011.
35. McGinnis AR. When courage was not enough: plains Indians at war with the United States Army. *J Mil Hist.* 2012;76(2):454–473.
36. Trudeau NA. Battle for the west: hard war on the southern plains. *Q J Mil Hist.* 2011:23(4):26–37.
37. Russell S. Army at Wounded Knee. http://armyatwoundedknee.wordpress.com/2013/08/27. Accessed 15 June 2015.
38. DeToledo JC, DeToledo BB, Lowe M. The epilepsy of First Lady Ida Saxton McKinley. *South Med J.* 2000;93(3):267–271.
39. Harris B. *First Ladies Fact Book.* New York, NY: Black Dog and Leventhal Publishers, Inc.; 2009.
40. Morris E. *Theodore Rex.* New York, NY: Random House; 2001.
41. Office of Medical History, US Army Medical Department. *Surgeon Generals. George Sternberg.* http://history.amedd.army.mil/surgeongenerals/G_Sternberg.html. Accessed 31 July 2015.
42. Trask DF. *The War With Spain in 1898.* Omaha, Nebr: The University of Nebraska Press; 1996.
43. Nofi A. *The Spanish-American War, 1898.* Philadelphia, Penn: Combined Books; 1996.
44. Kelly HA. *Walter Reed and Yellow Fever.* New York, NY: McClure, Phillips and Co; 1906.
45. Gorgas WC. The practical mosquito work done at Havana, Cuba, which resulted in the disappearance of yellow fever from that locality. *Washington Med Ann.* 1903;II:2–3.
46. Wintermute BA. *Public Health and the US Military: A History of the Army Medical Department, 1818–1917.* London, England: Routledge; 2011.
47. Gillet MC. Medical care and evacuation during the Philippine Insurrection. *J Hist Med Allied Serv.* 1987;42(2):169–185.
48. Linn BM. *The Philippine War 1899–1902.* Lawrence, Kans: University of Kansas Press; 2000.
49. Office of Medical History. US Army Medical Department. *The US Army Medical Department in the Aftermath of the San Francisco Earthquake and Fire of 18 April 1906.* http://history.amedd.army.mil/booksdocs/spanam/SFEQ/SFEQ1906.html. Accessed 15 June 2015.
50. Phelan H. Experience in the San Francisco disaster. *Mil Surg.* 1906;19(1):95.
51. Lister J. *On the Antiseptic Principle in the Practice of Surgery.* Vol. 38. Part 6 of 8. Harvard Classics. Bartleby.com. 2001. New York, NY: PF Collier and Son; 1909–1914.
52. Lister J. On a new method of treating compound fracture, abscess with observations on the conditions of suppuration. *Lancet.* 1867;89(2272):326–329.
53. Lister J. On the antiseptic principle in the practice of surgery. *Br Med J.* 1867;2(351):245–260.
54. Allen GA. Joseph Lister: a century of the antiseptic principle in the practice of surgery (August 12, 1865–August 12, 1965). *Arch Surg.* 1965;91(2):327–329.

55. Garrison FH. *Notes on the History of Military Medicine*. Washington, DC: Association of Military Surgeons; 1922.
56. Pasteur L, Jourbet J, Chamberland C. La theorie des germes et ses applications a la chirurgie. *Bull Academie Natl Med*. 1878;2eSer.VII:166–167.
57. Relman F, Relman D. Sequence-based identification of microbial pathogens: a reconsideration of Koch's postulates. *Clin Microbiol Rev*. 1996;9(1):18–33.
58. Wangensteen OH, Wangensteen S. *Rise of Surgery From Empiric Craft to Scientific Discipline*. Minneapolis, Minn: University of Minnesota Press; 1979.
59. Imber G. *Genius on the Edge*. New York, NY: Kaplan Publishing Company; 2011.
60. Brooks JJ, Enterline HT. The final diagnosis of President Cleveland's lesion. *JAMA*. 1980;244(24):2729.
61. Keefer BS. *Conflicting Memories on the "River of Death": The Chickamauga Battlefield and the Spanish-American War, 1863–1933*. Kent, Ohio: Kent State University Press; 2013.
62. McLaughlin R. *The Royal Army Medical Corps*. London, England: Leo Cooper; 1972.
63. Marble WS. Military support for Pershing's punitive expedition into Mexico 1916–1917. *Mil Med*. 1998;173(3):287–292.
64. Ramsay D. *Blinker' Hall Spymaster: The Man Who Brought America Into World War I*. Gloucestershire, UK: Spellmount; 2008.
65. Miller RG. Camp Furlong, the punitive expedition and the base of communications at Columbus, NM. *J Am Mil Past*. 2012;37:26–29.

Chapter Five

Forward Surgery in the Great War: A War of New Technologies

LANCE P. STEAHLY, MD

THE LEAD UP TO WORLD WAR I

AS THE PREVIOUS CHAPTER DISCUSSED, the Army Medical Department's healthcare system had evolved considerably since the US Civil War, the Indian wars, the Spanish-American War, and the "Punitive Expedition" into Mexico. By the time the US Army entered the World War in April 1917, a great many changes had occurred in the organization and deployment of Army medical assets, but many more needed to be made to address the coming significant medical and logistical needs.

Before discussing these needed changes, it is worthwhile to briefly recap the sizable casualties of this global conflict to lend context to the magnitude of the problem confronting the belligerents. If one considers that the war lasted from 1 August 1914 until 11 November 1918, it is difficult to grasp the magnitude of suffering sustained by the participants. In just one battle—the Battle of the Somme—1 million or more men were casualties. Some 14,000 British soldiers died in the first 10 minutes of the battle.[1(p5)]

In the Great War, as it was called then, some 60 million men were mobilized by all belligerents. Of that number, approximately 19 million were wounded and 7 million were killed.[2(p239)] The exact number of dead listed, however, varies depending on the source. Hastings cites figures showing 2 million military deaths for the Germans, 1 million for the British Empire (including 800,000 British), and 1.7 million for the French.[3(p561)] Jukes and associates list 325,000 casualties for the United States with 115,000 killed.[4(p346)] These authors cite 4 million wounded for Germany, 5 million wounded for the French, and 3.2 million wounded for the British Empire. However, the influenza epidemic of this period was estimated to have had 50 million worldwide deaths by contrast. Hence, the deaths from the influenza pandemic were more numerous than the deaths from the World War.[4(p346)]

After the opening maneuvers of 1914, the Western Front became an immobile battlefield, populated with artillery and trenches. Opposing sides used incessant artillery barrages, followed by desperate infantry actions, to gain little advance. The wounds sustained were largely due to artillery shells and shrapnel. The Eastern Front was a mobile front where maneuver for terrain was the characteristic. Gunshot wounds were most common there.

CHRONOLOGY OF THE WAR

The events precipitating World War I have been attributed to the assassination of the heir to the Austrian-Hungarian throne (and nephew to the Emperor), Archduke Franz Ferdinand, and his wife, Sophie Chotek. They were shot at Sarajevo by a 19-year-old Serbian on 28 June 1914.[5(p46)] As Clark points out, the Serbian organizations that were incriminated in the archduke's assassination were very secretive. Indeed, the head of the Serbian military intelligence regularly burned his papers.[6(p47)] Clark states that the murders of the archduke and his wife were "a transformative event, charged with real and symbolic menace."[6(p367)] Clark would argue that the events leading to war were so complicated with the myriad entanglements that the postwar blame apportioned to Germany and the Austrian-Hungarian empire was flawed.[6(p559)] As an example, Clark speaks of the Balkan Wars as causing changes in the relationships of the greater versus lesser powers. The French and Russian alliance caused the powers there to interpret the Sarajevo events in a way that moved the war footing forward. The assassinations did not allow the Austrian-Hungarian empire to reasonably negotiate with Serbia. As viewed by Clark, the Germans were not the only state to give in to hysteria as events moved forward. Clark sees the crisis bringing the war in 1914 to a reality was due to a shared flawed political culture.[6(p561)] Europe erupted into war 37 days later. As Clark pointed out in his book, *The Sleepwalkers: How Europe Went to War in 1914,*[6] the resulting war mobilized 65 million soldiers with over 20 million civilian and military deaths and 21 million wounded worldwide.[6(pxxiii)] Clark posits that no one country could be singled out as causing the war, but rather it was a result of a "shared political culture [which was] also multipolar and genuinely interactive."[6(p561)]

The British became involved in the war because of Germany's invasion of Belgium, which Britain was bound to defend by treaty. However, McMeekin in his book, *July 1914: Countdown to War,*[7] has a theme that the Treaty of Versailles accusations of war guilt unfairly single out Germany as the main warmonger. The placing of guilt had ramifications in terms of postwar reparations, territorial changes, and unilateral disarmament. He further argues that England would have eventually been involved due to its naval arrangements with France to protect the North Sea. He maintains that the invasion of Belgium just made it happen sooner.[7]

Germany's role in the conflict was only a part of the overall picture. McMeekin further argues that Germany's strategic position to prosecute a war in 1914 was not favorable.[7(p387)] He traces the regional instability involving Serbia, Austria-Hungary, and Russia as being a large factor leading to conflict. The Germans and the French were involved due to the understandings with Austria-Hungary and Russia, respectively, produced by the two Balkan Wars of 1912 to 1913, which could have erupted into a larger conflict.[3(p558),7(p388)] Russia had enough reason to start a war over Serbia in the Balkan Wars and at other times.[7(p384)] McMeekin points out that Germany had no interest in the Balkans in 1912 to 1913 or even 1914. He observes that the Austrians had an interest in curbing Serbia's influence in those years.[7(p385)]

The German High Command determined that France had to be beaten before the Russians could mobilize. The Germans believed that Russia would take an unusually long time to accomplish full mobilization due to poor transportation infrastructure and the huge size of the country.[5(p59)] However, the Russians had implemented the "Period Preparatory to War" before either Serbia or Austria had mobilized. This was a secret preliminary mobilization to give Russia more time to respond. Russia did not want its potential adversaries to know of the earlier mobilization plans because Germany and Austria-Hungary would expect a slow Russian mobilization in the war plans. The Russians' mobilization would be longer than, for example, Germany's, which had planned everything to the ultimate degree.

The Germans had planned for mobilization since the time of Bismarck by developing well-coordinated railroad infrastructure and excellent training of regular and reserve forces. The German Schlieffen Plan was a bold plan to defeat the French that seemed to work for a period of time. The plan anticipated Austria-Hungary and Italy as allies of the Germans. Further, the plan did not include Russian involvement. Soon, however, the warfare became more of a siege, rather than a war of maneuver.[5(p60)] McMeekin points out that recent research calls into question whether there was an inflexible Schlieffen Plan, or whether the invasion of Belgium was decided by General Helmuth von Moltke (the nephew of Moltke the Elder) in his role as Chief of the German General Staff.[7(p401)] Moltke the Younger probably modified any preexisting plan by a combination of planning and taking opportunities as they presented. Helmuth von Moltke the Younger replaced Schlieffen in 1906 and saw the fallacy of not planning for Russian involvement based upon his assessment of French and Russian cooperation. He also did not think Italy would side with Germany due to territorial issues with Austria-Hungary.[7(p401)]

McMeekin views as a mistake the German decision to invade Belgium 2 weeks before the German Army would be ready.[7(p401)] This decision did not follow even the modified Schlieffen Plan. Hastings in his book, *Catastrophe 1914: Europe Goes to War*,[3] notes that von Moltke (the less-than-talented nephew of the Elder) felt that Schlieffen's concept would be the key to German dominance over Europe.[3(p27)] Helmuth von Moltke the Elder wanted to deal decisively with France after the fall of Paris in the 1870 to 1871 War, but he was overruled by Bismarck.[3(p25-26)] General Alfred von Schlieffen devised his plan in 1905 after he became the Chief of the General Staff in 1892. The plan underwent modifications with various iterations up to the war's start.[8(pp15-16)]

After a series of mobilizations and declarations, Germany invaded Belgium on 4 August 1914. Britain, France, and Germany were in battle along the French borders in the last open movement of the war. In the Battle of Mons on 23 August 1914, the French and British were defeated. The Battle of the Marne stopped the German advance on Paris in September 1914. In September 1914, both sides moved to entrenchment with lines extending to the English Channel. The First Battle of Ypres lasted from 12 October until 22 November with heavy losses on each side (approximate casualties: British with 58,000, the French with 86,000, and the Germans with 134,000).[9(p259)] The Western Front became established. The Germans used poison gas on the Eastern Front on 3 January 1915.[9(p260)] Gas was used in the West by the Germans at the Second Battle of Ypres on 25 May 1915.[9(p260)] The Battle of the Somme began on 1 July 1916 and lasted until 19 November 1916. The Battle of Verdun ended on 18 December 1916 with the Germans pushed back.[9(p262)] The United States came to the conflict late for many reasons but the resumption of unrestricted submarine warfare by Germany was certainly a catalyst. America declared war on Germany on 6 April 1917.[9(p263)]

The Allies were mainly interested in having fresh American troops enter their lines to replace French and British casualties. General John Pershing, appointed as the American Expeditionary Forces (AEF) commander stubbornly held to the Americans serving under their own command. Pershing had the British and French help with the training of the new troops to prepare them for trench warfare. Pershing insisted that the American soldier be a marksman and participate in battles of movement. Pershing felt that a war of maneuver was the preferred route and that marksmanship was the most important skill.[10]

The American divisions were set up on the standard square pattern with two brigades each consisting of two regiments (each with three battalions of 1,200 men apiece). The American divisions were supplemented with an artillery brigade and three machine-gun battalions. The total division strength was 28,000 men per division.[8(p17)] Grotelueschen points out in his book, *The AEF Way of War: The American Army and Combat in World War I*,[11] that the American AEF division included two large infantry brigades, an artillery brigade of 5,000, and many support troops. The division at 28,000 officers and men would be twice the size of most German or Allied divisions.[11(p27)]

The German units were organized along the triangular pattern with three regiments (each with three battalions). The division had an artillery regiment (three or four battalions) and supporting units. The German divisions were smaller than the American division, having just 14,000 men in the German division. The Germans also had some specialized troops. In 1918, they had organized special elite units called *Stosstruppen* that could infiltrate trench systems in raids.[12(p9)]

British divisions officially numbered 13,000 men.[8(p12)] The British also had special troops for raiding, but they were not as well known as the German raiding troops. The French entered the war with a square 18,000-man division of four regiments. The German Army configuration was of two brigades (of two regiments each) of 12,000 men by the end of the conflict.[12(p18)]

On 26 October 1917, the Russians withdrew from the war after the Communist Revolution. German troops were then free to be sent to the Western Front. The Germans were anxious to use these extra forces before American manpower could affect the war situation.

Americans fought at such places as Belleau Wood, the Meuse-Argonne offensive, Chateau-Thierry, and Soissons. The Belleau Wood engagement was not well executed, unlike Soissons, which was well done. Pershing's emphasis on marksmanship paid off whenever the battles became fluid and out of the trenches. The Americans launched a successful 4-day offensive at St Mihiel on 12 September 1918. On 26 September 1918, the Americans started a successful offensive in the Meuse-Argonne.[10p33] The US Army had evolved into an effective force that tipped the scale against the Germans.

On 11 November 1918, an armistice was signed by the Allies and Germany, bringing hostilities to a close.[9(p264)] At the time of signing the armistice, the Germans assumed Wilson's Fourteen Points would form the subsequent treaty. The Treaty of Versailles was presented by the Allies for Germany to sign on 28 June 1919, but it incorporated none of

Wilson's points and instead imposed difficult obligations upon Germany. The reparations were especially harsh financially. The Germans were restricted to a small military force without submarines or air assets. In August and September 1919, Wilson brought the issue of ratification of the treaty and the League of Nations to the American people. The Senate did not ratify the treaty nor approve of the League of Nations.[5(p4)]

PIONEERING LEADERS OF THE WORLD WAR I MEDICAL EFFORT

The medical community stateside was keenly aware of the war in Europe and the looming possibility, indeed probability, of American involvement at some future time. In response to this awareness, many in this community began exploring what could be done to assist. Two physicians—Harvey Cushing and George Crile—were at the forefront of these efforts; their careers began in the decades leading up to an active American role in the global conflict. Their experiences prior to and after America's entry into the war parallel the gradual US involvement in the European conflict. The American people slowly came to support medical help for the Allies. Cushing and Crile helped immensely in calling attention to the need for military medical preparedness, which was not a popular stance.

Harvey Cushing

Cushing's life and accomplishments are chronicled in the detailed diaries from which he published selected excerpions, first in 1919 in his book *The Story of US Army Base Hospital No. 5*.[13] His 1936 book, *From a Surgeon's Journal 1915–1918*,[14] was a more complete work, drawing from nine bound volumes of personal diary. (Perhaps because Cushing's comments about the war are so descriptive, Peter Englund selected passages from his journal to mark Cushing's role as one of the 20 characters in *The Beauty and the Sorrow: An Intimate History of the First World War*.[15(p3)])

Cushing (Figure 5-1) spent 17 years at the Johns Hopkins Hospital in Baltimore, Maryland, under the direction of William Stewart Halsted (Figure 5-2), the Chief Surgeon at the Johns Hopkins Hospital and Professor of Surgery at the innovative Johns Hopkins University School of Medicine. Cushing initially came to Baltimore after a year as a surgical intern at the Massachusetts General Hospital in Boston. He started as Halsted's assistant resident. Cushing served as a resident physician from 1896 until 1900. He then studied in Europe in the 1900 to 1901 academic year. He was a faculty member at Johns Hopkins from 1900 until 1912, when he assumed a Harvard appointment.[16(p245)] Cushing was recognized as perhaps the most talented of Halsted's 17 chief residents. These talented men became Halsted's chief resident after years progressing through a complex pyramidal system to become the single leader of the house staff and a junior faculty member. Twelve of these men became professors, associate professors, or assistant professors of surgery in their own right.[16(p348)]

As Cushing progressed under Halsted, he essentially invented the neurosurgery specialty with the permission of Halsted. Halsted was interested in his residents taking over certain specialties. For example, he had an interest in the pituitary gland and encouraged

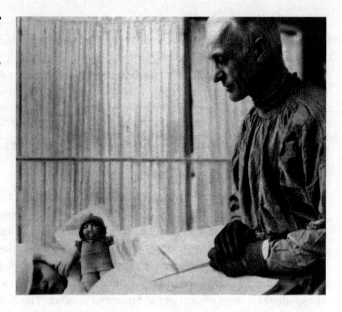

FIGURE 5-1. Harvey Cushing. Cushing was William Halsted's resident and later faculty associate (at Johns Hopkins Hospital in Baltimore, Maryland) who developed the specialty of neurosurgery with his mentor's encouragement. Cushing left to become the Professor of Neurosurgery at Harvard University in 1912, in part because Halsted would not give him a firm future commitment. Cushing's appointment came as a result of his success with General Leonard Wood's meningioma removal. Photograph courtesy of the National Library of Medicine, Image #B05024.

Cushing to study it. Cushing devised many of the procedures and instruments while largely limiting his work to neurosurgical concerns. He was known to typically spend many hours with his thorough operative notes, recapturing every detail of his surgeries, with particular focus on his failures.[17(p270)] As Imber discusses, Cushing was able to develop his skills while caring for most of Halsted's patients and taking responsibility for his teaching load because of Halsted's addictions (first to cocaine and then to morphine—both drugs were not illegal at the time) and long periods of absence.[16(pp229–241)] The situation with Halsted gave Cushing arguably more experience, but resulted in friction that became more of an issue as Cushing's stature advanced. A boost to his stature came in 1910, when he removed an intracranial meningioma from General Leonard Wood, then the Army Chief of Staff, with good recovery. Cushing's success with the case, in part, brought an offer of the Chair of Neurosurgery at the new Peter Bent Brigham Hospital and the Moseley Professorship in Surgery at Harvard. He left for Boston in 1912 when he was unable to get a clear commitment for his academic future from Halsted. Cushing felt that he had suffered under Halsted's erratic leadership and frequent absences.[16(p245)]

George Crile

George Crile's experiences were addressed in his 1947 two-volume set, *George Crile, an Autobiography*.[18] Crile graduated from Wooster Medical College (which later merged to form the Case Western University School of Medicine, located in Cleveland, Ohio) in 1887. He had joined the US Army Medical Reserve Corps in the Spanish-American War and served in Puerto Rico. Crile made valuable contributions to military medicine with his work that started in the Spanish-American War but continued through World War I. Indeed, Crile actually headed the first university *Ambulance* unit (which basically was a hospital unit in French terms), sailing in January 1915 for its 3-month service. By comparison, the Harvard unit was organized by Cushing and RB Greenough, and

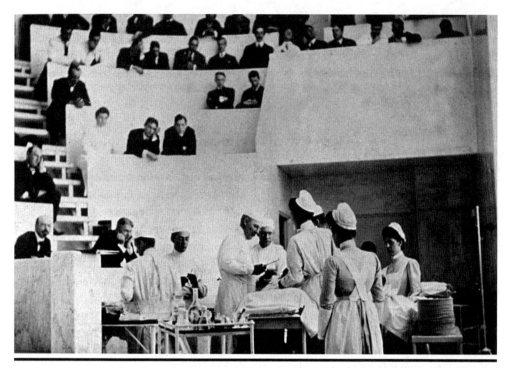

FIGURE 5-2. William Halsted. Halsted, the Johns Hopkins Hospital's famous Surgeon in Chief, is performing surgery in a hospital amphitheater ably assisted by his chief resident, Harvey Cushing, and his assistant resident Hugh Hampton Young. The operation is being observed by physicians and/or students seated in the background. There are also three nurses and two student attendants. Halsted introduced surgical gloves (shown in the photograph), originally intended to protect the delicate hands of his operating nurse, Miss Hampton (later Halsted's wife). Photograph courtesy of the National Library of Medicine, Image #A030435.

financed by William Lindsey of Boston.[14(p3)] The Harvard unit worked at the American Ambulance at the *Lycee Pasteur* in Neuilly, France.[19] Unlike Crile, Cushing did not actually head the Harvard unit (sailing in March 1915).[20(p418)] While Crile was the leader and the innovator, Cushing chose a passive role as a consultant with the 1915 Harvard unit traveling to various British hospitals (as part of the British Expeditionary Force [BEF])[14(p51)] to allow time to observe surgical techniques. At this point, Cushing was not interested in command per se. As an observer, Cushing only occasionally performed neurosurgery.[21] In 1917, Cushing was assigned to British Hospital No. 13, under the command of a British surgeon.[14(pp56–57)] He was later assigned to the No. 11 General (BEF) Hospital in May 1917.[14(p111)] When America entered the War, Cushing was assigned to Base Hospital No. 5. However, Roger I Lee, a Harvard colleague of Cushing's, was appointed as the Commander of Base Hospital No. 5.[14(p129)]

In contrast to Cushing, George Crile, a professor of clinical surgery at Case Western Reserve, held a reputation as a prominent surgeon with an interest in surgical research. His work with nitrous oxide-oxygen anesthesia reduced dependence on ether as an anesthetic agent. He also promoted the use of whole blood to treat shock. Crile described human direct artery-to-vein transfusion in an *Annals of Surgery* article in 1907.[22] He authored a 1909 book, titled *Hemorrhage and Transfusion: An Experimental and Clinical Research*,[23] discussing transfusion and shock. Crile became one of the founders of the Cleveland Clinic in 1921.[20] In recognition of his service, he was appointed as a Brigadier General in the Medical Reserve Corps after World War I.[24(p379)]

TREATMENT PHILOSOPHY

During World War I, the underlying philosophy of battle wound treatment differed among the various Allies. The British and the French gave preference in treatment to the wounded that had the best prospect of returning to combat. The Americans gave preference to the more seriously wounded; they also held that experience demonstrated that removal of traumatized tissues and fragments could wait as long as 12 hours. Hence the less severe wounds could wait.[25(p159)] The frequent artillery wounds received in the French farming countryside almost always resulted in infection with gas-forming bacteria.[25(pp159–160)] The British and French were convinced that early surgery was essential to deal with gas gangrene. Because of their awareness of the serious adverse potential of gas gangrene, the Royal Army Medical Corps placed emphasis upon a practice that made it a priority at the casualty clearing station to treat shock and to prevent infection.[26(p196)] This practice stabilized the patient before proceeding to any other treatment.

The difference in the Allies' underlying treatment philosophy had ramifications for hospital size, mobility, and location. Although originally mobile in concept, the British casualty clearing stations became located in groups to expand their capacity, thereby reducing their mobility. The French made their hospitals large and immobile, despite their role in developing mobile hospitals. The large size and immobility worked with static trench warfare, but not with battles of movement. The need for mobility of the hospitals highlights the need to protect the staff and patients from a mobile front and to position the care facility near the wounded to reduce transport distance and time, and thus expedite care.

The French had created the triage system of sorting patients based on their injuries and prognosis. To facilitate triage, the aid station moved with its battalions, although it had few medical supplies. At the battalion aid station, severely injured soldiers had their wounds lightly covered with iodine before the dressings were applied. Tetanus antitoxin was administered here and morphine was given for pain. The use of splints effectively reduced the amputation rates, which had previously been viewed as necessary in severe compound fractures, not unlike the situation dating back to the US Civil War.[9(pp240–241)] Compound fractures were immobilized with Thomas splints. (This is a long leg splint extending beyond the foot, consisting of rigid rods located on the lateral and medial aspect of the leg with a stabilizing ring that circumscribes the thigh. It can be adjusted to provide traction; it immobilizes the bones of the leg and makes transportation possible.) The splints were readjusted at the battalion aid station if they had been already placed in the field.[27(p105)] The amputation rate greatly declined with better splinting techniques for compound fractures.[9(pp240–241),27(p106)] Triage was adapted by the American Army from the French.

However, as already noted, the British and the French (unlike the Americans) placed the most emphasis on treating cases that could be returned to combat.[28(p1610)]

ORGANIZATION OF MEDICAL ASSETS IN THEATER

Ambulance Americaine Concept

American medical involvement in World War I began long before the United States officially entered the war on 6 April 1917. In March 1910, a group of American expatriates in Paris formed the American Hospital, a small facility located near the Boulevard Victor Hugo. There had been precedent established in the Franco-Prussian War of 1870 when a group of Americans living in Paris had solicited donations to establish a field hospital that became known as the American Ambulance (*ambulance* being a French military hospital).[21(pp678–685)] When World War I started in Europe in 1914, the American "colony" increased its support of the American Hospital Board—the administration of the *Ambulance Americaine*. Robert Bacon was the president of the Hospital Board and, fortuitously, was also the American Ambassador to France. Because there was historical precedent for American hospital help in the Franco-Prussian War, French approval for the role of the American hospital came with less delay than it had in the Franco-Prussian War.[21(p677)]

Because the Americans' intent was to treat wounded French soldiers, the French government offered the use of an unfinished school, named the *Lycee Pasteur,* for its *Ambulance Americaine* (or military hospital).[29(pp3–4)] The large school building was equipped to have a bed capacity of approximately 500 to 600 patients.[17(p270)] Physicians from American teaching hospitals volunteered to serve as the clinical faculty on a short-term rotating basis. In planned 3-month rotations, the *Ambulance*'s three wards were to be staffed by surgical personnel who were skimmed from the top American medical schools. These civilian medical units provided proactive preparation 2 years before the arrival of American military units.[21(p678)] A second *Ambulance Americaine* was established close to the front. It was financed by prominent New Yorkers and care was provided by physicians and staff rotating from the Columbia University College of Physicians and Surgeons in New York.[15(p3)]

In 1914, as already noted, the French government had offered to the American Hospital the use of the *Lycee Pasteur* (an unfinished French school) as its treatment facility. The new facility received its first patients on 6 September 1914. An ambulance unit was formed on 14 September 1914 to serve the original American Hospital in Paris, using Ford Model T cars converted to ambulances, each capable of carrying four patients.[29(pp4–5)] Later groups included the American Ambulance Field Service (formed by A Piatt Andrew, a prior Director of the US Mint and an Assistant Secretary of the Treasury).[24(p39)] Another group, formed by Richard Norton, an archeologist, was named the American Volunteer Motor-Ambulance Corps.[24(pp22–37)] A fourth group was formed by H Herman Harjes, an official of the Morgan-Harjes Bank in Paris. This group was termed the Morgan-Harjes *Ambulance Mobile de Premiers Secours*.[24(p14)] The Harjes group later came under the organization of the American Red Cross.[29(p45)]

All of these groups were financed through private donations. No American government funds were allocated prior to the 6 April 1917 Declaration of War. The success of the fundraising was attributed to the unique American flavor to the ambulance groups and the influence of upper class wealthy patrons, especially women.[21(p680)] The *Ambulance Americaine* hospital was also financed by private donations. The *Ambulance* held a popular position in the American press, which helped promote military medical awareness and started the idea of America's military medical preparedness.[21(p679)] The Cleveland unit, headed by Crile, was financed by Samuel Mather of Cleveland; the Harvard unit was financed by William Lindsay of Boston.[21(p679)]

During the 3-month rotation, Cushing visited with other units (French and British) and performed some neurosurgery. There were three university units rotating in the 3-month rotations. Cushing later visited the British No. 13 General Hospital in the middle of the Second Ypres combat.[14(p61)] The Second Battle of Ypres was the only major front launched by the Germans for the Flemish town of Ypres in Belgium's west. There had been the surprise German use of poison gas, the collapse of the Ypres Salient (a salient is a battlefield that extends into enemy territory), and the Germans' advance, accompanied by tremendous artillery barrages as they crossed the Yser River.[29(pp64-65)] Because he acted only as a consultant and not as the chief surgeon, per his own request, Cushing had this time available to visit these other units. Crile had selected and recruited Cushing and the Harvard unit to follow his Cleveland unit.[18(pp247-252)] Cushing took over the *Lycee Pasteur* from Crile's unit on 1 April 1915. Cushing also spent time with the French 2nd Army, where he visited with the French surgeon Alexis Carrel. Carrel was a major with the 2nd French Army at the time, but he had already helped devise the Carrel-Dakin treatment of wounds. The treatment involved the use of an antiseptic solution containing sodium hypochlorite. The wound was irrigated periodically with this solution for antisepsis.[14(p18)] Carrel and Cushing visited a British facility nearby, but Cushing was not impressed with how the medical care was provided because the emphasis was placed on treatment of patients who could return to duty first.[14(p19)]

When Cushing visited the British No. 13 General Hospital Royal Army Medical Corps during the Second Ypres combat, he also visited the No. 8 Field Ambulance, which was located in the area. It was at this time that Cushing had his first encounter with a British medical evacuation train.[14(p79)] In Cushing's description, the hospital train was made up of 23 cars carrying 250 stretcher cases and an additional 150 sitting cases. The trains carried 45 attendants, three doctors, and three nurses with an attached kitchen car.[14(p61)]

These medical hospital trains continued to evolve and by 1917, in British hands, the trains carried pharmacies, sterilization equipment, food units, and operating rooms that could rival a casualty clearing station. Serving on trains for surgeons, nurses, and attendants required some getting used to because of the delays (munitions and troops were given priority) and the movement of the trains, especially if doing surgery or another procedure. The nurses had to keep the wounded calm and even entertained during the delays, requiring some talent.[9(pp252-253)]

Cushing also traveled to England, where he stayed with Sir William Osler and Lady Osler at Oxford. Osler invited Sir Walter Morley-Fletcher, Secretary of the British Medical Research Committee, to discuss blood transfusions and plans for the project to send physicians and medical staff from 20 to 22 American medical schools to France to replace the original Harvard and Cleveland units.[30(p126)] During his time in England, Cushing described to his associates a French case in which he used a large magnet to remove a metallic foreign body from the brain, a process that was then relatively new in concept.[15(p50)] After his time in Europe, Cushing returned to the United States on a ship that traveled through the debris field where the *Lusitania* had recently been torpedoed by a German U-boat.[14(p77),15(p30)]

These American hospital units were officially neutral in their attitude, as outlined by George Crile in an article he wrote for the *Cleveland Medical Journal* in 1915.[31] This stance befitted America's status as a neutral country. During service in the *Ambulance Americaine*, treatment afforded to German prisoners was complicated by the requirement to guard them.[28] Allied sympathy became more apparent as the war progressed. Twenty-five United States Army medical personnel were placed with British units following the Balfour Mission to the United States in April 1917.[29(p38)] Lord Arthur Balfour had been sent by the British War Ministry to meet with the Council of National Defense in Washington. Balfour requested six base hospitals and 116 American surgeons from the War Department's medical assets.[30(p97)] The British had insufficient numbers of doctors in the military at the start of the war (before the civilian doctor population could be brought into the military) and by 1915 they had a shortage of surgeons, which impacted the staffing of the casualty clearing stations. The British subsequently had a marked shortage of civilian physicians at home due to the expanding military needs.[26(p43)] Ultimately, 1,649 American Army doctors would serve with the British Royal Army Medical Corps (RAMC).[32(p32)]

In response to the British requests of the Balfour Mission, Army Surgeon General William Gorgas sought the involvement of the American Red Cross in organizing base hospitals in France modeled upon military facilities. The Medical Reserve Corps was the first branch of the Army to be a reserve component. The Army had established the Medical Reserve Corps in 1910 to be better prepared for future conflicts and to avoid the mobilization problems of the Spanish-American War (where inadequately trained contract physicians and volunteer surgeons had to be used due to shortages of Regular Army surgeons).[33(p2)] No military training was required of the Medical Reserve Corps members. Few members opted to transfer to active duty because the opportunities were limited, in contrast to the opportunities available in the civilian world. Correspondence courses and joint training camps were established for Medical Reserve Corps officers. The correspondence courses were popular with the officers. The Medical Reserve Corps was ended in 1917 with the creation of the Officer Reserve Corps. Surgeon General Gorgas opposed this transition because the new corps included reserve officers of all branches, rather than just the medical officers, but Gorgas was not successful in his opposition.[26(p382)]

Originally a government body was formed in the United States by the National Academy of Sciences called the National Research Council (NRC). The NRC was succeeded by the Council on National Defense (CND). A rider to the Defense Appropriations Act of 1916 created the CND, which allowed Surgeon General Gorgas to be appointed as the member for medicine.[26(p379)] The CND oversaw the nation's preparations for the coming conflict.[26(p379)]

The National Defense Act of 1916 also helped the Army's Medical Department with the authorized expansion of the number of medical corps officers by 1,107 and also the authorized ratio of seven medical officers per 1,000 soldiers. Furthermore, it established a Veterinary Corps and allowed five Medical Corps officers to work with the Red Cross in preparation and planning for the coming war.[26(pp379–380)]

French Medical Assets

The French developed a mobile surgical hospital (called an *auto-chir*) and a mobile surgical unit (termed a *groupe complementaire*). The early models in 1917 had no hospital beds of their own so they functioned with evacuation hospitals. They added the needed bed capacity to their *auto-chir Plisson-Proust* model (type 1917), which normally occupied wooden troop barracks, when these were available, but could use their own tents (large and small *Bessonneau* models). They could use other buildings when they were available.[25(pp184–185)] Cushing wrote in his journal that he and Dr Alexis Carrel inspected an *auto-chir* in 1917.[14(p52)]

The *auto-chir* included an operating room truck, a radiography truck, a sterilizing truck, a truck for tents and bedding, and a kitchen truck. The radiography truck carried a gas-powered generator for lighting and other needs, while the operating truck carried operating tables and equipment. The trucks gave the unit the ability to follow the troops; they could be ready for service in only a few hours. The idea was that the *auto-chir* would use buildings as available and expand to 400 patients, at which time another *auto-chir* would start its tour. The *auto-chir* would have a staff of four surgeons and four assistants, four anesthetists (as they were then called), one bacteriologist and an assistant, a staff quartermaster, one radiologist, one pharmacist, 10 nurses, and 35 orderlies. The *groupe complimentaire* was a smaller unit carrying operating and radiography equipment used for specialized surgery, such as neurosurgery or orthopedics.[25(p186)]

British Medical Assets

American medical officers assigned to the British were placed in regimental aid posts and in casualty clearing stations (CCSs). If assigned to a CCS, they would be only a few miles away from the aid posts. As noted, the aid posts were the most dangerous assignments for the surgeons. Advanced aid posts were set up even closer to the action.

The British CCS was originally intended as a mobile hospital, which would be an intermediate between field ambulance units and the base hospitals. The Royal Army Medical Corps (RAMC) established three functions: (1) treat the sick and wounded not fit for transport, (2) evacuate patients that could travel, and (3) retain those who would be fit for duty in a few days.[26(pp195–196)] The CCS system ultimately performed more surgical operations than the stationary general hospitals. CCSs were often located a few miles behind the front lines on the Western Front as the war evolved from one of movement to one of static trench warfare. The Americans were part of a supplemental rotation. The CCS teams were often multinational, including teams from Canada, Australia, New Zealand, and South Africa, in addition to the British and the Americans.[26(p201)] Cushing said of his time at a CCS: "Life at a CCS alternates between pressure of work and no work at all. Both are killing."[14(p336)]

In 1916, the British sent surgical instructor teams to CCSs to impart new surgical techniques, including the use of the Dakins-Carrel antiseptic irrigating solution. In this tradition, the British also set up a training school (the British Service School in Leeds) specifically for American doctors assigned to the British Expeditionary Forces. The RAMC had an additional basic training school at Blackpool, England.[26(pp43,202)] After each major battle, the British would have need for more American medical staff due to their own medical staff casualties. (British doctors assigned to duty as regimental medical officers had a 1917 mortality rate of 40/1,000/per month.[25(p184)]) Thus, Americans would find increasing numbers attached to the CCSs.[32(p19)]

The British field organization started with the regimental aid post. The 16 stretcher-bearers were under the command of the regimental medical officer. They collected the wounded from the battle and brought them to the regimental aid post, which had been set up in some form of shelter close to the action. The next stop was the field ambulance, which included an advanced dressing station and the main dressing station. However, the field ambulance was seen by many as unnecessary because they felt the wounded should be taken directly to a CCS from the regimental aid post.[25(pp189–190,193)]

Over time, the CCS evolved in its functions. As previously noted, the CCS was designed to be a mobile hospital. A high incidence of gas gangrene spoke to the need for immediate surgery. As the war became static, the CCSs enlarged to become hospitals that handled most of the surgery on the Western Front. The surgeons in the CCS performed all types of procedures, as needed, using modern techniques and anesthesia.[9(p238)] There was, nevertheless, much argument as to the location near the action. Should the CCS be close in to the battle or further back to provide for safety? The CCS, in fact, was no longer mobile and was usually located near railheads. (The previous locations of CCSs are often marked now by proximity to military cemeteries.[25(pp198,278)] A list of CSSs in Flanders and France can be accessed online at http:// www.1914-1918.net/ccs.htm.) By 1917, the British had allowed for an exchange of surgeons between general hospitals and CCSs, so that the consultant surgeons in the general hospitals could provide advanced surgical care and teaching at the CCS. Also in 1917, the use of Carrel-Dakin (a hypochlorite solution) in surgical wound cleaning helped reduce infection rates. Most of the RAMC medical officers at the CCSs were not regular officers, although their commanders were often careerists.[26(pp129,165)]

American Medical Assets

Prior to US entry into World War I, much of the pharmaceuticals and surgical equipment came from Germany. In America, the drug and medical manufacturing resources were mobilized to meet the demand for medical and pharmaceutical equipment in the field and at home. Supplies such as bandages, tape, and disinfectants were produced and stockpiled as rapidly as possible.[27(p41)]

Medical care for the American soldier started with buddy or self-care, using the individually carried aid packet. Each soldier was issued a regulation first aid packet or a front aid pack. The first aid packet was a metal box containing several compresses, gauze bandages, and several safety pins with instructions. The front packs were used by medical units, but came in various types depending on the size of the dressings: Packet No. 1, red

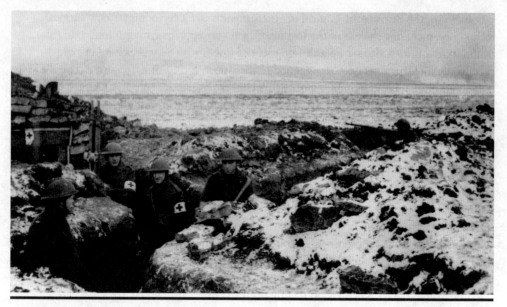

FIGURE 5-3. Dressing Station in American sector trenches. Initial treatment was rendered in the trenches at the dressing station. Photograph from the Army Nurse Corps Photograph Collection, Image #1999.91.191, courtesy of the Office of Medical History Research Collection, Army Medical Department Center of History and Heritage, Fort Sam Houston, Texas.

label (small-sized wounds); Packet No. 2, white label (medium-sized wounds); and Packet No. 3, blue label (large-sized wounds).[27(p117)]

The risk of tetanus was mitigated by a protocol that called for antitoxin treatment with even minor wounds. The antitoxin was usually given before reaching the field hospital. The battalion aid station was the usual place to give the tetanus antitoxin, but the field hospital gave it if not already administered.

Sanitary detachments carried the injured to the regimental aid station/battalion aid station after the sanitary troops applied bandages and splints. Company aid stations were more commonly used in trench warfare. The regimental aid station functioned mainly as a triage station. As battalion size was increased, the battalion aid station became essentially the same as the regimental aid station. The regimental aid station persisted in some situations, mainly as the location of the regimental surgeon with an administrative function.[28(p117)]

It was at the battalion aid station that sorting patients by the severity of their wounds ("triage") first transpired. And it was there that the first rudimentary treatment was given.[25(pp105,106)] The American battalion aid station's personnel performing this early treatment consisted of a medical officer (sometimes a dental officer), four to six enlisted Medical Department soldiers, two runners, and one or more litter-carrying squads supplied by the ambulance company.[25(p113)]

Dressing stations took patients from the aid station. Ambulance dressing stations were located at the point where ambulances could travel with some safety. Dressing stations (Figure 5-3) were located in a trench or any building in static trench warfare, although in more fluid combat they would be located in a tent. The dressing station's purpose was to give emergency treatment to casualties and ship them on to field hospitals. According to medical directives, surgery was to be confined to hospitals. Treatment elsewhere was to be limited to treating shock, hemorrhage, and the splinting of fractures. Probing of wounds for fragments or bullets was expressly forbidden.[25(p106)]

The evacuation hospital was the first surgical facility reached by the wounded. It operated alone or in conjunction with one or more mobile hospitals. The wounded were stabilized until they could be evacuated. The evacuation hospital did initial operations and also revised procedures done at forward facilities. The evacuation hospitals were usually located near rail lines. The evacuation hospital, the mobile surgical unit, and the mobile hospital were the main surgical resources.[34(pp111–112)]

The duration of time that postsurgical patients remained in the evacuation hospital depended on the situation and the nature of the wounds. It was policy that neurosurgical cases were kept 10 days to 2 weeks, while abdominal, knee, and thoracic injuries were kept up to 2 weeks. If the beds were needed, these patients would be evacuated sooner. It was estimated that 10% of the patients would be retained, while the rest would be moved.[34(p114)]

Evacuation hospital equipment assignments were modified in the period between 1912 and 1916. The modification involved increasing the amounts of equipment that had been previously intended for a field hospital. In the review of equipment, changes were made to place emphasis on equipment being durable, simple in design and function, and, especially, portable. The bed capacity was expanded from 324 to 450 by 1916. However, the changes were not sufficient to meet the challenge of the World War. The evacuation hospitals in 1917 were infrequently moved and the changes designed to ensure portability were not needed. The designated bed capacities were to prove inadequate in combat. The hospitals were enlarged in size and their equipment types were expanded and were of the more stationary design.[35(p290)] Field hospitals were increased in size to handle 216 patients in 1916. However, the equipment was reduced for the sake of transport.[35]

There were 21 American ambulance companies (of the 82 that were organized) in France by November 1918.[36(pp296–297)] The ambulance companies were now an integral part of the US Army under the direction of Colonel Jefferson Kean. Kean was a military officer assigned at the war's start to the American Red Cross. In 1917, he returned to the Army with the job of militarizing the American ambulance units. Unfortunately, not all of the drivers and units wished to be brought into the Army. Many wanted to remain in civilian capacities. After "converting" the units, the Army organized training facilities in the United States for Army drivers.[29(pp164–165)]

The Americans "discovered" the *auto-chir* amid their need for mobility. In 1918, the Chief Surgeon of the Allied Expeditionary Forces placed an order with the French manufacturer for 20 *auto-chir* units and a like number of the lighter complementary groups. The *auto-chir* was obtained from the French at *Fort De Vavnes*, located near Paris. Some of the hospitals were assembled on a polo ground near Paris (Hospitals No. 1, 2, 3, and 4) and later at the *Parc des Princes, Port St Cloud* (only 5 miles from *Fort De Vavnes*). The Americans planned to use the *auto-chir* to augment the surgical capability of the field and evacuation hospitals. Twelve mobile surgical hospital units were set up at the Paris Auto-Park. Mobile Hospital No. 5 (left for duty 20 September 1918) through Mobile

Hospital No. 12 (left for duty 23 January 1919 to provide care for occupation troops) were established for American use. The AEF had operational units numbered 1 through 11 and 39 (Base Hospital No. 39 provided the basis for the No. 39 Mobile Surgical unit and it was so named).[25(p187)]

The Army authorized a larger staff complement for the mobile hospitals than that of the French. A major of the Medical Department was to command. There were 10 captains or lieutenants, Medical Corps, authorized. One Sanitary Corps captain or lieutenant rounded out the commissioned complement. The senior NCO was a sergeant first class in charge of 17 sergeants (all Medical Department) and 62 privates or privates first class. There were 22 female nurses listed. The mobile surgical unit (corresponding to the *groupe complimentaire*) had a captain or lieutenant, Medical Corps, in charge. The enlisted group was headed by one sergeant first class leading three sergeants and eight privates or privates first class.[25(p187)]

Five of the first six mobile hospitals obtained their medical staff from base hospitals managed by the British. Base Hospital No. 2 (Presbyterian unit) supplied the staff for Mobile Hospital No. 2. Base Hospital No. 4 staffed Mobile Hospital No. 5. Base Hospital No. 5 (Cleveland, Ohio) staffed Mobile Hospital No. 6. The No. 10 Base Hospital supplied personnel for Mobile Hospital No. 8, while Base Hospital No. 21 (St Louis, Missouri) furnished operating staff for Mobile Hospital No. 4.[14(p66)] The mobile hospitals were run by the Americans, but were initially staffed in part by British personnel.

The mobile hospitals operated with evacuation hospitals or field hospitals, or operated independently. As an example, Mobile Hospital No. 39 (which had been a Red Cross base hospital, staffed by Yale personnel) was the first mobile hospital in action with American forces. It had tents and French-designed Adrian barracks to supplement the basic mobile unit. It participated in the area of the St Mihiel Battle of 1918 (involving the AEF, the French, and the Germans) with an expanded size of 524 beds.[25(pp191–193)] In his journal, Cushing described the first three mobile units planned along the lines of the French *autochir*, organized by Colonel (COL) JM Flint, of which the first was known as the Yale Mobile Unit. Cushing reported that No. 1 and No. 2 units had seen active service in the July 1918 offensive.[14(p66)]

Two operating rooms could provide for six teams. These hospitals were not standardized; each unit had flexibility in obtaining additional equipment or supplies that the commanding officer might desire. An example would be an ophthalmologist commander who wanted ocular equipment. The staff opinions of active unit mobile hospitals were gathered to determine what items were really needed. The new standardized equipment list items could be hauled on 20 3-ton trucks.[25(p189)]

The Army approach for mobile hospitals (Figures 5-4 and 5-5) envisioned dealing with the wounded along the lines of the French units previously discussed. The mobile hospital commander would be a major. The mobile hospital had fixed sterilization, radiology, and power generating plants, carried on two trucks. Other trucks carried tents and enough supplies to set up a 120-bed unit with six operating teams.[37(pp355–356)]

The mobile surgical unit also had trucks carrying equipment (such as a portable sterilizer and radiology equipment). The mobile operating room would have a portable light-generating plant along with supplies mounted on trucks. The mobile units ended up supplementing the field hospitals, but they did not carry organic setups for their own beds,

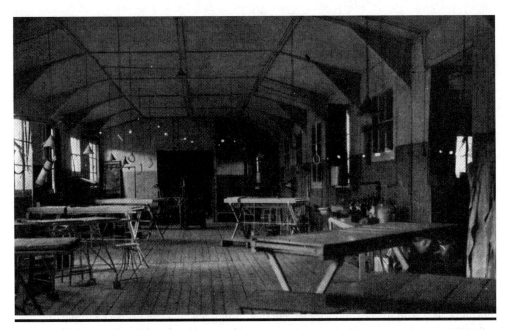

FIGURE 5-4. Operating Room, Mobile Hospital No. 39. Initially designated as Base Hospital No. 39, it was later set up as Mobile Hospital No. 39, which operated close to the troops. Photograph from *The Medical Department of the United States Army in the World War*, courtesy of the Army Medical Department Center of History and Heritage, Fort Sam Houston, Texas.

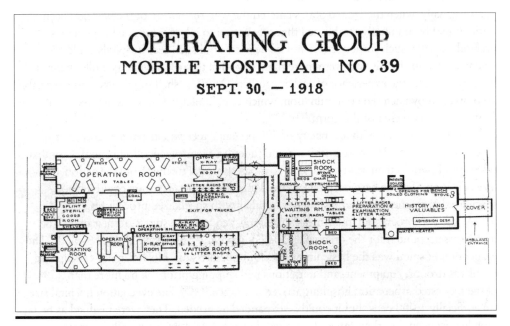

FIGURE 5-5. Mobile Hospital No. 39 Layout. The mobile hospital was designed to bring surgical care to the troops closer to their actual wounding. Photograph from *The Medical Department of the United States Army in the World War*, courtesy of the Army Medical Department Center of History and Heritage, Fort Sam Houston, Texas.

as did the mobile hospital. The commander of a mobile surgical unit was a captain. The mobile unit drew upon the surgical staff of the field hospital it was to augment.[37(p356)]

The plans for the mobile surgical units (complementary groups) called for 20 units. The equipment for these units was made in France. However, by the time of the Armistice, only 16 mobile surgical units were in operation. They were No. 1 through No. 12, and No. 100 through No. 103.[25(p199)]

Mobile hospital units provided a way to utilize specialty neurosurgical care. In many cases, Cushing noted that neurosurgeons were placed in command of surgical care in hospitals performing triage. The rush of patients and the ability to use local anesthesia for neurosurgery cases led to incomplete care, which in Cushing's view would include neurosurgery done too rapidly. Over time, the situation changed and he noted that by June 1918, only two neurosurgical teams were organized, one at Mobile Hospital No. 1 and the other at Mobile Hospital No. 2. The only penetrating wound of the head that survived in June 1918 came through those mobile hospitals that Cushing managed.[38(p755)] Cushing reported that special instruments for neurosurgery, such as rongeurs, drills, and "perforators," had to be obtained from French manufacturers because they were not available from Army sources. Most of the cases could be done under local anesthesia with morphine as a pain medication supplemental. Cushing felt that the British example of collecting several neurosurgical teams in a special hospital for head trauma worked best in a static situation. In his view, the use of two teams in the larger evacuation hospitals worked best for the Americans in situations such as the Meuse-Argonne operation. The patients would be later sent to specialized centers.[38(pp750,757)]

Originally, when the United States entered the war, the nature of the war had been static. It had been initially established that evacuation to a larger remote hospital was preferable. Later, such surgery could not be delayed until such rear hospitals could be reached. Wounds in this war were more than 80% due to shell fragments; bullet wounds were rare, unlike the experience of earlier conflicts.[39(p87)] The shell fragments were invariably accompanied by bacterial contamination, which could quickly lead to fatal infection if early forward surgery were not the norm.[39(pp87-90)]

The base hospital, with a capacity of 500 patients, received its patients from the evacuation hospital. The base hospital could function as an evacuation hospital if combat was close. It would then send its patients to a base hospital further from the action. Specialization of some base hospitals allowed improved care. The care could include specialized instrumentation and surgeons familiar with specialized procedures.[34(p86)]

As the war progressed, the Americans established more hospitals of their own. The Red Cross accounted for the organizing and equipping of 36 of the 42 base hospitals. The evacuation hospital was the basic unit to back up the division. However, due to shipping problems (troops, equipment, and munitions had shipping priority), no more than 25% of the requested evacuation hospitals arrived in France.[38(p290)] The evacuation hospital size was officially 1,000 beds, but it could be expanded as needed. They were planned as being mobile in concept but their large size limited that role.[35(pp161-163)] Eventually, organized professional teams, including surgeons and operating room staff from the base hospitals, were needed to fill out the professional staff of the evacuation hospital.[39(p28)]

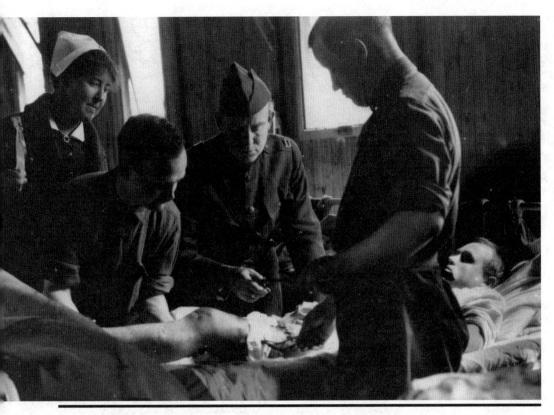

FIGURE 5-6. Badly wounded soldier receiving care at the Base Hospital, Johns Hopkins Unit, France. The Johns Hopkins unit was organized in Baltimore as Base Hospital No. 18. It set up at Saint Nazaire, France in 1917 and treated many patients until closure in 1919. It became Base Hospital No. 1 and later No. 101. Photograph from the office files of the Research Collection, US Army Medical Department Center of History and Heritage, Fort Sam Houston, Texas.

The field hospital was situated 3 to 8 miles from the front. The function and setup of the field hospital in static trench warfare could be different from the open warfare model. The static situation could mean a field hospital with fixtures and complete equipment. In fluid situations, field hospitals might not have the equipment and might be dedicated to evacuation. In other fluid situations, they could be found in good quarters and well-equipped.[27(pp100–101)] The field hospital at times had a mobile surgical unit attached to handle surgery for those that could not be evacuated.[27(p101)] The field hospital was never intended for major surgery on a regular basis; the mobile surgical or evacuation hospital was better suited for the task. Only the most serious cases were attempted at a field hospital, but if evacuation could not be done due to combat, then other cases were done. The field hospital sent patients to the mobile hospital and to the evacuation hospital. Base hospitals and general hospitals followed in the evacuation chain.[27(p81)] The evacuation hospital was generally located forward, not far from the field hospital, although exceptions were numerous depending on the fluidity of combat.[27(p107)]

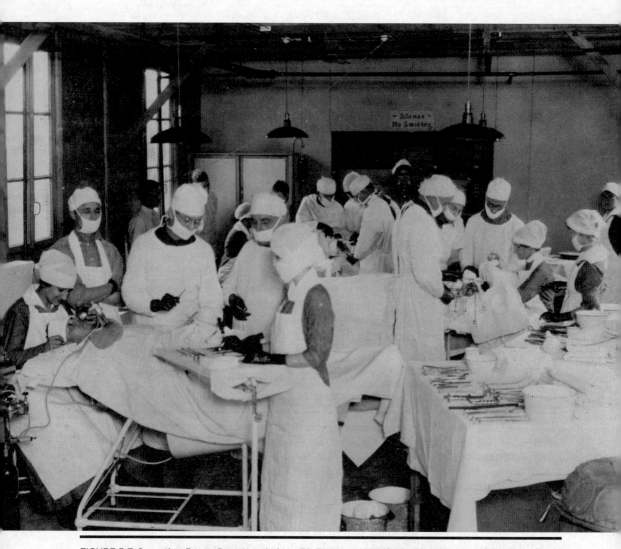

FIGURE 5-7. Operating Room, Base Hospital No. 52. Base Hospital No. 52 was initially organized at Camp Greenleaf, Georgia, and further organized at Camp Gordon, Georgia. It arrived at its station at Rimacourt, France on 8 August 1918, where it remained until it was closed in January 1919. The setup of the operating room was typical of a base hospital. Photograph from the office files of the Research Collection, US Army Medical Department Center of History and Heritage, Fort Sam Houston, Texas.

The organization of base hospitals and evacuation hospitals was detailed by the Army Surgeon General's Office. The hospitals that were to go overseas required the most careful planning. These plans called for the organization of the hospitals at one of the medical training camps. After 6 weeks of training, the hospital units would be moved to a cantonment area to be designated for further organization and training. At the conclusion of this process, the hospitals could be deployed. In 1918, when the American forces were involved in their heaviest fighting, urgent calls for more hospital units came from the AEF

Headquarters. The Surgeon General consolidated some of the units to provide a rapid deployment because it was difficult to find adequate personnel at all times.[40(pp351–353)]

Base hospitals (Figures 5-6 and 5-7) had 1,000 beds, with a colonel in command. The evacuation hospital was commanded by a lieutenant colonel, but also had 1,000 beds. Before the war, the evacuation hospital and base hospitals were to be 500 beds. During the war, however, the base and the evacuation hospital were increased to 1,000 beds, based on the expected flow of casualties. Because both hospital types could be expanded as needed, hospitals with several thousand beds were not that uncommon. The surgical service for the evacuation hospital would include a chief, 11 general surgeons, one orthopedic surgeon, one urologist, one neurosurgeon, one otolaryngologist, one ophthalmologist, and one oral surgeon. Two radiologists were attached.[40(p353)] The selection of a commander called for a person with "special administrative efficiency and the ability to command."[40(p353)] Following this scheme, 162 base hospitals and 59 evacuation hospitals were created in the United States. Of that number, 121 base hospitals and 40 evacuation hospitals were sent overseas. The end of hostilities allowed the remaining units still in the United States to be demobilized quickly.[40(p354)]

EQUIPMENT AND HOSPITALS

Ambulances

The first motorized Army ambulance was steam powered and placed at Washington Barracks, in Washington, DC, while a second steam unit was placed at the Army Military Academy at West Point, New York. The steam units were problematic because of operational and maintenance difficulties; animal-pulled ambulances returned until gasoline-powered ambulances were available. The Army contracted with the Keeton Motor Company for a 6-cylinder unit with special solid puncture-proof tires.[2(p362)]

In April 1917, the French requested that the Americans send 100 ambulance groups to serve with the French military. The ambulance groups had been militarized by that time and were known now as the US Army Ambulance Service. The section or group involved 20 ambulances and 45 men. This request was based on the work of the volunteer *Americaine Ambulance* groups with the French forces. The Ford Motor Company shipped 2,350 ambulances to France by October 1917. Fifty additional units were sent to Pennsylvania for training with the US Army Ambulance Service.[35(p363)]

Militarization of the American volunteer ambulance companies after America entered the war in April 1917 would involve administrative transfer into the US Army Ambulance Service. Because these units were taking care of French troops, they were brought into the US Army, but then reassigned to the French. The other volunteer organizations were assimilated into the military with varying degrees of success.[29(pp161–162,179)]

The Ford contract first involved the 1917-model body (the ambulance portions were to be added later), which was found to have many faults. These problems were redressed with the 1918-model body, which featured a wider wheelbase and extended body. The Hay-Dee 15-inch extension was incorporated into the body. The Army utilized the Fords but later used a longer body type. Although the Army used the Fords, it preferred the General Motors Corporation (GMC) ambulances for their larger size.[36(pp395-396)] However, the Fords did move best of the vehicles over rough and destroyed roads; the bigger GMC ambulances did best on improved roads.[36(pp265,290)]

General Motors had had the benefit of supplying vehicles for the 1916 Mexican-American conflict. However, the GMC ambulance they had provided was too light for Army purposes and a new model, the Model 16—a ¾-ton truck—was designed. A 1917 contract of 2,000 was expanded to 5,000 for 1918. The war ended before all could be assembled. Other companies were also contracted to build the ambulance, but no factories were built because the contracts were cancelled due to the end of the war.[39(pp337-340)]

Deployment of Base Hospitals

Surgeon General William Gorgas and Dr George Crile organized a simulated base hospital in Philadelphia, Pennsylvania, at the 1916 American College of Surgeons meeting. The simulation was to provide awareness of the need for surgical care in Europe and to provide training in setting up an operational facility.[2(p248)] A series of base hospitals was organized following the earlier model. These hospitals included the following units:

BASE HOSPITAL NO. 4

The experience gained in the early years started the formation of university base hospitals. Base Hospital No. 4 (Case Western Reserve, Cleveland, Ohio), led by George Crile, was the first American military unit in France, arriving on 25 May 1917. Base Hospital No. 4 was immediately assigned to help the desperate British manpower shortage by taking over the British General Hospital No. 9 in Rouen (1,240 regular beds and 300 crisis beds). Base Hospital No. 4 operated as the No. 9 General Hospital, British Expeditionary Force, for the entire period until it returned to the United States in 1919. The Lakeside unit was organized in August 1916 and mobilized in May 1917.[41(p2)]

BASE HOSPITAL NO. 5

At Boulogne, British General Hospital No. 13 was relieved by Base Hospital No. 5. Base Hospital No. 5 was organized by Harvey Cushing at Harvard University in February 1916 and mobilized in May 1917. It arrived at Boulogne, France, in May 1917, approximately a month after the United States formally entered the war. It was assigned to the British Expeditionary Force and was designated as British General Hospital No. 13, housed in a large city building until 1919. (The building had been the home of the Boulogne Casino.[13(p50)]) The Germans bombed Base Hospital No. 5 by plane, killing four Americans. Cushing received a message while he traveled to Camiers that among the dead was 1st Lieutenant William Fitzsimons, Medical Corps, US Army, the first American medical officer killed in action.[27(p2)]

Harvey Cushing and the Harvard unit sailed to England in 1917 on the SS *Saxonia*.[14(p103)] Cushing had previously been assigned to Base Hospital No. 5. Subsequently, he was assigned to the No. 46 Casualty Clearing Station at Mendingham from 22 July 1917 until 1 November 1917.[9(p166)] CCS No. 46 was one of three casualty clearing stations at Mendingham. Cushing wrote that the British were surprised by the Americans' use of nurse anesthetists because the standard in England called for physicians in the role.[13(p41)]

Harvey Cushing was asked to attend to the son of Sir William Osler who had been wounded by artillery shrapnel near St Julien. Second Lieutenant Edward Revere Osler (known largely by the name Revere) had served with the Royal Artillery since 1916. He had been taken to Casualty Clearing Station No. 47 at Dosinghem. Despite the desperate surgical intervention of a group of surgeons including Crile, Osler's son did not survive. (Cushing did not actually involve himself in the operation because there was no head trauma.[15(p197)])

Cushing's time with a British CCS was fruitful. He collected a series of technical reports of patients treated during the Passchendaele. (This was actually the Third Battle of Ypres, which transpired from 31 July until 6 November 1917. The British carried the Allied burden in the Third Battle of Ypres as they attempted to prevail over the Germans strictly by attrition rather than any grand tactical maneuver.[9(p263)]) Cushing perfected his *en bloc* bone resection under local anesthesia for his intracranial surgeries. He popularized the use of magnets to remove intracranial metal fragments and pioneered the use of dichloramine-T as a neurosurgical wound antiseptic.[42(pp283-294)] Crile recorded in his autobiography a visit with Cushing during which his younger subordinates complained that Cushing was too slow and deliberate for combat surgery. Crile said he advised them to let Cushing work at his own pace on select cases while they handled the larger burden.[18(p161)] Cushing was noted for his methodical pace and great care to detail in his operations and notes throughout his career. His style as a perfectionist with slow methodical technique could be attributed to his Halsted training.[16(p236)]

BASE HOSPITAL NO. 21

Also at Rouen, the duties of the British General Hospital No. 12 were assumed by Base Hospital No. 21. Base Hospital No. 21 came from Washington University at St Louis, Missouri. It was organized in July 1916 and mobilized in April 1917. It remained there until January 1919.[43]

BASE HOSPITAL NO. 12

While at Camiers, No. 18 British General Hospital was replaced by Base Hospital No. 12. No. 12 (the last to sail) was set up from staff at Northwestern University in Chicago, Illinois. It was organized in July 1916 and was mobilized in May 1917. British General Hospital No. 18 remained attached to the British Expeditionary Force until March 1919.[37]

BASE HOSPITAL NO. 10

At Treport, Base Hospital No. 10 replaced British General Hospital No. 16.[16(p683)] Base Hospital No. 10 was organized from the University of Pennsylvania, Pennsylvania Hospital (Philadelphia). It was organized in February 1917 and mobilized in May 1917. It was sent to Le Treport, where it was assigned to the British Expeditionary Force and operated under the auspices of No. 10 General Hospital, British Expeditionary Force. The No. 10 Base Hospital remained with the British Expeditionary Force until February 1919.

Initially, the university-anchored base hospital system provided a solid basis for excellent care of the Allied Expeditionary Force by utilizing the best available surgeons and their staffs. At the end of the war, 50 Red Cross Base Hospitals were set up in Europe.[25(pp92–93)] Cushing noted that the five original base hospitals assigned to the British Expeditionary Force treated more wounded than the 78 base hospitals in the American Expeditionary Forces, which he viewed as reflecting the more efficient British experience and organization. Cushing felt that the Americans did not wish to deal with this implied inefficiency of American versus British facilities officially. Unofficially, the senior medical officials saw no problem.[15(p73)]

Other Base Hospitals

Examples of some of the base hospitals to arrive later include the following:

Base Hospital No. 1 was organized at Bellevue Hospital, New York in September 1916 and was mobilized in November 1917. It eventually set up in Vichy, France where it took over a group of hotels used by the French as hospitals. It remained in operation in Vichy from March 1918 until March 1919.[37(pp629–655)]

Base Hospital No. 2 was the Presbyterian Hospital of New York City. It was organized in March 1917 and mobilized for duty in May 1917. Base Hospital No. 2 was assigned to British Hospital No. 1 at Etretat, France. It was there until February 1919.[37(pp629–655)]

Base Hospital No. 3 was organized at Mount Sinai, New York, in September 1916 and mobilized in November 1917. It was posted to Vauclaire, France, where it stayed until March 1919.

Base Hospital No. 6 was organized at the Massachusetts General Hospital, Boston, in March 1916 and mobilized in May 1917. It was sent to Bordeaux, France. It took over a French hospital, where it remained until March 1919.[37(pp629–655)]

Base Hospital No. 7 was organized at Boston City Hospital, Boston, Massachusetts, in December 1917 and mobilized in February 1918. It was set up at Loire, France, where it remained until early 1919.

Base Hospital No. 8 was organized at the Post-Graduate Hospital, New York, in November 1916 and mobilized in July 1917. It was sent to Savenay, France, where it functioned until January 1919.[37(pp629–655)]

The added American medical staffs greatly helped the British. By July 1917, American base hospitals sent doctors and staff to British casualty clearing stations. The British reported having insufficient surgeons on their own to perform frontline surgery. This shortage threatened planned expansion of surgery at the front.[33(pp43,202)] Many of the British surgeons were not surgeons in fact, but only had rudimentary surgical training. The Americans brought much needed skills and training to the CCSs.[9(p166)] The contribution of American military medicine was a significant gift to the Allies.

Medical officers were trained additionally at home. Soon after war was declared, the Army set up Army Medical Officer Training camps at the following locations: Fort Riley, Kansas; Camp Greenleaf, Georgia; and Fort Benjamin Harrison, Indiana, all of which operated until the end of the war (with the exception of Fort Benjamin Harrison, which closed in 1917 because it was deemed nonessential).[40(pp348–349)]

SIGNATURE WOUND OF WORLD WAR I

Early on, the surgeons of the Western Front were expecting the relatively uncomplicated gunshot wound of earlier conflicts. The woundings in World War I were complicated by contamination resulting in infection, gangrene, and shock. The type of projectile that caused the most problem came from artillery. Terraine, in his 1982 book *White Heat: The New War 1914–1918*,[46] gives artillery the credit for being the cause of "the greatest loss of life, the most dreadful wounds, the deepest fear."[44(p146)]

The German 7.7 cm, the British 18 pounder, and the French 75 mm were the most used artillery pieces in the light field gun category. The Americans used the French 75 mm field piece, even producing them under license in the United States. The French 75 mm threw a shell out to 8,400 meters. (A special dedicated shrapnel shell could travel 9,000 meters.[45(p14)]) The use of heavier artillery became more common as the war progressed. Artillery ranging from the 90 mm to the use of large naval guns mounted on railcars was seen.[45p14)] Upon impact, the high-velocity shells gave off splinters and parts of fuses, casings, or other parts that created unusually configured wounds.[45(pp14–15)]

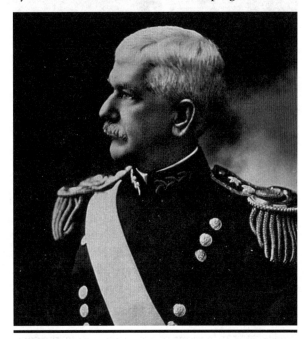

FIGURE 5-8. William C Gorgas. Gorgas was the Army Surgeon General from January 1914 until October 1918 (covering most of World War I). His work eradicating mosquitoes and yellow fever from Cuba and later in the Canal Zone brought him acclaim as a sanitarian. Photograph courtesy of the National Library of Medicine, Image #B029216.

OFFICE OF THE SURGEON GENERAL AND THE ESTABLISHMENT OF CONSULTANTS

William Gorgas (Figure 5-8) became the Army Surgeon General in 1914 after the unexpected death of the former Surgeon General, George H Torney. Gorgas had an illustrious background largely grounded in epidemiology, especially with reference to yellow fever. His largest challenge was in the area of administration and expansion of the medical care system. Gorgas was Surgeon General for most of the war.[39(p154)]

Interestingly, Merritte W Ireland (Figure 5-9), the Surgeon General during the latter part of World War I, had been assigned to the Fort Sam Houston Hospital, San Antonio, Texas, to treat casualties of the Punitive Expedition. He met Brigadier General (BG) John

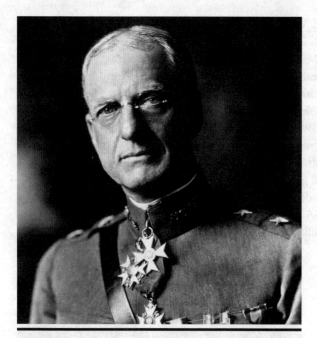

FIGURE 5-9. Merritte W Ireland. Ireland followed William C Gorgas as the Army Surgeon General. He remained in office until May 1931. Ireland had to deal with the drawdown of World War I and the influenza pandemic. Photograph courtesy of the National Library of Medicine, Image #B015407.

Pershing there. Pershing later made him the Assistant Chief Surgeon of the AEF. He promoted him to the Chief Surgeon's slot before recommending Ireland as a replacement for Surgeon General Gorgas in October 1918.[5] While Gorgas handled most of the World War, Ireland presided over the last phase of the war, the postwar occupation, and the influenza crisis.[39(p155)] After the war, Ireland's Army Medical Department produced a seminal 15-volume series titled *The Medical Department of the United States Army in the World War*,[27] which covered the activities of Army medicine in the period.

The AEF established a consultant system by General Order No. 88, on 6 June 1918. BG John MT Finney (Johns Hopkins) was named the Surgical Services Chief Consultant, with COL Harvey Cushing as the Neurosurgical Consultant and COL George Crile as the Consultant for Surgical Research. Their positions as consultants allowed them to advise the command concerning their areas of expertise.[42(p385)] The Surgical and Medical Consultants reported to the Director of Professional Services, who was COL William Keller. Consultants were appointed for each of the surgical services and for each of the medical services. (Interestingly, the Roentgenology Consultant fell under the Surgical Consultants listing.) The headquarters for the Professional Services Division was situated in Neufchateau, France.[46(pp63–64)] In terms of accomplishments, the consultant group arranged for some of the base hospitals to specialize in certain cases. This allowed the specialized consultants to be co-located with cases of their interest. For example, Base Hospital No. 20 dealt with tuberculosis cases while Base Hospitals No. 8 and No. 25 specialized in neuropsychiatric cases. Base Hospital No. 46 was devoted to neurosurgery patients. No. 115 concentrated on ophthalmic and maxillofacial cases. Finally, Base Hospital No. 9 was reserved for orthopedic injuries.[46(p65)]

Influenza Pandemic

The influenza and pneumonia pandemic of 1918 created havoc for the armies on both sides of the conflict, with significant losses of soldiers in a short time. The increased mortality in Army camps compared to the civilian population was due, in part, to close living conditions in military camps and mess hall areas. The Surgeon General's report was favorable in its reporting of the Medical Department's response and the dedicated response of its nurses, doctors, and enlisted members.[45(pp1033–1035)] Byerly, however, in the book *Fever of War*,[47] raises the question of whether the Army did all it could to deal with the pandemic.[47(pp154–155)] The flu infected over 1 million Army soldiers (26% of the Army troops). It accounted for 82% of the Army's deaths from disease.[44(p6)] Byerly points out that military leaders, medical officers, and the Federal Government all tended to downplay the significance of the influenza pandemic on the war. Byerly is of the opinion (not necessarily shared by others) that such attempts added to the complacency in responding to the crisis. Byerly's sense is that the military did not realize the impact of the pandemic upon war-fighting capability in further planning.[47(p11)]

SUMMARY: ADVANCES

Each war is said to have its own medical advances. The medical progress of World War I built on prior advances. The recognition of germ theory established new sterile techniques. Immunizations for tetanus and typhoid became available. New frontiers were being advanced in abdominal, thoracic, and neurosurgery that had been previously closed to the surgeon.[44(p1609)] World War I advances to remember include the use of whole blood transfusions, advances in shock treatment by transfusion (Crile's work), debridement (with antiseptic solutions) as a standard surgical technique in dealing with wounds, and, finally, advances in neurosurgical injury repair.

Orthopedics

A surgeon on the Western Front was required to deal with all types of procedures. World War I saw advances in orthopedic open reductions with internal and external fixation. The Army created a *Manual of Splints and Appliances* as the result of several "splint boards" convened to standardize the use of splints and to reduce the number of splints to 10.[35(pp554–555)] The Thomas splint was the best known of the available splints due to its ease of use. Improvements were made in splint application after surgery (considered a weak point) by the creation of hospital splint teams, which increased the productivity of orthopedic surgeons.[39(p584)]

Neuropsychiatry

Recognition and treatment advances were made in neuropsychiatric cases termed "shell shock." Much work in the war was directed to "war neurosis." Artillery was considered an important part of the etiology.[45(pp373–375)] The psychiatrists also described a neurasthenic version of the war neurosis, with an antecedent pattern of exhaustion.[45(p379)] Drugs were to be used as little as possible. The patient's morale was to be strengthened, always with a view to getting back to duty. The treatment was deemed a success if the soldier could be motivated to return to duty.[45(pp403–404)]

Neurosurgery

Cushing learned from his experience with the British that the mortality rate for head wounds could be reduced in half if soldiers were operated on in the forward area. He describes a 28% mortality rate in a British Casualty Clearing Station for his own cases versus a 45% rate in an American base hospital attached to the British Expeditionary Force.[38(p755)] The British adopted a plan to have several teams concentrated in one hospital for neurosurgery. The Americans felt it was preferable to have two teams located in evacuation hospitals along the lines of evacuation. As the levels of experience in neurosurgical procedures increased among specialized neurosurgeons, the Americans came to see the best results in larger centers with concentrated expertise.[38(p757)]

Neurosurgeons became aware of the impact of helmet design upon head wounds. The British helmet was seated too high to afford protection. The French Adrian helmet, which was produced quickly, was not adequate to prevent penetration of projectiles. The German helmet was better designed and was 30% stronger than the English and American helmets.[39(pp1-2)] Experimental versions of the American interpretation of the German design were made, but the war ended before production could be considered. In fact, versions of the reengineered World War I helmet were used through 1942 in the US Army. The German design also afforded greater protection of more of the head, especially the sides and the back of the head.[39(pp1-3)]

Plastic Surgery

Advances were made in plastic surgery to deal with the huge number of facial disfiguring wounds. Facial wounds were not that uncommon, even during the Civil War. Facial wounds were to be closed as soon as possible without excision of tissue unless necrotic. Mucous membranes were to be closed along with skin closure. Secondary plastic repair could be done for reasons such as an unsightly scar. There was collaboration between general surgeons, otolaryngologists, oral surgeons, ophthalmologists, and neurosurgeons in the development of new approaches to facial plastic surgery.[48(pp313-314)]

Radiographic Localization of Foreign Bodies

Radiographic localization of foreign bodies was used during surgical operations in World War I to find and remove projectiles and shrapnel. Fluoroscopic control was often used to facilitate such extractions.[40(pp258-259)]

Transfusions

Transfusion of blood was a truly life-saving innovation. Wright described the use of citrates to allow storage of blood in 1894.[30(p126)] Landsteiner reported blood groups in 1901. In 1906, George Crile reported direct transfusion from a donor radial artery to a donor cephalic elbow vein,[22(pp329-332)] and Jansky described blood group incompatibility in 1907.[30(p129)] In 1912, the first perioperative blood transfusion was completed at Massachusetts General Hospital. A paraffin collection vessel and delivery cannula (to discourage blood clotting) was used. The equipment was termed the Harvard Kimpton paraffin-coated transfusion apparatus.[15(p124)] By 1918, the British were providing transfusions in base hospitals and casualty clearing stations to an average 50 patients per day. In that year, all blood was citrated, but not all was typed and stored in blood banks. The level of understanding was incomplete in terms of incompatibility and treatment of transfusion reactions at this stage of development. As an example, Dr Archibald Lee of McGill University served in France from April 1915 until October 1916. In his series of eight soldiers receiving transfusions, six died, one had success, and one survived despite having a hemolytic reaction. The use of citrated-glucose enhanced blood transfusion, followed by the use of preserved blood in 1917 and 1918, reduced morbidity and mortality. However, the testing for blood groups and issues of incompatibility had to await future improvements after the war.[30(p130)]

Evacuation

The Army Medical Department used motor ambulance vehicles, trains, and canal barges in Europe to evacuate the wounded to treatment sites. Ships were used to transport the wounded to America. Trains were obtained from the French and the British. The plan to use ordinary modified boxcars was abandoned following the European finding that dedicated trains were superior. Nineteen British trains were delivered before the end of hostilities. The trains procured were not the more advanced British units featuring surgical capabilities. Two French trains converted from passenger units were also used in American service. Sixty barges were converted to American medical use. Barges were to be used for soldiers with compound fractures, and abdominal or chest wounds who would not be able to be transported by train. Ambulances were used extensively. The issue of spare parts for these vehicles called for a change in future shipping protocols. All spare parts were to be shipped in boxes with the ambulance. It was found that the ambulance should be shipped with its frame and body assembled.[49(pp317–348)]

The events of World War I encouraged many advances in techniques, medications, life-saving transfusions, and equipment such as motorized ambulances. As Garrison pointed out, "the forgotten principle of debridement . . . was revived by Lemaitre and HMW Gray and in this way the danger of infection between front and base was effectively bridged and thousands of lives were saved."[50(pp201–202)] Garrison noted that as the war neared its conclusion, evacuation hospitals were pushed closer to the front lines. His book, *Notes on the History of Military Medicine*,[50] summarizes nicely the many contributions of the noted military surgeons and the advances in military medical care during the World War.[50(pp200–202)] Inasmuch as history is often forgotten, many lessons learned from this great conflict had to be relearned for the next worldwide conflict,[50(pp283–294)] only a little more than 20 years away.

REFERENCES

1. Rubin R. *The Last of the Doughboys; The Forgotten Generation and the Forgotten World War*. New York, NY: Houghton Mifflin Harcourt; 2013.
2. Gabriel RA, Metz KS. *A History of Military Medicine*. Vol 2. *From the Renaissance Through Modern Times*. London, England: Greenwood Press; 1992.
3. Hastings M. *Catastrophe 1914: Europe Goes to War*. New York, NY: Alfred A Knopf; 2013.

4. Jukes G, Simkins P, Hickey M. *First World War: The War to End All Wars*. London, England: Osprey; 2013.
5. Winter J, Baggett B. *The Great War and the Shaping of the 20th Century*. New York, NY: Penguin Studio (Division Penguin Books); 1996.
6. Clark C. *The Sleepwalkers: How Europe Went to War in 1914*. New York, NY: Harper Collins; 2012.
7. McMeekin S. *July 1914: Countdown to War*. New York, NY: Basic Books; 2013.
8. Hart P. *The Great War: A Combat History of the First World War*. New York, NY: Oxford University Press; 2013.
9. Mayhew E. *Wounded: A New History of the Western Front in World War I*. New York, NY: Oxford University Press; 2014.
10. Stroock W. Doughboys' bloody baptism. *Mil Heritage*. 2014;16(1):27–33.
11. Grotelueschen ME. *The AEF Way of War: The American Army and Combat in World War I*. London, England: Cambridge University Press; 2006.
12. Perello P. Hindenburg's war: decision in the trenches, 1918. *Strategy & Tactics*. 2014;288:9.
13. Cushing H. *The Story of US Army Base Hospital No. 5*. Cambridge, Mass: The University Press; 1919.
14. Cushing H. *From a Surgeon's Journal 1915–1918*. Boston, Mass: Little, Brown and Company; 1936.
15. Englund P. *The Beauty and the Sorrow: An Intimate History of the First World War*. New York, NY: Alfred A Knopf; 2011.
16. Imber G. *Genius on the Edge: The Bizarre Double Life of Dr William Stewart Halsted*. New York, NY: Kaplan Publishing; 2011.
17. Craddock WL. Harvey Cushing: contributions to military surgery. *Mil Med*. 1994;159(4):268–274.
18. Crile GW, Crile G, ed. *George Crile, an Autobiography*. 2 Vols. Philadelphia, Penn, and New York, NY: Lippincott; 1947.
19. Cushing H. The Harvard Unit at the American Ambulance in Neuilly, Paris. *Bost Med Surg J*. 1915;172:801–803.
20. Lee JA, Weismann WD, Handy MA. George Washington Crile. *Current Surg*. 2005;62(6):415–418.
21. Rutkow BA. George Crile, Harvey Cushing, and the *Ambulance Americaine*: military preparedness in World War I. *Arch Surg*. 2004;139(6):678–685.
22. Crile GW. The technique of direct transfusion of blood. *Ann Surg*. 1907;46(3):329–332.
23. Crile GW. *Hemorrhage and Transfusion: An Experimental and Clinical Research*. New York, NY: D Appleton and Company; 1909.
24. American College of Surgeons: Division of Member Services. Feature: George Crile, MD, FACS (1864–1943). http://www.facs.org/archives/crilehighlight.html. Accessed 22 July 2015.
25. Lynch C, Weed FW, MacAfee L. United States, Surgeon General's Office. In: Weed FW, ed. *The Medical Department of the United States Army in the World War*. Vol 8. *Field Operations*. Washington, DC: War Department, Department of the Army, Office of The Surgeon General; 1923.
26. Whitehead IR. *Doctors in the Great War*. Barnsley, South Yorkshire, England: Leo Cooper; 1999.
27. Lynch C, Ford JH, Weed FW, eds. Medical service of the division in combat. In: Weed FW, ed. *Medical Department of the United States Army in the World War*. Vol 8. *Field Operations*.

Washington, DC: War Department, Department of the Army, Office of The Surgeon General; 1925: Chap 4.
28. Jessep JE, Ketz LB. Studies of the history, tradition, policies, institutions of the armed forces in war and peace. In: *Encyclopedia of the Army.* Vol 3. New York, NY: Charles Scribner; 1994.
29. Hansen AJ. *Gentlemen Volunteers: The Story of the American Ambulance Drivers in the First World War.* New York, NY: Arcade Publishing; 2011.
30. Hedley-White J, Milamed DR. Blood and war. *Ulster Med J.* 2010;7979(3):125–134.
31. Crile G, Rowland A, Littleton M, et al. A composite report of the three months' service of the Lakeside Unit at the American Ambulance. *Cleve Med J.* 1915;14:421–439.
32. Rauer M, Marble S, ed. *Yanks in the King's Forces: American Physicians Serving With the British Expeditionary Force During World War I.* Washington, DC: Office of Medical History, Office of The Surgeon General, United States Army. http://history.amedd.army.mil/booksdocs/wwi/AmericanArmyMCOfficersBEF.pdf. Accessed 21 July 2015.
33. Gorgas WC. *Inspection of Medical Services With the American Expeditionary Forces: Confidential Report to Secretary of War.* Washington, DC: Government Printing Office; 1919.
34. Jaffin JH. Medical support for the American Expeditionary Forces in France During the First World War. Thesis. Fort Leavenworth, Kans: Command and General Staff College; 1990.
35. Lynch C, Ford JH, Weed FW, eds. Evacuation hospitals, mobile hospitals, mobile surgical units, professional teams, convalescent depots, evacuation ambulance companies, mobile laboratories. In: Weed FW, ed. *The Medical Department of the United States Army in the World War.* Vol 8. *Field Operations.* Washington, DC: War Department, Department of the Army, Office of The Surgeon General; 1925: Chap 5.
36. Wolfe EP. Evacuation hospital. In: Weed FW, ed. *The Medical Department of the United States Army in the World War.* Vol 3. *Finance and Supply.* Washington, DC: War Department, Department of the Army, Office of The Surgeon General; 1928: Chap 17.
37. Ford JH, ed. Base hospitals. In: Ireland M , ed. *The Medical Department of the United States Army in the World War.* Vol 2. *Administration, American Expeditionary Forces.* Washington, DC: War Department, Department of the Army, Office of The Surgeon General; 1927: Chap 24.
38. Weed FW. Section III: Neurosurgery. In: Ireland M, ed. *The Medical Department of the United States Army in the World War.* Vol 11. *Surgery.* Washington, DC: War Department, Department of the Army, Office of The Surgeon General; 1927: Chap 1.
39. De Tarnowsky G. Surgery at the front. In: Ireland M, ed. *Medical Department of the United States Army in the World War.* Vol 11. *Surgery.* Washington, DC: War Department, Department of the Army, Office of The Surgeon General; 1927: Chap 4.
40. Case JT. Localization and extraction of foreign bodies under x-ray. In: Ireland M. *Medical Department of the United States Army in the World War.* Vol 11. *Surgery.* Washington, DC: War Department, Department of the Army, Office of The Surgeon General; 1927: Chap 8.
41. Rhoads TL. Principles of evacuation, I. The comprehensive plan. *Mil Surg.* 1924;54:296–297.
42. Ford JH, ed. Division of hospitalization (continued)—The professional services. In: Ireland M. *The Medical Department of the United States Army in the World War.* Vol 2. *Administration, American Expeditionary Forces.* Washington, DC: War Department, Department of the Army, Office of The Surgeon General; 1927: Chap 18.
43. Hanigan WC. Neurological surgery during the Great War: the influence of Colonel Cushing. *Neurosurg.* 1988;Sept 23(3):283–294.
44. Terraine J. *White Heat: The New War, 1914–1918.* London, England: Sidgwick and Jackson; 1982.

45. *United States Army in the World War 1917–1919: Reports of the Commander-in-Chief, Staff Sections and Services;* Vol. 25. C-in-C Report File Folder 319: Report Activities of Chief Surgeon's Office, 28 February 1919. Washington, DC: Center of Military History, US Army; 1991.
46. Annual Reports, War Department Fiscal Year Ended 30 June 1919. Report of the Surgeon General, US Army to the Secretary of War, 1919. Vol 1. (Letter of Transmission–Surgeon General Merritte Ireland); Washington, DC: Government Printing Office; 1919: 41.
47. Byerly CR. *Fever of War: The Influenza Epidemic in the US Army During WWI.* New York, NY: The New York University Press; 2005.
48. Pool EH. Wounds of the soft tissues. In: Ireland M. *Medical Department of the United States Army in the World War.* Vol 11. *Surgery.* Washington, DC: War Department, Department of the Army, Office of The Surgeon General; 1927: Chap 12.
49. Ford W. Medical Department transportation. In: Ireland M. *Medical Department of the United States Army in the World War.* Vol 11. *Surgery.* Washington, DC: War Department, Department of the Army, Office of The Surgeon General; 1927: Chap 17.
50. Garrison FH. *Notes on the History of Military Medicine.* Washington, DC: Association of Military Surgeons; 1921–1922: 201–202.

Chapter Six

World War II: Army Forward Surgery on a Worldwide Scale

LANCE P. STEAHLY, MD

INTRODUCTION

WORLD WAR II FOLLOWED in one generation after the end of World War I, which had been called the "war to end all wars." The immense scope of the fighting in World War II required unparalleled planning, preparation, and execution on the part of the military medical community. As Roberts noted in his book, *The Storm of War: A New History of the Second World War*,[1] World War II (quoting Gilbert) "lasted for 2,174 days, cost 1.5 trillion [dollars] and claimed the lives of over 50 million people."[1(p579)] The total casualty count for all of America's armed forces in World War II was 1,073,000 (dead and wounded). The counts varied by combat theater. For example, the Pacific (including Asia) Theater of Operations casualties were 27.6% of that total, of which 106,207 were killed in action (KIA) and 253,142 were wounded in action (WIA).[2(p675)] In the European Theater of Operations, the casualties were 52.4% of that total, of which 185,924 were KIA and 376,000 were WIA.[3(p543)] The remaining casualties of the war (approximately 150,000 KIA and WIA) were from lesser theaters of operation as well as training accidents and the like.

Rather than trying to cover all of the medical and surgical aspects of World War II, this chapter will focus on the narrower topic of Army forward surgery and its impact on care. As an example of forward surgery, the China-Burma-India (CBI) theater of operations will be examined in greater detail throughout this chapter because it required forward surgery in its simplest form to deal with the jungles and mountains, and lack of transportation.

Start of World War II

World War II began in Europe when Germany invaded Poland on 1 September 1939 in conjunction with the Soviet invasion from the east.[1] The Soviet Union and Germany had signed the Molotov-Ribbentrop Pact (a comprehensive nonaggression pact), which had a secret aspect dealing with the countries' respective roles in the coming Polish invasion. The Soviets were to invade and control the eastern portion of Poland, while the Germans were to invade and control the western part of the conquered nation.[1(p29)] The respective forces would meet at agreed upon demarcation points. The Germans (the

SD—*Scherheitsdienst*—and the feared Gestapo) and the Soviets (the NKVD—the People's Commissariat for Internal Affairs [secret police]) quickly set out to arrest classes of people that would be "problems" for the respective regimes. These groups included professional classes, Jews and Gypsies, military officers, and intelligentsia of all types. The secret accords also detailed proposed Soviet advances into Finland and the various Baltic states.[1(pp10,29)] France and Britain declared war on Germany on 3 September 1939 in response to the invasion of Poland. France and England had signed defense treaties with Poland in 1939. There was a lull in the fighting for 6 months until April 1940 (the so-called Phoney War or *Sitzkreig*), when Hitler occupied Denmark (9 April 1940) and invaded Norway. Denmark was taken originally as a prelude to the invasion of Norway. The country did offer some resistance, but its position was weak. The presumed reason for the lull was that the Axis powers were making preparations to expand the conflict to other countries and to stockpile more supplies, but required time. The Allies chose to delay any land offensives, although operations at sea continued. In rapid succession in 1940, the Germans then took over Holland (May), Belgium (May), Luxembourg (May), and France (June). In September 1940, Germany and Italy signed an agreement of cooperation with Japan. Germany and Japan had previously signed an Anti-Comintern Pact (the Comintern was formed by the Soviet Union to foster international communist revolution) in 1936, which Italy had joined in 1937. A military alliance resulted, first in 1939 between Germany and Italy, and further in 1940 with the merging of military goals for the three countries.[1(p5),4(p145)] Italy declared war on the then-Allies (predominantly Britain and France) on 10 June 1940[1(p70)]; Mussolini had already committed Italian forces to the invasion of Ethiopia and Greece.[1(p119)]

Although the war in Europe had started in 1939 with the German invasion of Poland, the United States did not enter the war then, nor during 1940, nor most of 1941. On 10 August 1941, in Placentia Bay off the coast of Newfoundland, the *Prince of Wales* carried Winston Churchill to meet Franklin D Roosevelt on the USS *Augusta*. Churchill had hoped that Roosevelt would declare war on Germany at this shipboard meeting. Roosevelt, however, did not agree to United States involvement at that point, presumably responding instead to America's isolationist sentiment.[5(pp62–68)] Hamilton suggests that it was Roosevelt's intent to dissuade the Axis powers from risking war with the United States by increasing America's deterrence through the showing of its military strength.[5(p35)] Unfortunately, Japan felt its endeavor to pursue a policy of expansion in the Pacific Rim area was threatened by the existence of the US Navy's Pacific Fleet, stationed in Hawaii. The United States finally entered the war following the Japanese attack on Pearl Harbor on 7 December 1941. Congress declared war on Japan on 8 December 1941.[4(p365)] The vote in Congress had only one dissenting member. On 11 December 1941, Germany declared war on the United States, as did Italy.[1(p193),6(p637)]

Army draftees then in service were extended on active duty even if they had completed their 1 year of service; Guard units scheduled to return to state control were immediately retained under federal control.[4(p635)] In April 1941, the War Department planned an operation, called "Rainbow-5,"[7(p46)] to station American troops in the British Isles, of which a portion were to be stationed in Northern Ireland. The first US Army units arrived in Belfast, Ireland, as early as March 1942. The shift of American troops to Northern Ireland would allow the British to move their troops from there to North Africa. By May 1942, the contingent included the 5th Corps (1st Armored Division and 34th Infantry Division).[8]

Start of the War for the Army Medical Department

In 1939 when Germany invaded Poland, the US Army had seven general hospitals and 119 station hospitals. The five general hospitals in the continental United States were: Walter Reed (Washington, DC), Letterman (San Francisco, California), Fitzsimons (Denver Colorado), William Beaumont (El Paso, Texas), and the Army and Navy Hospital (Warm Springs, Georgia). The two overseas general hospitals were Tripler General Hospital (Honolulu, Hawaii) and Sternberg General Hospital (Luzon, Philippines).[9(p2)] The Surgeon General had determined by 1934 that even the peacetime hospitals were inadequate in terms of size and state of the equipment. Little concrete progress was made by 1939, despite planning efforts, due to the limitation of Congressionally appropriated funds. The amounts of appropriated construction funds were only enough to allow for maintenance of existing structures.[9(p3)] The only medical equipment the Army had as backup was stored after World War I and was, at best, of 1918 vintage. Many pieces of equipment were obsolete or close to it. The fiscal limitations consistent with the Depression-era constraints prevented the Army from incorporating the newest technology.[9(p6)]

The 119 station hospitals were designed to deal with the less serious cases, referring the more complicated ones to one of the seven general hospitals. Based upon the Army's experience in the Civil War, the Spanish-American War, and World War I, the Army Surgeon General had a vision of how wartime medicine should be conducted. Hospitals in communication zones (ie, "back home") were designated either station or general hospitals and were considered "fixed." However, in combat zones, there were three classes of hospitals, categorized as: (1) the evacuation hospital, (2) the surgical hospital, and (3) the convalescent hospital. They were considered "mobile hospitals" because they were able to mobilize and physically move; they were to be assigned to field armies.[9(p4)] The surgical hospital could function in the army area much like an evacuation hospital or in the division area as an emergency treatment facility. The surgical hospital in the division treated shock, gave transfusions, treated complex fractures, and generally stabilized the soldier for evacuation to the rear, where the evacuation hospital functioned.[9(p5)]

Medical Officer Training

Although still considered peacetime (even after the invasion of Poland), the Army's various medical branches began some measures to enlarge their numbers in anticipation of a possible mobilization. As an example, the Officer Basic Course for physicians was shortened from 5 months to 3 months in 1940 and was to be expanded to be given twice a year. This shortened course was designed to increase the physician numbers coming into the service and for Regular officers who had not attended the Medical Field Service School, at Carlisle Barracks, Pennsylvania. An expanded class of 111 doctors was graduated in 1940 (the previous largest class had been in 1935 when 81 graduated).[10(p36)]

In preparing for possible conflicts, the Army could look to manpower from the Regulars, the Reserves, and the National Guard. In peacetime, the Army maintained a small professional element, including physicians assigned to the Medical Corps, dentists assigned to the Dental Corps, veterinarians assigned to the Veterinary Corps, and administrative staff with the Medical Administrative Corps. The Army had a Medical Department Reserve, which had professionals with the same qualifications as the Regular group. In the Reserves were many physicians from World War I with military medicine and military administrative experience who had stayed in the Reserves. These physicians were able to be placed in leadership roles due to their awareness of military ways. The Reserve officers performed 2 weeks of duty yearly and took medical extension courses.[9(p2)] The Medical Department of the Army National Guard placed emphasis on field training. In 1939, physicians numbered 1,098 for the Regular component, 15,198 for the Reserves, and 1,085 for the National Guard.[10(p3)]

In 1940, the initial training for the Regular Medical Corps officer was a 4-month Basic Graduate Course at the Army Medical Center (Walter Reed, Washington, DC) followed by a 5-month course at the Medical Field Service School (MFSS) (Carlisle Barracks, Pennsylvania).[10(pp5-6)] The MFSS trained enlisted and officers in matters of administration and field medicine.[10(p4)] The students of the MFSS also participated in the 1940 spring corps and Army maneuvers in Louisiana, termed "The Louisiana Maneuvers." The corps phase was held at Fort Benning, Georgia. Half of the MFSS students were assigned to medical battalions and the other half to regimental medical detachments. The students then switched their assignments during the Army phase of maneuvers, which was held in the Sabine River area of Louisiana. By all accounts, the students showed more interest than the assigned physicians. The MFSS staff felt that the time would have been better spent doing field work near the Carlisle Barracks, Pennsylvania home base.[10(p36)] The officers of the maneuver units had been pulled from hospitals and were inexperienced in command. The Army's modest assessment of their performance in the maneuvers was described as "creditable" in after-action reports.[10(p35)]

The Army started a partial mobilization as part of the limited emergency in the fall of 1940, drawing upon its Regular, Reserves, and National Guard constituents. The Selective Training and Service Act of 1940, starting in September, made medical personnel subject to the draft. Some professionals joined with the threat of being drafted, in many cases to proactively deal with the inevitable and also in the hope of gaining some advantage in terms of assignment. The act was extended for an additional year after the summer of 1941. During the year of partial mobilization, Medical Corps officer strength (physicians) was expanded from 2,000 to 14,000. A 1-month refresher course for National Guard and Reserve officers was begun.[10(pp36,39)] The Army introduced the Army Specialized Training Program to provide training in engineering, science, and medicine for enlisted soldiers. The Army used this program to expand the supply of physicians available for military service. The supply of trained Reserve physicians was used up by the end of 1941. The Army Medical Corps was expanded to 47,000 physicians by August 1945. There were sufficient numbers of older physicians (some of whom deferred their retirements) to treat the home civilian populations.[10(pp42-43)]

The new military physician students first participated in the corps phase at Fort Benning, Georgia. Eight faculty members from the MFSS came with the students. The

Army started a 1-month basic course in December 1940 as a refresher course for Reserve and National Guard. Extension courses by mail remained available for Reserve officers, but not the Regulars.[9(pp36–37)]

In an attempt to ensure that it had enough military physicians, the Army also contracted (through the efforts of the National Research Council) with civilian institutions to provide specialized training for medical officers. In 1942, the Mayo Clinic (Rochester, Minnesota) and the Johns Hopkins Hospital (Baltimore, Maryland) were the initial training institutions. By late 1942, specialized training was given at 15 institutions in 12 areas of specialty work. Many courses were cancelled in late 1943 and by June 1944 there were only remaining courses in neurosurgery, radiology, physical therapy, anesthesiology, and surgery/medicine. The civilian courses were reduced because of shortages in the Medical Corps officers needed to staff military facilities rather than being involved in training in civilian facilities.[10(p60)] However, a special course in anesthesiology for portable surgical hospitals was held from 7 August to 4 September 1943. This type of instruction was critical because the anesthesiology course was designed to train personnel to use the limited anesthesia equipment in the portables. The portables seldom had trained anesthesia personnel and relied on physicians/surgeons who could do double duty.[10(p71)]

Deployment of Medical Assets

In 1942, the most immediate need for troops and medical assets was in the South and Southwest Pacific. In the aftermath of the Japanese victories in the Pacific at the expense of the Allies, urgency was placed on building up American assets in a largely neglected theater. Australia was in grave danger and combat augmentation was needed despite the fact that Europe would soon claim the most attention. In the first 6 months of 1942, the Surgeon General sent to Australia the following: two evacuation hospitals, two surgical hospitals, and four general and 14 station hospitals. Two each of evacuation, surgical, and station hospitals were sent to other islands in the Pacific. The field hospital was created in early 1942 to provide for a smaller and more mobile hospital in the Pacific than the smallest other type of hospital (the 250-bed station hospital).[9(p144)]

By the mid-point of 1942, the emphasis began to turn away from the Pacific and toward North Africa and later Europe. The British were anxious that Europe become the priority because Hitler was the most direct threat for that region.[9(p160)] Toward the end of 1942 and the first half of 1943, US Army hospital units were sent to North Africa and England. However, the Army Inspector General found that the casualty rates for North Africa were less than anticipated and that more than enough beds were available there. The planners had estimated that more casualties would result, hence accounting for the increased number of beds available.[9(p216)]

In early 1942, Northern Ireland also received one general and one station hospital. To support the deployed troops in Iceland (which had replaced British troops earlier) one general hospital was dispatched to Iceland.[11(pp8,10)] Hospital facilities were established by the Army in Greenland, which served all service branch personnel there.[11(p18)] Medical facilities were also established in 1942 in Newfoundland, at Gander and at Fort Pepperrell.[11(p23)] American bases were set up in the early war years extending from the Arctic Circle of Canada to the Azores.[11(p7)]

Two general and three station hospitals were sent from the continental United States to England. Other hospitals were sent to India and to Canada in 1942 to provide care for the builders of the Alcan highway, which was seen as a critical defense need to allow rapid transport of troops and supplies in the event of a Japanese invasion of the American/Canadian/Alaskan mainland.[12(p143)]

American forces were dispatched to Iceland to free up British troops for use elsewhere. Six thousand men of the US Army's 5th Division arrived to supplement 4,100 US Marines. Most of the hospital beds were in the Reykjavik (the capital) area. Three station hospitals came initially in 1942. Later in that year, six more station hospitals and one general hospital arrived in Iceland to deal with the increased number of soldiers.[11(p12)] (If captured, Iceland could be used by the Germans as an additional base to thwart Allied convoys bearing arms and supplies to Russian north ports.) By August 1943, troops were moved to England and the medical support was reduced in Iceland to reflect the changes. By 1945, only the 92nd Station Hospital remained in Iceland.[12(pp195–204)]

Forces were also sent to Greenland. There were ultimately four station hospitals in Greenland. That area was important as a potential German base, which could threaten Canada and the United States. It also had a role as an air base and refueling point on the Atlantic routes.[12(pp190–192)]

In Bermuda, the 221st Station Hospital was the main facility. Bermuda was a British possession off the American Atlantic coast, which had potential use as a German base close to the American mainland. Again, British troops could then be spared for use in the Middle East after the American troops arrived.[11(p8)]

In 1942 there were also discussions under way concerning the proposed invasion of France to drive the Germans out. General George Marshall favored an early cross-Channel invasion while Prime Minister Churchill and Field Marshall Alan Brooke, Chief of the Imperial General Staff, urged caution and delay in such plans. The British view did hold as President Roosevelt was also influenced by the force of Churchill's personality (and arguments). Marshall and Admiral King, the Navy's Chief of Naval Operations, implied that a Pacific first approach might be the result of the British position. President Roosevelt sided with the caution of the British and a continued Europe first commitment. The evolving plan for "Operation Bolero" included sending 30 divisions (1 million soldiers) to England by late 1942 or at least by early 1943.[9(p150)] The Surgeon General estimated at least 100,000 beds would be needed to support Bolero alone. The timing of an Allied invasion proved controversial throughout the war. The Soviets were always pushing for another way to take pressure off their own forces on the Eastern Front. The final consensus was to delay, with a tentative date of 1 May 1944 (even then the date had to be delayed a month due to the shortage of LST [landing ship, tank] landing craft).[1(p465)]

MAJOR COMBAT THEATERS

The Pacific Theater: Difficult Times

The Japanese had been involved in China since the 1931 invasion of Manchuria, which was part of Japan's overall plan to expand its domain and acquire additional raw materials.

The Japanese seized French Indochina in September 1940. The Japanese then captured the oil, tin, and rubber-containing Dutch East Indies (now Indonesia). The attack on Malaya began on 8 December 1941. (The Malayan coast is in the South China Sea with Singapore lying off the southern tip of the Malay Peninsula.) Singapore was considered the most heavily defended British colony. Singapore fell to the Japanese on 15 February 1942. The Japanese could utilize the natural resources of its conquests to supplement its own meager supplies on its island nation.[1(p190)]

As previously mentioned, Japan regarded the United States as its main impediment in its quest to control the Pacific Rim region. Events heated in the Pacific when the United States put an embargo on the sale of scrap metal to Japan, in an attempt to interfere with the acquisition of these materials. The Japanese decided that the time was right to strike at the Pacific Fleet. The attack on Pearl Harbor on 7 December 1941 started at 0600 and was over at 1000. Because the American aircraft carriers were out to sea, the Japanese did not launch their third wave attack for fear of the carriers engaging them in battle.[1(pp191–192)] Japanese attacks on Malaya, Hong Kong, Guam, the Philippines, Wake, and the Midway Islands followed within days.[1(p193)] Wake Island was first attacked on 11 December and a final time on 23 December. Hong Kong was attacked shortly after Pearl Harbor; the 15,000 Commonwealth troops finally surrendered on 25 December 1941. Thailand was taken on 8 December 1941. The fall of Singapore on 15 February 1942 involved the surrender of 130,000 troops.[1(pp200–205)] In the span of just 2 months, the Japanese had made inroads in their overall invasion plans.

General Douglas MacArthur had been the US Army Chief of Staff[1(p208)] until he retired in 1935. MacArthur then received an offer to go to the Philippines as its military advisor. In 1936, MacArthur was made a field marshal in the Philippine Army, while remaining on the US Army retired lists. He was recalled to active duty in the US Army with the coming of war. His 130,000-man force, consisting of 22,400 Americans and 107,600 non-Americans (Philippine forces and forces of the colonial powers of the British, Dutch, Portuguese, and Australians)[1(p208)] had a formidable task given the Japanese naval, air, and army resources in the region.[1(p207)]

The Japanese successfully destroyed most of MacArthur's air assets at Clark Field on the first day of the invasion on 8 December 1941 (18 of 35 B-17 bombers were destroyed, as well as 56 fighters out of 90). By 23 December, MacArthur had abandoned Manila, moving to the Bataan Peninsula and later the island fortress of Corregidor. MacArthur faced upward of 200,000 Japanese troops,[1(p208)] including the 43,000 14th Army soldiers landed on Lingayen Gulf in the Philippines on 22 December 1941 under General Homma.[10(p93)]

Following the Japanese conquests in the Far East and the looming loss of the Philippines, General George Marshall, who had been appointed as the Army Chief of Staff, promoted (with President Roosevelt's concurrence) MacArthur back to the four-star rank (he had returned to his two-star permanent rank in retirement) he had held as the former Army Chief of Staff. Furthermore, Marshall suggested to President Roosevelt that he order MacArthur's withdrawal from the Philippines and award him the Medal of Honor as a symbolic act for the American people. The troops were not complimentary, referring to MacArthur as "Dugout Doug."[13(p82)]

Subsequently, MacArthur was ordered by Marshall (again for President Roosevelt) to Australia on 11 March 1942.[4(p711)] Bataan, just west of Manila, was surrendered by General Jonathan Wainwright (who was left in command by MacArthur) to the Japanese on 9 April 1942.[1(p209)] However, some Americans and Filipinos refused the order to surrender and instead slipped away into the surrounding terrain to form an impromptu guerilla force to continue fighting the Japanese.

The infamous "Bataan Death March" began on 10 April 1942. Seventy-eight thousand troops (12,000 Americans and 66,000 Filipinos) were marched over 60 miles with horrific losses. Of the 78,000 troops who began the march, between 7,000 and 10,000 Filipinos died, as well as 500 to 700 Americans.[1(p209)] The exact numbers lost on the Bataan Death March vary as some Filipinos were able to escape and blend in to the native culture. The Japanese held in contempt the Filipino troops who had been loyal to the Americans. Indeed, the Japanese were described as using Filipino troops and civilians for bayonet practice, which accounts for their greater losses.[1(p209)] The Japanese also executed many along the way who could not keep up with the 5-day march pace. Some were shot execution style while others were bayoneted or shot randomly.[9(pp172–173)] Many more died in the camps to which they were marched. Exact losses at the various prison camps maintained by the Japanese are largely approximations based on estimates and prisoner information. As documented in postwar trials, the conditions at all Japanese prisoner camps were horrific.[1(p209)]

On 6 May 1942, Lieutenant General (LTG) Jonathan Wainwright surrendered the remaining part of the Philippine Islands not already held by the Japanese.[1(p209),6(p713)] The troops had only 3 days' water supply left when he surrendered. Wainwright, a West Point graduate and a friend of MacArthur's, had been the North Luzon commander and became the Philippine commander with the evacuation of MacArthur. Wainwright remained in Japanese captivity until the end of the war.[9(p87)]

Malaria was a problem for the Filipino-American forces well before their capture. Malaria was a serious handicap to military operations, with shortages of quinine for prophylaxis. It is estimated that 24,000 cases of malaria (among the 130,000 troops) afflicted the Filipino and American troops at the time of their surrender in 1942.[9(p503)] The battle for the Philippines including Bataan and Corregidor cost the Americans 2,100 casualties (900 killed and 1,200 wounded) and, of course, the 12,000 captured. The Japanese sustained 4,000 casualties (1,900 killed and 2,100 wounded) as well.[1(p209)] (General MacArthur and his forces returned to the Philippines with the Leyte invasion on 20 October 1944 but it was May of 1945 before all Japanese organized resistance had stopped.[9(p92)])

By early 1942, the Allied fortunes had fallen in land engagements. The war against the Japanese moved to the sea and demonstrated the importance of the aircraft carrier. The Battle of the Coral Sea was not a clear victory for the Americans, although the Battle of Midway, which followed, was such a victory. The Battle of the Coral Sea, on 7 and 8 May 1942, was fought some 800 miles to the northeast of Queensland, Australia, in the Coral Sea. The Americans lost the aircraft carrier *Lexington* while the Japanese lost a light cruiser and had two carriers damaged. The Japanese plan to take Port Moresby in New Guinea was abandoned as a result of the stalemate during the Battle of the Coral Sea.[1(pp251–252)]

The Battle of Midway took place 1 month after the Battle of the Coral Sea and was a decisive turning point in the effort to control the waters of the Pacific Theater of Operations. The naval battle was near the Midway Atoll west of Hawaii—actually midway between Japan and the mainland of the United States, between 4 June and 7 June 1942.[1(p256)] The Japanese lost four carriers to one for the United States. The American carrier *Yorktown* was also damaged. The US success at the Battle of Midway made the 7 August 1942 Guadalcanal invasion (the first American land invasion) possible by freeing up naval assets from imminent threat. However, the Australian and American ships off Guadalcanal were forced to leave when threatened by Japanese naval assets.[1(p257)] (The carrier *Yorktown* and an escorting destroyer were sunk by a Japanese submarine on the way back to Pearl Harbor for repairs.[1(p256)])

Guadalcanal is an island near Telavi in the Southern Solomon group. The Japanese established a seaplane base at Telavi and later started an airfield at Guadalcanal, from which the Japanese could threaten the sea lanes to Australia. On 7 August 1942 this initial Guadalcanal invasion began with 18,700 troops deploying to Guadalcanal. The US Marines were led by Marine Major General (MG) Alexander Vandergrift. The Marines made amphibious landings also on the neighboring islands of Telavi and Gavuth.[1(p257)] Unfortunately, the American naval forces sustained a night attack, in what became known as the Battle of Savo Island, on 7 and 8 August,[1(p258)] while still unloading the Marines' equipment and supplies. The escort withdrew, leaving the Marines to fend for themselves.

In that Battle of Savo Island, three American cruisers and one Australian cruiser were sunk by the Japanese.[1(p258)] These events are well recounted in Newcomb's 1961 book, *The Battle of Savo Island*.[14] The Japanese air assets from Rabaul (in New Britain, Papua New Guinea) had a fairly free hand to attack the Marines. The limited air power of the defending "Cactus Air Force" (the assembled Allied planes in the Guadalcanal area) was no match. On 13 October 1942, after 2 months of fighting, Army troops reinforced the Marines at Guadalcanal.[1(p259),15(p717)] The arrival of Major General Alexander Patch and Army Regular troops caused the Japanese to finally evacuate the island. Guadalcanal losses for the Japanese were approximately 25,000 dead, while for the Americans it was 1,490 dead (mostly Marines) and 4,804 wounded.[1(p259)]

The Japanese had previously created problems in the American-owned Aleutian Island chain off the coast of Alaska. The Japanese had raided the Dutch Harbor Naval Base in the Aleutians with an air attack on 3 June and 4 June 1942. Losses at Dutch Harbor consisted of burning oil tanks and damage to the hospital and a barracks ship. The Japanese had taken the islands of Kiska (6 June 1942) and Attu (7 June 1942).[16(p722)] Almost a year later, on 11 May 1943, Army forces invaded the Aleutian Islands at Attu, off the coast of Alaska. Attu was briskly defended by the Japanese who were heavily dug in. The Americans sustained almost 3,929 casualties (580 killed), while the Japanese were exterminated except for 28 prisoners. The extent of Japanese involvement so close to the Alaskan mainland enhanced the importance of building the Alcan Highway as a military road to speed troops and supplies to the North.[16(pp722–723)]

Elsewhere in the Pacific Theater of Operations, the Army would play varying roles in a largely Navy sphere of operation in the follow-up to Guadalcanal. Kwajalein, Saipan, Tarawa, Guam, Luzon, Iwo Jima, and Okinawa would be other famous battle islands in the drive toward the main Japanese islands.

The China-Burma-India Theater of Operations

World War II involved many distant and diverse theaters of operation that required different types of engagement. For example, the Japanese saw India as a source of British manpower and resources and planned to take India with a view to connecting with the Germans in the Middle East.[1(p188)] The Japanese were moving toward India, the jewel of Britain's Empire, until the May 1942 monsoon, which was so severe that it disrupted Japan's plans. The Japanese took over Burma in May 1942. Burma and Thailand were to be part of the Japanese Greater East Asia Co-Prosperity Sphere. This Sphere was designed to tap the resources of these counties for the Japanese benefit.[1(p188)] Previously the Japanese had taken operational control of the Vichy French-held territory of Vietnam in an agreement with Vichy (in 1940). The Japanese invaded Thailand (8 December 1941). The Thai government then signed an alliance (21 December 1941) effectively giving the Japanese occupation of the country.[1(p260)]

Britain was unsuccessful in 1942 and 1943 in conventional warfare in its attempts to retake the Arakan, the coastal province of Burma, and Akyab Island, off the coast of Burma with an important airfield. Hence, the British adapted a unique version of irregular warfare (long penetration jungle fighting) that was the innovation of British Brigadier General (BG) (later MG) Orde Wingate.[1(p260)] An epic personality, Wingate was an unconventional officer employing irregular, but successful, techniques (such as hit-and-run tactics and ambushes where the enemy least expected) against the Japanese in Burma. Wingate's forces (3,000 men[1(p262)]) known as the "Chindits," were composed of Indian, Gurkha, and British troops who engaged the Japanese far behind their lines.[1(p260)] (The origin of the term "Chindit" is uncertain. Some feel that it may be Wingate's version of the Burmese *chinthe* [lion] but only Wingate knew and he did not report it.[1(p260)]) The Chindit expeditions in 1943 and 1944 created much press publicity for their courageous raids. The reporters based in India (but not embedded with the units) popularized the tales of extraordinary human endurance. The public found encouragement in their dramatic episodes.

As with the other theaters of operation, the China-Burma-India (CBI) theater had many casualties for the medical service to tend to. The forward surgical support for the wounded soldier had been well founded in World War I. The more refined forward surgery concept of World War II was exemplified in its most elemental form by the portable surgical hospital. The most "colorful" of the portable surgical hospitals was the Seagrave Unit headed by Lieutenant Colonel (LTC) Gordon S Seagrave.

GORDON S SEAGRAVE AND THE SEAGRAVE UNIT

Seagrave was born in Rangoon, Burma, to a family of Baptist missionaries. In fact, he was the fourth generation of missionaries, although he was the first to be a doctor. He graduated from Johns Hopkins University School of Medicine in Baltimore, Maryland, in 1921. Seagrave then completed an internship at Baltimore's Union Memorial Hospital before he and his wife came to Namkham (in the Shan States of the northeastern part of Burma) in 1922.[17(p10)]

Over the years, he developed a hospital, sponsored by the Baptist Mission, caring for native Karen, Kachin, and Shan people. (Seagrave enjoyed some fame after he was the subject of a *Life* magazine article, with photographs in 1943.[18(p23)]) As he noted in his books, *Burma Surgeon* (1943)[19(p35)] and his later *Burma Surgeon Returns* (1946),[17(p10)] he had provided dedicated care to these people in the local native tradition, honoring the family as the caretaker. Entire families would literally camp out with their family member patient and provide some of the simpler care.[20(pp357–358)] By 1942, his hospital had a 100-bed capacity. Interestingly, he had set up an in-house program to train native girls as nurses. It started with 11 students but he later expanded it to 19. Seagrave's "Burmese nurses" were not Burmese at all, but instead represented the Shan, Karen, Kaelin, and a number of other ethnic groups.[17(p10)] His nurses called the chain-smoking surgeon "Doctor Cigarette."[17(p11)]

The British hoped to reestablish control of Burma, while the Chinese were concerned with the loss of the Burma Road (which was a major supply route for China), and to that end the Chinese had positioned the 6th Army in the Eastern front.[21(p33)] The British under the command of Lieutenant General (LTG) Sir William Slim (14th Army Commander) requested that Seagrave provide medical care for the Chinese 6th Army, then operating in eastern Burma in the First Burma Campaign. The Chinese 6th Army was one of the Nationalist Chinese more elite units.[22(p36)] However, the Chinese had few medical supplies and their medical organization was almost nonexistent.[22(p103)] Seagrave organized his unit as a civilian mobile surgical hospital.[23(p288)] Seagrave and his staff of American and British ambulance drivers and British medical professionals took care of the Chinese. Seagrave found that the Chinese were in such poor condition that they required immediate medical attention.[22(p104)]

After Americans, in the form of LTG Joseph Stilwell and his military forces, arrived in Burma in February 1942,[17(p32)] Seagrave had a decision to make about joining the military effort. He could remain a civilian or he could become a military physician. Some in his Baptist missionary circle were critical of the decision that he reached. Seagrave said in his *Burma Surgeon Returns*, "I am a conscientious objector. I detest war . . . in the face of what Germany and Japan have done to the world, the pacifism that will choke over the idea of wearing a uniform in a reconstructing group is something the world can do without."[17(p120)] Seagrave also noted that, "All my life, I've been my own boss, often to the consternation of the American Baptist Burma Mission."[17(p110)] He continued, "When you are actually fighting and hoping to wipe something bad out of the world, the Army is the only place to be."[17(p110)]

Seagrave asked to be under American command after Stilwell arrived in Burma. Stilwell (called "Vinegar Joe" behind his back, reflecting his caustic personality[24(p1)]) had been appointed in 1942 by President Roosevelt and Chief of Staff General George Marshall as the Commander of American forces in the CBI and as the concurrent Chief of Staff for the Chinese leader Chiang Kai-shek.[1(p265)] Stilwell's staff surgeon, Colonel (COL) Robert

Williams, swore Seagrave in as a major in the US Army Medical Corps on 21 April 1942. Williams followed the now-Major (MAJ) Seagrave's recommendation to split Seagrave's repurposed missionary unit in order to care for both the 5th and 6th Chinese armies.[23(p288)] Stilwell agreed to his request. Seagrave was joined by Captain (CPT) John Grindlay, who had graduated from Harvard Medical School in 1935. Subsequently, he completed a year at Dartmouth's Mary Hitchcock Hospital as a pathology fellow and then another year at Hitchcock Hospital as a rotating intern. Grindlay then trained in surgery at the Mayo Clinic and earned an MS in surgery from the University of Minnesota. Grindlay became the head of surgical services for Seagrave's unit.[21(p28)]

Seagraves's medical supplies largely came from American Red Cross stocks at Lashio in Burma.[22(p104)] Grindlay had been sent from the American Military Mission, the military part of the American Embassy in China that provided assistance and distributed Lend-Lease shipments to China. CPT Donald H O'Hara, a dentist, also joined the unit. He had the misfortune to be allergic to rice, which due to shipping limitations necessarily formed part of the American rations available. O'Hara had come directly from the United States.[23(p288)]

General Joseph "Vinegar Joe" Stilwell

The war was not going well for the Allies in Burma during the period from March to May of 1942. The Japanese had defeated the British and Chinese armies and rolled the respective armies toward India (British) and back to China (Chinese). General Stilwell had sent part of his headquarters out of country by plane while he stayed with the rest. Stilwell actually did not have many American troops in his command. Most of his troops were Chinese units that he had been training. His headquarters unit was American (100 officers and enlisted soldiers), largely in an advisory, rather than command and control, sense. He famously declined to get on the evacuation plane, offering no reasons for his decision. Two Army Air Force colonels had been sent by General Hap Arnold who told them to "rescue" Stilwell.[25(p292)] It was because of this refusal that air advocates said that "Walking Joe" did not understand airpower.[25(p293)]

Because the Japanese were closing in on his forces, Stilwell had to leave quickly. He led a party, including Seagrave and his nurses, to Imphal, India, a journey of over 600 miles. The group numbered approximately 100 people, which included 18 officers and six enlisted personnel. Seagraves's unit, with 19 Burmese nurses and two civilian doctors, provided the medical support. An English Quaker ambulance unit of seven (the Friends Ambulance Unit) joined the group and helped with the provision of medical care, specifically the transport of patients. The remaining members of the *ad hoc* group consisted of some British officers, an American missionary, and some Malayan and Burmese porters and cooks.[25(p293)] COL Williams served as the headquarters detachment medical officer with the group.[25(p290)] Stilwell later added a group of 15 British commandos who were independently evacuating from Northern Burma. He also hired a Chinese pack train that his party came across. The mules were used to carry items that an additional hired contingent of 60 local people "carriers" could not transport.[25(p295)] Seagrave's unit also created extensive good will by their treatment of Burmese villagers they encountered along the march. This good will was confirmed by the natives' willingness to serve as porters and guides.[24(p11)]

Stilwell set the jungle march rate at the standard Army 105 steps a minute as infantry soldiers are taught. He kept the pace himself and was disgusted that many of the "soft" members of the group fell out from fatigue or heat exhaustion. Stilwell first had to grant a 5-minute rest per hour.[25(p296)] Later Stilwell had to increase the rest period to 10 minutes per hour as malaria and dysentery took their toll on many of the marchers. Making matters worse, COL Williams' supply of medicines was stolen at one point under suspicious circumstances (probably by a member of the party; the medications were not recovered). Williams called for more rest stops due to the sickness. Stilwell reportedly said to him, "Dammit, Williams, you and I can stand it. We're both older than any of them. Why can't they take it?"[24(p6)] Stilwell was in good physical shape despite his 59 years of age.[26(p96)] Seagrave's nurses, ages 17 to 22, kept the unit going with their good cheer and singing[20(p60)] hymns, favoring "Onward Christian Soldiers."[23(p39)] The personal diary of Grindlay[16] details the arduous nature of the "walk out" as well as the courage of the participants. Grindlay kept up the 30 miles per day pace, which he credits to the efforts of Seagrave's nurses.[21(p29)] Finally, largely due to Stilwell's force of personality, the group made it to India without loss of life. The exodus took 3 weeks of moving through the jungles and mountains of north Burma.[23(p298)]

Stilwell described the earlier defeat that made necessary the trek to reporters as "a hell of a beating and it's humiliating as hell."[23(p290)] Stilwell's frank comments were in contrast to those of the British Major General Sir William Slim, who had taken his troops on a roughly parallel 600-mile trek with two divisions with reduced strength of several thousand troops.[26(p96)] Slim tried to give the event a favorable spin by speaking in terms of "strategic withdrawal." (In Burma, Slim was a corps commander in charge of the Burma Corps [consisting of the 1st Burma Division and the 17th Indian Infantry Division] under the command of General Sir Harold Alexander. Slim went on to command a joint English and Indian Army that eventually retook Burma in 1945.[1(p567)]) The Burma Corps of the British Army had sustained 13,000 casualties overall, of which 9,000 were missing in action. Stilwell reported in his *Stilwell Papers* that many of the missing were lost or Japanese prisoners of war.[26(p97)]

Stilwell's plan, once he reached Imphal, India, was to train Chinese troops of the 6th Army (an elite Chinese force) there to retake the northern part of Burma. Seagrave and his unit helped screen and treat the Chinese troops for various diseases and disabilities. Over the course of a few months, his unit vaccinated the thousands of Chinese troops against diseases such as smallpox, typhoid, and cholera with vaccines shipped from India.[27(p326)] At Ramgarh, India, Seagrave treated the damaged Chinese 22nd and 38th Divisions, which formed the main Stilwell forces there.[27(p138)]

CPT Grindlay became the head of surgical services under Seagrave at Ramgarh after the "walk out."[17,21(p36)] The unit remained there until mid-1943, when it moved to northwest Burma. The unit provided medical care to Chinese and American construction units working on the Ledo Road, which was to be a replacement for the captured Burma Road to supply China. Seagrave later established a hospital at Tagap Ga to be followed by other units down the Ledo Road.[21(p37)] Grindlay told the Surgeon General that every jungle combat unit needed a mobile surgical unit. He felt there were enough restless surgeons to form teams if there were too few portables.[24(p324)]

By late 1942, Stilwell had some 32,000 Chinese troops in training. Stilwell was ultimately successful in his plan to train the Chinese to improve their combat readiness, despite opposition from the British, Claire Chennault, and Chiang Kai-shek. Chennault had resigned his Army commission to form a nascent air force for the Chinese to engage the Japanese. Chennault ultimately became a major general, in charge of the US Army Air Forces' 14th Air Force in China. Chennault and Stilwell were in constant disagreement over the role of airpower in the CBI Theater.[1(p268)] Chiang Kai-shek resisted Stilwell's more aggressive plans for utilization of the Chinese troops. Chiang and the Communists were more interested in keeping the other side from advancing its agenda. In the end, Chiang tied up Japanese troops, but was not able to take out the Communist Chinese.[1(p268)] The British were leery of armed Chinese troops in India because they might have some effect on the possibility of an Indian rebellion (which did not occur) to secure Indian independence. In some cases, the British detained fervent nationalists. Nonetheless, India supported Britain in World War II, adding many troops that served in all theaters. Furthermore, the Indians did not wish to use Chinese troops to retake Burma because it had been among British possessions. The British were concerned that Indian troops would support indigenous fervor for independence.[10(pp314,315)] Marshall's support was critical to the success of using Chinese armies to defeat the Japanese in Northern Burma.[28(p66)]

Stilwell had been appointed by Chiang as his Chief of Staff (but he had no real control in this position)[18(pp86–87)] and by Marshall as the Commanding General of the US Army Forces in China. He was no stranger to controversy. His contentious relations with the Nationalist leader Chiang Kai-shek centered on Stilwell's view that the leader was more interested in fighting the Chinese Communists than the Japanese. Stilwell's vision of how things should go in the China-Burma-India theater didn't correspond to those of General Chennault, Chiang, or the British. Stilwell has been accused of favoring Chiang merging his forces with the Communists to fight the Japanese. Stilwell did propose at one point that the Nationalists operate with the Communist 8th Route Army, to no success.[23(pp388–389)] Neither the Chinese Nationalists nor the Communists were as interested in fighting the Japanese as they were in keeping the other side down and jockeying for position once the war ended. The Nationalists and the Communists were more interested in fighting each other. (Because the Communists were ultimately the winners of the struggle in 1949, both Stilwell and General Marshall were subsequently incriminated in the 1949 loss of China by such notables as Herbert Hoover.[29(pp352–353)])

Stilwell had graduated from West Point in 1904. He stood 32nd in a class of 124 and ranked as a lieutenant of cadets.[25(p15)] In 1911, while stationed in the Philippines, Stilwell had his first contact with China, touring the country as a revolution took place installing Sun Yat-sen as president.[25(pp37–41)] Stilwell was a World War I veteran of some distinction. Over the following 20 years, he had assignments that alternated between the United States and China, becoming fluent in Chinese as a consequence. In World War II, Stilwell hoped for the command of troops in the invasion of North Africa, but deferred to Marshall's selection.[25(p86)] Stilwell had diverse roles including the role as Commanding General of American forces in India, Burma, and China. He also had the job of controlling Lend-Lease material to be dispersed in theater. As General Albert Wedemeyer, Stilwell's successor, later learned, the position in China was an impossible one due to the ongoing Nationalist-Communist struggle for power and the corruption of the Nationalist regime.[30(pp109–130)]

MERRILL'S MARAUDERS

On 6 January 1944, 3,000 men formed the group known as the 5307th Composite Unit ("Provisional") (code named "Galahad").[27(p293)] It was organized into three battalions with 700 pack animals total for the battalions. Each battalion had three combat teams. An air supply section was set up to provide the planned air supply for the troops, as well as for casualty evacuation.[27(pp293–294)] COL Charles N Hunter led the volunteer unit for several months before General Stilwell appointed a new commander, Brigadier General (BG) Frank D Merrill, in June 1944. Soon thereafter the unit was dubbed "Merrill's Marauders."[27(p293)]

The "Marauders," an all-volunteer unit, were all physically fit and ready for a risky mission. They were expected to handle up to 3 months of jungle fighting. They were also expected to be in poor physical condition at the end of this period, and thus would require prolonged rest and healing. No replacements were anticipated.[27(p294)] They actually spent 4 months in the jungle. They evacuated their sick and wounded to clearings in the jungle where light planes could evacuate a few men at a time for treatment.[27(pp294–295)]

The new unit marched 100 miles from Ledo to Shingbwiyang, where newsmen met them. This was the route through the mountains and jungles to deal with the Japanese as part of their first combat mission.[27(p295)] Merrill's men stayed in the Burma jungles striking the Japanese for 4 months, suffering innumerable trials and privations. The diseases were numerous outside of battle injuries. The malaria rate was extremely high, despite Atabrine prophylaxis, to the extent that operations were impaired.[27(p296)] The Marauders also suffered from many diseases including dengue fever, dysentery, diarrhea of various diseases, neuropsychiatric conditions, and numerous skin conditions.[27(p323)] Amebic and bacillary dysentery were both common.[27(p392)] Scrub typhus was also a serious medical problem.[27(p393)] The Marauder's long trek of over 700 miles, including the 100-mile initial trek, compounded their exhaustion. Indeed, Merrill sustained a myocardial infarction during the strenuous march. Although Atabrine discipline was enforced, its use fell. The men's morale was low because they were overcome by the pressures to continue the mission, as well as disheartened by the tough restrictions on evacuation and relief. As the morale fell, Atabrine discipline fell further.[23(p395)]

Air evacuation was critical to the Marauder mission. The Marauders were evacuated when possible from jungle clearings or even sand bars in rivers. Light planes (L-1 and L-5 planes) could get in and then out of such isolated areas. They would take the injured to landing strips where C-47s could land. The C-47s flew the casualties to the 73rd Evacuation Hospital or the 20th General Hospital, both located at Ledo.[23(p307),27(pp325–326)] A disadvantage of the longer land evacuation route to larger hospitals was that some patients could have been restored to duty more quickly if treated at a more forward facility. Combat Command directing the Marauder combat had no mobile evacuation hospitals but did improvise using the Seagrave unit and the 25th Field Hospital. The 400-bed 25th Field Hospital was able to function like three portable surgical hospitals by dividing itself into hospital sections. One such hospital section took over a Seagrave unit and treated 460 cases in 8 days at Taipha Ga.[27(p324)]

The medical situation in the China-Burma-India theater was more complicated than in the Pacific. Troops in the Pacific did not have to endure the long periods of remote fighting behind enemy lines. They could be resupplied by sea while the troops in the China-Burma-India theater relied on air supply because the rough trails (and nonexistent roads) precluded other means. Supplies were obtained through British channels in Karachi, Pakistan, and other locations.[23(pp507–508)]

North Africa/Sicily/Italy Prelude to the European Continent

By 1943, the Americans had shifted their focus to the European area of operations as part of the "Europe First" decision. Britain, led by Prime Minister Churchill, was pushing for the defeat of Hitler as the priority before Japan. The Soviet Union put pressure on the Allies to relieve German pressure on Soviet troops by occupying the Germans elsewhere. President Roosevelt adopted this plan, although the US Chief of Naval Operations, Admiral Ernest King, felt the Pacific should be the priority. The emphasis on Europe had been decided at the highest levels. In part, this was driven by the fact that the Germans had quickly defeated the French forces and occupied the country. The British Expeditionary Force (BEF) withdrew from the Continent to the port area of Dunkirk, where their troops were evacuated. However, the British left most of their arms and equipment behind. The French surrendered on 22 June 1940. The Vichy French were allowed some autonomy until the Germans occupied the whole of France in November 1942.[1(p77)] The French colonies of North Africa remained loyal to the Vichy French regime. Hence, the initial Allied combined operations were directed to North Africa where "Operation Torch" was to take place. General Bernard Montgomery (later Field Marshal) had just won his victory at El Alamein in North Africa on 8 November 1942. The British needed a real land victory to restore the morale of the Commonwealth. The Germans' *Afrika Korps*, depleted of resources, men, and munitions, was soundly defeated,[1(p300)] and provided this much needed morale boost.

MG Dwight D Eisenhower commanded the overall invasion force for Operation Torch on 8 November 1942. The operation consisted of an amphibious landing on Algerian and Moroccan beaches facing Vichy French forces.[3(p645)] Atkinson saw the North African operation as being very important. He pointed out that the North African invasion surpassed all other operations in World War II for its risk, complexity, and daring. It was also the first joint English and American operation.[3(pp50–51)]

Allied landings in Sicily on 7 August 1943 began the race to Messina between Patton's and Montgomery's forces. Once at Messina, Patton's troops won the race, but the Allies found that the Germans had already evacuated to Italy proper.[4(p651)] The collapse of Sicily had the effect of hastening the end of Mussolini's rule, despite the fact that a large German force was able to be evacuated to mainland Italy to fight again.[1(p376)] The 5th US Army, under the Command of LTG Mark C Clark, landed near Naples on 9 September 1943. The amphibious landings were planned for the Bay of Salerno (south of Naples), which was the most northern point that airpower could be concentrated at this point in the war.[1(p378)] The Battle of Salerno, as the landing was called, ran from 9 to 16 September 1943, with a strong German defense of the beach.[4(p652)] The Germans had concentrated their resources in a bid to defeat Clark, which almost succeeded.[1(p378)] Indeed, LTG Clark came close to ordering the withdrawal of the 6th Corps at Salerno.[1(p380)] The Allies had 15,000 casualties (out of 170,000 troops) at Salerno, as opposed to only 8,000 for the Germans.[1(p381)] Italy surrendered to the Allies on 18 September 1943. The Allies met difficult resistance going toward the North.[3(p653)] For example, the advance up the Apennine Mountains to reach the Po Valley was challenging, in part because of bad weather. However, the Germans used the 80-mile wide Apennine Mountains to help in their rearguard actions, while making great use of mines and booby-traps in villages.[1(p382)] The situation in Naples was poor with disease, starvation, and corruption rampant. With rain, snow, and temperatures at an all-time low, disease was an Allied problem (pneumonia, trench foot, fevers, jaundice, and dysentery).[1(p382)]

There were four battles of Monte Cassino involving a wide variety of Allied troops from many countries, holding up the Allied advance for 4 months.[1(pp390,393)] The great monastery hill of Monte Cassino was the strongest part of the heavily fortified German Gustav Line that bounded Mount Cairo. The town of Cassino surrounded the base of the 1,700-foot high peak where the abbey was located.[1(p386)] The capture of Monte Cassino (although resulting in the destruction of the abbey) was necessary to break through the Gustav Line.[1(pp388–389)]

The landing at Anzio (a small port used for holiday travels in peacetime that is located 30 miles south of Rome[1(p393)]) and the resulting conflict were much criticized, especially by the British War Cabinet.[1(p397)] The Allied losses were high and the whole operation was stalled by the Germans. The German leadership of Field Marshal Albert Kesselring was hard to match. He was the German general with ultimate charge of the forces in Italy. Rommel reported to Kesselring in North Africa and in Italy. He was an infantryman who transferred to the *Luftwaffe* after its creation. Kesselring had a native genius for tactics.[1(p378)]

Not all of the action in Italy was on the ground. The Germans bombed the American ship *John Harvey* in the harbor at Bari, Italy, on 2 December 1943. Mustard gas had been introduced into the European Theater by the United States in case the Axis Powers used gas; the *John Harvey* was part of that plan, which was kept strictly classified for years. The mustard gas on board the ship mixed with oil on the surface of the water.[3(pp653–654)] The horrific burns that resulted were not acknowledged to medical providers to be gas-related for a number of weeks. During the interim period, medical personnel thought that they were dealing with exposure because the gas was diluted enough to escape detection. There were 800 casualties hospitalized, of which 628 were ultimately attributed to mustard gas exposure. Fifty-nine deaths were listed as a direct result of gas exposure. The majority of the casualties were American and many were merchant seamen. The injured were wrapped in blankets while still in contaminated clothing. The majority of the injured were hospitalized in British hospitals because the American hospital equipment had been destroyed in the bombing.[11(pp350–351)]

The Americans also considered using mustard gas and phosgene in the Pacific against the Japanese. Apparently Generals Marshall and MacArthur supported the recommendation of the Anglo-American Lethbridge Commission to use these materials. President Roosevelt, however, did not allow the measure to progress.[1(p568)] The Germans did not use gas because Hitler was opposed to its use in combat, based on his World War I experience in the trenches.

The Americans were not involved in fighting on the Eastern Front, other than providing copious supplies and equipment under the Lend-Lease Program. The Germans had made remarkable progress in the early invasion of Russia in July and August 1941. The Germans would later be slowed into the spring of 1942 by the defense of Leningrad. The terrible Russian winter weather also slowed down any German advance. However, the German loss of Stalingrad on 2 February 1943,[1(p343)] and the tactical draw at Kursk[1(p520)] 5 months later, turned the tide fully against Germany on the Eastern Front. The success of the Soviets did, consequently, affect the fighting in the West being waged by the Americans, the British, and the Free French. The Soviets were persistent in their demands for the Allies to mount a second front against the Germans to take pressure off the Soviets. The struggles on the Eastern Front had been epic in proportions. For example, the Stalingrad campaign ran from 17 July 1942 until the German surrender on 2 February 1943. Out of an estimated quarter million German troops in the city, only 90,000 remained to surrender at the end of that battle.[1(p343)] The Germans lost approximately 20 German divisions and several divisions of Allies at Stalingrad.[1(p344)] Kursk, which is situated 315 miles south of Moscow, was the site of the German Operation *Zitadelle*, an epic tank battle (only 5 months after the surrender at Stalingrad) between the Soviets and the Germans. Although losses were high for both sides, the Germans withdrew after 2 months of combat during July and August 1943.[1(pp417,427–428)]

The European Continent

The Allies moved on to Sicily after North Africa. As already noted, the Allied campaigns on the Italian mainland were to follow with the 1943 amphibious landings at Salerno (south of Naples). Italy capitulated and Mussolini was killed. Although the Germans in Italy were under the able generalship of Field Marshal Albert Kesselring, the Allies ultimately prevailed.

Army operations in Europe were focused on the impending amphibious landings upon the well-defended coastline. Roberts, in his *Storm of War*, states that a significant defeat in the invasion of Normandy in 1944 "would almost certainly have had the effect of the United States abandoning the Germany First policy and turning to the Pacific War instead."[1(p461)] In preparation for the invasion, the Allies mounted two Fortitude operations, which were elaborate deception operations started years prior to the planned date of the invasion.[1(p463)]

General Eisenhower had been chosen to be the Supreme Commander of the Allied Expeditionary Force in December 1943. His headquarters was located in London, which was the central planning site for the invasion. The original plan was to invade as early as May 1944, but the LST landing craft used at Anzio, Italy, had to be brought to England. Hence June 1944 was the new target with the actual date depending on the weather. The loss of an LST at Slapton Sands in a preinvasion exercise further strained the landing craft availability.

After much planning and preparation, the invasion of the Continent began with Operation Overlord and D-Day on 6 June 1944. After the success of D-Day, the Allies began pushing forward, finally crossing the Rhine River into Germany in March 1945.

The Germans launched a nearly successful counteroffensive at the Ardennes in Belgium. However, the evitable momentum of Allied troops and the Soviets pushing in from the East sealed Germany's fate.

STRUCTURE OF FORWARD SURGERY IN WORLD WAR II

Full-Sized Surgical Hospitals in Combat Environments

In actual practice, the 400-bed surgical hospital operated largely in the Mediterranean and Southwest Pacific area, in part to supplement the surgical capacity of field and evacuation hospitals. Organized under Table of Organization and Equipment (T/O&E) 8-231, this unit consisted of two hospitalization units and one mobile surgical unit. The mobile surgical unit had integral transport. Interestingly, the two hospitalization units could each field 200 beds and could operate independently of one another.[9(pp280–281)]

The World War II evacuation hospital was usually about 400 beds (which was smaller than the World War I evacuation hospital, which could range above 1,000 beds, as needed). In Europe, the 1st Army prior to "Operation Overlord" (the Normandy Invasion) had organized 10 such 400-bed evacuation hospitals and a 750-bed evacuation hospital.[31(p109)] The field hospital provided forward surgical support by sending a platoon with surgical teams closer to the actual combat. In Europe, the field hospital platoon provided most of the forward emergency surgery, drawing upon the experience of the World War I mobile surgical unit.

The Pacific Theater of Operations and the China-Burma-India Theater of Operations were similar in that they both presented medical difficulties unlike that of the European Theater of Operations. Supply difficulties (especially in the CBI) were constant. The environmental conditions for the fighting were extraordinary. The mountains, jungles, and rain were found in the Pacific and the CBI, although many Pacific islands had relatively even terrain. The common thread in the Pacific and CBI theaters is that the conditions were hard to endure and conducive to disease. Tropical diseases such as malaria were rampant, which added to the burden presented by combat casualties.

Portable Surgical Hospitals in Constrained Environments

Creation of the portable surgical hospital (PSH) was a direct response to the need for small mobile units to fit into the CBI and Pacific theaters. In New Guinea and Papua, the dense jungle and terrain made larger unit operations difficult. The standard evacuation hospitals of 400 to 750 beds were too large and cumbersome for the task at hand. The mobile surgical hospital described in Field Manual (FM) 8-5, *Mobile Units of the Medical Department* (1944),[32] consisted of a headquarters and three subordinate units. The three units included one mobile surgical unit and two hospitalization units.[32(p418a)] The one mobile surgical unit was to hold "sufficient integral transport for its own movement, together with the necessary facilities for messing, supply and technical operations."[32(p423a)] Evacuation, field, and surgical hospitals could not be where they were needed due to their inherent lack

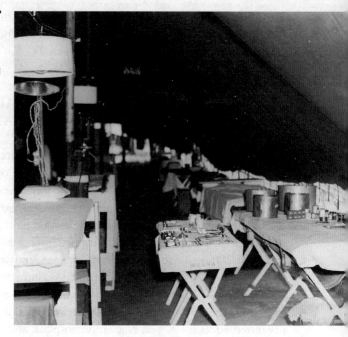

FIGURE 6-1. The interior of a portable surgical hospital showing the limited surgical equipment that had to be carried every step of the way. Improvised instrument and tray tables are shown. The portable surgical hospital had five operating room tables for the three surgeons, which allowed greater efficiency and the ability to handle more cases. The recovery period was geared to evacuate the patient by ground or air as soon as the tactical situation allowed. The wounded soldiers needing immediate surgery were taken to the portable surgical hospital. The less immediate surgery cases were taken to the clearing station located about 2 miles away from the portable surgical hospital. Photograph courtesy of the AMEDD Center of History and Heritage, Image #MU-WWII-LL-012.

of mobility. Furthermore, division clearing stations were not intended to provide emergent surgery.

The 12 January 1942 version of Military Field Manual 8-5, published by the War Department, made no mention of portable units, other than field hospitals.[33] FM 8-5, as amended 20 April 1944, discussed the portable surgical hospital in detail.[32] It was described as a mobile 25-bed unit that would "support the surgical service of a task force or division engaged in jungle or amphibious warfare."[32(p417)] It would also provide "surgical care to the sick or critically wounded for whom transportation to the rear would be fatal."[32(p417)] Other functions outlined included provision of temporary hospitalization, pending arrival of larger units, and to support division clearing stations.[32(p417)]

FM 8-5 (per the 1944 amendment) also spelled out the deployment from land to amphibious operations. Of note, it pointed out that the portable surgical hospital (PSH) was to be "employed in areas where the terrain is such that . . . all equipment must be hand carried, and all patients must be evacuated by litter."[32(p418a)] The PSH finds "its primary usefulness in jungle warfare."[32(p418a)] In amphibious operations, the PSH are "moved on landing craft."[32(p418c)] After landing, the portable surgical hospital would set up in a "sheltered area or near a route of evacuation."[32(p418c)] The equipment would be "limited to bare essentials."[32(p418c)]

The *Military Medical Manual*[34] was published by the Military Service Publishing Company of Harrisburg, Pennsylvania, in a nonofficial format to introduce medical officers to medicine in the military, in preparation for their deployment to austere locations. It provided the young doctor with listings of Army tactics, organization, and procedures in a more readable format. The 1941 4th edition of the *Military Medical Manual*[35] mentioned only the 400-bed surgical hospital in the Army's inventory. The 1941 *Mobile Units of the Medical Department,* which was published by the Medical Field Service School, also listed only the 400-bed hospital.[36] The 1944 edition of the *Military Medical Manual* presented more detail about the portable surgical hospital[34] (Figure 6-1). (Of interest, Carlisle Barracks, the location of the Medical Field Service School [the training center for military medicine] had been the home of General Hospital No. 31 in World War I. The Medical Service School began classes there in June 1921. Carlisle Barracks is currently the home of the Army War College.)

Organization of the Portable Surgical Hospitals

COL Percy J Carroll (later brigadier general), the Chief Surgeon of the US Army Forces Far East and of the US Army Services of Supply, conceived of the need for the PSH. In a 1944 article, COL Augustus Thorndike, Medical Corps, reported that Carroll discussed the PSH concept with his surgical service as early as June 1942. Carroll saw the PSH as a temporary solution to an operational necessity because evacuation in jungle warfare was problematic.[37(p79)] Carroll at first split the hospitals in Australia into smaller units that were mobile. He tried various configurations of personnel and equipment to reach the desired portable setup. These units were to be scattered around Australia in expectation of the Japanese invasion (which never came). The Japanese had landed on 8 March 1942 on the northeast coast of New Guinea.[1(p210)] The Japanese forces advancing toward Port Moresby, New Guinea, were repulsed at the otherwise indecisive Battle of the Coral Sea with the sinking of one Japanese light carrier and the damage of two additional carriers. The Japanese withdrew as their resources and supply lines were stretched too far. Hence, the threatened Japanese push toward Australia was halted permanently.[1(p252)]

Carroll noted that the difficult terrain, with mountains and jungle swamps in New Guinea and Papua, would call for smaller combat units and thus the need for small and mobile units to provide surgical/medical care. It is noteworthy that Carroll saw the PSH as a compromise method to offer emergency surgical care in the difficult jungle settings of the Pacific and the CBI theaters. Carroll envisioned that the portables would be replaced by larger hospitals as the war logically progressed. He felt that larger hospitals would be brought in as the combat situation stabilized, the areas were secured, and the need for evacuation lessened. However, Carroll felt the need for portables would remain in many diverse areas, including remote areas of Burma, the Philippines, and some Pacific islands with rugged terrain. These more remote locations would not be sites for larger hospitals. When combat commenced in these areas, the need for surgery close to the combat called for innovation because evacuations were hard in such conditions.

The PSH was envisioned as a way to provide surgery on a smaller scale in jungle and amphibious operations. Carroll initially had an adequate supply of well-trained surgeons in Australia to assign to the new portables. (Unfortunately, the degree of surgical training for later assignees would not meet this standard. There was a tendency at higher command levels to assign the best trained surgical talent to the larger hospitals. The thinking was often that such talent would be wasted on small remote operations such as the portable surgical hospital.) Once stabilized, the wounded could be transported to larger

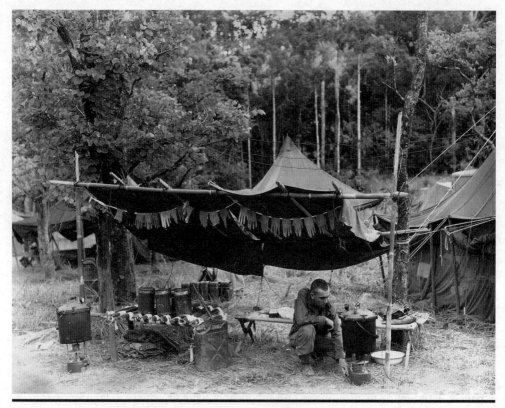

FIGURE 6-2. Portable Surgical Hospital. Gloves are being sterilized in the portable sterilizer units. Gloves washed hanging out to dry. All parts of the portable surgical hospital had to be hand carried. Photograph courtesy of the AMEDD Center of History and Heritage, Image #MU-WWII-LL-015.

facilities.[38(p541)] Hence, the PSH was created to provide a truly mobile alternative to the 400-bed evacuation hospital. Due to the European Theater of Operations priority of the Combined Chiefs of Staff, and the emphasis on the Southwest Pacific area (MacArthur) and the Central Pacific area (Nimitz) drives, the CBI theater was given a very low priority for much of the war for resources and manpower, thereby reducing the number of medical units to service combat operations there (Figures 6-1 through 6-3).

In some locations, the Army Medical Department used existing structures for hospitals. For instance, the Lend-Lease Program allowed the United States to provide aid (food, oil, and various materiel) to its Allies, especially England and the Soviet Union. The British, in a "reverse Lend-Lease," provided leases on facilities/bases, some of which were used by the Army Medical Department, in the Commonwealth and provided some equipment (such as Spitfire fighters) to the United States.[1(pp87,130)] Other facilities were created to meet the medical needs. In Europe and the Mediterranean, for example, the Corp of Engineers crafted hospitals using Nissan huts (a prefabricated corrugated steel building loosely based on a British building of the World War I era) or local materials. Existing buildings in Europe were often modified for hospital use once the invasion gained territory.[38(p542)]

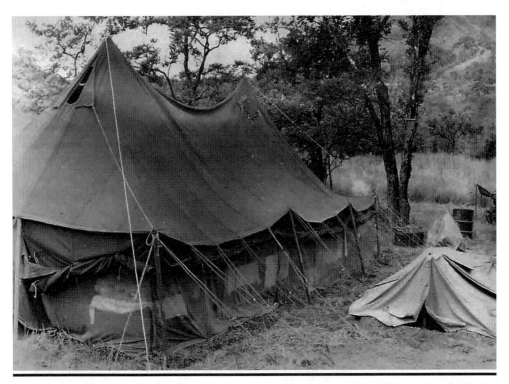

FIGURE 6-3. Portable surgical hospital tent. Note the covered dugout in front of the larger tent for shelter during raids. The staffing of the portable surgical hospital was to consist of four medical officers. Three were to be surgeons, of which one would be the commander. The fourth physician was to be an internist and anesthetist combination. In addition, there were to be 33 enlisted men, including 15 medical technicians and five surgical technicians. Photograph courtesy of the AMEDD Center of History and Heritage, Image #MU-WWII-LL08.

Portables' Table of Organization and Equipment

As usual, the Army set up a T/O&E for the portable surgical hospitals (T/O&E No. 8-572S) on 4 June 1943.[39] The inevitable changes started with Change No. 1 to 8-572S on 2 September 1943.[40] Change No. 2 to the T/O&E came on 7 December 1943.[41] The final T/O&E 8-572 for portable surgical hospitals came on 14 December 1944.[42] T/O&E 8-572 describes the concept of the portable surgical hospital as a mobile 25-bed unit "designed to furnish definitive surgical care in areas where it is impractical to use larger, more specialized medical units."[42(p418a)] The document spoke to the necessity to hand carry all equipment, while the personnel would be on foot carrying patients on litters as needed.[42(p418a)] It is an "independent, self-contained unit"[42(p415a)] placed under the direction of "the division, task force or Army commander, depending upon the unit to which it is attached."[42(p415a)]

The *Medical Field Manual*[32(p419f2)] stated that the hospital's movement depended on the personnel carrying the organizational equipment, with loads not to exceed 40 pounds per man. It pointed out that the organic motor transport would not be sufficient to transport the portable surgical hospital. Native bearers were to be used if the unit required them.[32(p419f2)]

Staffing of the Portable Surgical Hospital

The staffing of the portable surgical hospital was to consist of four medical officers. Three were to be surgeons, of which one would be the commander. The fourth physician was to be an internist and anesthetist combination. In addition, there were to be 33 enlisted men, including 15 medical technicians and five surgical technicians. Exhibit 6-1 delineates the specific tasks of each individual.

The portable surgical hospital had five operating room tables for the three surgeons, which allowed greater efficiency and the ability to handle more cases. The recovery period was geared to evacuate the patient by ground or air as soon as the tactical situation allowed[43(p61)] and the patient was stable enough for the trip.

A smaller number of personnel helped in the mobility of the portable surgical hospital. Early on, the overall few numbers of personnel and medical units limited the support available. As an example, in 1943, 25 portable surgical hospitals were requested to support the Chinese Armies in northern Burma, but only five were received. These units were more likely to have obstetricians and pediatricians assigned than surgeons. The lack of experienced and trained surgical talent was a continuing problem in the Pacific and China-Burma-India theaters of operations.[25(p298)] The commentaries from the time show that the Army did not appreciate the difference between a medical officer designated to do surgery versus one trained to do surgery.[44(p755)] An *Army Medical Bulletin* article in 1943 stressed that personnel for these Portable Surgical Army Hospital units must be young and vigorous. It recommended that officers be under 35 years of age while enlisted should be under 30 years of age.[45(pp7-8)]

An Example of the Use of the Portable Surgical Hospital: The Buna Campaign

Australian and American units in 1942 attacked the Japanese beachhead at Buna as part of the campaign to dislodge the Japanese from New Guinea and protect Australia from invasion by the Japanese. The Americans planned to set the stage for the Buna Campaign (Buna, New Guinea, November 1942–January 1943) by using three regimental task forces of the 32nd Division in the attack. The 126th Infantry Combat Team, the 127th Infantry Combat Team, and the 128th Infantry Combat Team were all deployed. The 114th Engineer Battalion accompanied the 127th. Their engagement ran from November 1942 until February 1943. The 107th Medical Battalion and the 19th Portable Surgical Hospital accompanied the 126th Infantry Combat Team. The 127th was serviced by the 3rd Portable Surgical Hospital, the 4th Portable Surgical Hospital, and the 5th Portable Surgical Hospital.[46(pp1-3)] The 128th was accompanied by the 14th Portable Surgical Hospital and the 18th Portable Surgical Hospital. The choices for PSH placement were determined to be best near a trail close to the front. An area 1,500 yards (less than a mile) behind the front was safe enough to protect the hospital, its patients, and staff from the enemy, yet close enough to the front to be effective as a forward surgical element.[46(p23)]

The Owen Stanley Mountain Range in New Guinea was a natural obstacle and a hurdle for the Australian and the American forces there.[47(p209)] The 32nd Division, a unit composed largely of National Guard units, was under the command of MG Edwin Harding. The 32nd Division ultimately was composed of three infantry combat teams

EXHIBIT 6-1. **PERSONNEL AUTHORIZATION FOR A PORTABLE SURGICAL HOSPITAL**

RANK	NUMBER OF POSITIONS	TITLE
COMMISSIONED OFFICERS: Total 4		
Major/Captain	1	Hospital Commander/Surgeon
Captain/1st Lieutenant	2	Surgeon
1st Lieutenant	1	Internist/Anesthetist
ENLISTED: Total 33		
Technical Sergeant	1	Chief Clerk
Staff Sergeant	1	Mess and Supply Sergeant
Sergeant	2	Medical Sergeant
Technician, Grade 4	1	Cook
Private First Class	1	Cook's Helper
Medical Technicians		
Technician, Grade 2	4	Medical Technician
Technician, Grade 5	3	Medical Technician
Private First Class	3	Medical Technician
Private	5	Medical Technician
Surgical Technicians		
Technician, Grade 3	1	Surgical Technician
Technician, Grade 4	1	Surgical Technician
Technician, Grade 5	1	Surgical Technician
Private First Class	1	Surgical Technician 1
Private	1	Surgical Technician 1
Technician, Grade 5	1	Clerk/Typist
Technician, Grade 5	1	Carpenter, Construction
Technician, Grade 5	1	Driver, Light Truck
Private First Class	1	Driver, Light Truck
Private	1	Driver, Light Truck
Private First Class	1	General Clerk
Private	1	Basic Clerk

Note: The rank of Technician, Grade 3, was approximately equivalent to a staff sergeant; a Technician, Grade 4, was approximately equal to a sergeant; and the Technician, Grade 5, was roughly equal to a corporal.

(regimental task forces), each with a portable surgical hospital assigned. In the Buna Campaign, the 2nd and 9th Portable Surgical Hospitals were also attached, but remained in the rear near Dobadura to act as an evacuation hospital.[46(p23)] Unfortunately, the 32nd Division was felt to be undertrained; they were also lacking equipment such as artillery, grenade launchers, and flamethrowers.[47(pp213–215)] Because the division was not making progress addressing these shortcomings, MacArthur relieved Harding (a rare event for

MacArthur) and replaced him with MG Robert Eichelberger. (MacArthur had come to recognize that the Australians were right that there was a lack of leadership.[47(pp218–219)])

Eichelberger brought effective leadership to the 32nd Division. For example, he made sure the troops had dry shoes and a hot meal before starting an offensive. He also had a medic check each man's temperature in one company and found that all had a fever. The soldiers were all in poor condition with torn and rotted clothing, waterlogged and ruined boots, and little hot food to eat. Not surprisingly, the morale was low.[47(p221)]

The Buna Campaign was where the first portable surgical hospitals proved their worth. The combat was fought in jungle swamps. Malaria was rampant before Atabrine was valued and was available. There were between 900 and 1,400 "fever" casualties (most were known to be malaria) per 1,000 troops[43(p9)] in the Buna Campaign alone (out of a high mean strength of 10,650).[43(Table 3)] Because the level of combat was low and the numbers of troops involved was limited, thus limiting wounded casualties, the malaria issue was paramount to the medical community. The medical cases were led by malaria, followed by "exhaustive states," gastroenteritis, dengue fever, acute upper respiratory diseases, and typhus fever.[43(p26)]

The Buna portable surgical hospitals were close to the action. The portables were organized out of a station hospital and attached one to each combat team.[43(p22)] The medical setup for the 32nd Division's three regimental task forces included three portable surgical hospitals, a clearing platoon, and a clearing company for each task force.[9(pp22–23)] The Japanese frequently provided strafings and bombings, especially to the portables (the 14th and the 22nd), which were located on the coast. The 22nd Portable Hospital had previously been loaded into a boat with three other boats off Cape Sudest. When the Japanese attacked, they sank all the boats and thus all of the portable's equipment.[47(p9)]

LTC Warmenhoven, the division surgeon for the 32nd Division, described conditions of these portable surgical hospitals. He said that "Portable hospitals were not portable after their first set up in practically all cases."[46(p24)] Warmenhoven noted that a 40-pound load was all that could be carried by a man over a jungle trail. He recorded a "tendency to acquire tentage."[46(p24)] LTC Warmenhoven stated that the pyramidal tent was the tent of choice for him. It could be easily moved and set up.[46(p28)] He mentioned that the heavy pyramidal tent and the small wall tent were difficult to carry while the tentage allowed by the Table of Basic Allowance (TBA) of the portable hospital was not heavy enough to work at night under blackout conditions. The ward tent required motor transport. Hence, the portable surgical hospital was not moveable with the required tentage, unless moved by motor transport.[46(pp24–25)] Warmenhoven placed emphasis on the importance of waterproofing supplies and equipment, while giving the Japanese credit in their waterproofing efforts. He spoke of using the Hydran Burners with thermos equipment, instead of field ranges (unless mounted on vehicles), in combat. The idea was to guarantee at least two hot meals a day for the hospital troops.[46(p29)]

The battalion aid station operated as close to the combat as possible, which varied between 200 to 1,000 yards (usually 300 yards distant).[46(p23)] The wounded were carried by the regimental detachment to the portable surgical hospital along jungle trails. In the Buna Campaign, the distance between the portable surgical hospital and the battalion aid station was kept to a 20- to 30-minute on foot litter carrying time, depending on the terrain. The wounded soldiers needing immediate surgery were taken to the portable surgical hospital. The less immediate surgery cases were taken to the clearing station, located some 2 miles away from the portable surgical hospital.[46(p23)] The terrain was rough and the aid men acting as litter carriers periodically came under fire.[46(p24)]

In surgery, sodium pentothal anesthesia was used universally.[46(p26)] Blood plasma was used frequently; the plasma was started at the aid station. The surgery was done in tents set up in an as aseptic a situation as possible. The patients were kept in tents to be protected from the sun and rain. Work at night was carried out by flashlight to keep nearby Japanese soldiers from acquiring a target in the dark. The wounds were debrided, with sulfonamide powder spread topically (sulfa drugs were available then). Plaster of Paris immobilization for fractures was utilized. The postoperative patients remained at the portable surgical hospital for 24 to 48 hours before they were further evacuated by native carriers to a field hospital in the rear. This trip could last up to 8 hours. At the field hospital they were air evacuated through a gap in the Owen Stanley Mountains to Port Moresby, New Guinea. They were subsequently evacuated by hospital ship or air to a general hospital in Australia. The prompt and high-quality care at the portable surgical hospital allowed for good outcomes.[44(pp34–54),47(p77)]

In 19 days of the Buna Campaign, 560 patients were treated, with 389 of those being wounded, and the rest suffering from various diseases endemic to the combat area. Two hundred and two of the wounded were operated on. The operations frequency ranged from three to four per day to as many as 25 per day.[46(p10,Table1)]

Warmenhoven, following the Buna Campaign, opined that the "portable hospitals attached to the division during the Buna Campaign proved to be of tremendous value . . . it would be hard to give an exact estimate of the number of lives . . . saved by their emergency surgery and heroic work performed near the front lines."[46(p28)]

To gain an appreciation of the scope of casualties that the medical department had to care for, it is important to note that in the Buna, Gona, and Sanananda battles, of the 35,000 Australians and Americans involved, over one-third were killed, wounded, or sick. In Buna alone, the 32nd Division lost two-thirds of its strength (586 killed, 7,000 ill, and 1,954 wounded).[47(p225)]

Portable Surgical Hospitals in Other Locations

The Buna Campaign discussion delineated in some detail the functioning of a portable surgical hospital in austere conditions. These same conditions were encountered elsewhere. For instance, in Burma, a number of American medical units arrived in portable surgical hospitals in late 1943 to support the Chinese armies. This included the 42nd, 43rd, and 46th Portable Surgical Hospitals; the 25th Field Hospital; and the 803rd Medical Air Evacuation Transport Squadron.[25(p307)]

Unlike the CBI (especially Burma), the Pacific battles were varied as to duration, intensity, and casualties. Army medicine was significantly involved in the care of the wounded. The Navy and Navy medical personnel were obviously involved in this care as well, due to the insular nature of the theater. Naval resources were especially heavily involved in various phases of evacuation because the Army deferred to the Navy in that regard.

The American troops were taken aback by jungle warfare in the beginning of the war. Marston, in his book *The Pacific War Companion*,[48(p10)] comments that by 1944, the Americans (and the Australians) had learned a great deal about jungle warfare. Bougainville, in the northern Solomon Pacific Island group, was the scene of American Marines landing on 1 November 1943.[48(p11)] It came to be characterized by epic diseases, with malaria and a wide assortment of tropical diseases, including scrub typhus, dengue fever, filariasis, influenza, and intestinal parasites.[22(p194)] In the Bougainville campaign, the Navy controlled all planning and actual evacuation from the beachhead.[22(p193)] The Australians took over control of Bougainville and New Guinea, which allowed MacArthur to focus on the coming Philippine invasion.

Other areas also saw combat operations. In the Marshalls, Kwajalein was in reality an easy campaign, as was Eniwetok.[23(p227)] The Marshall Islands were invaded by American troops on 31 January 1944, to be followed by the Admiralty Islands on 29 February 1945.[48(p12)] At Eniwetok, the Navy cleared an entire deck of the transport USS *Wharton* to be used as hospital space, which fortunately was not required. The Army set up a clearing company and a portable surgical hospital that worked with Navy personnel jointly.[23(p232)] The Gilberts were dire in intensity and casualties, and Saipan in the Marianas (15 June 1944) was heavily defended. The attack on the beaches was difficult. In the subsequent battles, the Japanese often held the jungle trail routes to collecting stations, which made evacuation difficult. Guam was invaded on 21 July 1944.[48(p11)]

In the invasion of the Philippines starting with the 9 January 1945 landings on Luzon, the 8th US Army conducted 51 amphibious landings on several dozen islands. In these battles, portable surgical hospitals reinforcing clearing companies performed most of the forward surgery. Later, in the Philippines, the role of the portables was diminished by the openness of the terrain. For example, in the 24th Division, two portables were combined by the division surgeon to form an extra clearing company. While in the Central Plains of Luzon, some portables functioned as surgical teams attached to medical battalion collecting companies.[23(p347)] Yet, in the more remote jungle areas of Luzon, the portables were of great value. For instance, in May 1945, a portable was doing surgery after a 5-day trek into the Luzon mountains.[23(p348)]

The Battle of Leyte, Bataan, the recapture of Corregidor, and the Battle of Zig-Zag Pass on Luzon were featured 8th Army operations. COL Frank McGowan, the Consultant in Surgery, 8th US Army, reported that in the Battle of Leyte in the regions of Ormoc Corridor and the area of Cariaga, the entire surgical care of the wounded soldiers was done by two portable surgical hospitals and clearing companies. The two evacuation companies were 15 to 20 miles away, due to the mountainous terrain. In the follow up to the Subic Bay landings (the Battle of Zig-Zag Pass), two portable surgical hospitals did most of the forward surgery in their location 2 to 3 miles from the front.[49(p565)] In the invasion of Corregidor, the forward surgical care was provided by a regimental medical detachment, which jumped with the parachute troops, and one portable hospital, which was landed by water. The parachutists (503rd Parachute Regiment) had 182 injured from the jump itself (of 2,100 jumping), many with compound fractures.[49(p571)]

McGowan also reported that the small units in the 8th Army handled the majority of the frontline surgery despite the fact that their surgeons were generally not well trained. He noted that the certified and more experienced surgeons were to be found at the general and evacuation hospitals. McGowan made a plea that in combat more experienced surgeons be assigned to the receiving areas for the casualties.[49(p566)] COL Robert Williams, General Stilwell's staff surgeon,[23(p287)] when setting up the portable surgical hospitals in Burma, found that the staffing had many "pediatricians, general practitioners, and obstetricians but a minimum of trained surgeons."[23(p298)] This was a problem that continued for all CBI and Pacific operations. Condon-Rall and Cowdrey noted the scarcity of competent surgeons and reported that in the South Pacific Area, 90% of the replacement medical officers had neither field training nor combat experience.[23(p186)] Besides the personnel training and experience issue, McGowan decried the lack of equipment for the portables, especially because they performed the majority of surgeries in theater. McGowan tried to attach them to separate clearing companies reinforced with surgeons. Being assigned to a portable surgical hospital was not without risk; McGowan reported that in the campaign for Mindanao in the southern Philippines, the Japanese ambushed a portable surgical hospital, destroying its equipment and bayoneting the commander.[49(p567)]

At Mindanao, in the Philippines, collecting companies served as hospitals, in contrast to the use of portable surgical hospitals in New Guinea as collecting companies, because they often had to hold patients for a period greater than 2 weeks.[23(p350)] The Chief of Surgery in the Philippines assigned one general surgeon and one orthopedic surgeon, along with six surgical technicians, to flexible surgical teams. In general, as the battles moved away from isolated islands and jungles, the portables were needed less.[23(pp345–347)] However, on Luzon, as late as 1945, portables were still in use.[23(p322)]

LEVELS OF CARE

The levels (echelons) of care started at the unit level of care, with self-care and buddy care starting in the field. The scheme continued with the corpsman, then followed by treatment at the battalion or regimental aid station. The next level of care was at the division level, provided by the organic division medical battalion, including collecting and clearing companies. The next level fell to the field army with the field and evacuation hospital.

Field Hospitals

The field hospital was created in early 1942 to provide for a smaller and more mobile hospital in the Pacific Theater of Operations.[50(p144)] It had a headquarters and three hospitalization units that could function by themselves (as 100-bed units). The field hospital had organic tents to provide a mobile unit. The field hospital could function in isolated areas because it had its own transportation assets. When augmented by surgical personnel, it became a mobile hospital to support airborne or ground troops.[23(pp144–145)]

The field hospital was organized with 22 officers, 18 nurses, and 227 enlisted men. The headquarters of the field hospital had four commissioned officers, three nurses, and 19 enlisted men. It was further divided into three identical hospital units with each having six commissioned officers, five nurses, and 67 enlisted men.[23(p67)] The nurses held "equivalent ranks" to officers until June 1944, when they were commissioned as regular officers.[23(p67)]

Reflecting the versatility of the concept, the field hospital could function as one 400-bed hospital or three 100-bed units.[50(pp644–645)] In reality, the field hospital's units worked closely with the division clearing company to provide more definitive care for the division. (The lack of surgery teams in the field hospital [set up that way due to lack of surgical personnel] was one of the reasons for creation of the Mobile Army Surgical Hospital [MASH] later in the period. The Mobile Army Surgical Hospital had an expanded complement of 41 nurses and 16 medical officers to handle 60 beds, while the World War II field hospital had five Medical Corps officers and five nurses for the 100-bed hospital unit.[51(p68)])

Sometimes there were personnel problems in the field hospitals. For example, the ETO Anesthesia Consultant, COL Ralph M Tovell, described the situation in which the auxiliary surgery group had poor relations with the personnel of a field hospital in the Normandy area (1944). He attributed the problems to a lack of authority for the commander of the facility to ensure cooperation. He referred the matter up the chain for resolution. Guidance was issued that the commander had the authority to coordinate separate units under the same roof.[52(p608)]

In a 1945 interview with COL Paul Streit, who was a surgeon with the Central Pacific Base command, he observed that each division in Europe had an evacuation hospital and a field hospital. However, in the Pacific, one field hospital served a division. Streit commented that the field hospital had to function as an evacuation hospital as well as a field unit. Inasmuch as the field hospital had insufficient staff, surgeons and anesthetists had to be added to the field units before they were deployed.[53(pp4–5)]

COL Streit said that air transportation was key to holding down the mortality rate in the Pacific islands' operations. At Iwo Jima, he notes that it was 6 days after landing before a field hospital was set up due to the level of combat. Casualties were taken to the LSTs, where surgery was performed before they were evacuated to the Marianna Islands for more definitive surgery. After the 7th day, C-54 transport aircraft were able to land and to evacuate the wounded.[54(p5)] COL Streit commented that the Japanese on Iwo Jima used less artillery than in other theaters of operations and hence there were fewer large shrapnel wounds.[53(p7)]

Portable Surgical Hospitals

LTC William J Shaw, who ultimately became the division surgeon for the 41st Division, 6th Army in New Guinea, gave an interview in September 1944, which well illustrates the lot of the surgeon in 1942 New Guinea. Such interview encounters provide a remarkable opportunity to see the 1942 experience from an individual's vantage point. Shaw was an early American arrival to Australia in March of 1942. After 9 months of training in Australia, Shaw was sent with the 41st Division to Biak Island (a coral reef) off the northwest coast of New Guinea. Assigned to the division were an evacuation hospital and three portable surgical hospitals, one designated for each regiment. In addition, there was a clearing company along with two collecting companies. In the difficult terrain of New Guinea, he reported that it could take 20 native bearers taking turns to carry one patient over a 4-mile trail. A clearing hospital served as a base hospital. Shaw said patients presenting with multiple woundings were common. The portable surgical hospitals did the complex surgeries with a 2% death rate.[55(pp1-2)] Less serious cases were performed at the clearing hospital.[55(pp1-2)] Plasma was used at the portable surgical hospital but whole blood was available only at the clearing hospital. The hospitals there used nitrous oxide, thiopental sodium, and regional anesthetics. Disease became more of an overall issue for the medical staff because woundings were not that frequent.[55(pp1-6)]

While the Navy and Marines had been the predominant US forces in the Pacific, the Army was most extensively engaged in the Middle East, Africa, and Europe. The relatively more environmentally friendly theaters did not feature the rough jungle terrain with its disease threats. Hence, somewhat different medical assets were required. The evacuation hospital was the most common iteration.

Evacuation Hospitals

The evacuation hospital was defined as a 400-bed or a 750-bed hospital. The 400-bed unit was semimobile with 25% of organic transport (trucks). The evacuation hospital was designed to be moved in 8 to 10 hours after the patients were first moved. It could then set up in a new locale in 4 to 6 hours. However, the 750-bed hospital was really immobile because in reality it had no organic transportation assets and the hospital personnel were not trained to break down and relocate for facility moves.[50(pp632-633)] The 750-bed evacuation hospital was designed to have a complement of 47 commissioned officers, 52 nurses, a warrant officer, a dietitian, and 380 enlisted men. The evacuation hospital was intended to provide major definitive surgical and medical treatment as near to the front as possible. The evacuation hospital could then evacuate patients as needed to a general hospital in the rear echelon.[51(p67)]

The 750-bed evacuation hospital was seen by many as being too large and fixed to be of great value. The bed capacity could certainly be utilized, but the smaller 400-bed configuration was seen as more flexible and easier to provide command and control. COL William A Shambora, Commander of the 1st Medical Group and the 9th Army Surgeon (as of June 1944) was the officer-in-charge of medical operations for Europe in the 1st Medical Group area.[56(p291)] COL Shambora was known to have this opinion of the larger evacuation hospital. He went to some lengths to avoid attachment of such a hospital from the European Theater Services of Supply (where they were usually placed).[51(p27)]

In Europe prior to the Overlord Invasion, the 1st Army planned one convalescent hospital; five field hospitals (small, nonsurgical for resuscitation); 10 400-bed evacuation hospitals; one 750-bed evacuation hospital; various ambulance, collecting, and clearing companies; one medical gas treatment battalion; one medical laboratory; one medical depot; and one auxiliary surgical company.[57(p61)] As the invasion progressed, the 3rd Army had 11 evacuation hospitals and one field hospital to work with those of the 1st Army. Up to the end of July 1944, 1st Army had attached 22 evacuation hospitals and six field hospitals, which provided medical/surgical support for 16 divisions.[57(p72)]

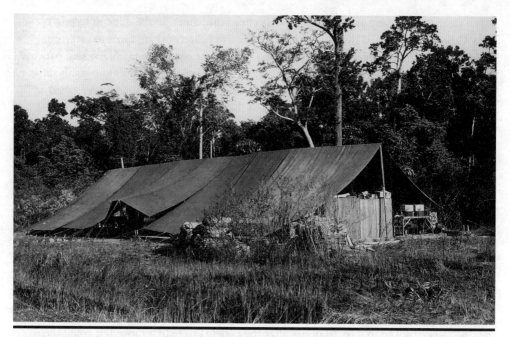

FIGURE 6-4. Surgical tent of an evacuation hospital set on an abandoned concrete platform in the Palawan, Philippine Islands, 1943. Photograph courtesy of the AMEDD Center of History and Heritage, Image #MU-WWII-LL-016.

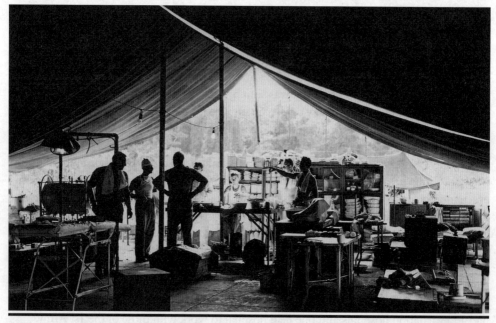

FIGURE 6-5. Operating room of an evacuation hospital in the Pacific. Note the autoclave, the surgical scrub table, the operating room table, and supplies with the concrete floor. Photograph courtesy of the AMEDD Center of History and Heritage, Image #MU-WWII-LL-017.

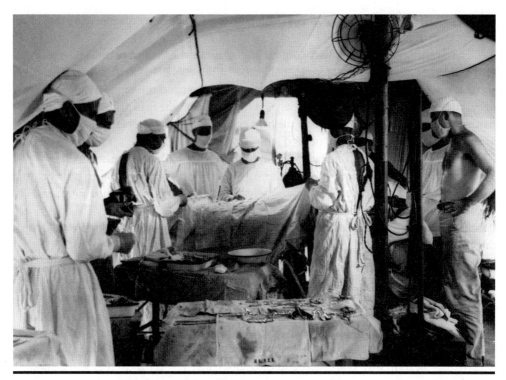

FIGURE 6-6. Colonel Williams, Chief of Surgery of the 99th Evacuation Hospital (at the head of the OR table), Mindanao, Philippines, May 1945. Note that the operation was proceeding under tentage. The evacuation hospital was not mobile because it had no organic transportation for movement. Photograph courtesy of the AMEDD Center of History and Heritage, Image #MU-WWII-B1-001.

On the beaches during the Overlord Invasion, surgery was done in the clearing stations of the amphibious battalions. However, as soon as field hospitals were established, surgery was transferred there. The field hospitals operated like evacuation hospitals. Auxiliary surgical teams were pressed into service to deal with the surgical load at the field hospitals. The field hospitals, operating close to the lines, saved many who could not have been transported. The field hospitals were too large to be considered mobile, but, due to their smaller size, could be located more forward than the evacuation hospital.[50(p97)] Evacuation hospitals were situated as close to the front as safety allowed. The evacuation hospitals had problems of surgical backlog also requiring auxiliary surgery unit help. Auxiliary surgery teams numbered from the usual three to four to the maximum of eight. The one 750-bed evacuation hospital generally operated without auxiliary teams except during overload situations that occurred during intense combat[57(p99)] (Figures 6-4 through 6-6).

Auxiliary Surgical Groups

A 1944 article, titled "Surgery at the Front," discussed the formation of auxiliary surgical groups to complement portable surgical hospitals in providing emergent care. The analogy of these groups was to firemen who were always on call to put out fires.[54(p2)] Army

Surgeon General Norman Kirk hailed these innovations as reducing the mortality rate once soldiers were admitted for care.[58(p3)]

The Army established auxiliary surgical groups under the War Department T/O&E 8-571, titled *Auxiliary Surgical Group*, published 13 July 1942.[59] Sixty-one surgical and shock teams of four to six personnel were established to expand the surgical capability of evacuation and field hospitals. The surgical teams were in the field army, designed partly to offset the lack of surgeons in the field hospitals. Because they couldn't function independently, they could not be utilized in the field alone.[57(pp78-92)] These units were tried out initially in North Africa and later used in Europe.[57(pp78-92)] There were no auxiliary surgical groups in the Pacific and China-Burma-India theaters of operations to provide command and control of the placement of needed surgical teams, unlike their European counterparts. After recommendations from the surgical consultant, however, the Southwest Pacific Area organized surgical teams to facilitate the temporary meeting of those needs on the battlefield.

The auxiliary surgical groups had about one-half of their staff in general surgical teams, while the rest were in specialty teams doing neurosurgery, chest, nerve, and maxillofacial work.[60(pp1-3)] The teams were listed as Team EA General Surgery, EB Orthopedic Surgery, ED Maxillofacial Surgery, EE Neurosurgery, and EF Thoracic Surgery. These teams had one officer, one nurse, and three enlisted men in their group. Team EC was a shock treatment team with one officer, one nurse, and three enlisted men. Team EG was a gas treatment team with one officer and three enlisted. These teams were situated under a headquarters to form an auxiliary surgery group. Field Manual 8-5, dated 12 January 1942, addressed the purposes of the mobile units of the Army Medical Department.[60] Change No. 2, dated 20 April 1944, addressed changes to these units, including the surgical group and the portable surgical hospital.[61]

As an example, mobile surgical units of the 3rd Auxiliary Surgical Group were set up with one surgical truck and three Proco Surgical Units (self-contained surgical units manufactured by the Proco Company). These units augmented field and evacuation hospitals. They had two operating tables and their own instruments and supplies. The mobile surgical units used in the ETO were of two types: (1) the "USA" type with a 2½-ton van with a 1-ton trailer attached and (2) the "ETO" type with three 1½-ton trucks and a 250-gallon water trailer. The operating room tent (USA type) was double-walled and air-conditioned. These hospitals worked better with evacuation hospitals than field hospitals because the latter had heavier surgical capacity.[62(pp22-25)] The use of surgical teams from surgical auxiliary groups to augment the role of the field hospital was discussed in a military publication that showed abdominal injuries, chest wounds, and fractured femurs were the primary surgeries done.[58(pp44-45)] The 5th, 45th, and 91st Evacuation Hospitals did use the mobile units early in the war. These units fell into disuse as hospitals became more numerous and personnel shortages made filling the staffing needs of the mobiles difficult.[58(p80)]

In the 3rd Auxiliary Surgical Group, it was established that the team surgeon would handle all phases of surgical care in a field hospital, while in an evacuation hospital, the chief of surgery would have these responsibilities. Additional written instructions to hospital commanders reminded them that the teams were meant to work as a team and not to be dispersed, as had happened in North Africa. The field hospitals depended entirely on auxiliary surgical teams for their surgical care so they had first call on these teams before an evacuation hospital could receive their services.[58(p3)] The 3rd Auxiliary Surgical Group fielded 25 general surgery teams, nine specialty teams, and 15 nurse teams.[58(p58)]

The 3rd was put to the test in the invasion of Europe in 1944. Its combat experience in the Mediterranean Theater was for 3 months in 1943, with only half of the group.[63(p1)] The deployed group (North Africa) returned to England in November 1943, where the two separate groups were joined together. The procedure established was that only after the operating field hospitals had their surgical staffing filled would the evacuation hospitals be able to tap into surgeons.[58(p3)]

In the invasion planning, four surgical teams were to be with each of the three medical battalions and two each with each of the airborne medical companies.[58(pp9–10)] The purpose of the teams with the airborne units was to do forward major surgery from the start because evacuation of casualties wouldn't be possible until the ground troops joined up with the airborne.

FORWARD SURGERY AS EXPERIENCED BY INDIVIDUAL PHYSICIANS

Major Albert Crandall, Medical Corps, Surgeon, 3rd Auxiliary Group

Crandall wrote an account of his experiences as a surgeon in the 3rd Auxiliary Group and in the 1st Airborne Surgical Team. Crandall graduated in 1933 from the University of Vermont. He was inducted into the Army in 1942 and attended the Medical Field Service School at Carlisle Barracks, Pennsylvania. He volunteered for overseas duty and was assigned to the 3rd Auxiliary Surgical Group. Crandall crossed the Atlantic on the *Queen Mary* (converted to carry troops), arriving in Scotland in December 1942. He was then sent to various British facilities to observe and help as needed. Crandall described his surgical group as consisting of 30 teams. Twenty of the teams were general surgery. Four teams each comprised neurosurgery and thoracic surgery. He said at times there were also maxillofacial and orthopedic teams.[64(pp1–2)]

With his assignment to the 1st Airborne Surgical Team, Crandall described training in orientation to airborne techniques. The group worked to be able to field a working surgical team without resort to evacuation. Crandall's group was the first to be assigned to an airborne unit. For the Normandy Invasion, Crandall's unit equipment was loaded on a trailer, which was thereafter placed in a glider. The Americans used the Waco GG4A unit (made of wood, fabric, and a metal frame), which was smaller than the English Horsa glider. All gliders were towed by C-47 "tugs" (DC-3). The gliders were a load-capacity expander allowing the C-47 to carry more material and men, much like a truck pulling a trailer. A C-47 aircraft could tow and then release the glider closer to the landing area to allow a quieter approach and the ability to carry larger loads than could be accommodated in a transport aircraft alone.[64] The gliders proceeded as a group and tried to land in the same general area. Crandall's Waco glider landed near Hiesville in Normandy on 6 June 1944. He received injuries in the landing, including to his neck and right eye. His auxiliary surgical group treated 125 casualties at the landing sites and 250 to 300 more at their station set up. More personnel arrived so that they were able to run five operating tables continuously. They were able to start evacuations 3 days later, on 9 June 1944.[64(p5)]

Crandall was west of Bastogne when his unit was captured by a German Panzer unit. At one point, they were loaded into railway cars, which were subsequently strafed by Allied fighters. The prisoners were marched into Germany proper, suffering from the cold; some even had frostbite. Crandall also described his experiences in various prisoner of war camps.[64(pp9–14)] He commented that the Russians who liberated them treated the Americans badly.[64(p15)]

1st Lieutenant Frank Davis, Medical Corps, Medical Officer LST 496 on D-Day, Normandy Invasion

An interview with Davis (dated 24 November 1944) is of interest because he was the officer-in-charge of medical service for LST 496 on D-Day. Davis had been classified as a general surgeon and an orthopedic surgeon in the Army way (he was a general surgeon who could do orthopedics). He had been a medical resident in Baltimore before his Army experience.[65(p1)] His LST, like the others, was to transport troops to the Continent and to return to England with casualties. Davis had two surgical technicians assigned to him on the LST. His LST landed troops at Omaha Beach. He soon had the DUKWs (not an acronym, but rather refers to a landing craft with wheels that could go onto the beach) returning with casualties. Davis had 20 Navy corpsmen to help with the litters. On the LST, Davis had two Navy surgeons and a Navy Chief Pharmacist Mate to help as a surgical assistant. Davis commented that the Army surgical technicians had never scrubbed on a major surgery case.[65(p2)] His LST could hold 250 litter cases. Upon the ship's return to England, Davis had divided the cases into nontransportable, transportable, and ambulatory cases. The nonambulatory cases were transported only a mile for definitive treatment while the transportable were sent 30 miles inland. He described his Navy corpsman as his only death when an elevator fell on him.[65(p4)] Davis also described an episode in which his LST hit a mine left by a German E-boat (S-boot or *Schnellboot*). There were significant casualties. Davis sustained several fractured vertebrae, which required his ultimate evacuation back to the continental United States[65(p4)] (Figures 6-7 through 6-9).

Captain Willis P McKee, Medical Corps, 326th Airborne Medical Company, 101st Airborne Division–D-Day Invasion

Captain Willis McKee was assigned to the 101st Airborne Division, specifically the 326th Airborne Medical Company, prior to D-Day in Europe. The airborne plan was for him to have 15 enlisted men and 85 containers filled with medical equipment. Captain McKee parachuted in and ended up near Hiesville, Normandy, with 10 men and only five containers full of supplies and equipment with which to perform major surgery. He (unlike many others) did land close to his deployed area. The later arriving gliders carrying

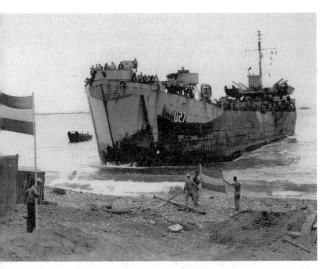

FIGURE 6-7. [Top] LST (Landing Ship, Tank) coming on to the beach, Italy, 1943. The LST was a key asset for the Anzio Invasion in Italy, and later in the Normandy Invasion. The invasion date for "Operation Overlord" (the cross-Channel invasion of Europe) had to be delayed due to a shortage of LSTs (two were lost in Operation Tiger near Slapton Sands, England, May 1944) while waiting for such landing craft to be redeployed to England from Italy. Photograph courtesy of the AMEDD Center of History and Heritage, Image #MU-WWII-LL-004.

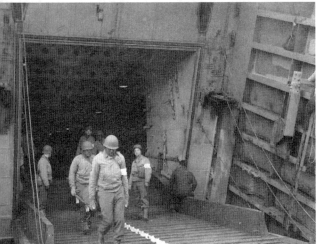

FIGURE 6-8. [Middle] Patient being off-loaded from an LST (Landing Ship, Tank) on litter, 14 April 1944, Pacific Theater of Operations. The LST was an essential feature of Operation Overlord (the cross-Channel invasion of Europe). An LST displaced more than 1,600 tons when empty and was somewhat longer than a football field. The LSTs were constructed in the United States in inland points on the Ohio River. The LST could carry 20 tanks, 30 large trucks, or 2,100 cargo tons, and sleep 350 soldiers. Due to the LST's flat bottom, it could come right up to the beach to disembark its cargo. Photograph courtesy of the Office of Medical History, Uniformed Services University of the Health Sciences, Image #OMH-USUHS-0452.

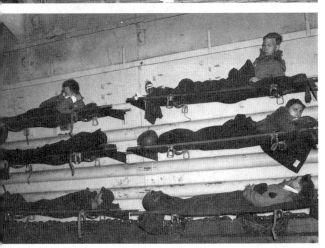

FIGURE 6-9. [Bottom] LST (Landing Ship, Tank) carrying wounded on litters attached to the ship walls. The LSTs' construction program was begun in 1942 for Operation Bolero, an early invasion of the Continent. The North African invasion used existing LST numbers. The Pacific and Europe theaters of operations were in competition for these essential landing crafts. Photograph courtesy of the Office of Medical History, Uniformed Services University of the Health Sciences, Image #OMH-USUHS-0456.

additional medical people and supplies/vehicles landed safely and their personnel were also soon performing surgery. He described glider casualties consisting of limb fractures (legs, arms, and hips) and skull fractures. He also described small arms wounds and shrapnel wounds. Penicillin was not authorized for McKee's unit due to its limited production and availability at this point in the war. The surgeons had to make do with traditional sulfa drugs, including the granulated powders sprinkled onto recent woundings.[66]

FORWARD SURGERY IN VARIOUS COMBAT THEATERS

Overlord + Invasion of Europe

Overlord was the code name given to the invasion of France, while Neptune was the code name for the naval aspect of Operation Overlord.[1(p464)] The invasion was finally launched on 6 June 1944 as the weather prevented going forward on the planned June 5th date. The overall great size of the landing at Normandy was impressive in terms of the logistical planning, gathering of troops, landing craft, and supplies. On the first day, 154,000 Allied troops landed, with 24,000 of them coming by parachute and glider.[1(p465)]

The LST was an essential feature of Operation Overlord (as well as the Anzio Invasion, Operation Torch with the invasion of North Africa, and later in the landing in the South of France after D-Day). An LST displaced 1,625 tons when empty and was 327 feet long.[67(p18)] The LSTs were constructed in the United States in inland points on the Ohio River. They were launched sideways into the Ohio River and sailed down the Mississippi into the Gulf of Mexico. The LST could carry 20 tanks, 30 large trucks, or 2,100 cargo tons. The LST had bunks for 350 soldiers. Due to the LST's flat bottom (drawing only 4'–7' when loaded), it could come right up to the beach to disembark its cargo.[67(p19)] The LSTs' construction program was begun in 1942 for Operation Bolero, or an early invasion of the Continent.[67(p20)] The North African invasion used existing LST numbers. The Pacific and European theaters of operation were in competition for the landing crafts. Further, LST production was halted and many yards were ordered to work on sections of destroyers and escort craft for convoys.[67(p21)]

No invasion on the scale of the Normandy operation had been planned or carried out up to 1944.[68(p42)] As Nigel Lewis, in his book *Exercise Tiger*,[68] observes, prior rehearsals such as Exercise Beaver (27–31 March 1944) were not successful. There was mass confusion and unit structure broke down. Hence, Operation Tiger was to be a most realistic dress rehearsal for the coming invasion. Slapton Sands (at Lyme Bay) not far along the coast from Plymouth, England, was picked because the beach conditions were most similar to the Normandy coastline.[68(p43)]

Exercise Tiger was to involve 25,000 men who would be on their LSTs for the time required to make the actual invasion run. Three hundred thirty-seven ships were to be involved and the plan would have two phases like the real one. The first phase would be the engineers clearing the beach obstacles, to be followed by the second wave, which would be the landing of the reinforcing troops.[68(p43)] The mixed American and British command had potential dangers not recognized before the exercise began, which included failure to coordinate operations to deal with external threats. Even the simplest measure of common radio frequencies so that the commands could communicate was neglected.[68(pp46–47)]

The 261st Medical Battalion participated in "Exercise Tiger" from 22 April until 1 May 1944 at Slapton Sands.[68(pp11–13)] Unfortunately, German E-boats (the English called these E-boats while the Germans termed them S-boot for *Schnellboot*—fast boat) of the German *Schnellbootwaffe* attacked the eight LSTs at 0200 on 27 April 1944. The 5th and 9th *Schnellboot* flotillas were based at Cherbourg, France. These swift craft could run at 37 to 40 knots per hour, in contrast to the 12 knots of the American LSTs. These S-boots carried two torpedoes and cannon/machine gun armament.[68(p52)] The German boats on 27 April 1944 came upon the eight LSTs and a British frigate. The LSTs were carrying Jeeps, DUKWS (amphibious vehicles), weapons, and supplies. The German attack resulted in the loss of LST 507 (and damage to two other LSTs) and the loss of 197 sailors and 400 soldiers.[69(p145)]

On one LST, Medical Teams 2 and 3 treated the casualties (18 casualties including an LST captain and his executive officer).[68(p12)] The loss of even LST 507 in this situation negatively impacted the coming invasion. The shortage of LST landing craft presumably delayed the invasion and postponed the invasion of the South of France, which at one point had been envisioned as a simultaneous invasion thrust with Normandy. The American admiral in charge of Operation Tiger subsequently killed himself.[68(p145)]

Over 100 bodies of officers privy to the Overlord Invasion plans (the so-called "bigoted") were not initially recovered, increasing anxiety that the Germans had abducted survivors from the sea. It took a month to recover all the missing bodies. The bodies of the dead were secretly dealt with while the next of kin were not notified of their deaths until after the invasion, when they were designated casualties of the invasion (casualties were reported starting in mid-June 1944). The incident did not receive public awareness until 1988.[69(pp61–78)]

The medical teams had different experiences in the Normandy Invasion on 6 June 1944. Utah Beach was comparatively calm while Omaha Beach was chaotic. On Utah Beach, some 23,000 men landed with only 210 killed or wounded. On Omaha Beach, the 1st Division and the 29th Division sustained over ten times the casualties as on Utah Beach.[1(pp473–474)] On both beaches the teams were behind schedule in setting up operations, as could be anticipated. In particular, the cliffs at Omaha were more of an obstacle than had been considered.[63(p30)]

Despite a heavy naval bombardment (which turned out to be too brief to neutralize the German guns), the Germans still were able to focus heavy fire on Omaha Beach. After the first 2 hours, the landings at Omaha were halted due to the casualties and heavy fire. The Navy ordered the supporting American destroyers to get in close to the beach and provide bombardment. Twelve destroyers provided fire to support the Army Rangers who were assaulting the cliffs of the Pointe du Hoc.[68(pp24–25)]

The English and Canadian beaches, termed Gold, Juno, and Sword, had no cliffs and received more naval bombardment.[1(p476)] The loss of the majority (27 of 29) of the modified M4A3 Sherman DD (duplex drive) tanks, which were designed to float (with waterproofed canvas shells[63(p31)]), kept the Americans on the beaches longer than planned. The tanks sank when the waves came over their waterproof screens.[1(p475)]

The casualty losses on D-Day were less than anticipated due to such interventions as early surgery. As an example, the early surgery on the beach at Omaha allowed the teams to operate on 900 wounded soldiers before the regular hospital units arrived.[63(p3)] In the case of Omaha Beach, a recommendation after the fact was that the surgical teams at Omaha would have been more useful if they had been stationed on ships rather than being on the beach, concerned with their own safety due to the constant fire that made care difficult.[63(p31)] The 1st Engineer Special Brigade performed definitive surgery in its clearing hospital on Day 2 of D-Day. Two field hospitals arriving on the beaches from the 1st Brigade were used as evacuation hospitals. The first airstrip for evacuation was opened on D+4; 12 patients were air evacuated that day.[68(p69)]

The losses at D-Day included 9,000 Allied casualties. Of the number that were killed (4,572), 2,500 were Americans, 1,641 were British, and 359 were Canadian.[1(p477)] There were also 37 Norwegians, one Belgian, 13 Australians, and 19 Free French. The losses were considerably less than what had been anticipated (or feared).[1(p477)]

Combat/Medical Care Across France/Belgium

It was 11 months from D-Day to the German surrender.[1(p491)] The Allies carried out Operation Anvil in the South of France on 15 August 1944 as a diversionary tactic to tie up German troops that would otherwise be diverted to the north.[1(p491)] (As noted earlier, Anvil had to be postponed due to a shortage of landing craft. It had been envisioned as a simultaneously landed diversionary tactic to keep German troops engaged in the south, while Operation Overlord was carried out in the north. Due to the delay until 15 August, the Germans had largely withdrawn from the region to respond to the Normandy invasion.[1(p469)]) The 21st Army Group was to advance through Belgium. They would pass to the north of the Ardennes. Of Bradley's 12th Army Group, Hodges was sent north of the Ardennes, while Patton moved to the Saar.[1(p499)]

The British-led Market-Garden Operation didn't work out as envisioned, due to poor planning and strong German opposition in the area. Its implementation diverted manpower, petroleum, and supplies from Patton. The result was that Patton, closing on the Rhine, could not cross it for 6 months, which meant his forces remained static along the Rhine. The Germans used the period to reinforce the Siegfried Line.[1(p502)] On 16 December 1944, the Germans launched their Ardennes offensive.[1(p504)] The surrounded forces at Bastogne were relieved by Patton's 3rd Army, which had linked up with the 1st Army by 8 January 1945.[1(p507)]

At Bastogne, the 101st Airborne Division and parts of the 9th and 10th Armored Division sustained significant casualties. The weather, with constant snow and fog, precluded air evacuation; furthermore, the perimeter was held by the Germans.[60(pp415-426)] On December 26th, two surgical teams were flown to Bastogne by glider. The 101st Airborne Medical Company had been captured by the Germans; thereafter care was delivered by echelon medical staff, which consisted of medical staff from the various divisions put together to function as a medical company.[70(p10), 71] The most reliable figures for casualties at Bastogne are for the 101st Division for the period 15 December until 26 December, which lists 704 battle casualties, as well as six other injuries and 573 "disease" cases (including 84 neuropsychiatric cases).[70(pp11–12)] The 101st Airborne Division reported 33 deaths in the period 19 December until 31 December.[60(p424)] In a 2-day period of 27th to the 29th of December, all Bastogne hospitalized patients, numbering 964 at the time, were evacuated by ambulance.[60(p422)] The military doctors had no instruments or supplies for major surgery. A medical hospital platoon with an attached surgical team was rushed into Bastogne when the siege was lifted[60(pp416–426)] by Patton's 4th Armored Division on 26 December 1944.[1(p507)]

A surgeon, Dr Henry M Hills, was flown in by glider to Bastogne with surgical instruments and supplies, and set up an operating room. Hills was a West Virginia orthopedic surgeon who had participated in the D-Day landings. He volunteered to go into Bastogne (for which he later received a Silver Star) to provide medical help. Originally he said the plan was to parachute, but as he had no experience with that, the plan was changed to a glider insertion.[72] He supplemented the battalion aid surgeons, who were not really surgeons, per se, but had been trained as anything from a family doctor to a pediatrician. Additional medical supplies were dropped by air. The whole blood didn't survive the air drop, but the supply of plasma was adequate.[72(p4)] Three days later additional surgical teams and supplies arrived. With the lifting of the siege,[72(p23)] ambulances of the 614th Medical Group arrived to evacuate some of the patients. Meanwhile, surgery continued with 50 major operations performed (and three deaths sustained).[72(p2)]

The field hospitals of the 1st Army had been operating in the 1st Division, acting to provide surgery for the nontransportable wounded. Other wounded or sick were sent to evacuation hospitals, which were kept mobile in the 1st Division area. They could be advanced when another unit was filled or the front moved.[73(p132)] After the breakthrough at St Lo, the 1st Army evacuation hospitals had a surplus of lightly wounded that had not received surgery. A decision was made to establish the 77th Evacuation Hospital in the rear of 1st Army to free up the hospitals.[73(p132)] The approach to the Siegfried Line (which was the German reinforced line with tank obstacles and mines to protect German territory) slowed the mobility needs for the hospitals.

The German lines were reached in September 1944. The contest for the Hurtgen Forest ran from September to December 1944. The combat in the Hurtgen Forest was part of the entire Siegfried Line campaign. In the campaign as a whole, the 1st and 9th Army together suffered 57,095 casualties. For the period 15 June to 31 December 1944, the 1st Army sustained 47,039 of the total, which included 7,024 killed, 35,155 wounded, and 4,860 missing.[74] The 9th accounted for the rest of the casualties, which included 1,133 killed, 6,864 wounded, and 2,059 missing.[74]

In January 1945, the 1st US Army Medical Service was evacuating because of shortages of materials and adverse weather conditions, including snow and ice, that prevented vehicles from being able to turn around. Medical facilities could not be erected in fields because they quickly became impassable to vehicles.[73(p144)] In a push to gain sufficient medical bed space, the 45th Evacuation Hospital and the 5th Evacuation Hospital were set up together at Spa. The 4th Convalescent Hospital was subsequently moved to Spa. In February 1945, experiments were made using light planes in evacuation due to the icy roads, which were impassable for ambulances.[73(p147)] Some outfits, such as the 1st Medical

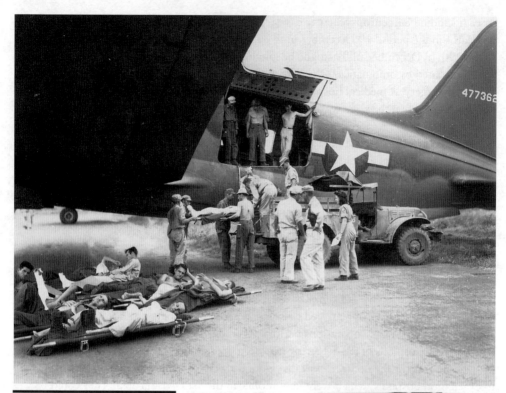

FIGURE 6-10. [Top] Wounded being loaded into aircraft for evacuation. As the war progressed, the Army preferred to use air evacuation, rather than ships. The C-43 Commando (shown here) and the C-47 (DC-3) workhorse were the primary planes. The C-54 (DC-4) was used late in the war for air evacuation. Air transportation was key in holding down the mortality in the operations in the Pacific islands and Europe. Photograph courtesy of the AMEDD Center of History and Heritage, Image #MU-WWII-LL-055.

FIGURE 6-11. [Bottom] Ambulatory evacuation patient being helped up plane's ladder. Photograph courtesy of the AMEDD Center of History and Heritage, Image #MU-WWII-LL-054.

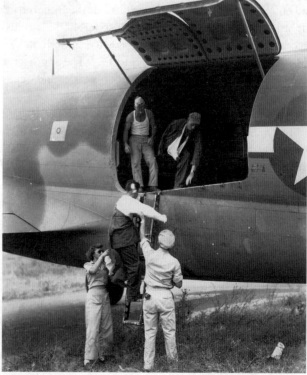

Group, in the short period between 27 February and 11 March 1945, moved five times (average of one move every two to five days), reflecting their flexibility.[73(pp59–60)] The 1st Medical Group received two auxiliary surgical teams and two shock teams from the 5th Auxiliary Surgical Group to handle casualties from the Roer River crossing[58(p47)] (Figures 6-10 and 6-11).

North African Campaign Surgery

Medicine and surgery in North Africa were less rushed because the casualties were fewer than anticipated. The plans for Operation Torch were developed by General Mark Clark and his staff. The Allies were to assault the Moroccan and Algerian coasts on 8 November 1942.[11(p108)] Algiers surrendered first, due to previous contacts with the French and the presence of Admiral Jean-Francois Darlan, the Vichy naval military commander second to the authority of the Vichy President Marshal Henri Petain. In planning for Operation Torch, there were to be three commands in the form of eastern, western, and central task forces. The Eastern Task Force going into Tunisia had the most medical assets of the three task forces. The Eastern Task Force, commanded by MG George Patton, took Algiers, which surrendered with little resistance.[11(pp108–109)] There were few casualties on the actual day of invasion but later most casualties were from bombing raids and land mines.[27(p111)] The Central Task Force, commanded by MG Lloyd Fredendall, experienced more casualties than in the taking of Algiers, due to more determined French Vichy resistance. The Western Task Force, commanded by the British LTG KAN Anderson, made three separate landings on the Atlantic side. This force sustained the most casualties of any (694 casualties of which 603 were combat wounds and 91 were fatalities).[11(p119)]

The Western Task Force had provisional hospitals at Safi and Mehdia. The 750-bed 8th and the 400-bed 11th Evacuation Hospitals came to Casablanca. The 400-bed 91st Evacuation Hospital came to the same region later. These evacuation hospitals were operated as fixed units.[11(pp119–120)] In the Oran region, the 48th Surgical, the 38th Evacuation Hospital, and the 77th Evacuation Hospital were joined by the 750-bed 9th Evacuation Hospital. The 1st Battalion 16th Medical Regiment lost all of its equipment with a ship sinking. The Eastern zone medical care was handled by the British forces in the Eastern Zone turned toward Tunisia.[11(p120)]

The Kasserine Withdrawal ended with the Germans defeating troops under the command of MG Fredendall (leading to his relief and replacement by MG Patton). The 200-bed 48th Surgical Hospital did demonstrate that it could evacuate its patients, dismantle, and move in less than 5 hours. In contrast, evacuation hospitals couldn't move because they had no organic transport[11(p127)] (Figure 6-12).

Sicily and the Mediterranean

Sicily was the next selected target after North Africa.[11(p147)] In the invasion of Sicily, on 10 July 1943, the British and Canadians landed at the southern tip of the island. The Americans landed to the left of the British on a 70-mile strip of beach on the southern shore. There were no fixed hospital assets in Sicily and only one 400-bed evacuation hospital due to shipping limitations. A 750-bed evacuation hospital did make it to Sicily by

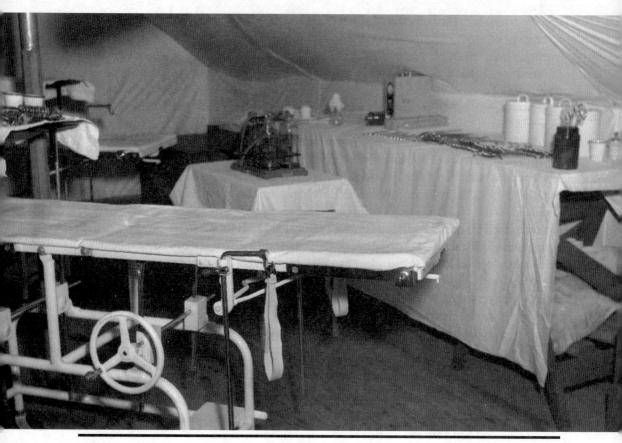

FIGURE 6-12. Operating room in the 59th Evacuation Hospital, Casablanca, North Africa, February 1943. Photograph courtesy of the AMEDD Center of History and Heritage, Image #B2-02-014.

late August but with its equipment at sea, it worked out of an existing Italian facility.[11(p164)] The wounded were therefore evacuated to Africa. The 15th Evacuation Hospital was able to expand to 950 beds by incorporating parts of a clearing hospital.[11(p164)] Evacuation of the wounded to Africa was evenly delegated to air and sea routes[11(p167)] (Figures 6-13 through 6-18).

FORWARD SURGERY IN OTHER MILITARIES

The experiences of other countries' armies' medical care can be useful in planning and executing one's country's own care. In World War I, the United States' close work with the British medical care system, including the rotation of a large number of American surgeons through their casualty clearing stations, clearly benefitted the implementation of the US military healthcare system. The French had much to teach in World War I in the design and use of mobile surgical facilities and in the use of the motorized ambulance, as discussed in the previous chapter.

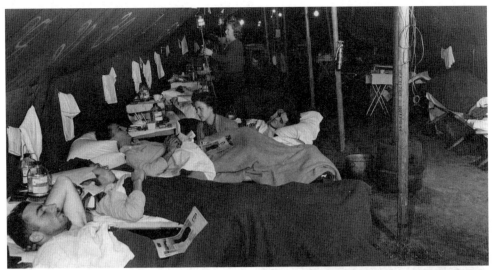

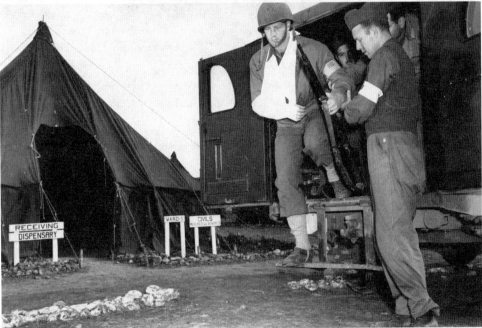

FIGURE 6-13. [Top] This is a postoperative ward of the 27th Evacuation Hospital in France, November 1944. The ward is composed of three ward tents connected end-to-end with a 60-patient capacity in the ward. Photograph courtesy of the AMEDD Center of History and Heritage, Image #B1-11-38.

FIGURE 6-14. [Bottom] A patient is being helped out of an ambulance in North Africa, 1943, after having a shrapnel wound in his arm dressed at an aid station. He is being delivered to the receiving dispensary of an evacuation hospital for treatment. The World War II evacuation hospital was usually about 400 beds (which was smaller than the World War I evacuation hospital, which could range above 1,000 beds, as needed). Photograph courtesy of the AMEDD Center of History and Heritage, Image #B2-01-02.

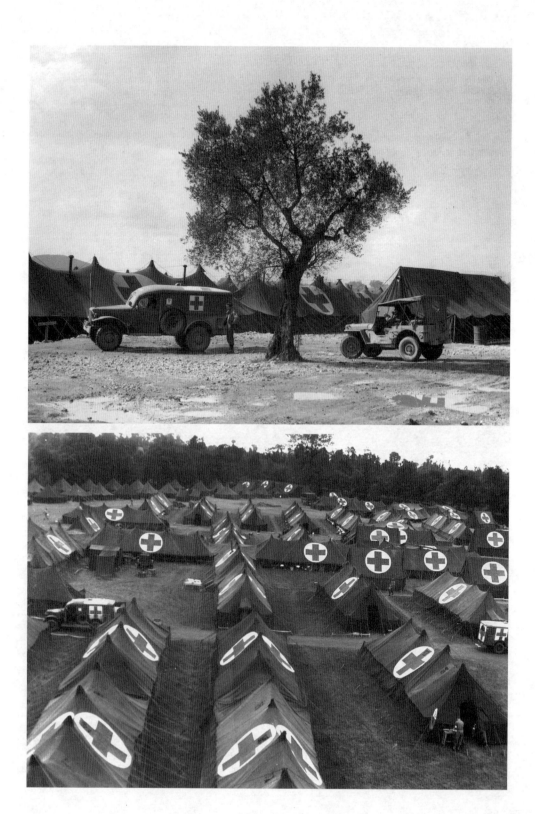

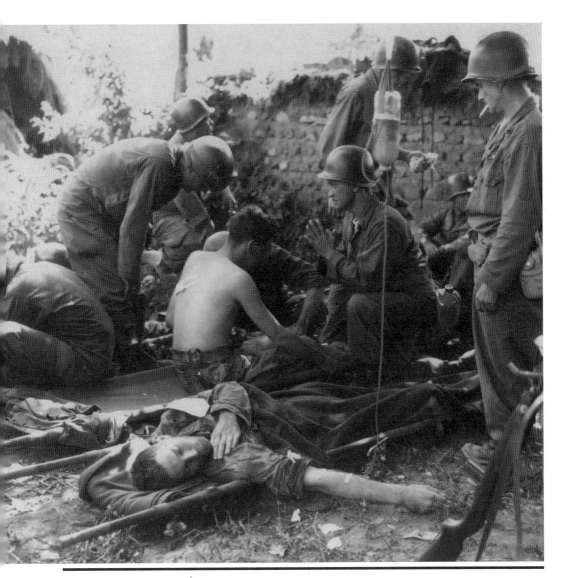

FIGURE 6-15. [Top Left] Army ambulance at the entrance to the 8th Evacuation Hospital, Teano area of Italy, March 1944. Note that the "red cross" symbols on the tents were visible from the air. Photograph courtesy of the AMEDD Center of History and Heritage, Image #MU-WWII-B1-002.

FIGURE 6-16. [Bottom Left] World War II, European Theater of Operations, France. 2nd Evacuation Hospital, with 750 beds. Note that the deployed tents are all marked with red crosses to be seen from the air. Later in the war, the Allies gained air superiority, making enemy bombing and strafing raids on hospitals like this one less likely. Photograph courtesy of the AMEDD Center of History and Heritage, Image #B1-11-31.

FIGURE 6-17. [Top Right] World War II, European Theater of Operations, France. Note the medics and chaplain working with casualties. Chaplains offered spiritual comfort to the injured and sick, but also often pitched in doing active care. Photograph courtesy of the AMEDD Center of History and Heritage, Image #B1-11-29.

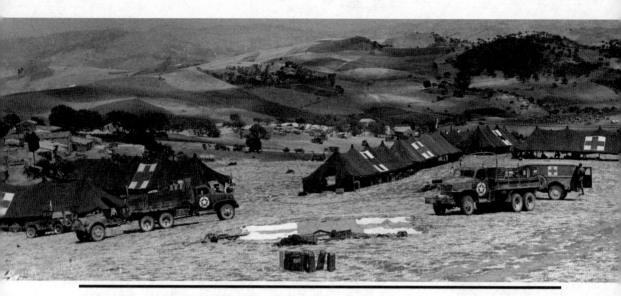

FIGURE 6-18. Tents of the 11th Field Hospital (2nd Platoon), Italy, August 1943. Note the 2 1/2-ton trucks, one pulling a water tank. Tents were deployed over the hillside. Tents were very commonly used for hospital facilities in all theaters of operations. Photograph courtesy of the AMEDD Center of History and Heritage, Image #MU-WWII-B1-003.

Spanish Civil War Forward Surgery

The Spanish Civil War, which lasted from 1936 until 1939, has been considered a testing time for the newer weapons and tactics of the supporters of each side. The Germans and the Italians supported the Nationalists, while the Soviet Union was the supporter of the Republican side. Britain, France, and the United States remained nominally neutral. The mobile surgical team concept was used in the war. Transfusions, the use of sulfa antibiotics, and the utilization of the tetanus vaccine were milestones in military medicine that were used extensively, depending on supplies. Many lessons in battlefield surgery were learned in this conflict.[75(p252)]

German Forward Surgery

The German Army has been always impressive in its ability to organize and plan; that admiration must be extended to the medical side. The German (Prussian) Army in the 1870–1871 Franco-Prussian War had dedicated litter bearers and ambulances. It utilized the railroads for evacuation. World War I medical and surgical care was excellent until logistical problems reduced medical supplies and medicines.

In World War II, the German military surgeon received intensive training at the Army medical schools. After a few months of medical training, the trainee would be posted as a medical officer's orderly. He would then receive basic infantry training for 8 months. The trainee would then attend the Berlin Military Medical Academy. Lectures at the Charité Hospital were next. The trainees took state examinations and then spent a year in the clinics. The trainee wrote a doctoral dissertation after which examinations followed. They were only then sent to the line with a rank of *Leutnant* (lieutenant) (*Assistenzarzt*). In wartime, the training was necessarily shortened.[76(p8)]

All German battalions, regiments, and divisions had variable manning levels, depending on the circumstances. The basic battalion was made up of several companies of 100 to 200 men. The battalion had a doctor with two corpsmen at the troop bandaging station. The division, which could vary from 10,000 to 20,000 men, had 16 doctors and 500 medical corpsmen.[76(p15)] There were typically two medical companies, of which one was horse drawn and the other was motorized. In the companies, the main bandaging station was led by the surgeon.[76(pp8–11)]

German field hospitals were usually located some 20 kilometers (12 miles) behind the front. They were set up to handle 200 patients, but could be expanded to handle another 300 if needed. A surgery team with two to three surgeons could handle 30 severely wounded, or 60 to 120 less severely wounded, in a 24-hour period. The evacuation of the wounded would extend back to reserve hospitals in Germany.[76(pp8–10)]

The first-line medical attention was given by a medical officer and medics at the VD (*Verwundetennest*—equivalent to an aid station). The next step in the move was a litter transport to the TV (*Truppenverbandplatz*—a troop clinic), which was analogous to the American battalion aid station. After the wounded were stabilized, they were taken to the HV (*Hauptverbandplatz*—a higher level troop surgical and triage center), which performed clearing and hospitalization details. The HV was located to the rear. It was operated by the division *Sanitaets Kompanie*. Two surgeons could be augmented by six to eight more as casualty load developed. Major surgical operations were done at this level.[76(pp8–11)]

British Forward Surgery

The Army Surgeon General detailed consultants to Britain to learn of its experience with preparing for and caring for casualties. The British had been in combat since 1939 and many of their innovations from World War I had been improved upon. The casualty clearing station of World War I fame was in operation but the new advanced surgical center (ASC) would supplement its function as an advanced surgical facility close to the front.[75(p253)]

The British had found that the great distance from a forward aid station to the casualty clearing station and then again to the general hospital mandated the creation of the ASC. The purpose of the ASC was to provide surgical care in the combat front lines. It was to be attached to a casualty clearing station or a field dressing station. The ASC was self-sufficient and could be moved to the area of greatest need. The ASC could deal with all areas of surgery and handled 15% of the overall surgery cases.[75(p253)]

SURGEONS GENERAL OF THE WORLD WAR II ERA

Charles Ranson Reynolds (1 June 1935–31 May 1939)

Reynolds graduated from the University of Michigan in 1895. He was a contract Army surgeon in 1900 and served in the Philippines. In World War I, he began his overseas service as a surgeon at Base Hospital No. 2. Later in the war, he was promoted to colonel and served in various staff positions. He directed his attention to frontline treatment issues and medical evacuation problems.[77]

Reynolds became the Surgeon General on 1 June 1935. As the threat of war increased, Reynolds was able to oversee some increase in medical officers and the reopening of medical internships in Army hospitals. He also oversaw the renewed emphasis on training at the Medical Field Service School. He was succeeded by James Magee on 1 June 1939.[77]

James C Magee (1 June 1939–31 May 1943)

Magee graduated from Jefferson Medical College (Philadelphia, Pennsylvania) in 1905. Interestingly, Magee worked as an Army contract surgeon from September 1907 until July 1908, at which time he was selected as one of the first lieutenants in the newly created Medical Reserve Corps. Magee completed the Army medical school course in Washington, DC, after which he was appointed a first lieutenant in the Regular Army Medical Corps in 1909.[78]

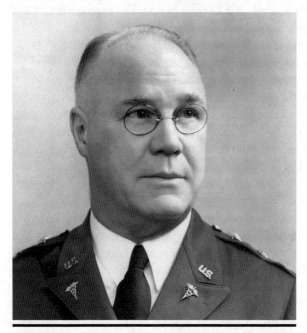

FIGURE 6-19. Surgeon General James Magee, US Army. Magee was selected as Army Surgeon General in June 1939 to replace Major General Charles Reynolds, who had completed his term of office; World War II started in September 1939 in Europe. Magee had to contend with changes in the reporting of his office. The Surgeon General and his office were moved from a direct War Department staff relationship to be subordinate to the Services of Supply. In addition, the personnel treating the Army Air Force were moved to a newly created Air Surgeon's Office. Photograph courtesy of the National Library of Medicine, Image #SGV2.

His service prior to World War I involved time in the Philippines with campaigns against the Moros and with the Punitive Expedition with Brigadier General Pershing in search of Pancho Villa after the Mexican irregulars attacked a United States community. Magee went to France in 1917 with Base Hospital No. 12. He was moved to an administrative post in France with the Services of Supply.[78]

Magee was selected as the next Army Surgeon General in June 1939 to replace MG Charles Reynolds, who had completed his term of office. As previously noted, World War II began in September 1939 in Europe. Magee had to contend with changes in the reporting of his office. The Surgeon General and his office were moved from a direct War Department staff relationship to be subordinate to the Services of Supply. In addition, the personnel treating the Army Air Force were moved to a newly created Air Surgeon's Office.[79] Magee worked to have direct access to the Chief of Staff of the Army, rather than going through the Chief, Services of Supply (direct access was finally granted in 1944). Magee laid the foundation for worldwide medical supply, hospitalization, and evacuation to meet the expanding theaters of war[80] (Figure 6-19).

Norman T Kirk (1 June 1943–31 May 1947)

Kirk graduated from the University of Maryland in 1910. He served with Pershing's Punitive Expedition into Mexico and also in the Panama Canal Zone. He spent World War I at the Medical Officer's Training Camp at Fort Oglethorpe, Georgia. In 1919, Kirk switched his specialty from general surgery to orthopedics. He went on to serve at a number of hospitals, including Sternberg General Hospital in the Philippines. He was selected as the Surgeon General in 1943 because General Marshall did not want Magee appointed to another term. Marshall preferred Alfred Kenner, but he was not chosen; Kirk was the compromise candidate.[81]

Kirk is credited with taking surgery to the men at the front. The mobile hospitals and the use of trained medical aid men at the front were singled out for praise. Under his guidance, his office reported that 15 million patients during the period of World War II (1941–1945) were admitted to the 692 hospitals overseas and the 65 general and 13 convalescent hospitals in the United States[81] (Figure 6-20).

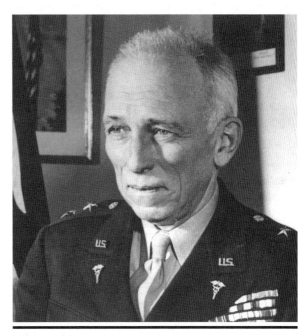

FIGURE 6-20. Surgeon General Norman T Kirk. He was selected as the Surgeon General in 1943 because General Marshall did not want Magee appointed to another term. Kirk is credited with taking surgery to the men at the front. The mobile hospitals and the use of trained medical aid men at the front were especially singled out for praise. Under his guidance, his office treated 15 million patients during the actual period of World War II. Photograph courtesy of the National Library of Medicine, Image #B030267.

MEDICAL ADVANCES IN WORLD WAR II

Surgical recommendations were made by COL McGowan, the Surgical Consultant for the 8th Army, in his report to the Surgeon General. These recommendations were echoed by other surgeons. He commented that in abdominal wounds gastric drainage was routine. He suggested liberal use of plasma and blood for support and the use of wire sutures. In chest injuries he suggested earlier diagnosis of hemothorax, as well as more liberal use of thoracotomy as needed.[49(p577)] The following discussion details other medical advances in World War II.

Anesthesia for the Wounded

In the official history of World War I, George Crile, a surgeon, wrote the section on anesthesia because there was no anesthesia representative on the Surgeon General's consultant list. In the "Great War," a nitrous oxide and oxygen combination was used primarily.[82(p53)] Ether and chloroform gave better muscular relaxation; however, the ease of use and quick recovery without many side effects made both ether and chloroform valued. Abdominal surgery requiring greater muscular relaxation could be supplemented by regional anesthesia.[82(p54)]

A number of anesthetics were available to provide anesthesia, including thiopental (Pentothal Sodium), ethylene, and ethyl chloride. Beecher, the Surgeon General's Anesthesia Consultant during World War II, noted that not all agents could be used in the interests of standardization. He also noted that the shortage of qualified personnel to deliver anesthesia called for agents that could be administered safely by nurses and physicians with limited anesthesia experience.[82(p57)] Hence, World War II anesthesia was limited to ether, thiopental sodium, and procaine hydrochloride (Figure 6-21).

To compensate for the shortage of trained personnel, a limited 6-month course was begun in 1939 at the Mayo Clinic to train one anesthesiologist at a time for 6 months, to be followed by another officer for another 6 months.[82(p57)] Army medical officers were to give anesthesia. Nurses gave inhalational anesthetics in Army hospitals mainly. Regional anesthetics were usually given by the surgeon. As the war progressed, the most able anesthetists were assigned to combat areas, at least in theory. Beecher observed that the evacuation hospital required the most personnel in the forward area. The field hospital was staffed by four auxiliary surgical teams with a physician anesthetist assigned to each team.[82(p58)]

The portable Heidbrink and McKesson equipment was used by the Army to deliver anesthesia. Henry Beecher designed a portable machine that was improved in configuration. It was small enough to be carried by hand and it had a feature that thoracic surgery could be done without using compressed oxygen, thereby conserving it.[82(p63),83(pp602–608)]

Because the Army combat focus had shifted to a "Europe first" plan, the increased number of troops to be stationed in England required that some English medical assets be utilized. The use of anesthesia in England for the United States Army Air Forces and Army units stationed there in the lead up to D-Day required the adaptation of American machines to use British gas cylinders (to save shipping). The plan was that the more serious cases would be evacuated to England for more definitive surgery until a strong foothold on the Continent could be achieved and more Allied medical assets could be based there. Training was set up to include lectures and practical work in British hospitals in 1943.

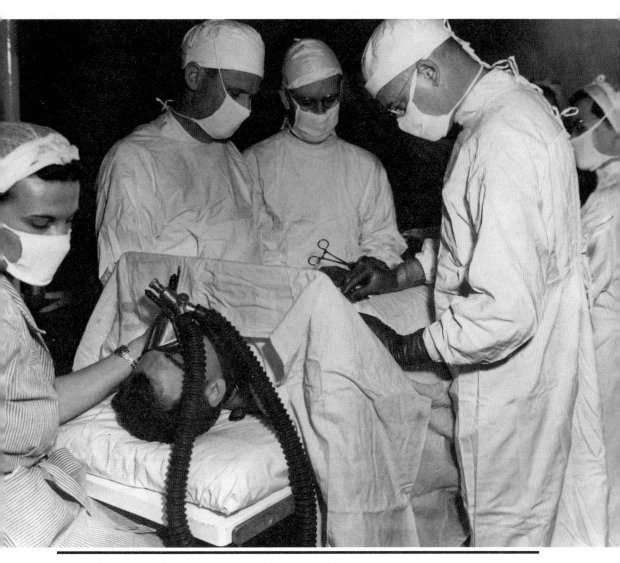

FIGURE 6-21. 11 August 1944, Major James H Spencer Jr, Chief Surgeon, operating on a patient in the 280th Station Hospital, Audely, England. Note the nurse anesthetist administrating face-mask anesthesia. Photograph courtesy of the Army Nurse Corps Photograph Collection, Image #B2-02-07.

This instruction was later taken over by Americans proficient in anesthesia. Shortages of portable anesthesia machines were present in North Africa because the British could not supply enough machines.[83(p601)] Cyclopropane and ethylene were not used in North Africa due to flammability of the former and difficulty of supply for both. In the North African casualties, it was determined that seriously wounded soldiers needed little premedication, if at all. Morphine was used sparingly as a preanesthetic because the drug might still be around in the circulation from the dose given in the field. Endotracheal intubation was

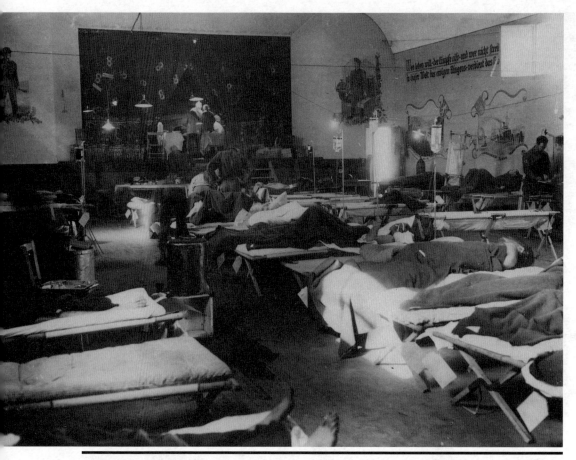

FIGURE 6-22. World War II, European Theater of Operations, 60th Field Hospital. Note the use of an existing building by the field hospital. The patients are awaiting surgery, which is being conducted on the stage at the rear. St. Max, France, 3 October 1944. Photograph courtesy of the AMEDD Center of History and Heritage, Image #B1-11-34.

used for all cases over an hour in length and in all cases of intracranial, abdominal, or facial wounds.[82(pp77–78)]

As Beecher pointed out, there were too few trained anesthetists even for the civilian world in peacetime America. The military supply of anesthesia personnel reflected that shortage at the start of the war. The Army anesthetist shortage appeared in the North African theater first because it was the site of the first prolonged fighting between the Americans and the Axis powers (Germany, Hungary, Bulgaria, Romania, Croatia, Italy, and Japan).[82(p57)] Hence, in an effort to improvise, anesthesia training was initiated in short schools and in on-the-job training. Regional anesthesia improvements included the addition of epinephrine hydrochloride in certain cases to reduce the amount of procaine used. Vasoconstrictors had to be avoided in surgery of tissues such as genitals, fingers, and noses to prevent tissue sloughing[82(pp66–67)] (Figure 6-22).

Improvements in Vascular Surgery

World War II saw a large number of arterial wounds due to the larger number of shell wounds with shrapnel. These patients were sent to vascular centers in the United States (Zone of the Interior). The Mayo General Hospital (Vascular Center) in Minnesota and the DeWitt General Hospital in Virginia were the main centers in terms of activity. The centers concluded that extirpation of the lesion and the maintenance or restoration of the arterial continuity in the surgical repair of aneurysms and arteriovenous fistula were the preferred treatments. Previously arterial ligation was the usual treatment.[84(pp267,300)] Specialized vascular centers were established initially at Ashford General Hospital, White Sulphur Springs, West Virginia, and Letterman General Hospital, San Francisco, California. The vascular activities at Letterman were transferred in 1943 to Torney General Hospital, Palm Springs, California.[84(p2)]

During the conflict at the Siegfried Line in 1944, the 45th Evacuation Hospital set up a vascular clinic to improve the treatment of patients with main vascular injury to the extremities. One surgical team from the 3rd Auxiliary Surgical Group was attached to the 45th to facilitate this treatment.[84(p160)] Other facilities devoted special care to vascular injuries at this point.

Treatment of Shock and Advances in Transfusion Methods

The thoughts about shock that were accepted at the start of conflict in Europe included (1) the onset of traumatic shock came from a reduction of the circulating blood volume and (2) the main treatment was a replacement of blood volume by transfusion.[79(p43)] These improvements in the understanding of shock and the use of whole blood transfusions were an area of significant advance in World War II. (The Germans did not develop a blood bank system. Indeed, they had no method of storing blood. They did use only direct transfusions from the donor to the recipient. The Germans had an aversion to the transfusion of more than 1,000cc [1 liter], apparently on doctrinal grounds.[79(p256)])

Plasma was embraced at the start of the war because there was no effective overseas blood program and the value of whole blood in the treatment of the wounded was not appreciated. Plasma was much easier to maintain and to ship without special time constraints.[79(pp48–49)] Dried plasma was selected as a blood substitute. A package was designed that was 50cc in size to facilitate the use of plasma; it was soon seen that a larger size was needed.[79(p133)] Three million packages of plasma were produced in 250cc size and another three million were packaged in the 50cc size.[79(p133)] Liquid plasma was developed for use in hospitals in the Zone of the Interior (continental United States).[79(p134)] Albumin, in the form of serum albumin transfusion, was useful in that it was immediately available for use, not requiring rehydration. Its storage required less space than the plasma supplies.[79(p140)]

In the Southwest Pacific Area Command, COL McGowan reported the use of whole blood increased with improvements in blood storage and packaging. For example, blood was supplied at Leyte in a package of 16 units with 17 pounds of cracked ice. McGowan had reaction-free tubing, which matched the ease of using plasma. The consultants for orthopedics and general surgery stressed the use of whole blood when possible.[49(p573)]

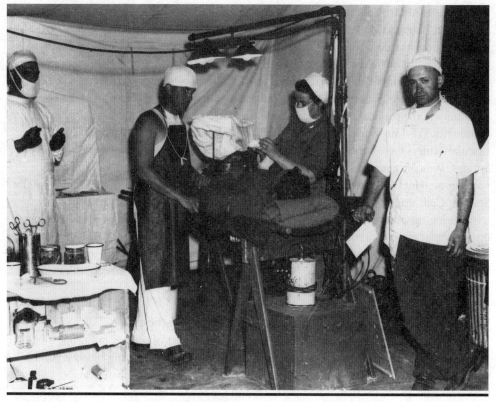

FIGURE 6-23. World War II clinical nursing. Operating room scene in a field hospital. Photograph courtesy of the AMEDD Center of History and Heritage, Image #B2-02-44.

The need for whole blood readily became apparent in North Africa as casualties mounted. The safe storage of whole blood was felt to be for only 5 days at the time.[79(p50)] However, one surgeon reported use of blood over 30 days of age without problem.[79(p50)] In May 1943, the Subcommittee on Blood Substitutes of the War Department recommended the use of whole blood be adopted by the armed forces in a speedy manner.[79(p54)] The British found in North Africa that the use of plasma in severe wounds was not able to replace the use of whole blood.[85(p55)] The British at the Battle of El Alamein (May 1942) attempted large-scale combat casualty transfusion.[79(p54)] COL Edward D Churchill became the Surgery Consultant in North Africa in March 1943. He concluded after a review of the data that whole blood was the agent of choice. Four months later, a central blood bank was set up in the theater. LTC Candict W Carter, of the Surgeon General's Surgical Consultant Division, stated that by July 1944, the value of whole blood was recognized for both the Zone of the Interior (the continental United States) and combat areas[79(pp71–72)] (Figures 6-23 and 6-24).

Improved Survivability in Thoracic Surgery

In World War II, 80% of chest wounds were caused by artillery shell fragments, and the remaining 20% from bullet wounds.[86(p54)] As the war progressed, more men recovered

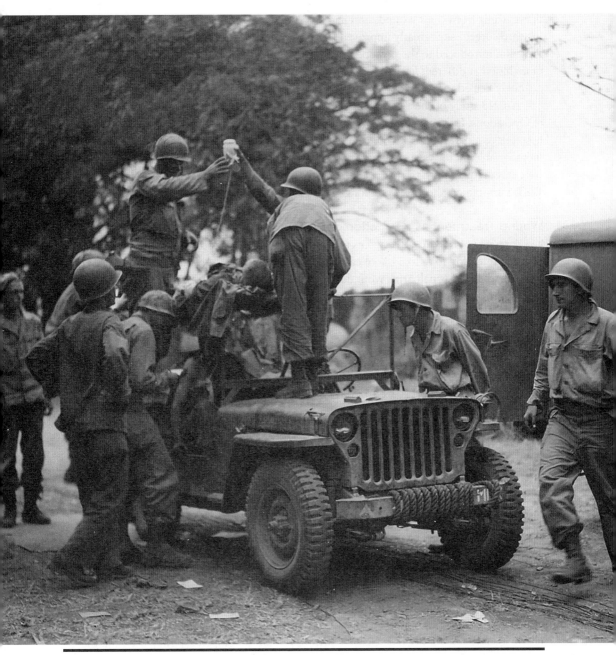

FIGURE 6-24. Jeep carrying patient receiving plasma. The 4-wheel-drive Jeeps were often used for evacuation of the wounded. Plasma was used at the start of World War II because there was no effective overseas blood program and the value of whole blood in the treatment of the wounded was not appreciated in the early part of the war. Plasma was much easier to store without any special time expiration dates. Dried plasma was selected as a blood substitute and featured even greater storage and transport capability over the liquid version. Photograph courtesy of the AMEDD Center of History and Heritage, Image #MU-WWII-LL-039.

uneventfully from chest wounds and had less surgery at fixed facilities. The surgery at forward surgery sites greatly improved. The indications for thoracotomy were established. Penicillin introduced to the postoperative scene helped recovery. Thoracotomy required more blood at different levels of complication. The improved availability of whole blood definitely helped recovery.[87(p303)]

A 1943 study of chest wound patients was initiated in the Mediterranean Theater of Operations. It showed that thoracotomies were performed unnecessarily in forward hospitals as a part of initial wound surgery. The study also showed that indications for thoracotomies in forward surgery facilities could be clearly defined. Procedures and practices were standardized with the net result that as part of this study, patients were followed until 1961 with soldiers showing good long-term results following thoracotomy.[88(pp441–443,525–527)]

Wound Treatment as a Function of Ballistics

A review of the causative agents in wounding revealed interesting findings. Small arms fire accounted for 14% to 31% of casualties, depending on the theater of operations. The Pacific had 30.7% small arms woundings, compared to 23.4% in Europe. (Artillery and mortar fire accounted for 65% of casualties in Europe and the Mediterranean but only 47% in the Pacific.[89(p76)])

A variety of weapons accounted for the small arms ballistic woundings. The Americans used the M1A1 Thompson submachine gun (.30 caliber). Many of the earlier M1928 A1s were also carried, especially by paratroops. The M1903 Springfield Rifle, of World War I fame, was still used by many troops, even on D-Day. The M1917 A1 heavy machine gun was used by the infantry. The M3 "grease gun" submachine gun could be made much more cheaply than the Thompson and was preferred in close quarters. The main infantry weapon was the M1 Garand. The carbine M1A1 had a folding stock and a 15-round magazine, which was popular. The British used the Lee-Enfield No. 4, Mk.I, and the Sten gun in .303 caliber. The Germans used the MP40 submachine gun and the MG42 machine guns. The Kar98k Mauser rifle with the 7.92 Mauser rifle cartridge was the standard German arm. Later in the war, the Germans developed and fielded the first assault rifle— the FG-42 Type II *Fallsschirm Jagerewehr*. The main change from World War I was the availability of automatic weapons on an increased level for the troops, with a concurrent increase in lethality.[90(pp43–47)]

Development of Various Pharmaceuticals

One of the most important areas in forward surgery for World War II was the use of antibiotics. Prior to World War I, Germany was the world leader in developing pharmaceutical chemicals. The German firm Bayer had developed aspirin (acetylsalicylic acid) in 1899. The Germans developed Novocain and the synthetic antimalarial Atabrine in the period from 1900 to the 1920s. Tannic acid and gentian violet, which was sometimes mixed with sulfa powder, were used for burn treatment. Paul Ehrlich, a German and the winner of the 1908 Nobel Prize for his work, introduced Salvarsan and Neosalvarsan against syphilis in 1910. A treatment for venereal disease such as syphilis and later gonorrhea had obvious importance for the militaries of all nations.[91(pp15–16)] The development of penicillin brought great effect against the ravages of syphilis.[92(p6)] Antibiotics in the form of the sulfonamides were used in the Spanish Civil War and their use was ensured for World War II.[75(p254)] The Spanish Civil War involved active participation by the Spanish, Germans, Italians, and the Russians. All of the participants from outside Spain used the war as a testing ground for new techniques, equipment, and medicines. Tetanus vaccine developed by the Pasteur Institute in 1931 was used in the Spanish Civil War for the first time.[75(pp253–254)]

Sulfa drugs were developed in the 1930s and marked a pivotal move of industrial pharmaceutical research and production from Germany to America, France, and England.[91(pp8–9)] Penicillin was produced by a critical English-American cooperative venture in 1942. Bayer Laboratories, of the firm IG Farben, introduced Prontosil, which was the first sulfonamide drug, in 1932.[91(pp15–16)] Sulfa medicines were available at Pearl Harbor. The military used sulfa for a wide range of diseases. Actually, penicillin was often used as an addition to sulfas rather than replacing them. Sir Alexander Fleming published his original *British Journal of Experimental Pathology* article reflecting his 1928 discovery of penicillin.[93(p226)] Sir Howard Florey placed penicillin in clinical use. He had significant help at the Rockefeller Foundation. Because the British had difficulty manufacturing penicillin in quantity at Oxford, the British then worked with the US Department of Agriculture at the Northern Regional Research Laboratory in Peoria, Illinois. In the quest for a better mold, a laboratory technician in Peoria brought in a cantaloupe from a market infected with an interesting fungus identified as *Penicillium chrysogenum*.[94(pp93,95–99)] Production increased each year after 1943. The pilot use in troops was done at Bushnell General Hospital (Utah) and at Halloran General Hospital (New York).[94(p106),95(pp64–67)] In December 1945, Sir Alexander Fleming, Dr Ernst Chain, and Sir Howard Florey were awarded the Nobel Prize for their work on the discovery of penicillin.[94(p119)]

COL Cutler, the ETO Chief Consultant in Surgery, received a crate from the Merck and Company of New Jersey at a US Army Air Forces base containing the first penicillin in quantity. Cutler took the shipment to the 2nd General Hospital in England. He worked with Professor Florey in its use, storage, and recovery from the urine of patients due to its scarcity. The use of penicillin was restricted to gangrene, serious infections including osteomyelitis, eye infections (used in ointment), and "septic hands."[57(pp68–69)]

Penicillin proved to be the most effective antibacterial agent used by military surgeons. The ability to mass produce penicillin saved many lives. For example, in 1943, there was just enough penicillin for 100 cases. In the next year, the penicillin production was increased to 3 billion units per year, which was enough to treat the Allied casualties. Although the Germans had been foremost earlier in the century in pharmaceutical research, they did not have access to penicillin.[75(p254)]

Treatment of Burns/Plastic Surgery

The Chief Surgeon in the European Theater of Operations made the plastic surgery service responsible for treating burns that might require skin grafting. The Army Surgical Research Unit was the first hospital set up as a burn center, which would become a model for burn centers in the future.[57(pp539–540)] Plastic surgery was considered a new specialty in World War II. A Consultant in Plastic Surgery was appointed. Cases that were to be considered in the realm of plastics were defined, including burns, maxillofacial injuries, and injuries requiring skin grafts or flaps.[57(p521–522)] There were 10 burn centers in different locations in England.[57(p543),85(p176)]

Mobile Surgery Units

In 1943, COL Elliott C Cutler requested that MG Paul R Hawley, the ETO Chief Surgeon, request that Washington assign auxiliary surgery teams to the ETO. Cutler believed that optimal care could be best given by bringing the surgeon to the wounded soldier. In February 1943, he attended a conference featuring MG David C Monro, Royal Army Medical Corps, and the consulting surgeon to the British Army. At this meeting, the experience of the British in Libya and their move away from casualty clearing stations and forward units in favor of mobile surgery teams were discussed. In North Africa, the British had field surgical units and later mobile surgical units. He stated that the surgeons used should be skilled and that fixed equipment in vehicles was not satisfactory because a single bullet to the radiator could stop the vehicle (the World War I Mobile Surgical Hospitals and the French *auto-chir* also illustrate this point).[96(pp78–79)]

Later, COL Cutler assigned MAJ Robert Zollinger, Medical Corps, of the 5th General Hospital (later colonel and Senior Consultant in General Surgery), to work up plans for a mobile surgical unit. Cutler stipulated that Zollinger should not have any vehicles with fixed installed equipment, that the tents and equipment were to be for a mobile surgical unit, and that the unit have enough materials and lighting to handle 100 major surgeries or 200 minor cases.[96(p80)]

Significant advances in forward surgery were made in World War II. Although many lessons learned in World War I had to be relearned for this next war, the roles of the portable surgical hospital and the auxiliary surgery groups were important. The need for increased mobility and the need for talented surgeons brought about the Mobile Army Surgical Hospital (MASH) of the next conflict. Although this chapter did not cover the spectrum of World War II medicine and surgery, the increased importance of forward surgery was highlighted.

For forward surgery in its basic form, the 70 portable surgical hospitals received campaign credit during World War II. The Pacific theater counted 52 portable surgical hospitals, with 18 listed for the China-Burma-India theater. The six portable surgical hospitals utilized in the European theater were too late for combat, but received occupation service credit.[97]

The amphibious operations were carried out on varied terrain from coral atolls (Kwajalein) to large land masses (the Philippines). The evacuation hospital could not be employed in the small coral atolls and were used on larger targets. However, the portable surgical hospitals were perfect to support smaller landings and to provide support to division clearing companies in amphibious operations.[98(p61)]

THE WAR ENDS

VE (Victory in Europe) Day was on 8 May 1945. Hitler had committed suicide on 30 April 1945 in his bunker in a besieged Berlin along with his wife Eva Braun (married prior to their suicide). Joseph Goebbels, the Propaganda Minister, committed suicide with his wife after they had murdered their children.[1(p560)] Mussolini had met his end at the hands of Italian people on 28 April 1945.[1(p405)] Before his suicide, Hitler had removed Reichmarshal Herman Goering as his successor. Goering was captured shortly thereafter and stood trial after the war (but committed suicide from a secreted cyanide capsule[1(p510)]). Berlin surrendered on 2 May 1945; the remaining German forces capitulated on 8 May 1945. Hitler had designated Grandadmiral Karl Donitz as his successor.[1(p559)]

The Japanese surrendered on 14 August 1945.[1(p577)] The atomic bombing of Hiroshima, followed by the atomic bombing of Nagasaki, helped persuade the Japanese to capitulate. However, the entry of Russia into the Pacific War had had a more immediate effect. The surrender of the Japanese on the USS *Missouri* was presided over by General of the Army Douglas MacArthur. The ceremony was conducted on the ship in Tokyo Bay.[1(p577)]

Even with the end of the war, it was clear that the Soviet Union was following its own agenda. All of the countries taken over by the Soviets from the Germans were to remain in the Soviet sphere. The stage was being set for additional conflicts for which the Army Medical Department had to prepare.

REFERENCES

1. Roberts A. *The Storm of War: A New History of the Second World War*. New York, NY: Harper Collins; 2011.
2. Costello J. *The Pacific War: 1941–1945*. New York, NY: Harper; 2009.
3. Pogue FC. *The United States Army in World War II: The European Theater of Operations: The Supreme Command*. Washington, DC: Center for Military History; 1989.
4. Atkinson R, D'Este C, Hastings M, et al. *On War: The Best Military Histories*. Leesburg, Va: Weider History Group and the Pritzker Military Museum; 2013.
5. Hamilton N. *The Mantle of Command: FDR at War, 1941–1942*. New York, NY: Houghton Mifflin Harcourt; 2014.
6. Bluhm RK, ed. *US Army: A Complete History*. Arlington, Va: The Army Historical Foundation; 2004.
7. Matloff M, Snell EM. Strategic planning for coalition warfare 1941–1942. British-American plans. January–November 1941. In: *United States Army in World War II*. Washington, DC: US Government Printing Office; 1980. Chap 3.
8. Greenfield KR, ed. *United States Army in World War II. United States Armed Forces in Northern Ireland*. Washington, DC: Center for Military History, US Government Printing Office; 1960. Chronology section.
9. Smith CM, ed. *United States Army in World War II. The Technical Services. The Medical Department: Hospitalization and Evacuation, Zone of the Interior*. Washington, DC: Center for Military History, Office of the Chief Military History; 1989.

10. Mullins WS, ed. *Medical Department of the United States Army in World War II. Administrative Series; Medical Training in World War II*. Washington, DC: Office of the Surgeon General; 1974.
11. Smith CM. Medical service in the Atlantic defense area. In: Wiltse CM. *The Medical Department: Medical Service in the Mediterranean and Minor Theaters*. In: *United States Army in World War II. The Technical Services*. Washington, DC: Department of the Army, Office of the Chief of Military History; 1987 [first published 1965].
12. Hoff EC, ed. *Preventive Medicine in World War II*. Vol 8. In: Lada J, ed. *United States Army in World War II. The Medical Department*. Washington, DC: Department of the Army: Office of The Surgeon General; 1976.
13. Manchester W. *American Caeser: Douglas MacArthur: 1880–1964*. New York, NY: Back Bay Books (Little Brown); 1979.
14. Newcomb RF. *The Battle of Savo Island*. New York, NY: Henry Holt and Company; 1961.
15. LeTourneau R, LeTourneau D. *Operation KE: The Cactus Air Force and the Japanese Withdrawal From Guadalcanal*. Annapolis, Md: The Naval Institute Press; 2012.
16. Seipe S. *Ghost in the Fog: The Untold Story of Alaska's World War II Invasion*. New York, NY: Scholastic Press; 2011.
17. Seagrave GS. *Burma Surgeon Returns*. New York, NY: WW Norton; 1946.
18. Editor. *Life* visits an Army Hospital in Burma. *Life*. 1 November 1943: 23.
19. Seagrave GS. *Burma Surgeon*. New York, NY: WW Norton and Company; 1943.
20. Editor. Review of *Burma Surgeon Returns*. *JAMA*. 1946;122(6):357–358.
21. Lathrop AK. Dateline Burma. *Dartmouth Med*. 2004;28(3):28.
22. Romanus CF, Sunderland R. China-Burma-India theater. Stilwell's mission to China. In: *United States Army in World War II*. Washington, DC: Center of Military History, United States Army; 1987.
23. Condon-Rall ME, Cowdrey AE. The China-Burma-India challenge. In: *The Medical Department: Medical Service in the War Against Japan*. In: *The United States Army in World War II. The Technical Services*. Washington, DC: US Army Center for Military History; 1998.
24. Tuchman BW. The retreat from Burma. *Am Heritage Mag*. 1971;22(2):6.
25. Tuchman BW. *Stilwell and the American Experience in China*. New York, NY: The Macmillan Company; 1971.
26. Stilwell JW, White TR, ed. *The Stilwell Papers*. New York, NY: Sloane and Associates; 1948.
27. Stone JH, ed. *Crisis Fleeting; Original Reports on Military Medicine in India and Burma in the Second World War*. Washington, DC: Office of The Surgeon General, Department of the Army; 1969.
28. Young KR. The Stilwell controversy: a bibliographical review. *Mil Affairs*. 1975;39(2):66.
29. Hoover H. *Freedom Betrayed: Herbert Hoover's Secret History of the Second World War and Its Aftermath*. Stanford, Calif: Hoover Institution Press; 2011.
30. McLaughlin J. *General Albert C Wedemeyer: America's Unsung Strategist in World War II*. Havertown, Penn: Casemate Publishers; 2012.
31. First United States Army. *Report of Operations 20 October 1943–1 August 1944*. Washington, DC: Office of Medical History, Office of The Surgeon General; 2004.
32. War Department, US Army. *Medical Field Manual: Mobile Units of the Medical Department*. Washington, DC: War Department; 1944. Field Manual 8-5, as amended Change 2.20. April 1944.
33. War Department, US Army. *Medical Field Manual: Mobile Units of the Medical Department*. Washington, DC: War Department; Field Manual 8-5. 1942.

34. War Department, US Army. *Military Medical Manual*. Harrisburg, Penn: The Military Service Publishing Company; 1944.
35. War Department, US Army. *Military Medical Manual*. Harrisburg, Penn: The Military Service Publishing Company; April 1941.
36. War Department, US Army. *Mobile Units of the Medical Department*. Carlisle Barracks, Penn: Medical Field Service School; 1941.
37. Thorndike A. Surgical problems in the Buna campaign. *Bull US Army Med Dept*. 1944:77–81. http://cdm15290.contentdm.oclc.org/cdm/ref/collection/p15290coll6/id/1373. Accessed 30 November 2015.
38. Developments in military medicine during the administration of Surgeon General Norman T Kirk. *Bull US Army Med Dept*. 1947;7(6):594–646;520–562,541.
39. War Department, US Army. *Portable Surgical Hospital*. Washington, DC: War Department; Table of Organization and Equipment, No. 8-572S. 4 June 1943.
40. War Department, US Army. *Portable Surgical Hospital*. Washington, DC; War Department; Table of Organization and Equipment, No. 8-572S. Change 1. 2 September 1943.
41. War Department, US Army. *Portable Surgical Hospital*. Washington, DC: War Department; Table of Organization and Equipment, No. 8-572S. Change 2. 7 December 1943.
42. War Department, US Army. *Portable Surgical Hospital*. Washington, DC: War Department; Table of Organization and Equipment, No. 8-572. 14 December 1944.
43. Pattillo DA. *Portable Surgical Hospitals in the North Burma Campaign: Lessons for Providing Forward Surgical Support to Nonlinear Operations in Airland Operations* [thesis]. Fort Leavenworth, Kans: Command and General Staff College; 1993.
44. Thorndike A. Surgical problems in the Buna campaign. *Bull US Army Med Dept*. 1944;79.
45. Editor. The portable surgical hospital. *US Army Med Bull*. 1943;69(October):7–8.
46. Warmenhoven S. *Medical Department—32rd Infantry Division Papuan Campaign*. In: *Medical Department, United States Army in World War II*. http://history.amedd.army.mil/booksdocs/wwii/PapuanReport/default.html#PAPUAN. Accessed 30 November 2015.
47. Perry M. *The Most Dangerous Man in America: The Making of Douglas MacArthur*. New York, NY: Basic Books; 2014.
48. Marston D. *The Pacific War: From Pearl to Harbor to Hiroshima*. University Park, Ill: Osprey Publishing; 2012.
49. McGowan FJ. Surgical manpower. In: Rankin FW, ed. *Activities of Surgical Consultants*. Vol 1. In: Coates JB, ed. *Medical Department United States Army in World War II*. Washington, DC: Department of the Army, Office of The Surgeon General; 1955: Chap 19.
50. Smith CM. Providing hospitalization for theaters of operations. In: *The Medical Department: Hospitalization and Evacuation, Zone of the Interior*. In: *United States Army in World War II. The Technical Services*. Washington, DC: Office of the Chief Military History, Office of The Surgeon General, Department of the Army; 1966: Chap 8.
51. Hall DE. *From the Roer to the Elbe with the 1st Medical Group: Medical Support of the Deliberate River Crossing* [thesis]. Fort Leavenworth, Kans: US Command and General Staff College; 1992.
52. Tovell RM. Anesthesia. In: Carter BN, ed. *Surgery in World War II: Activities of Surgical Consultants*. Vol 2. In: Coates JB, ed. *Medical Department, United States Army*. Washington, DC: Office of The Surgeon General, Department of the Army; 1964; Chap 10.
53. Streit PH. Report of the 61st Medical Battalion, Annual Report for 1944, Medical Department Activities in the Pacific Ocean Areas. http://history.amedd.army.mil/booksdocs/wwii/StreitCenPacrev.htm. Accessed 30 November 2015.

54. Editor. Surgery at the front. *Bull US Army Med Dept.* 1944;75(4):1–3.
55. Shaw WJ. Report of Medical Department Activities in New Guinea. 2 September 1944. http://history.amedd.army.mil/booksdocs/wwii/Shaw41ID.htm. Accessed 30 November 2015.
56. Cosmas GA, Cowdrey AE. *Medical Services in the European Theater of Operations*. In: Smith CM, ed. *Medical Department US Army in World War II. Technical Services*. Washington, DC: Center for Military History; 1992.
57. Cutler EC. The chief consultant in surgery. In: Carter BN, ed. *Surgery in World War II, Activities of the Surgical Consultants*. Vol 2. In: Coates JB, ed. *Medical Department, United States Army in World War II*. Washington, DC: Department of the Army, Office of The Surgeon General; 1964: Chap 2.
58. Operation Overlord. Annual Report to the Surgeon General from the Third Surgical Auxiliary Group for the Year 1944. In: Smith CM, ed. *The US Army in World War II. The Medical Department Medical Service in the European Theater of Operations*. Washington, DC: Surgeon General's Office, Army Medical Department; 1962.
59. War Department, US Army. *Auxiliary Surgical Group*. Washington, DC: War Department. Table of Organization and Equipment 8-571; 13 July 1942.
60. War Department, US Army. *Mobile Units of the Medical Department*. Washington, DC. War Department, Department of the Army; Field Manual 8-55. 12 January 1942.
61. War Department, US Army. *Mobile Units of the Medical Department*. Washington, DC: War Department, Department of the Army; Field Manual 8-55. Change No. 2. 20 April 1944.
62. Author unknown. Surgery at field hospitals. *Bull US Army Med Dept.* 1944;83(12):22–25.
63. Staff. Lost enemy action. *Naval History. (USNI)1.* 2014;28(3):31.
64. Report of Medical Department Activities in European Theater of Operations. Crandall AJ. Interview 8 June 1945. http://history.amedd.army.mil/books.html. Accessed 30 November 2015.
65. Experiences of 1st LT Davis, MC–Medical Officer LST 496 on D-Day. http://history.amedd.army.mil/booksdocs/wwii/Overlord/DavisDday.html. Accessed 30 November 2015.
66. Narrative by Captain Willis P McKee, Medical Corps, 326th Airborne Medical Company, 101st Airborne Division–D-Day Invasion. http://history.amedd.army.mil/booksdocs/wwii/326thAirborneMedCo101stABDiv/CPTMcKee326thABMedCoDDay.html. Accessed 30 November 2015.
67. Symonds CL. Normandy's crucial component. *Naval History.* 2014;28(3):17–23.
68. Lewis N. *Exercise Tiger*. New York, NY: Prentice Hall Trade; 1990.
69. Small K. *The Forgotten Dead: Why 946 American Servicemen Died off the Coast of Devon in 1944 and the Man Who Discovered Their True Story*. London, England: Bloomsbury Publishing; 1988.
70. 101st Airborne Division Annual Report 1944. http://history.amedd.army.mil/booksdocs/wwii/101stABNDIVSurg1944/101stABNDivSurg1944.htm. Accessed 20 September 2015.
71. Hall DE. "We Were Ready": Health Services Support in the Normandy Campaign. http://history.amedd.army.mil/booksdocs/wwii/Overlord/Normandy/HallNormandy.html. Accessed 30 November 2015.
72. Henry M Hills Jr, MD. http://www.zoominfo.com/p/Henry-Hills/917498145. Accessed 30 November 2015.
73. First United States Army. Annex 11. Report of Operations 1 August 1944–22 February 1945. Medical Section Report–Surgical. Washington, DC: Department of the Army; 1945.
74. The Fight for the Hurtgen Forest, 11 September 1944–15 December 1944. http://history.amedd.army.mil/booksdocs/wwii/HuertgenForest/HF.htm. Accessed 30 November 2015.
75. Gabriel RA, Metz KS. *A History of Military Medicine*. Vol 2. *From the Renaissance Through Modern Times*. London, England: Greenwood Press; 1992.

76. Buchner A. *The German Army Medical Corps in World War II: A Photo Chronicle*. Atglen, Penn: Schiffer Publishing; 1999.
77. US Army Medical Department. Office of Medical History. *Surgeons General. Charles Ranson Reynolds*. http://history.amedd.army.mil/surgeongenerals/C_Reynolds.html. Accessed 30 November 2015.
78. Engert RM. (Revised 2001 Greenwood JT.) *James C. Magee–Surgeon General for the period 1 June 1939–31 May 1943*. Washington, DC: Surgeon General's Office. 1964 (revised 2001).
79. Kendrick DB. The blood program. In: Rankin FW, ed. *Activities of Surgical Consultants*. Vol 1. In: Coates JB, ed. *Medical Department, United States Army in World War II*. Washington, DC: Department of the Army, Office of The Surgeon General; 1962: Chap 6.
80. US Army Medical Department. Office of Medical History. *Surgeons General. James Carre Magee*. http://history.amedd.army.mil/surgeongenerals/J_Magee.html. Accessed 30 November 2015.
81. US Army Medical Department. Office of Medical History. *Surgeons General. Norman T Kirk*. http://history.amedd.army.mil/surgeongenerals/N_Kirk2.html. Accessed 30 November 2015.
82. Beecher HK. Anesthesia for men wounded in battle. In: DeBakey ME, ed. *General Surgery*. Vol 2. In: Coates JB, ed. *Medical Department of the United States Army Surgery in World War II*. Washington, DC: Department of the Army, Office of The Surgeon General. 1955; Chap 3.
83. Beecher HK. An easily transportable anesthetic apparatus for anesthesia with or without compressed oxygen. Especially designed for positive pressure anesthesia in thoracic surgery under military conditions. *War Med*. 1942;2: 602–608.
84. Freeman NE, Shumacker HB Jr. Arterial aneurysms and arteriovenous fistulas: maintenance of arterial continuity. In Elkin DC, DeBakey ME, eds. *History of Surgery*. In: Coates JB, ed. *Medical Department, United States Army: Surgery in World War II*. Washington, DC: Department of the Army, Office of The Surgeon General; 1955; Chap 8.
85. Naythons M. *The Faces of Mercy. A Photographic History of Medicine at War*. New York, NY: Random House; 1993.
86. Berry F. General consideration of chest wounds. Berry F, ed. *Thoracic Surgery*. Vol. 1. In: Coates JB, ed. *Medical Department, United States Army Surgery in World War II*. Washington, DC: Department of the Army, Office of The Surgeon General; 1963: Chap 2.
87. Burford TH. Reparative surgery. In: Berry FB, ed. *Thoracic Surgery*. Vol 1. In: Coates JB, ed. *Medical Department, United States Army Surgery in World War II*. Washington, DC: Department of the Army, Office of The Surgeon General; 1963; Chap 12.
88. Brewer LA. Long term (1943–1961) follow-up studies in combat induced thoracic wounds. In: Berry F, ed. *Thoracic Surgery*. Vol 1. In: Coates JB, ed. *Medical Department, United States Army Surgery in World War II*. Washington, DC: Department of the Army, Office of The Surgeon General; 1965: Chap 11.
89. Beyer JC, Arima JK, Johnson DW. Enemy ordnance material. In: Beyer JC, ed. *Wound Ballistics*. In: Coates JB, ed. *Medical Department, United States Army in World War II*. Washington, DC: Department of the Army, Office of The Surgeon General; 1962: Chap 1.
90. Morgan M. Forgotten guns of D-Day. *Am Rifleman*. 2014;162(6):43–47.
91. Lesch JE. *The First Miracle Drugs: How the Sulfa Drugs Transformed Medicine*. New York, NY: Oxford University Press; 2007.
92. Budd R. *Penicillin: Triumph and Tragedy*. New York, NY: Oxford University Press; 2007.
93. Fraser I. The doctor's debt to the soldier. *J Royal Army Med Corps*. 1971;117:64–67.

94. Jacobs F. *Breakthrough: The True Story of Penicillin*. Originally published Dodd, Mead and Company. 1985 and reissued as An Authors Guild BackInPrint.com. Linçoln, Nebr: Universe, Inc; 2004.
95. Fleming A. On the antibacterial action of cultures on a penicillin with special reference to their use in the isolation of B. Influenza. *Br J Exp Path*.1929;10:226.
96. Bricker EM. Plastic surgery. In: Carter BN, ed. *Surgery in World War II, Activities of the Surgical Consultants*. Vol 2. In: Coates JB, ed. *Medical Department, United States Army in World War II*. Washington, DC: Department of the Army, Office of The Surgeon General; 1964: Chap 8.
97. US Department of the Army. *Unit Citation and Campaign Participation Credit Register*. Washington, DC: Headquarters, Department of the Army; DA Pamphlet 672-1, with Changes 1–4; July 1961.
98. Willis JN, Menaker GJ. Medical aspects of amphibious operations in Pacific Ocean areas. *Bull US Army Med Dept*. 1945;4(1):61–68.

Chapter Seven

Forward Surgery in the Korean War: The Mobile Army Surgical Hospitals

SCOTT C. WOODARD

INTRODUCTION

NAPOLEON'S SURGEON TO THE IMPERIAL GUARD, Dominique Jean Larrey, in Europe and the Army of the Potomac's Medical Director, Jonathan Letterman, in the War Between the States were both faced with a similar dilemma—how to quickly render surgical aid to the wounded soldier in combat. Their struggle has continued to plague the surgeon in modern times. The critical challenge is balancing the close proximity of surgical care near the front lines where the wounded need it most, with the need to not become a casualty as well. The military surgeon must weigh his ability to protect himself and save others to fight another day.

Popular culture's most highlighted medical story of the Korean War is the Mobile Army Surgical Hospital (MASH). Hollywood wove the tale of the MASH through the movie and television series, M*A*S*H. However, one actual MASH surgeon, Dr Otto F Apel Jr, cautioned that, "the interpretation [presented by the movie and television series] is several times removed from the reality it purports to depict. . . . The artistic presentation is always four or five times removed from reality."[2(p93)] He did add, however, that the appearance of irreverent attitudes and lighter moments often depicted had basis in truth.[2(ppxi–xiii,122–123)] Intended originally to be close to the fighting front, the MASH was equipped to move on its own[3–6] (Table 7-1). The light scale of medical services provided reflected this efficient mobility. As combat on the peninsula matured, becoming large and stalled, the MASH evolved into a stationary

> [I]N EVERY NEW WAR THE SAME STUPID MISTAKES ARE MADE AGAIN AND SOLDIERS LOSE THEIR LIVES AND LIMBS, BECAUSE THE DOCTOR WAS IGNORANT OF PAST EXPERIENCE. I CANNOT OVER EMPHASIZE THE NEED TO STUDY MILITARY MEDICINE AND SURGERY. [1(P716)]
>
> Colonel Edward D Churchill
> US Army

TABLE 7-1. **MASH MOVES BY YEAR**

Unit	1950 No. of moves	1951 No. of moves	1952 No. of moves	1953 No. of moves
8055th	(9 Jul–31 Dec) 14	(1 Jan–31 Dec) 9	(1 Jan–31 Dec) 0	(1 Jan–1 Feb) 0
8063rd	(18 Jul–31 Dec) 23	(1 Jan–31 Dec) 9	(1 Jan–31 Dec) 0	(1 Jan–1 Feb) Unknown
8076th	(2 Aug–31 Dec) 7	(1 Jan–31 Dec) 9	(1 Jan–31 Dec) 0	(1 Jan–31 Dec) 1
1st 8209th	(26 Sep–31 Dec) 4	(1 Jan–31 Dec) 4		
8209th		(22 May–31 Dec) 2	(1 Jan–31 Dec) 0	(1 Jan–1 Feb) 1
2nd 8225th		(15 Apr–12 May) 1		
8225th		(13 May–31 Dec) 2	(1 Jan–31 Dec) 2	(1 Jan–1 Feb) 0
8228th		(15 Jun–31 Dec) 0	(1 Jan–31 Dec) 2	(1 Jan–1 Feb) 0

Data sources: Annual reports of Medical Department activities for each MASH unit, National Archives II, Suitland, Maryland, boxes 144, 146, 239, 240, and 241.

facility with more capabilities. Initially, the unit was formed to provide surgical capabilities for one division. It transformed through the course of the war into a multidivision and multinational all-purpose hospital.[7(pp88–89)] For example, as early as November 1950, the 1st MASH transformed from a 60-bed to a 200-bed capacity hospital. There was an expansion in workload (medical cases in addition to surgery) without a commensurate increase in personnel. Rapid patient evacuation was the only means of keeping up with the workload.[8(pp115–116)]

WORLD WAR II: PRELUDE TO MOBILE ARMY SURGICAL HOSPITALS

The MASH story began before the well-known fictional account of "Hawkeye" Pierce and the comedic 4077th in Korea. The idea was actually quite old. The experience of Americans in France during the "War to End All Wars" saw the emergence of this idea.

In World War I, hospital equipment and mobile surgical teams were transported, together with their equipment and tentage, in trucks across the front.[7(p69)]

In World War II, the European and North African theaters of operation generally employed linear battlefields where combat support and combat service support units provided services by doctrine along fairly defined battle lines in the mountains and fields of the European continent and the deserts of Africa. The intent was to bring definitive care to the seriously wounded in far forward areas through auxiliary surgical groups. Close attention was paid to the selection of individuals to compose surgical teams within the groups, balancing the need for varying specialties, as well as the requirement of healthy young men capable of performing major surgery of the abdomen, chest, and extremities. The theory of bringing well-trained surgeons to the critically wounded, rather than the older method of evacuating the seriously wounded far to the rear for definitive surgical care, was proven logical and sound. This helped reduce the mortality and morbidity among the troops wounded in the combat zone. Because chest and abdominal wounds formed the majority of wounded cases, it was emphasized that the specialist must also be a good general surgeon.[9(pp385–386)]

The other side of the conflict in Asia is contrasted in the surgical support provided in World War II to the Pacific and China-Burma-India theaters of operation where the jungle canopy and island combat made the fight nonlinear. Here portable surgical hospitals bore the brunt of front line definitive surgery. They lacked generators, electrical illumination, refrigerators, suction apparatuses, and resuscitation equipment. Because of this, the portable surgical hospital could not operate independent of clearing companies and reinforcement by surgical teams.[9(p573)]

INTERWAR YEARS (1948–1950)

After defeating the Axis powers, the United States Army Medical Department improved upon the knowledge gained in Africa, Europe, and Asia. Immediate far forward surgical care to front line troops was obtainable and proven in all theaters of operation.

Of the five MASH units between 1948 and early 1950 (Exhibit 7-1), none were in the Far East.[10] Prior to the Korean conflict, the MASHs were organized under Tables of Organization and Equipment (T/O&E), but were not ready for deployment. The

EXHIBIT 7-1. **INTERWAR YEARS (1948-1950)**

The five MASH units were as follows:

Unit	Location	Assignment
1st	Fort Lewis, Washington	VI Army
2d	Fort Bragg, North Carolina	III Army
3d	Fort Meade, Maryland	II Army
4th	Munich, Germany	EUCOM
5th	Heidelberg, Germany	EUCOM

Source: *Station List, World Wide, US Army Medical Department Units,* 31 January 1950, National Archives II, Suitland, Maryland, box 239.

1948 T/O&E called for a self-mobile, 60-bed holding capacity, tented surgical hospital. It contained the headquarters and headquarters detachment, preoperative and shock section, operating section, postoperative section, pharmacy, radiography section, and holding ward. Authorized personnel were 14 Medical Corps officers, 12 Army Nurse Corps officers, two Medical Service Corps officers, one warrant officer, and 97 enlisted soldiers. To meet the need of far forward surgical intervention, the physicians included a commander, radiologist, two anesthesiologists, an internist, four general medical officers, and five surgeons.[7(pp69–70)] Typical of postwar drawdown, this organizational table was how the unit was supposed to be staffed, not how a unit might actually be staffed. For example, Fort Bragg's 2nd MASH's 1949 Annual Report of Medical Activities detailed the inadequacies they faced as they "stood up" the new unit and implemented the T/O&E approved on 28 October 1948. With a skeletal crew of only 22 enlisted men, two administrative officers, and one warrant officer, the unit struggled to support a maneuver exercise and conduct its medical proficiency training. The unit equipment was fielded, but the personnel were slow in arriving. In the report's closing remarks, the 2nd MASH commander requested that all incoming personnel not be raw recruits, that the aptitude test results for those to be assigned in the future be increased, and that medical noncommissioned officers be utilized when filling the authorized slots because this was such a "specially trained organization."[11(pp3–4)]

MASH Table of Organization Review (1948)

During the MASH T/O&E review, at least one agency within the Medical Department reported on several mistakes and made recommendations to the Army Field Forces in Fort Monroe, Virginia. The observation of inadequate personnel and support equipment came from the Surgeon General's Office and only addressed organizational and equipment issues pertaining to supply and field operations. No clinical review was documented.[12]

Mobile Striking Force (1948)

The Office of The Surgeon General, Deputy for Plans, focused on unit allocations to support divisional forces during the interwar years. As early as 1948, the intent for the newly created "Hosp, Surg" T/O&E 8-571 was to support a division-sized element. As the correspondence described, one surgical hospital would support one division in combat whether the total Army was 18, 20, 22, or 25 divisions strong. However, it noted the future requirement to identify whether the units would be procured from the Regular Army, National Guard, or the Organized Reserve Corps.[13]

As with all branches of the armed forces at the time, contingency plans to counter the perceived threat of Soviet aggression were instituted within the Medical Department through its support of the Mobile Striking Force of 1948. Initially, the minimum service support for this contingency operation was 60 days of overseas combat service. Each task force was configured to deploy as a divisional element. The medical portion supporting this Mobile Striking Force contained six "Med Hosp, Surg, Mbl" with a T/O&E 8-571 dated August 1945. However, even though the "intended" MASH included specialty surgical teams for far forward care, the Mobile Striking Force, in addition to the six MASHs, had 18 medical detachments with labels such as neurosurgical, orthopedic, shock, surgical, and thoracic.[14]

MEDICAL FIELD SERVICE SCHOOL (1950–1951)

The concept of far forward surgical care had been proven in war and staffed during peace. What were young officers attending the Medical Field Service School, the predecessor of the United States Army Medical Department Center and School, at Fort Sam Houston in San Antonio, Texas, learning about the newly formed MASH unit? A student "special text" reiterated the allocation of one MASH per division and emphasized there were currently 12 in the inventory.[15] This publication devoted one paragraph to one of the most critical medical units in an unexpected war merely months away:

> Mobile army surgical hospitals are mobile units of the *field army medical service* [emphasis added] designed primarily to provide adequate facilities near the front for major operative procedures necessary to save life or limb, and which cannot be postponed until the casualty reaches an evacuation hospital; and to relieve clearing stations immediately of nontransportables in order to prevent the immobilization of such stations through the accumulation of casualties that cannot be immediately evacuated.[15(p193)]

During the 1951 Army Medical Service Organized Reserve Corps and National Guard Instructors' Conference at the Medical Field Service School, Captain (CPT) RL Devine, Medical Corps, relayed his experience in treating frontline casualties. As if foreshadowing reports typical of conditions on the peninsula, he spoke of the extreme difficulties in traversing the harsh terrain, whether in attempting evacuation or resupply. Operations and support discussions concerning the MASH followed along doctrinal guidelines, just as the earlier referenced student special text had delineated.[16(pp49–58)] This would hold true in the early phases of the war, but as the mission changed and the front began to stabilize, so too the character of the MASH changed (Exhibit 7-2).

EXHIBIT 7-2. MASH UNITS AND NOMENCLATURE

Throughout the war, the MASH changed numerical designations and nomenclature

Unit	Numeric Change	Numeric Change
8055th		43rd
8063d		44th
8076th		45th
1st	8209th	46th
2nd	8225th	47th

Prewar	Mobile Army Surgical Hospital
1950	Mobile Army Surgical Hospital xxxx Army Unit
1953	Surgical Hospital (Mobile Army)

Sources: (1) Eighth United States Army Annual Report, Army Medical Service Activities, 1950, National Archives II, Suitland, Maryland, boxes 195–196; (2) Eighth United States Army Annual Report, Army Medical Service Activities, 1951, National Archives II, Suitland, Maryland, box 196; (3) Eighth United States Army Annual Report, Army Medical Service Activities, 1952, National Archives II, Suitland, Maryland, box 197; and (4) Eighth United States Army Annual Report, Army Medical Service Activities, 1953, National Archives II, Suitland, Maryland, box 198.

KOREAN WAR

The joyous and peaceful years after the Allied victory in World War II soon transformed into the uneasy and fearful years of the Cold War. The Soviet Union, the United States' former ally, was perceived as building Communist satellite-nations within Eastern Europe in preparation for a war against the forces of Western democracies. The perception gained momentum with the Soviet Union's successful atomic bomb test in 1949. That same year, the Communist forces in the Chinese revolution established the People's Republic of China. On 25 June 1950, Democratic People's Republic of Korea (North Korea) forces, supported by fellow Communist China (in word) and the Soviet Union (in deed), invaded the Republic of Korea (South Korea). The United States immediately moved troops from Japanese occupation duty to block the Communist invasion. With this move, the United States spearheaded a United Nations (UN) force composed of 21 countries to combat the aggressive action of North Korea.[17(pp445-446)] Thus, the local conflict became an international effort.

Post-World War II had been marked by the rapid demobilization of the military as the United States had traditionally done in all previous wars. The United States Army Medical Department was no exception (Exhibit 7-3). From June 1945 until June 1950, the Army lost 86% of its wartime officer strength and 91% of its enlisted strength.[7(p8)] This was difficult by itself. With the initiation of what President Harry S Truman agreed to describe as a "police action" (a quickly realized misnomer) in Korea, the results were disastrous. A dangerously small military poised against a large-scale enemy force was a recipe for failure. The nation, and subsequently the Army, had made no plan for partial mobilization or limited war.[7(p3)]

Unlike the Axis Powers in the European Theater of Operations in World War II, the North Korean People's Army and Chinese Communist Forces were not signatories to the Geneva Convention. Indeed, the medical "red cross" now became the aiming point for enemy soldiers.

EXHIBIT 7-3. RAYMOND W BLISS, SURGEON GENERAL (1 June 1947–31 May 1951)

Raymond W Bliss replaced Norman T Kirk as Surgeon General of the Army in June 1947 during a time of transition for the recently victorious US Army. A former surgical student and subsequent instructor at Harvard College, Bliss eventually served as the Chief of Operations Service in the Surgeon General's Office in World War II. It was here that he made a reputation for himself in the art of planning medical support that entailed patient evacuation and distribution, and the establishment of specialized hospitals. When the war ended, he was Assistant Surgeon General. During the interwar years, Bliss' focus was on preparing for the next conflict and providing specialized training for new physicians. Army hospitals began offering residency training, emphasizing clinical and preventative medicine, research and pathological study. From this desire to enhance the professionalism of the Medical Service, Major General Bliss incorporated civilian consultants in the training hospitals. The early ability of the Army Medical Department to react strongly to the rapid chaos early on the Korean Peninsula exemplifies his judgment in equipping the surgeons in accomplishing low death and high recovery rates, and high morale.[1]

Source: (1) Heaton LD. Raymond W Bliss. *Mil Med*. 1966;3(5):458–459.

Medical units were specifically attacked and, therefore, the red cross was covered and medics carried M-1 rifles, just like their infantry counterparts. In this environment, medical organizations now surrounded themselves with armed troops whenever possible.

Korean War (1950)

Colonel (COL) Chauncey E Dovell, the Eighth Army Surgeon, reported that the activities of the Eighth Army in the last 6 months of 1950 were "highlighted by many events which have both cheered and tested the spirit of the entire army."[3(Preface)] There was the UN breakthrough from the Naktong River in September, the pursuit of the Communist forces up the Korean peninsula, and finally the victorious entrance of UN troops in the North Korean capital of Pyongyang in October 1950. In opposite measure were the devastating reverses suffered in the very beginning of the conflict by the 24th Infantry Division and Task Force Smith, the Naktong Bulge penetration in August, the entry of Chinese Communist Forces in October, the 1st Marine and 7th Infantry Division's bitter fighting in the Changjin Reservoir ("Frozen Chosin") in November and December, and finally, the death of the Eighth Army commander, Lieutenant General (LTG) Walton H "Bulldog" Walker, at the end of December 1950.[17(pp661–662)]

Shortages of personnel, equipment, and supplies, and the lack of trained medical units characterized the medical problems present since June 1950, the beginning of the war. Therefore, centralized control was important in distributing the scarce resources across the combat zone. As doctrine had dictated, the MASH was utilized in direct support to the combat division. But the Army's 400-bed evacuation hospital could not properly function on the peninsula because of the lack of transportation, an inadequate road and rail network, and the volatile tactical situation. Under COL Duvall's direction, the MASH was "organized" to provide surgical care for all patients, not just nontransportables. The MASH now became a small 200-bed capacity (a 140-bed increase) evacuation hospital providing care to the division in addition to its intended surgical role. In some instances, the MASHs exceeded 400 patients a day.[3(p5)] There were three MASHs to support four United States infantry divisions and other United Nations forces until 26 December 1950. By the end of the year, when all medical assets from X Corps were transferred to the Eighth Army, there were four MASH units in support of seven divisions and attached United Nations troops. As a recommendation in his annual report, Dovell urged the US Army to develop an authorized unit, similar to the *de facto* MASH units struggling in Korea, to be planned and activated to cover the current needs in Korea.[3(p5)]

The MASHs organized for Korea were not intended for any extended service. They were actually filled utilizing a Table of Distribution (TD), today referred to as a Table of Distribution and Allowances (TDA).[7(p69)] The theory developed by the Surgeon General in the United States and the reality in the Far East Command were not one and the same. This rapid adjustment to the critical needs on the ground manifested itself within the field surgical ward. It was described by a real-life MASH surgeon, Dr Richard Hornberger, in his fictional account from the novel *MASH*.[18] His character explained,

This is certainly meatball surgery we do around here, but I think you can see now that meatball surgery is a specialty in itself. We are not concerned with the ultimate reconstruction of the patient. We are only concerned with getting the kid out of here alive enough for someone else to reconstruct him. Up to a point we are concerned with fingers, hands, arms, and legs, but sometimes we deliberately sacrifice a leg in order to save a life, if the other wounds are more important. In fact, now and then we may lose a leg because, if we spent an extra hour trying to save it, another guy in the preop ward could die from being operated on too late.[18(p195)]

The 8055th MASH relayed critical elements to rapid field surgery in their *1950 Annual Report of Medical Department Activities* emphasizing triage techniques to quickly weed out nonsurgical cases coupled with the use of radiographs and lab work to quickly move patients into vital surgery. Most patients were evacuated in 2 to 3 days following recovery in the postoperative ward. Unfortunately for the 8055th, their medical technicians (corpsmen) and operating room technicians, enlisted strength, was only 65%.[19(pp2-4,7-8)] On-the-job training was the only measure to fill the gap created by the lack of these qualified personnel. From this gap in specialty skills, it is logical to conclude the huge emphasis made in assigning and maintaining nurses in this type of unit.[19(pp14-15)] The report conveys that,

> Corpsmen are not a suitable replacement for nurses, as demonstrated by the experience of this unit. At least this hospital has not found an adequate substitute for nurses during the short periods when operations were carried on without them. This is especially true in surgery where they are considered the most essential.[19(p13)]

According to its annual report, the 8063rd MASH began to feel the strain of not having enough enlisted soldiers on hand. Cold weather affected the radiographic developer, but was mitigated once better heaters were used. During the 23 moves in 1950, women were transported by helicopter because of the security issues en route to each destination. In reviewing the types of surgical cases, the commander recommended additional orthopedic surgeons because 60% of all surgical cases required orthopedic interventions.[20] More generator power was requested. This continued to be a common theme throughout all the MASHs in theater for the entire conflict. Tent heaters had to be used in the operating room to manage the extreme cold of the winter; insect screens had to be requested to combat the vermin that came from open windows in the summer. This time of the war was particularly difficult. The annual report noted that the local civilian population was starving and resorted to taking the hospital's food waste for any kind of nourishment. Air evacuation was cited as excellent. By continuously locating near airfields, patients could be evacuated to the rear when defenses were overrun in order to prevent capture. In closing, the 8063rd commander commented that the medical troops needed overall "tightening" up in military discipline and training.[20]

During the first move of the 8076th MASH in combat that August 1950, the unit worked through the night while fighting off "guerilla" attacks. They were operational and ready to receive casualties the very next day. Their own mess sergeant was their

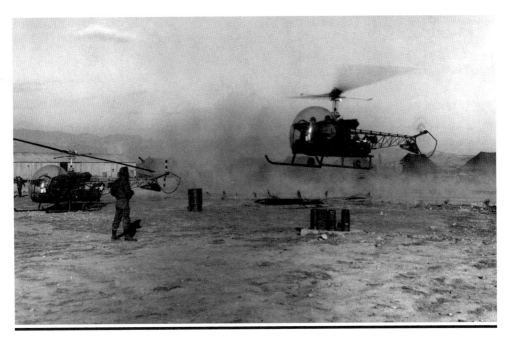

FIGURE 7-1. Captain Joseph W Hely of St Louis, Missouri, 2nd Helicopter Detachment, 2nd Logistical Command, lands a Bell H-13 at his detachment headquarters following an evacuation from the front (31 December 1950). Note the litters covering patients like a "casket," and skids replacing the wheeled landing gear. Photograph courtesy of the AMEDD Center of History and Heritage, Army Nurse Corps Photo Collection, Korean War, Box 25, Item #B4-04-02(1).

first patient. In November, American forces were surprised by the intervention of the Communist Chinese Forces, and had no cold weather gear for fighting. Over the course of 6 days the 8076th admitted 1,836 patients, 661 in one day.[21(pp1–2)]

The casualty flow matched the intensity of the cold where temperatures ranged from 20 to 30 degrees below zero Fahrenheit. Some of these patients froze to death while waiting transport into the hospital after the ambulances dropped them off. Shelter within the canvas was not always sufficient. Patients froze inside the hospital confines, too. The chaos of battle, and its subsequent injuries, was always exasperated by the elements.[21(pp2–3)]

It was during this particular time in November 1950 that the tactical situation necessitated the order to "bug out" in advance of the Communist Chinese Forces. The roads were clogged with retreating UN vehicles and personnel. After all means of evacuation had been exhausted, 40 patients remained that required transport. Unable to move, one doctor and several corpsmen stayed with the remaining patients while the MASH rapidly escaped under orders to move. Fortunately, 4 hours later the entire group was rescued before capture by enemy forces.[21(p3)]

In that same move from Kunuri to Pyong-yang along a designated route, Lieutenant Colonel (LTC) Kryder Van Buskirk, just promoted earlier that month, decided that the prescribed left turn at a fork was unsafe and chose to continue along the right. This decision saved the 8076th MASH and its patients from disaster. Every unit that took the

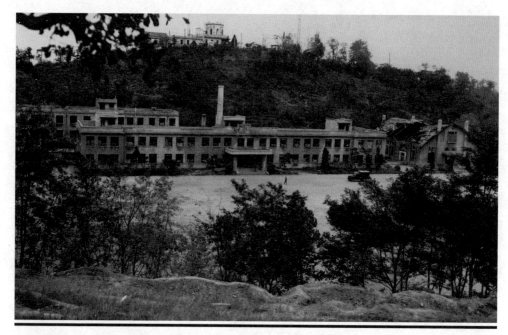

FIGURE 7-2. The Korean civilian hospital in Inchon, Korea, was operated by the 1st MASH and had little or no supplies initially (3 October 1950). Fixed facilities were much better than canvas tents and were utilized whenever possible. Photograph courtesy of the AMEDD Center of History and Heritage, Army Nurse Corps Photo Collection, Korean War, Box 25, Item #B4-03-02(1).

left turn encountered a Communist Chinese roadblock and the soldiers were killed or taken prisoner. Van Buskirk's unit continued to experience enemy attacks.[21(p3)] In response, he fashioned a 10-man guard section that he felt did not disrupt the medical shifts.[22(p2)]

Several recommendations were made to improve orthopedic sets for this particular type of field environment. Additionally, there were several recommendations made to improve the surgical procedures included in Technical Bulletin Medical 147 (TB Med 147), *Notes on the Care of Battle Casualties*.[23] Those included specific procedures for intraabdominal wounds, chest wounds, and wounds of the genitourinary tract.[22(pp2,6–7)] In the area of environmental controls, much dissatisfaction was heaped upon the assigned gas-powered space heaters, which were referred to as "gadgets rather than as functional pieces of equipment."[22(p3)] In fact, one had been converted to run using an electric motor. Litter and blanket exchanges worked well with the train system, but not within the air evacuation platform. Because of the extreme cold, each patient had six blankets during evacuation to the rear, but the helicopters could not exchange the patient blankets with six more blankets from their supply stock upon their delivery. It was commented that "too much cannot be said in praise of the helicopters"[22(p3)] (Figure 7-1) in getting patients in remote and inaccessible locations on the front lines quickly transported to the MASH, therefore, minimizing shock and delay in surgical intervention. The standard method of evacuation from the regimental area was by ground evacuation in wheeled ambulances accompanied

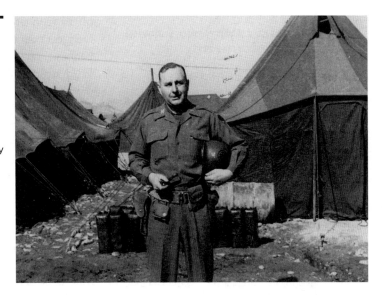

FIGURE 7-3. Colonel Thomas N Page, Eighth Army Surgeon, in Joju, Korea (March 1951). In a note to his mother, he remarked how much weight he had lost. Photograph courtesy of the AMEDD Center of History and Heritage, Thomas N Page Collection, Box 1, Image #2010.11.5.

by medics, unless distance or medical condition dictated a quicker response with rotary-winged aircraft. Hospital trains were used to move patients throughout Korea. Fixed-winged aircraft were used to move patients out of the combat zone to Japan. However, these airplanes were utilized to transport within the peninsula at times as well.

The 1st MASH (later designated the 8209th in 1951) arrived late in September 1950. The hospital began caring for enemy prisoners of war while awaiting the arrival of its equipment. Because of this, this treatment became pure "clinical medicine" inasmuch as there were no supplies. The hospital at one time set up in an old school (Figure 7-2). One can only imagine the frustration of the early days in Korea as described in the annual report,

> The abysmally insanitary conditions and revolting nature of the gangrenous and maggoty wounds and accompanying complications were of such nature as to stir all concerned to their utmost endeavor to relieve the suffering. It was an experience which impressed each and every member of the unit with the value of the supplies and equipment which are ordinarily taken for granted in our modern medicines.[24(p8)]

They finally became fully operational as a MASH late in the year, 27 December 1950. Compared to the textbook and academic training they had undergone in the United States, in combat they became fully functional on patient movement, unloading, and set-up.[24(p9)]

Korean War (1951)

The following year, 1951, the new Eighth Army Surgeon's report from COL Thomas N Page (Figure 7-3) to the Surgeon General (Exhibit 7-4) was much more upbeat. The Army Medical Service had suffered and succeeded along with their fellow soldiers in the Eighth Army under General (GEN) Matthew Ridgway. As COL Page reported, many of the problems faced in the early days of the war no longer existed. The UN regained the

> EXHIBIT 7-4. **GEORGE E ARMSTRONG, SURGEON GENERAL (1 June 1951–31 May 1955)**
> Unique to most physicians, George E Armstrong began his career as an enlisted member of the National Guard. Upon commissioning, he rose through the ranks obtaining vast experience in the Philippines and China during the interwar period and World War II where he eventually served as the Theater Surgeon, China Theater. Before his appointment as Major General and The Surgeon General, he was the Deputy Surgeon General for 4 years under Major General Raymond Bliss.[1] Some of the highlights of his tenure were the remarkable decrease of the death rate from World War II's 4.5% to Korea's 2.3%. Helicopters and their use in medical evacuation became an integral part of the medical field organization. Surgical Research Team investigations and progress in vascular surgery marked the increased knowledge gained from focused research as witnessed to an 80% arterial repair success rate compared to the previous 50% in World War II.[2]
>
> Sources: (1) Biographical Files (Armstrong GE), 2010.7.1, AMEDD Center of History and Heritage, Archival Repository, Joint Base San Antonio-Fort Sam Houston, Texas; and (2) Armstrong GE. Military medicine in Korea. *US Armed Forces Med J* [USGPO, Washington, DC]. 1954:1–7.

offensive in late January, including the great counterblow to Communist Chinese Forces at Chipyong-ni in February, the UN stood its ground at the 38th parallel in June that began the truce talks, and battles such as Heartbreak Ridge beginning in August ensured the lines were held through the year. The Chinese had taken Seoul in January, but the aforementioned UN offensive directly reclaimed Seoul in March. Fierce fighting and testing of the lines characterized the combat, but UN forces under the direction of GEN Ridgway (after GEN Douglas MacArthur's recall in April), held fast the new cease-fire line. From this movement in leadership, LTG James A Van Fleet assumed command of the Eighth Army.[4(Preface),17(pp662–663)]

The previous staff policy of centralized administration began to change as Page better utilized the abilities of various staff members upon his appointment in July. Surgical consultants, as well as those in medicine and neuropsychiatry, were assigned. This further raised the standard of medical professionalism of the Eighth Army and began the remarkable record of surgical intervention, primarily in neurosurgery, displayed in the MASH on the battlefields of Korea. Research teams in surgery and cold injury arrived to work with the MASHs to fully capitalize on newly developing techniques in modern medicine. Through the latter part of the year a concerted effort was made to move the MASHs closer to the front lines of the fighting, usually 10 to 20 miles away. This balanced easy access for the wounded and still allowed surgeons to operate with a "fair margin of safety."[4(p24)] Because the MASH received the greatest casualty load, relatively inactive hospital staffs in the rear were moved to augment the heavily burdened MASHs. As a matter of concern for Page in his annual report, certain individuals, presumably from higher headquarters in the continental United States, visited "supposedly to check"[4(Preface)] on conditions in the field. Inasmuch as these individuals were inexperienced in field service, he stated that the "desirability of continuing this somewhat extravagant policy becomes questionable."[4(Preface)]

The pace and movement of the MASH in 1951 was a replication of the experience from 1950. The introduction to the MASH operations in the 1951 annual report is exactly the same as the earlier annual report of 1950. But now there were five US MASHs

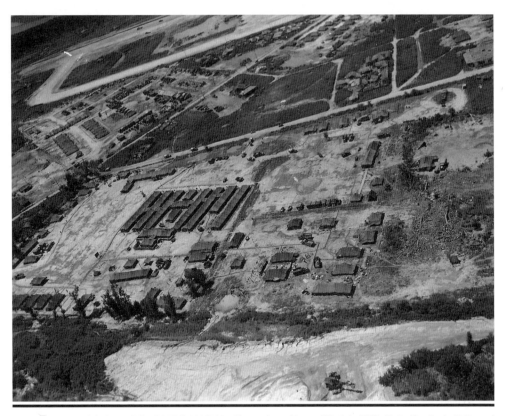

FIGURE 7-4. Aerial view of the 8076th MASH in Chounchon, Korea (29 July 1951). Note the Basic "U" used to build the tented hospital. It was here that the core functions were established—preoperative, postoperative, and surgical wards. Photograph courtesy of the AMEDD Center of History and Heritage, Thomas N Page Collection, Box 4, Image #8A/854-9/FEC-51.

and a Norwegian Mobile Surgical Hospital (60-bed capacity) in support of US and UN troops. One MASH, with the exception of the higher medical professional personnel, was held in reserve. Standards were established as these MASHs developed through the year. They disassembled, loaded on vehicles, and were ready to depart with a 6-hour notice. After arrival at their new destination, they were operational within 4 hours. Each MASH operated five surgical tables in a shift with a highly organized system of managing shock patients. A ground ambulance platoon was attached to each MASH to facilitate the rapid evacuation when postoperative recovery was complete. Additionally, four helicopters were attached to each MASH. They, in turn, were utilized for resupply, rapid patient delivery to the MASH, and comfortable (compared to a bumpy ground) evacuation from the MASH.[4(p5)]

Through Page's direction, auxiliary surgical and neurosurgical teams were assigned to augment and aid the "extremely busy and somewhat overworked"[4(p24)] mobile surgical hospitals. The surgical cases followed the flow of battle. The hospitals were crowded with Allied and enemy wounded personnel during the winter and early spring. The situation changed in late spring and summer following the slackened intensity of fighting and, therefore, the flow of wounded was sporadic. However, after the ceasefire negotiations seemed to be failing in September and October, the flow of wounded mirrored the pace of fighting on the front.[4(pp23-24)]

CPT Samuel L Crook, detachment commander of the 8076th MASH, described in an after-action interview the utilization of the basic "U" and split operations of his MASH developed by the previous hospital commander, LTC Kryder Van Buskirk, and the current hospital commander, LTC John L Mothershead (Figure 7-4).

The hospital is moved in two phases. In Phase I, the tents housing Registrar, Receiving, and Holding are taken down. The laboratory, the pharmacy, and the admitting functions of Receiving are moved into the Pre-operative ward. The tentage which has been struck is then moved to the new location with half the personnel of Pre-operative, Post-operative, Surgical, Central Supply, and one receiving clerk. This tentage is erected at the new location to form the Basic "U," consisting of Pre-operative, Post-operative, and Surgical. Central Supply functions, which consist of sterilizing instruments and dressings, are carried out in the surgical tent.

At one point, therefore, there are two completely functioning hospitals. The hospital in the rear continues to admit patients until the forward installation is ready to operate. When the advance unit opens to patients, the rear installation ceases to receive. When all its patients have been evacuated, the rear unit moves up and joins the advance hospital as Phase II of the move. Tentage brought up is added externally to the Basic "U" in the new location.[25(pp4-5)]

Dr Otto F Apel Jr, chief surgeon at the 8076th MASH, wrote of his experience as a medical eyewitness from 1951 to 1952. As relayed earlier, the MASH was still in its infancy. Unlike the end of the war, the MASH was still truly mobile during the second year of fighting. Within Apel's first year with the 8076th, the unit moved about every 3 weeks, just as described by CPT Crook.[2(pp49,57)] In addition to constant movement, continuous sustained operations characterized the busy MASH. Upon his arrival, Apel operated for 72 hours on combat casualties and had to cut off his boots due to the swelling in his feet.[2(pp36-37,39)] The 8055th Table of Distribution increased their manpower strength and equipment. Patients flowed from the front lines 20 to 50 miles away into the MASH within an hour to an hour and a half from the time of injury. Plasma and whole blood were the agents used to fight shock, using intraarterial transfusion and positive pressure oxygen inhalation. It should be noted that there was discussion within the surgical community as to whether intraarterial transfusion was more beneficial than the traditional intravenous method in the resuscitation of the wounded. Studies conducted by the Surgical Research Team later in 1952 to 1953 at the 46th Surgical Hospital (formerly the 8209th MASH) determined "no definite conclusions"[26(p64)] could be drawn. Sometimes surgical staff had to conduct surgery before the shock was controlled, but a large percentage of patients improved quickly from the surgeons finding the source of bleeding and stopping it. The radiograph was a critical tool in identifying foreign objects and became the policy of the unit for all battle

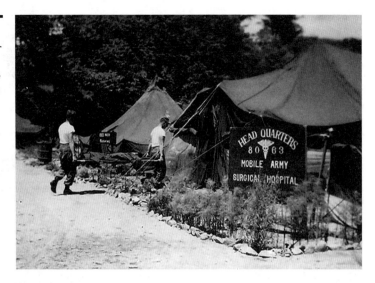

FIGURE 7-5. A litter patient is presented for triage at the entrance to the 8063rd MASH (1951). Note the results of fewer moves reflected in the "garden." Photograph courtesy of the AMEDD Center of History and Heritage, Joseph Hely Collection, Box 2, Image #2010.11.13.

casualties to have radiography performed to simplify the work of the surgeons. The old authorization tables were created in 1948, but now the 8055th was transforming to new authorizations and steadily increased their size. In the first part of 1951, the hospital was all in canvas tents. But by December, the preoperative, operative, and postoperative wards were in prefabricated buildings. Across the board Japanese products were cited as inferior in quality and this caused major problems in the upkeep of the hospital and, in medical products specifically, hurt patient care. Patients also were referenced as reasons to adopt electric heaters because of the noise and maintenance required from the poorly performing gas heaters then on hand. One could minimize the importance of heat for the staff because winter clothing was on hand; however, it was often the wrong size.[27(pp2–5,11–13,18–20)] This would continue to plague the MASH staffs throughout the theater and the war.

In an endorsement for the 8063rd's annual report for 1951, COL Page acknowledged the poor quality of Japanese procured equipment and supplies and mentioned that they were being replaced. While acknowledged throughout the theater for its benefits, the radiography equipment had problems from the heat of the summer. The 8063rd commander insisted that visits from the radiological consultant be longer and more often because they did not have their own radiologist assigned to the MASH.[28(End4)] Ironically, the leadership of the 8055th argued the radiologist should be deleted from the authorization the following year because there were no problems in interpretations among the technicians.[29(p10)] With the increased equipment, a pattern emerged where units remarked that the current level of equipment and supplies on hand was beyond the capability of relocating the hospital in one move (Figures 7-5 and 7-6). With the addition of a neurological team, the lack of enough generator power was troublesome for the daily operations of the MASH because it could not carry the full load of the hospital when it was operating at its maximum capacity. The first part of the year, strangely enough, saw the preponderance of all the illness (sick; noncombat wounded) cases within the unit for the entire year. By the command's own admission, there was no explanation for this. By late

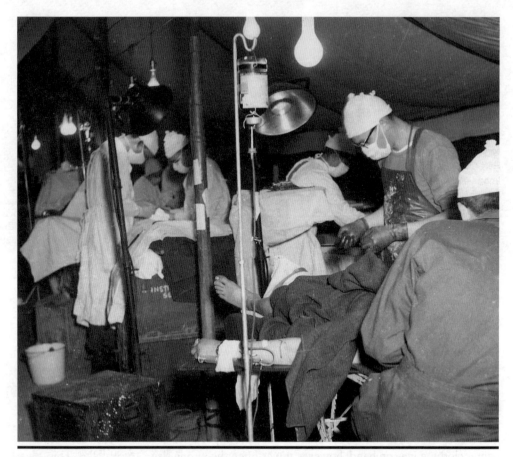

FIGURE 7-6. Operating room of the 8063rd MASH (1951). Note the wooden floors improved the environment, but limited directional lights and single bulbs still provide lighting. The procedure in the foreground appears to be on a surgical table and the background shows several instrument set boxes holding up a litter replicating a surgical table. Photograph courtesy of the AMEDD Center of History and Heritage, Thomas N Page Collection, Box 2, Image #2010.11.5.

June 1951, however, the first cases of hemorrhagic fever discovered and properly diagnosed in the war were seen at Kachae-Ri. For epidemic hemorrhagic fever, this was the beginning of a long battle for UN forces with this disease, first identified in 1939 by the Japanese in Manchuria. The unit praised and benefitted from the clinical consultant program instituted by the Far East Command and Eighth US Army Korea Surgeon. The 8063rd commander specifically lauded the benefits to general surgery, ear-nose-throat surgery, and oral surgery. He did, however, request that the visits should last at least 2 to 3 days.[28(pp5,8–9,11–13)]

Throughout the year, the 8076th was 5 to 10 miles from the front. The weather was a constant aggravation where the rain and mud oftentimes would not allow the tent stakes to stay in the ground, and thus the tents collapsed under the deluge (Figure 7-7). The hospital had to resort to placing its vehicles under the tents to keep the tentage up.[21(pp4–5)] In the opinion of the 8076th's command in 1951, the guard section was inept in its duties,

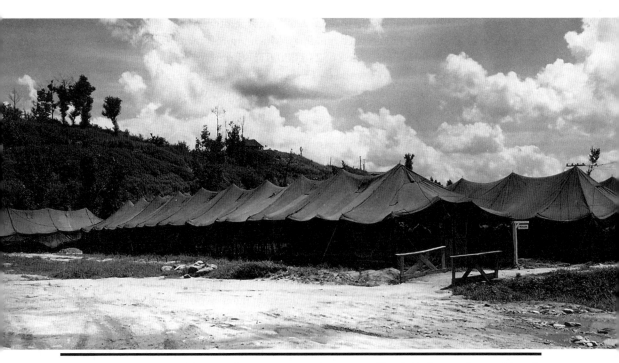

FIGURE 7-7. Ground view of the 8076th MASH in Chounchon, Korea (29 July 1951). Note the condition of the road network approaching this section of the hospital. Rain and mud proved to be constant environmental challenges. Photograph courtesy of the AMEDD Center of History and Heritage, Thomas N Page Collection, Box 4, Image #8A/854-8/FEC-51.

with average or below average intelligence. In LTC Maurice R Connolly's opinion, they were of poor quality, possessed low morale, and had a slovenly appearance while on guard duty. In his assessment they were not fulfilling their mission based upon the numerous thefts and penetration of the perimeter and he, therefore, disbanded the group. Instead of a permanent group, most enlisted soldiers rotated through the duty, but this soon affected MASH operations. A newly formed guard section was created under better selection criteria and supervision and proved to be worthwhile.[30(pp5–6)] The 8076th's interaction with the Communist Chinese Forces was not at an end. There was an enemy clearing company overrun by UN forces and 200 wounded Chinese were admitted to the hospital within an hour. One Chinese nurse stayed with the patients for 1 month, taking care of them.[21(p6)]

Within the clinical realm, the preoperative and shock treatment sections were combined with great results and remained so, even though the new Table of Authorization separated them. More gas heaters were converted to electric-motor-operated heaters. The hospital had to improvise in making operating room and orthopedic tables, surgical lights, and scrub sinks. Several feats of improvisation and ingenuity were detailed in drawings of these recommendations that included a portable version of an operating room table, an operating lamp that moved (original one did not bend), a surgical scrub sink with a heater, and a transtracheal anesthesia apparatus.[30(pp6,8,12,77–80)]

By late December 1951, the preoperative and postoperative wards, as well as the operating room, were in prefabricated buildings. Much improvement to temperature control was evidenced through the use of 250,000 BTU (British thermal units) blowers used in the hospital (when the motors worked). Cases of suspected epidemic hemorrhagic fever were immediately evacuated to the rear. Because of the high suspicion of disease, not all of those evacuated were shown to have this illness.

The unit focused on efforts to improve the clinical practice of the MASH and again made recommendations to the newly revised Technical Bulletin Medical 147, now titled *Management of Battle Casualties*.[31] Specifically, the report addressed treatment and intervention in intraabdominal, intrathoracic, and neck wounds, as well as vascular injuries and anesthesia. Supplies requisition continued to be problematic with several needed articles marked "not in stock." With the construction of five prefabricated hutments to house the hospital, the basic-U plan for the 8076th MASH, in practical terms, became immobile.[30(pp8,16,18–19,21–24,28,33)]

It is interesting to note that the 1951 annual report recommended a "mobile surgical platoon" that could keep up with division clearing stations. Initially the mobile surgical platoon would stay with the main hospital. Evacuation flights would come directly from regimental clearing stations. Because of inadequate road networks between the MASH and division clearing stations, the idea of this mobile surgical platoon was born. In concept and design, it foreshadowed the current forward surgical team concept. According to the plan, the surgical platoon would

> leave the main hospital and attach itself to the Division Clearing Station. The platoon would use the facilities of the clearing station for shock, pre-op, and x-ray. (For many years the need of a portable x-ray for the Division Clearing Station has been evident, and would be necessary for *our concept*). It would set up a two table operating room, work-room and a small anesthesia recovery ward. The two surgical teams would select only those cases who obviously would not live to reach the main hospital, and would not stock-pile a group of cases. Most of their work would probably be during the hours of darkness when the helicopters can not (*sic*) evacuate direct to the main hospital.[30(p42)]

It was in 1951 that the 1st MASH was redesignated to be the 8209th MASH.[32(p1)] Evacuation was primarily through fixed-wing aircraft and train, while helicopters were used in emergencies, simultaneously solving the problem of prompt refill of a depleted blood supply. Most reports of the MASH described the challenges of balancing security and the mission. The 1st actually had a Raider platoon—elite volunteers who fought irregular warfare—assigned to the hospital to provide security. Like the year previously, abandoned buildings were used when available. At one time the surgical suite occupied a former bank building. Blankets became a problem during exchanges with aircraft. During one operation, the MASH went through about 1,000 blankets per week and had to begin using staff blankets to keep patients warm.[33(pp1–2,4–5)] The 8209th staff served as consultants to the Korean Army and civilian hospitals. Interestingly, the 8209th never used their holding

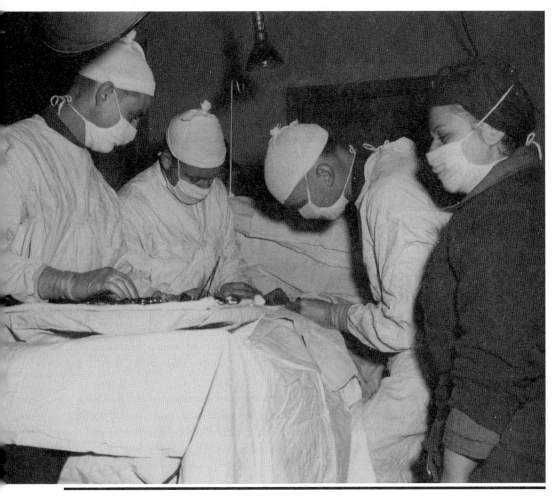

FIGURE 7-8. A team from the 1st MASH performs surgery on a wounded soldier in Inchon, Korea (14 February 1951). Left to right are: Corporal Bob Crain of Los Angeles, California, surgical technician; Lieutenant Junior Grade Bruce Meiers of Berlinger, California, Navy surgeon; Captain John J Wilsey, Newark, New York, surgeon; and First Lieutenant Marie Smarz of Shelton, Connecticut, Army Nurse Corps. Note what appears to be a vehicle light serving as an improvised surgical lamp. Photograph courtesy of the AMEDD Center of History and Heritage, Army Nurse Corps Photo Collection, Box 25, Image #B4-03-02(1).

section during this time because patients did not stay long. At each location, patients were rapidly evacuated, enabling the hospital to "leap frog" to the next position. The forward hospital received the more severely injured patients, while the rear hospital took the overflow of the lightly wounded. Before each move, patients were evacuated from the two functioning sections of the MASH conducting split operations. Extra duty details were performed by the staff.[32(pp4–5)]

Field expediency dictated replacing the issued light sets with improvised lights in the operating room (Figure 7-8). Like the other MASHs, the equipment authorized exceeded the power generation system that was available. Furthermore, gasoline engine heaters were notoriously inoperative (nine of 12 were out at one time) and were replaced with electric motors. This, of course, only strained the already overburdened generators.[32(pp6–7)]

As the year progressed, morale was enhanced through numerous outdoor recreational activities that included baseball, softball, volleyball, horseshoes, and swimming parties. Nightly movies were shown in the tent theater that held 400 people, which also made for the perfect venue for a United Service Organizations tour stop. It was no wonder the 1951 annual report cited these amenities as a reason for a significant reduction in depression among the staff.[32(p8)]

The 8209th 1951 annual report noted that the incoming enlisted personnel were so poorly trained that only a small percentage could be used immediately upon their arrival. For example, out of the 70 new soldiers who arrived in 1951, 43 had to be given other temporary jobs before being allowed to practice their "trained" skill set. A medical society, which included medical personnel from a supported division, met weekly. Here they followed up cases, reviewed patient care summaries from patients transferred to Japan, and produced medical papers. By year's end all sections were still in tents with frames and floors except for the prefabricated buildings containing the preoperative ward, operating room, postoperative ward, and the combined admissions, dental, optical, refraction, and pharmacy sections.[32(pp11–12)]

After its arrival to the peninsula from Japan, the 2nd MASH became operational in April 1951 with about 95% of the authorized 10 days of supplies. However, they had to request additional material to transform from a 60-bed to a 200-bed hospital. With only a little over a month in combat, the hospital was redesignated as the 8225th MASH. While most of the unit was under tentage with dirt and tarp floors, winterization brought wooden and concrete floors, walls, wooden frames and doors, tent liners, and, most importantly, Herman Nelson heaters. The Admission and Disposition Sections morphed into an Outpatient Clinic. Like other MASH units, they had to evacuate any head, neck, and eye injuries for a lack of the specialty to treat those injuries. With the exception of small burns, no plasma was administered, but rather whole blood was given to treat shock. During the summer months (when the war raged in the heat), there was a great demand for intravenous fluids and blood. Until July, there were actually four Navy doctors on the surgical staff.[34(pp2–7,9)] The presence of Navy doctors in Army units was indicative of the severe shortage of medical personnel in the Far East Command. Army interns and residents from hospitals in Japan, and Navy residents, had filled the gaps in field units facing the North Koreans and eventual Communist Chinese early in the war.[7(p140)] A cold-injury ward was created and physicians collaborated with the Army's Cold Injury Research Team in the care and in research of these patients. It was policy to radiograph every combat wound, which assisted the surgeon in debridement, and the film was then transported with the patient during evacuation. But this created a scenario where two of the six radiography technicians' blood count displayed evidence of excessive radiation exposure.[34(pp12–13)]

The triage effort between the preoperative section and the operating section was critical and several recommendations were made based on the unit's experience: (a) there was a great need for more anesthetists; (b) there should be at least two orthopedists; (c) acute head injuries should be dealt with in the MASH; and (d) the MASH should have well-trained surgical teams where the commander was a surgeon and provided policy and consultative advice. During heavy patient flow, the dentist was used as a surgical assistant. Defective Japanese equipment was lamented, with examples describing syringes breaking, intravenous bags leaking, and plaster of Paris falling apart. The problem of not having enough generator power was evident once again. Blood was good only because of the transport by helicopter and fixed wing aircraft. Clothing for hospital staff was abysmal. When patients no longer needed items, staff used their boots and clothing. There was also a period of clothing issuance where sizes were just too small. For the lack of proper uniforms, women were issued male clothing.[34(pp10,16–17)]

The year 1951 was the first year for the 8228th MASH. COL Page described it as the only replacement MASH in the Eighth Army. Initially the unit was composed of a small cadre: two medical service corps officers and four to six carefully selected enlisted soldiers. Toward the end of the year they were busy unloading equipment from the train and using replacement personnel as guards, some of whom had transferred from other MASHs. Within the barbed wire containing the newly arrived hospital equipment, two-man patrols were required to keep vigilance against theft. Making good use of their time and consulting with the other MASHs, the unit began realistic training and had 95% of their medical equipment along with 85% of the technical services equipment by year's end.[35(pp1–4)]

Korean War (1952)

The fighting stalemated and resembled the entrenched defenses of World War I as peace talks slowly drug on through April 1952. Enemy prisoners of war held in UN hands began rioting in April, with the rioting lasting through June. This even included an enemy prisoner of war patient riot in two field hospitals. General Mark Clark became the third Korean War commander of the Far East Command when he replaced Ridgway in the summer. The casualty flow, in turn, mimicked the steady waiting in which the two forces engaged in bearing down upon one another. When battle cries and horn blasts erupted from the Chinese Communist Forces on hilltops, the wounded flowed once again through the MASH.[5(pp1,3–4)] As the war pressed on and the battle lines became fixed, so did the MASH. Concrete and wooden buildings replaced the canvas tents of earlier months. Specialized surgical consultants and research teams began to develop and improve the status of care and surgery on the front lines.

The Eighth Army Surgeon, Brigadier General (BG) L Holmes Ginn Jr (Figure 7-9), in his annual report for 1952 again lamented the shortages of personnel. Of the 139 field-grade Medical Corps officers authorized by T/O&E in country, only 36 were present. Fortuitously, the battle lines remained relatively static. Only two of the six US Army MASHs moved the entire year. MASHs began to establish permanent residence and construct temporary buildings or were issued prefabricated buildings (tropical shells with insulating kits) to provide better care and comfort to patients. Few individuals on duty in a 1952 MASH in Korea had ever seen their unit move. In contrast to the first 2 years of combat in Korea, the MASHs functioned within their authorized 60-bed capacity for

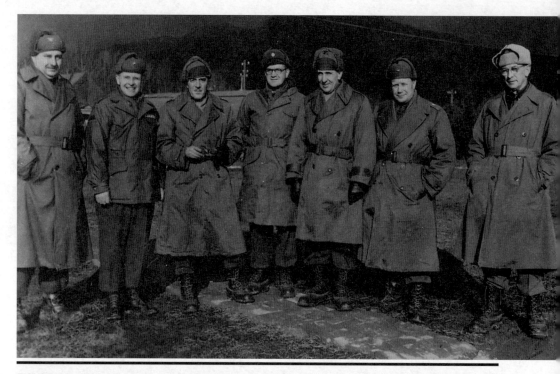

FIGURE 7-9. Major General George E Armstrong, US Army Surgeon General, visits the X Corps Headquarters in Chounchon, Korea (22 January 1952). Standing left to right are: Colonel Thomas N Page, Eighth Army Surgeon; Brigadier General Lawerence E Dewey, IX Corps Chief of Staff; Major General Armstrong; Lieutenant Colonel Francis L Carroll, IX Corps Surgeon; Brigadier General Earl E Standlee, Army Field Forces Surgeon; Brigadier General William E Shambora, Far East Command Surgeon; and Colonel Holmes Ginn, incoming Eighth Army Surgeon. Photograph courtesy of the AMEDD Museum Photo Collection, Korean War, Volume 2, Image #KW-0309.

priority surgical patients. The 8055th was the only exception.[5(pp1,4–5;AnnexIV,pp7,26)] Because battle injuries remained constant, disease and nonbattle injuries "accounted for the preponderance of our hospitalization,"[5(p1)] according to Ginn. The 8228th MASH became host to the onslaught of teams researching Eighth Army hemorrhagic fever cases. Moving from field conditions to a fixed facility in Seoul with 62 concrete-floor Quonset huts,[36(p6)] the 8228th became the logistical and support center for hemorrhagic fever in Korea. As cases of hemorrhagic fever decreased in the winter and cold weather injuries increased, the 8228th emerged as the consolidated center for the treatment of cold injuries[5(pp4–5;AnnexIV,pp7,13)] (Figure 7-10).

A stabilized combat situation, coupled with a lack of resources, resulted in each MASH beginning to develop its own specialization, similar to the 8228th. Neurosurgical detachments were stationed with both the 8209th MASH, in the east, and 8063rd MASH, in the west. It is interesting to note Ginn's knowledge of the auxiliary surgical groups in World War II in his annual report. He stated the past concept was sound and could also work in Korea, if only the staff were available. In his opinion, the use of "professional

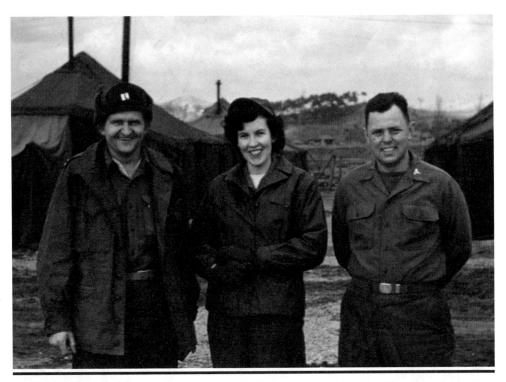

FIGURE 7-10. Doctors' tents serve as the background for a reunion of University of Pennsylvania Nursing School colleagues now with a Surgical Research Team (February 1952). From left to right are: Captain Howard, Medical Corps; 1st Lieutenant RE DeLaney, Army Nurse Corps; and 1st Lieutenant Scott, Medical Corps. Photograph courtesy of the AMEDD Center of History and Heritage, Army Nurse Corps Photo Collection, Box B24, Image #B4-02-03.

service detachments," as he called them, however, were much diminished because the MASH was organized as a fully staffed surgical hospital superseding the field hospital platoons that performed the priority surgery at forward locations in the past. Significant reductions in infections were seen because minor surgical cases and debridement were properly handled at the division clearing stations. Now priority surgery could be done more quickly at the 60-bed MASH instead of waiting along with all other surgery patients in the 200-bed MASH.[5(p5;AnnexIV,p26,Section2;AnnexVI,pp1–2)]

From 1952 to 1953, Dr Mel Horwitz served in the 8055th MASH and 8225th MASH (later designated 8225th Army Surgical Hospital, Mobile).[37(p212)] As discussed earlier, the lack of hospital movement reflected the stationary warfare of the third year of fighting.[7(pp88–89,167)] Dr Horwitz worked in a more mature MASH with prefabricated buildings and new equipment, in correlation to the stagnated front lines.[37(p99)] Just as the experiences of Drs Apel and Horwitz differ, so does the MASH differ according to the time and place.

The biggest "medical lesson to remember" that unfolded in 1951 and came to resolution by 1952 was the debate on medical specialization versus field medical education.

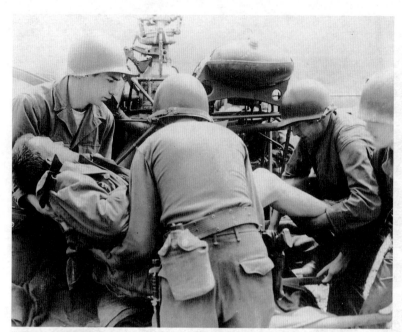

FIGURE 7-11. Medics from the 23rd Infantry Regimental Collecting Station, 2nd Infantry Division, load a casualty onto a Bell H-13 litter for air evacuation near Sangchon, Korea (14 April 1951). Photograph courtesy of the AMEDD Center of History and Heritage, Thomas N Page Collection, Box 4, Image #X/FEC-51-12427.

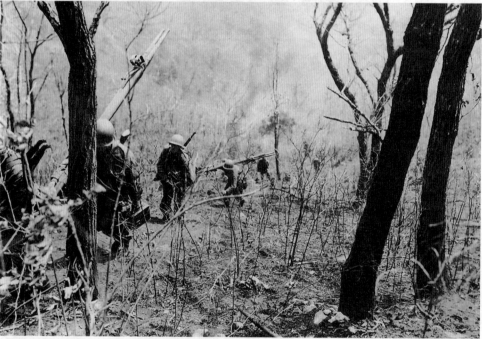

FIGURE 7-12. Medics from Company A, 32nd Infantry Regiment, 7th Infantry Division, climb Hill 902 carrying litters in preparation to evacuate the wounded from Companies A and B to the division clearing station for further treatment (23 April 1951). Note that the "red cross" is not displayed on the uniforms to identify medical personnel. Photograph courtesy of the AMEDD Center of History and Heritage, Thomas N Page Collection, Box 3, Image #X/FEC-51-13264.

In competition with the civilian medical community during the interwar years, US Army Medical Department officials had emphasized the opportunities to specialize in a particular field of medicine in order to attract more physicians. The result was that there was no interest in field medicine, but only specialties. Doctors were supplemented with Medical Service Corps (healthcare administrative) officers who were versed in procedural paperwork and field/combat operations. This concerted effort, in effect, halted the training of young medical officers in combat medicine after World War II. Clinical expertise and military medicine/field expertise were not the same. The lack of combat acumen for physicians proved to be disastrous, resulting in preventable soldier and doctor deaths.[7(pp34–35,189,191)] The leader in condemnation for the condition of Army field medicine was BG Crawford F Sams, former Chief of Public Health and Welfare in Korea. Sams had extensive experience as a "field soldier" and physician. (In March 1951, for instance, he led a three-man special operations "commando-type" infiltration mission into Wonson, North Korea, to determine whether intelligence reports of bubonic plague were true, but determined they were not.[7(pp175–176,188)])

BG Sams blamed the current program of placing recently graduated medical residents fresh from the halls of a hospital directly into a battalion aid station for the amateurish state of military field medicine (Figures 7-11 and 7-12). There was no field or tactics training. His son-in-law, a battalion surgeon, was killed defending his patients in November 1950. He painfully recalled how his son-in-law was not prepared for his assignment, had fired a weapon for the first time just months before, and was "largely ignorant of field procedures, organizations, and weapons."[7(p188)] Sams rightly argued in June 1951:

> Our younger men were thrown into combat without a day's training—similar to taking a boy out of a drugstore and saying "I'll give you a gun—go fight the Koreans." We did this to our young doctors. They were pulled out of the specialty programs, arrived in Japan, because we had nothing else; given field equipment which they had never seen before, told they were going to be assigned to field units the names of which meant nothing to them. Those young men, within five days after their arrival, were being shot at by the enemy. . . . That, I think, was one of the most disgraceful things in the military service. And still, a year later, we are almost in the same fix insofar as the men who are physically in the forward echelons are concerned at this time.[7(p189)]

Professional medical experience was common, but unfortunately, command rank and military experience were not.[7(p234)] Dr Apel received no military field medicine training prior to reporting to Korea and pointed out that there was no remedy for lack of experience. He painfully remarked how he and his fellow physicians did not know how to establish a defensive perimeter, had no field manuals, and did not know tactics. Everything they did to survive in combat was from figuring it out by themselves.[2(pp15,35)] Improvements and recommendations were implemented to correct the obvious problems within the training of the Army Medical Department at the Medical Field Service School under Sam's direction as the Assistant Commandant.[7(pp195–196)] By the end of the first year of fighting, better field training was initiated for officers and enlisted personnel.[7(pp192–195)] A clear example of this change is evidenced by Dr Horwitz's 8 weeks of field medical training at Fort Sam

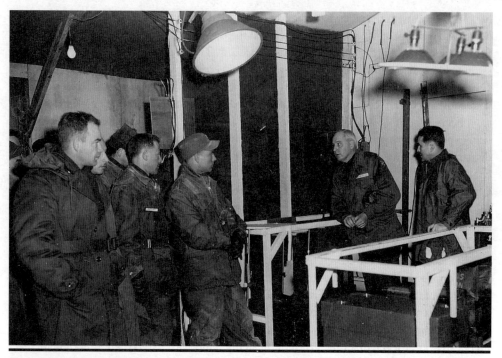

FIGURE 7-13. Students from the first class of the Seoul Branch Medical Field Service School listen as the commander of the 44th MASH, Colonel WS Cornell, explains the function of the Neuro Surgical Ward (22 February 1953). Note the improved facilities—hardened structure, bug screens, built up tables, and three surgical lights configured together. Photograph courtesy of the AMEDD Museum Photo Collection, Korean War, Volume 2, Image #KW-0450.

Houston, Texas, in 1952 prior to reporting to Korea,[37(p7)] compared to Dr Apel's complete lack of field training in 1951.[2(p35)]

Paralleling the changes taking place at the Medical Field Service School under Sams' leadership, Ginn instituted a tough in-country training program for officers and enlisted medical personnel in Korea in 1952 (Figure 7-13). He stated,

> Field training with a division, is an indispensable ingredient of [the medical officer's] education, especially if he is in the regular service, no matter how rarified and sacrosanct his MOS [military occupational specialty]; . . . along with knowledge and skill, a young medical officer must be taught a sense of mature responsibility toward his patients which comes from experience and from living with his mistakes.[7(pp196–197)]

The 8055th treated shock as it had previously and also emphasized that in surgery the type of agent or technique in anesthesia was not as important as the manner used.[29(pp2–4,7–9)] Looking with modern lenses, the 1952 annual report's discussion of surgical preparation seems strange, but the message is delivered with all seriousness: "We feel that the wounded man is entitled, if feasible, to undergo surgery while asleep."[29(p7)] Some of the problems

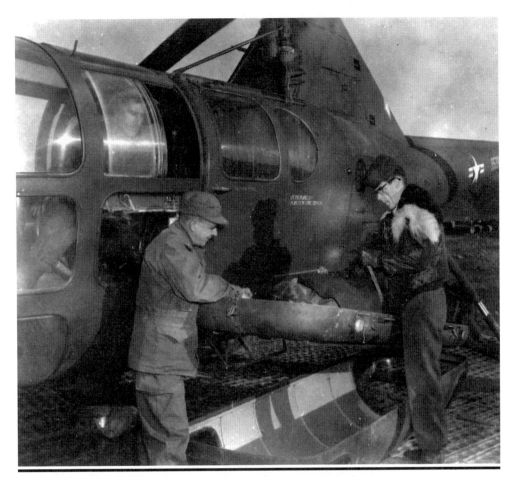

FIGURE 7-14. Chaplain (Captain) Thomas L Doyle (left) from Lowell, Michigan, and Airman First Class Peter J Farpell (right) from Albany, New York, tend to a casualty just arrived from the front lines in an Sikorsky H-5 rescue helicopter at the 8055th MASH (20 November 1952). Note the litter cover lying on the ground has a transparent viewing area, removing the "casket" experience of early Korean War evacuations. Photograph courtesy of the AMEDD Museum Photo Collection, Korean War, Volume 2, Image #KW-0400.

affecting the radiograph's ability to assist the surgeon were the great fluctuations in temperature, which affected the quality of the film development. It was noted, however, that the films were good enough for a general surgeon to interpret and the command recommended replacing the authorized radiologist with another general surgeon.[29(pp9–10)] This was the opposite opinion held by the 8063rd commander just the year before[28(p4)] (Figure 7-14).

By December, the headquarters detachment and mess facility were in prefabricated buildings, following the earlier preoperative, operative, and postoperative wards transitions. Japanese products, again, accounted for complaints of inferior quality. And again, winter clothing was on hand, but not the right size. The unit was challenged with getting replacements into the hospital. Enlisted soldiers with medical specialties were diverted to fill administrative jobs to keep the unit functioning. The quality of the soldiers also affected the performance. Of the 132 enlisted personnel, only 53 were high school graduates. Low morale concerning promotion and rotations was countered with interventions such as building a club tent, Red Cross reading and game room, hosting unit parties, and showing movies every night.[29(pp11,14–20)]

The Far East Command's endorsement of the 8063rd annual report supported the units' request for improved radiographic capabilities and facilities to continue the essential task of identifying foreign bodies. This ability, combined with the presence of a neurological team, would greatly increase favorable outcomes for the battle casualties arriving at the MASH.[38(End,pp1–2)] Ground and air ambulance evacuation means were "heartily recommended"[38(p2)] to continue in providing care to and from the hospital. Interestingly, the commander was severely critical of his medical counterparts because of their insistence in transferring ambulatory patients for radiography, labs, and general medical illnesses. LTC WS Cornell's comments echoed BG Sams' concerns from 1951 when he lamented,

> A misunderstanding seems to exist on the parts of the medical officers in forward echelon stations as to the capacity of the MASH. The function of this unit as stated in the Service Regulations is to treat emergency surgical conditions and the unit is not in a position to administer any more or better treatment of non-surgical conditions than is available in the division clearing stations. This fact should be made apparent to the medical officers of these installations.[38(p4)]

Additionally, the report warned it would be stressed under sustained action because of its current minimum staffing. The command had to train its nurses in anesthesia because of want of an anesthesiologist and had to train its surgical technicians with on-the-job training because they were unprepared out of the schoolhouse. Because the laboratory was still in tentage, reagents froze and the blood box overheated. This was corrected once the lab moved into a prefabricated building. The pharmacy also found it hard to keep medicines and liquids from freezing, but this also was remedied after moving into a tropical shell. Two and a half years of wear and tear were taking its toll on the vehicles of the unit. There was a considerable record of waiting for vehicle parts and the return of unserviceable vehicles. Recreational outlets such as swimming, softball, and ice skating, and entertainment through movies and United Service Organizations shows helped to improve morale.[38(pp5,7,10–11)] The radiograph was emerging as a critical piece to the ability of surgeons to properly identify and remove the elements of battle that damaged their young patients, but the machines in the MASH were not adequate. This knowledge and plea was supported by the report's citing Dr Eldridge Campbell in the March 1952 *Symposium on Treatment of Trauma in the Armed Forces*,

> Prior to debridement of a wound of the brain or spinal cord, it is essential to ascertain the location of in-driven bone, skull and rock fragments. Plain films, even of good quality, are inadequate. Good stereoscopic views are necessary, since not only the

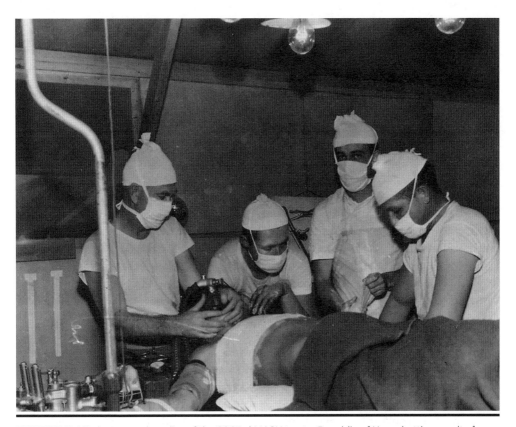

FIGURE 7-15. US doctors and medics of the 8063rd MASH treat a Republic of Korea battle casualty from the Battle of White Horse Mountain (8 October 1952). Note the standard surgical lights are now configured to hang from a movable structure above. Photograph courtesy of the AMEDD Museum Photo Collection, Korean War, Volume 2, Image #KW-0361.

depth and exact location but even the identification of many small shadows can be determined only in this manner. This technique was not available in World War II, and thus far not in the Korean conflict. This can and should be adopted without delay.[38(p12)]

Not surprisingly, the 8063rd commander states that most personnel in the unit were "not used to the rigors of Army life and life in the field."[38(p15)] Within the realm of clinical experience, the hospital made improvements in vascular repair by using clamps fashioned after Potts arterial anastomosis clamps. These clamps and subsequent training program came about directly from the general surgery consultant from the Far East Command. The treatment of severe burns and traumatic shock were improved through the use of polyethylene tubing for continuous intraarterial and intravenous fluid administration. Because the forward aid stations were using less morphine, patients were now able to go into surgery much sooner than they had in the past because the complications with anesthesia were far less. The unit now had eight tropical shells, concrete floors, and framed tents[38(pp18–19,22–23)] (Figure 7-15).

The 8076th began the transition from a surgical hospital mission to a *de facto* area medical support-type hospital. The care they began to provide was equal to the evacuation and station hospitals in other locations throughout the peninsula. Because of the lack of increased authorizations of enlisted personnel, the command utilized indigenous labor in support of the Post Exchange, sanitation requirements, and utilities details. The security requirements of the enlisted personnel affected the surgical, preoperative, and postoperative sections' efficiency. There was obviously an institutional memory within the organization, enough to gain notice in the annual report and admit their current situation was not as bad as it had been in 1950 and 1951. It was acknowledged that the current fleet of vehicles, 24 in all, was not enough to move the hospital personnel and equipment. The winterizing and improvements of the MASH had created a larger and more spread out unit. Tents were replaced with wooden frames and new tentage, liners, and wooden and cement floors. The postoperative, preoperative, and surgical wards were all in prefabricated buildings. The prefabricated structures also bought comfort to a new chapel/theater, enlisted day room, garage for the motor pool, and an officer's mess. (Half-way through the year these separate dining facilities were established for the enlisted and officers. This was considered "more desirable" according to the annual report.[39(Encls1–2,10)]) In fact, the summer brought about a change of attitude, if not mission.

> Prior to this everyone was too occupied in work, keeping warm and moving to be very much concerned about the adequacy of latrines and quarters, the suitability of the Enlisted Men and Officers Clubs, etc. Now a concerted effort was put forth to improve the living conditions and the recreational activities in order that personnel could derive some comfort from their fairly comfortable surrounds. In conjunction with the improvement program, a training program was also put into effect for the first time in the history of the unit. Paper work, reports and red tape in general commenced to increase to an extent that times the expression "police action" seemed a vague term as applied to the general situation as far as the 8076th was concerned.[21(p7)]

Along the lines of health of the command, three cases of hemorrhagic fever were diagnosed after some staff members were walking and hunting in a surrounding brushy area, which was soon put off-limits. Those three and the other 13 cases were evacuated to the 8228th MASH. The unit received only 67 cold injuries compared to 400 from the previous year. This decrease was attributed to the improved tactical situation, better cold weather protection, and education of the troops. The first half of the year US soldiers made up the surgical cases, but the second half were mostly Republic of Korea soldiers. Unfortunately, the higher morbidity rate for the South Koreans was directly attributed to the slower Republic of Korea Army evacuation system because it delayed arrival to definitive surgical intervention. Noteworthy surgeries included abdominal cases with thoracotomies, fractures, vascular injuries, and amputations.[39(Encls3,5–6)]

A team from Walter Reed Army Medical Center trained staff on vascular surgery, focusing on the repair of peripheral arteries. Verbal approval was given for the Potts-type arterial clamps, but the unit was presently still awaiting their receipt.[39(Encl6)] It appears the clinical practice of fashioning on-hand clamps to replicate the clinically preferred Potts clamps was making the rounds as also documented earlier in the 8063rd.[39(p19)] Dr Apel told of paying a silversmith to make a clamp based upon his own hand drawing while he was on rest and relaxation leave in Japan.[2(p162)]

These surgeons all knew they were in a unique time and opportunity. Across the command, the doctors agreed that, "the experience gained as a result of being assigned to a MASH has no counterpart in the Army or civilian life."[39(Encl7)] There was an added note for nursing. The command supported 6-month rotations back to Japan citing "at best the field conditions under which they are required to live in is considerably harder on females than males."[39(Encl7)] Thus, nurses were authorized to request a rotation back to Japan after being in Korea for 6 months. On the enlisted side, an influx of less intellectual and technically trained personnel toward the latter part of the year was troublesome. This, combined with their concerns for points and promotions, produced low morale. The MASH replicated the usual on-the-job training for the enlisted, but the doctors and nurses started a formal professional training program. Of interest to note, it was recommended that the dental technician be taught operating room techniques in order to assist the maxillofacial surgeon. The technician's skills in the dental chair were good, but lacking in the operating room.[39(Encls7,12)]

The 8209th served as a 200-bed surgical hospital in the beginning, but transformed into the 60-bed MASH variety by October. The hospital provided neurosurgical support and had the Surgical Research Team of the Army Medical Service and Graduate School assigned the entire year. Much medical literature and research was produced during this time. In fact, the annual report, consisting of only three pages, seems to suggest that the Surgical Research Team was the *de facto* reservoir of any official record of unit history and clinical research. On-the-job training occurred, but the unit lacked an anesthetist, a recurring theme in the anesthesia story of the war. Interestingly, it was noted that one-third of the intravenous fluids were lost due to the glass bottles breaking in shipment. The commander ended his terse report suggesting the MASH may finally move because it was "somewhat far behind [the] Division which it supports"[40(pp1-3)] some 8 miles forward.

The 8225th functioned in its prescribed manner until 18 May. Then it was closed for training until 24 September. During this training phase, the unit practiced individual military and branch training, field training, and use of medical equipment. Technicians were also sent on temporary duty to other medical units to receive required training. During this time there was terrible flooding, so there was plenty of opportunity to exercise the evacuation plan of the hospital. Once the training cycle was complete, the MASH temporarily occupied an old rice paddy that required draining while waiting for improvements on the final destination just 700 yards away. Once the site was properly prepared, the entire hospital moved piecemeal into the new location. For several hours there were patients in the operating room at both locations simultaneously. The division clearing station was now 7 miles away and ground ambulances traversed the evacuation route. Oftentimes, however, helicopters travelled straight from front line battalion aid stations. The airstrip was 1 mile away. Priorities were set for determining further evacuation requirements. It was deemed that wounds of the spinal cord, brain, and eye requiring specialized care warranted evacuation to a higher-level care, while those presenting with only minor wounds could be further transported to evacuation hospitals for care. In November, the Eighth US Army in Korea Surgeon directed that all minor battle casualties be given surgery in the clearing stations. This filtered out many patients normally bound for the MASH.[41(pp1–3,Encls2–3)]

The 8225th's annual report described the advantages of collocating the administration and disposition, preoperative, and radiography sections in the same building. This collocation eliminated crossing over other sections and improved the electrical distributions and prevented "bottlenecks." This proximity also enabled the radiograph's use in finding all debris in battle wounds early in the process.[41(pp3–5)]

Problems with supplies and personnel still existed, however. The pharmacy reported the arrival of smallpox vaccine after its expiration date. The laboratory technicians' skills were found lacking and on-the-job training ensued. This situation may have contributed to the US Armed Forces–Far East Command arguing against the use of fresh whole blood within the MASH in its endorsement memo for the report. The higher command insisted that a mistake would be fatal and the dangers outweighed the advantages.[41(End,p6)]

There was gradual improvement in some areas. In reviewing the layout, the two hospital sites described in the 8225th's annual report provide examples of this improvement to MASH facilities in the theater, compared to the crude canvas of earlier years. The first operating room was a prefabricated building with wooden floors containing two standard field-operating tables, two litter frames, and one cast table for the five operating room tables. The lights were a three-cluster arrangement of 100-watt bulbs that moved on a cable and slide. These were augmented with truck lights running off the truck's batteries. Once the hospital occupied the well-prepared site, an additional field-operating table replaced a litter frame. Now the operating room was in a prefabricated building, but with concrete floors. Two portable lamps replaced the old truck lights. Curtains were even arranged on cables between patients, which enabled surgery on an unconscious patient to be private, and not intimidate the adjacent patient only receiving local anesthetic administration.[41(p7)] However, the lack of nurses caused operating room technicians to function as nurses if one nurse supervised. But sometimes there were no nurses at all.

Efficiencies were incorporated that saved numerous staff hours and are interesting to read in light of today's advancements, which have incorporated some of them or used the method to alter modern practices. These included:

- a glove powdering box limiting the dust in central supply;
- suspended drapes and intravenous bottle holders allowing draping and decreasing the number of poles on the floor;
- cast cart at surgical table saving time in walking;
- leg traction holder within the ceiling allowing surgical preparation at table;
- prep stands at surgical table allowing for consolidation of all items for surgical preparation;
- lighting that allowed movement of the lights over a cable system;
- portable intravenous stands allowing blood to be given in transit while attached to the litter;

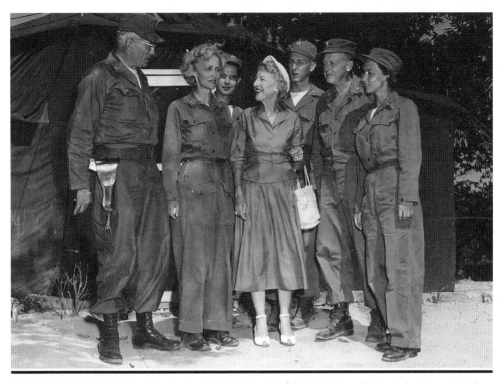

FIGURE 7-16. Visitors like Maurine Clark, wife of the Far East/United Nations Commander, General Mark Clark, were able to visit because the MASHs began to remain in place as the battlefields became stagnant (12 August 1952). Here Mrs Clark is visiting the hospital staff of the 8228th MASH. Photograph courtesy of the AMEDD Museum Photo Collection, Korean War, Volume 2, Image #KW-0335.

- sterile mimeographed supply check list allowing for item listings with levels for rapid reference;
- card index of unsterile supplies allowing for a quick reference and standardization;
- procedure book providing more MASH-centric surgical procedures readily available; and
- prepacked lockers and cases allowing for rapid mobility.[41(pp8–9)]

Beginning in September, the 8225th started to train all enlisted technicians in nursing because the 60-bed MASH had only two nurses. The eventual intent was to train and increase the enlisted medical proficiency in order for them to operate without nurse supervision at all.[41(pp11–12)] The Eighth Army Surgeon reported it as "entirely successful."[5(AnnexIV,p7)] This is interesting in light of the 1950 annual report from the 8055th arguing the opposite, that "corpsmen are not a suitable replacement for nurses,"[19(p13)] and emphasizing the incredible reliance and importance of nurses in the MASH.[19(p13)]

The 8228th MASH was unlike any of the other MASHs on the peninsula. The first 4 months of 1952 were dedicated solely to training. On 7 April, the 8228th was designated as the primary hemorrhagic fever center and on 27 November, it was also designated as the primary facility for cold weather injuries. Their first move entailed 33 trucks and 25 trailer loads over 3 days in March. As the hemorrhagic fever center, surgical supplies were not needed, but more laboratory and ward spaces were needed. The second move, in November 1952, took 7 days with 132 patients distributed among 17 ground ambulances and five helicopters. The MASH occupied 60 new prefabricated buildings with sidewalks, enough space for 500 beds and a detachment of 200 (Figure 7-16). There was no canvas tentage for the entire hospital. Because of the mission, treatment was medical rather than surgical. The medical officers were internists. Most were experienced with extensive residency training. Surgical technicians became medical technicians. On-the-job training related to hemorrhagic fever was conducted.

The mission change affected the ability to get the right types of supplies, which required letters of justification because the MASH was only authorized those items integral to surgical care. Some drugs had to be pulled from other installations in Korea by the medical depot trying to fulfill the new requirements. The commonly recurring saga of inferior Japanese products still emerged, even within this pristine MASH, but it was limited to light bulbs. Clothing in the wrong sizes continued to be a prevalent problem. One interesting note on equipment sustainability is seen where Japanese stapling machines were issued to the hospital, but only American staples were available through the supply system. In the spirit of redistributing desperately needed equipment, the unit received authorization to turn in unnecessary equipment needed elsewhere.

Along the lines of the clinical investigations, the clinicians knew the vector for hemorrhagic fever was an arthropod. Soon the center was conducting studies on rodent ectoparasites such as ticks, fleas, and mites (chiggers). As of the 1952 annual report, studies were looking into the theory that chiggers were the vector for hemorrhagic fever.[36(pp1–6;AppC,pp1–3)]

Korean War (1953)

The closing events of the Korean War only covered the first 7 months of 1953. The earlier stalemate following the deadlocked truce talks continued on through the beginning of the year. General (GEN) Maxwell Taylor replaced GEN Van Fleet as the Commander, Eighth Army, in February. Not all the battle lines were quiet, however. Veterans from Pork Chop Hill that April, and the subsequent savage fighting through May, would testify to an eventful "stalemate" while peace talks were negotiated. On 27 July 1953, a little over 3 years from the North Korean invasion of South Korea, a ceasefire agreement was finally signed that ended the fighting.[17(p664)]

In June, the 30th Medical group assumed medical service support to the Eighth Army. The medical units that had previously provided third-echelon medical care to the Eighth Army were organized under this new structure and commanded by BG Paul I Robinson. There were six MASHs in country, with one listed as inoperative. Following the armistice, additional equipment was assigned to the MASH to meet the increased demands of providing support to newly repatriated prisoners and maintaining the health of the populace in the devastated countryside. With this new command structure came a new name for the MASH—the "Surgical Hospital, Mobile Army." However, everyone still

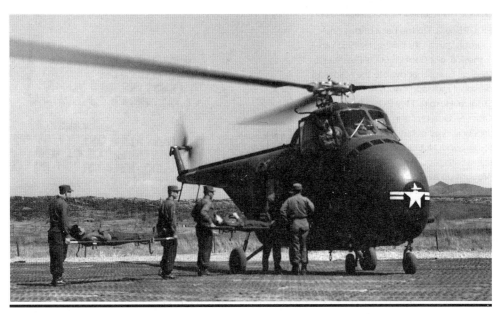

FIGURE 7-17. Members of the 45th MASH conduct a mission rehearsal for the exchange of sick and wounded prisoners on a Sikorsky H-19 helicopter in support of Operation Little Switch to begin the next day (19 April 1953). Photograph courtesy of the AMEDD Museum Photo Collection, Korean War, Volume 1, Image #KW-0173.

called it the MASH.[6(pp1–2,4–5)] As discussed earlier, the MASH moved into fixed facilities, in the words of Robinson, "so that hospitals could render more effective Medical and Surgical type care."[6(p4)] And he added, "With the construction of semi-permanent buildings the fire hazard in the Surgical Hospitals has been decreased."[6(pp4–5)]

A shortage of personnel plagued the 8076th as it sought the ability to handle additional duties and, again, local nationals were used to fill these positions. The "mobile" hospital now had 19 vehicles on hand, even less than the previous year's warning that there were too few to adequately carry out their mission, and again declared they would not be adequate to perform their mission when they transferred their excess and reached their authorized 14 vehicles.[42(Encls2,9)] A good news story clinically, the final report of the 8076th MASH noted that,

> [t]here has been a change in the form of new incoming men in our surgical service from a professional viewpoint and also enlisted men for our operating room. Both of these changes have brought well trained men to our service and should be adequate for the performance of good work, carried out in a logical and well supervised manner.[42(Encl6)]

It appears that the ebb and flow of training had come back to producing better-trained medical personnel after the strained effort to get many medical men into the battle very quickly. Medical services were in abundance over surgeries due to the stagnant front.

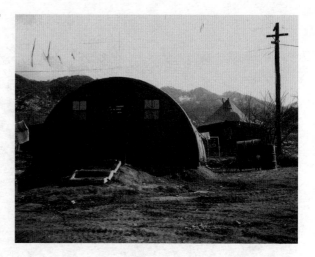

FIGURE 7-18. On the back of this photograph (circa late 1952/early 1953) anesthesiologist Captain Louis Eisenberg, Medical Corps, handwrote the following personal message, "46th A. S. H. [Army Surgical Hospital] My BOQ [Bachelor Officers' Quarter] is in rear—Nurses Janeway type of hut [Quonset Hut] in foreground. Notice Diesel oil drums on stand with rubber hose into tent. Oil brought up every day by KSC's [Korean Service Corps]." Photograph courtesy of the AMEDD Center of History and Heritage, Louis Eisenberg Collection, Box 1, Image page #2010.11.30.

Because of this move to general medicine, the command actually requested two more general duty medical officers to supplement their authorizations.[42(Encls6–7)]

The MASH continued to train 4 hours every week on required subjects such as guard duty, security of the unit, physical training, close order drill, firefighting and prevention, military courtesy, and air-raid precaution, augmented with subjects related to management of battle casualties for the doctors and nursing staff (Figure 7-17). With the transfer of excess equipment, the 200-bed 8076th MASH was transforming into the 60-bed 45th MASH.[42(Encls8–9)] The 45th practiced tearing down and then resetting the new unit for patients within 5 hours.[21(p9)]

During "Operation Little Switch" in April, the first prisoner exchanges occurred and 213 UN patients were seen at the MASH. It was a relatively short visit; each patient averaged about 40 minutes in the hospital. In August, a section of the hospital was sent forward to provide direct surgical support to the 40th Infantry Division, while the remaining portion supported "Operation Big Switch," treating five UN patients and 15 Korean People's Army and Communist Chinese Forces soldiers. Most injuries to the enemy, however, were from stone-throwing civilians. The unit conducted split operations, once again, during September through October, in order to move forward. The heavy winds whipping through rugged mountainous terrain pounding the tents tethered to soft ground helped to ensure a rapid transition to Quonset huts to replace the old canvas[21(pp9–10)] (Figure 7-18).

The 8209th made the move alluded to in the previous year's report and conducted a two-phased move closer to its supported divisional elements in January (Figures 7-19 and 7-20). The new location was much better because it was off from the main supply route, avoiding the usual dust, and was more dispersed. However, any plans to dig drainage and latrines were postponed until the ground thawed later in the summer. The Surgical Research Team of the Medical Service and Graduate School was still assigned there.[43(p1)]

The 8225th MASH continued on with its normal surgical care of nonevacuated battle casualties, but now had the mission of training enlisted technicians to replace nurses. The

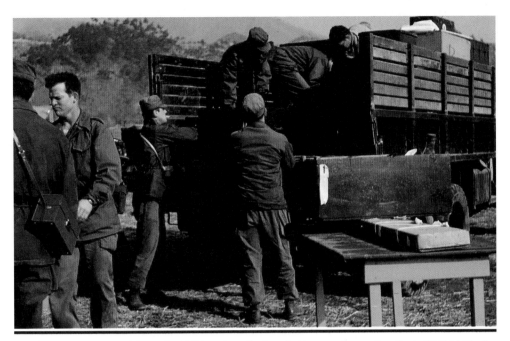

FIGURE 7-19. Members of the 46th MASH pack up the hospital to move forward on the battlefield (April 1953). It was at the 46th MASH, converted from the 8209th MASH in February 1953, where the Surgical Research Teams conducted studies 8 to 10 miles from the front. Photograph courtesy of the AMEDD Center of History and Heritage, Louis Eisenberg Collection, Box 1, Image page #2010.11.30.

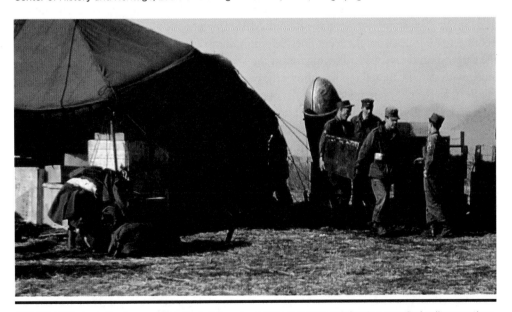

FIGURE 7-20. Jumping forward, the Central Supply section is shown conducting a typical split operations move on the battlefield (April 1953). Note the rice stalks along the ground to mitigate mud and dust. Photograph courtesy of the AMEDD Center of History and Heritage, Louis Eisenberg Collection, Box 1, Image page #2010.11.30.

60-bed configuration only had two nurses authorized and this was obviously a strain within the operating room and elsewhere. Medical officers often had to serve and nurse in the postoperative sections. The commander emphasized the importance of incoming enlisted personnel possessing high intellect and scores to fulfill the task of replacing nurses in the MASH.[44(pp3-7)]

The 8228th MASH continued to serve as the hemorrhagic fever and cold weather injury centers. All suspected cases of hemorrhagic fever were evacuated there for confirmation and treatment. A medical clearing company was assigned and became the convalescent and rehabilitation section of the hospital. Five more prefabricated buildings were added, bringing the total hospital building count to 65, which included eight 20' x 108' wards. All surgical cases were transferred to the 121st Evacuation Hospital and only minor procedures were performed at the 8228th. In the first part of the year the Army Surgeon General MG George Armstrong, Far East Command Surgeon MG William Shambora, and BG Ginn were presented with the preliminary results of the hemorrhagic fever research. Outdoor sports and military formations were conducted for the convalescents and this therapy was found to be productive. Universal praise was given to the educational teaching within the hemorrhagic fever center and the quality of training coming out of the Medical Field Services Staff School.[45]

The Surgical Research Teams

The Surgical Research and Renal Insufficiency Teams were lauded with praise. Through their efforts every department of the hospitals improved as they encountered various combat medicine problems.[6(pp3-4)] The major research unit was established at the 46th Surgical Hospital (formerly the 8209th MASH) where most of the studies took place, about 8 to 10 miles from the front lines. Monthly statistics of patients were compiled by the surgeons and reviewed, allowing for on-the-spot improvement to patient care. This, along with data in annual reports, shows the evolving patient statistics through the war (Table 7-2). Results were pulled from the operating room records and statistical data sheets that were part of the patient's charts upon admission. The more active Western Front hosted the vascular surgical unit located at the 43rd Surgical Hospital (formerly the 8055th MASH).[46(pp5-6),47(p4)] Surgeons from the Surgical Research Team instructed at each hospital. Immediate results of the work done through primary arterial repairs and vein grafts resulted in amputation rates falling sharply after arterial injuries. For example, following popliteal anastomosis, the amputation rate fell from World War II's 72% to approximately 20% in the Korean War.[46(pp9,17)] The research work was primarily performed from the summer of 1952 through the winter of 1952 to 1953. The liver function study was one part of the entire effort and took place simultaneously with all the other research. It documented this ideal clinical setting, a relatively immobile front line, providing a picture of conditions in the mature MASH:

> The casualties usually arrived at the hospital between 3 and 5 hours after wounding with range of 1 to 9 hours. The soldiers were all young and previously healthy. As a generalization, the more severely injured men were selected for study. Shortly after

injury, the casualty was treated at the battalion aid station. When needed, plasma, albumin or dextran was administered along with tetanus toxoid and penicillin. The casualty was then evacuated to the forward Surgical Hospital for definitive therapy where this study was begun. . . . Detailed clinical records were maintained throughout the period of study. Blood, 10 to 20 days of age, was used almost exclusively after the casualty reached the hospital. Operations were performed under pentothal, nitrous oxide, oxygen and ether anesthesia.[48(pp149–150)]

Another study conducted from May to August 1953 provides an additional snapshot of events at the mature MASH (Figures 7-21 and 7-22). Even though the survey was a short one, it appeared to replicate the previous 15 months of experience at the MASH. Of 250 battle casualties, except for open fractures where ground ambulance was the mode of transportation, approximately half of all casualties were evacuated by helicopter. From the data collected, it is apparent that the length of time in surgery for abdominal and thoraco-abdominal wounds was greater than all other types of wounds. For patients with abdominal wounds and those requiring amputations, an average of 3.5 liters of blood was given in the first 24 hours following their battle injury. And finally, the feared "gut wound" of so many wars before had an 82% survival rate.[49(pp9–12)]

Each war presents different circumstances that affect the casualty rate, and therefore, mortality rate. In relation to casualty care at the MASH, the last year of the Korean conflict was almost ideal. The battle line was stable, the UN forces had air dominance, and the hospital was close to the front. Because of shorter evacuation times and the availability of helicopters for evacuation, more patients were evacuated than would have survived in the past. This created a situation where more seriously wounded casualties were present at forward surgical hospitals. Survivability was improved because of the shorter evacuation times, large administration of resuscitative fluids before and after surgery, and the routine use of antibiotics.[49(p20)]

It was the opinion of the lead author, then-Major Curtis P Artz, who had been a member of the Surgical Research Team assigned to the 46th Surgical Hospital (formerly the 8209th MASH),[49(p1)] that the "greatest single difference in the management of casualties in Korea appears to be the large quantities of blood administered throughout resuscitative periods."[49(p20)] In the 46th Surgical Hospital from January 1952 to August 1953, the overall fatality rate for the 4,671 casualties admitted was 2.4%. Of the 402 abdominal wounds, the casualty rate was 12.6%.[49(p1)] These results also coincide with the statistics bearing out the cumulative results of the Korean War showing the fatality rate was a "new low of 2.5 percent compared to the 4.5 percent experienced in all of World War II."[50(p83)]

In laying out the ideal surgical team during the *Course on Recent Advances in Medicine and Surgery* at the Army Medical Service Graduate School in April 1954, Artz argued there should be two groups, each able to perform 12-hour shifts.[51(pp237–239)] Each group should have a team captain, a deputy supervised by the chief surgeon, and both should possess the most experience in battle casualty management among the other surgeons. He believed they should both visit the evacuation hospital to monitor follow-up care. The relationship between the chief surgeon and his deputies would mimic that

TABLE 7-2. PATIENT STATISTICS BY UNIT AND YEAR

Patient Statistics	1950	1951	1952	1953
8055th	(9 Jul 1950–31 Dec 1950)	(1 Jan 1951–31 Dec 1951)	(1 Jan 1952–31 Dec 1952)	(1 Jan 1953–1 Feb 1953)
Admission	8,577	29,579	15,012	510
Surgical Patients	1,516	5,751	5,689	292
Surgical Procedures	2,280	8,245	12,421	610
8063rd	(18 Jul 1950–31 Dec 1950)	(1 Jan 1951–31 Dec 1951)	(1 Jan 1952–31 Dec 1952)	
Admission	5,173	20,359	10,125	
Surgical Patients	1,008	Not reported	Not reported	
Surgical Procedures	1,048	5,416	4,787	
8076th	(2 Aug 1950–31 Dec 1950)	(1 Jan 1951–31 Dec 1951)	(1 Jan 1952–31 Dec 1952)	(1 Jan 1953–1 Feb 1953)
Admission	9,008	21,408	8,253	155
Surgical Patients	Not reported	Not reported	Not reported	Not reported
Surgical Procedures	Not reported	5,176	2,917	74
1st 8209th	(26 Sep 1950–31 Dec 1950)	(1 Jan 1951–20 May 1951)		
Admission	95	6,642		
Surgical Patients	Not reported	Not reported		
Surgical Procedures	282	Not reported		
8209th		(1 Jan 1951–31 Dec 1951)	(1 Jan 1952–31 Dec 1952)	(1 Jan 1953–1 Feb 1953)
Admission		8,806	9,360	416
Surgical Patients		2,128	Not reported	273
Surgical Procedures		2,400	9,485	350

TABLE 7-2 CONTINUED. **PATIENT STATISTICS BY UNIT AND YEAR**

Patient Statistics	1950	1951	1952	1953
2nd				
8225th		(15 Apr 1951–12 May 1951)		
Admission		1,409		
Surgical Patients		Not reported		
Surgical Procedures		Not reported		
8225th		(13 May 1951–31 Dec 1951)	(1 Jan 1952–31 Dec 1952)	(1 Jan 1953–1 Feb 1953)
Admission		8,108	3,155	328
Surgical Patients		Not reported	Not reported	318
Surgical Procedures		2,312	1,541	Not reported
8228th		(15 Jun 1951–31 Dec 1951)	(1 Jan 1952–31 Dec 1952)	(1 Jan 1953–1 Feb 1953)
Admission for Hemorraghic Fever		0	1,936	21
Confirmed Hemorraghic Fever		0	885	3
Admission for Cold Injury		0	193	105
Evidence of Cold Injury		0	170	85

Data sources: Annual reports of Medical Department activities of each MASH unit, National Archives II, Suitland, Maryland, boxes 146, 239, 240, and 241.

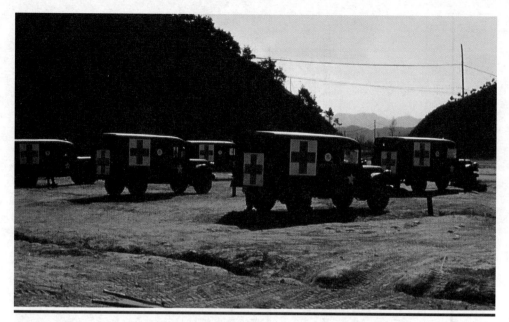

FIGURE 7-21. Captain Louis Eisenberg, Medical Corps, commented that these vehicles were the "new ambulances" for the new 46th MASH (February 1953). They appear to be Dodge M43 ambulances. Photograph courtesy of the AMEDD Center of History and Heritage, Louis Eisenberg Collection, Box 1, Image page #2010.11.30.

of the teaching professor conducting training with two assistants. With adequate rest, many operative procedures without an assisting surgeon could be performed with the aid of one or two capable operating room technicians. In cases with multiple wounds, two surgical teams could operate on the same patient—one team on the upper body while the other team performed on the lower body. This decreased the time required for surgery and anesthesia, thus benefitting the patient.

The chief surgeon should be a more experienced Regular Army officer trained in the principles of resuscitation and combat surgery. Oftentimes the most junior were sent forward and the more senior surgeons remained in the rear, but this was not the most ideal situation for the patient. In fact, Artz believed all Regular Army surgeons should be thoroughly trained in trauma with a subspecialty in forward surgery. His insistence that "Young career surgeons in the Regular Army should always be given an opportunity to gain experience in forward surgical hospitals"[51(p239)] seems to advocate the flip side and positive reason for pushing surgeons to the front versus the policy of reluctantly sending surgeons into combat for 90-day rotations to limit the effect on patient care back at the home station. Finally, as COL Page had implied in 1951, MAJ Artz emphasized that a surgical consultant visiting the MASH was better used for 2 weeks instead of 1 to 2 days so that his "knowledge could be better utilized if he actually performed some surgery and, by first-hand experience, became extremely familiar with the problems of the particular institution he visited."[51(p239)]

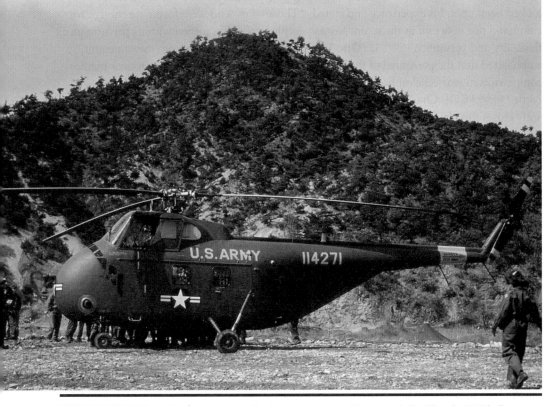

FIGURE 7-22. While routine/nonurgent patients were evacuated by ground, the Sikorsky H-19 helicopter was one of the workhorses for rapid evacuation of urgent wounded (March 1953). Note this is the same helicopter pictured before in the Operation Little Switch rehearsal at the 45th MASH. Photograph courtesy of the AMEDD Center of History and Heritage, Louis Eisenberg Collection, Box 1, Image page #2010.11.30.

Ironically, the Eighth United States Army Surgeon's Annual Report for 1953 notes less time for research was available as the war ended. Staff members found themselves occupied with promotion, courts-martial boards, and so forth. Now the fixed/garrison MASH had to train for combat and began to participate in field exercises to train the surgeons in the practice of military surgery.[6(pp3–4)] The MASH had come about full circle.

CONCLUSION

The innovations seen in the Korean War MASH were not effectively matched in the civilian world for another 15 to 20 years. The combined effort in trauma management through rapid helicopter evacuation, enlisted medics (paramedics), and advanced methods in the treatment of shock would be the model for future modern metropolitan trauma centers.[7(p209)] LTC Kryder Van Buskirk, previous commander of the 8076th MASH, looked back upon his experience and stated, "Those of us who were fortunate enough to command this new unit in the recent Korean conflict are well satisfied with its performance, flexibility and versatility."[52(p31)] Dr Otto F Apel Jr, a MASH surgeon from the same unit, emphasized that the personnel of the MASH were particularly different from their medical compatriots in rear-echelon hospitals. MASH members saw, smelled, and heard the battle.[2(ppxii–xiii)] COL Charles L Leedham, Medical Consultant in the Far East Command, aptly closes this chapter in forward surgery,

> These hospitals were, to me, the most remarkable field installations of the Army. The number of lives and limbs saved because of the MASH's special location and function cannot be comprehended unless one could see such a unit during a military operation when the flow of wounded was heavy. Many a veteran now living owes his life or one or more of his limbs to these units. Really emergency life-saving surgery was done here. The job they did was a truly outstanding one, while their accomplishments were rarely paralleled.[53(p23)]

REFERENCES

1. DeBakey MJ. History, the torch that illuminates: lessons from military medicine. *Mil Med*. 1996;161:711–716.
2. Apel OF Jr, Apel P. *MASH: An Army Surgeon in Korea*. Lexington, Ky: University Press of Kentucky, 1998.
3. Eighth United States Army Annual Report, Army Medical Service Activities, 1950, National Archives II, Suitland, Maryland, boxes 195–196.
4. Eighth United States Army Annual Report, Army Medical Service Activities, 1951, National Archives II, Suitland, Maryland, box 196.
5. Eighth United States Army Annual Report, Army Medical Service Activities, 1952, National Archives II, Suitland, Maryland, box 197.
6. Eighth United States Army Annual Report, Army Medical Service Activities, 1953, National Archives II, Suitland, Maryland, box 198.
7. Cowdrey AE. *The Medics' War*. Washington, DC: US Army Center of Military History; 1987.
8. Westover JG, ed. *Combat Support in Korea*. Washington, DC: US Army Center of Military History; 1987.
9. Coates JB, ed. *Activities of Surgical Consultants*. Vol 1. Washington, DC: Office of The Surgeon General, Department of the Army; 1962.
10. Station List, World Wide, US Army Medical Department Units, 31 January 1950, National Archives II, Suitland, Maryland, box 239.
11. Annual Report of Medical Activities (1949), 2nd Mobile Army Surgical Hospital, 3 March 1950, National Archives II, Suitland, Maryland, box, 144.
12. Memorandum: T/O&E 8-57 IN (sic), Mobile Army Surgical Hospital Review, 11 August 1948, National Archives II, Suitland, Maryland, box 40.
13. Memorandum: Tentative Troop Bases of the 18, 20, 22, and 25 Division Forces, 18 July 1948, National Archives II, Suitland, Maryland, box 40.
14. Memorandum: Mobile Striking Force Troop Basis (Tentative), 29 April 1948, National Archives II, Suitland, Maryland, box 40.
15. Special Text 8-10-1, *Medical Service in the Theater of Operations*, National Archives II, Suitland, Maryland, box 157.

16. Transcript of Proceedings: 1951 Instructors' Conference, National Archives II, Suitland, Maryland, box 157.
17. Fehrenbach TR. *This Kind of War*. New York, NY: The MacMillan Company; 1963.
18. Hooker (Hornberger) R. *MASH*. London, England: Cassel Wellington House; 2004.
19. 1950 Annual Report of Medical Department Activities, 8055th, National Archives II, Suitland, Maryland, box 146.
20. 1950 Annual Report of Medical Department Activities, 8063rd, National Archives II, Suitland, Maryland, box 240.
21. Unit History, 45th Surgical Hospital (8076th AU): 19 July 1950–19 July 1954, National Archives II, Suitland, Maryland, box 144.
22. 1950 Annual Report of Medical Department Activities, 8076th, National Archives II, Suitland, Maryland, box 240.
23. War Department. *Notes on the Care of Battle Casualties*. Washington, DC: War Department, Technical Medical Bulletin 147; March 1945.
24. 1950 Annual Report of Medical Department Activities, 1st, National Archives II, Suitland, Maryland, box 239.
25. 8076th MASH, After Action Interviews, 3rd Historical Detachment (EUSAK), National Archives II, Suitland, Maryland, box 347.
26. Sako Y, Artz CP, Howard JM, Bronwell AW, Inui FK. Experiences with intra-arterial and rapid intravenous transfusions in a forward surgical hospital. In: Howard JM, ed. *Battle Casualties in Korea: Studies of the Surgical Research Team*. Vol 3. *The Battle Wound: Clinical Experiences*. Washington, DC: Army Medical Service Graduate School, Walter Reed Army Medical Center; 1956.
27. 1951 Annual Report of Medical Department Activities, 8055th, National Archives II, Suitland, Maryland, box 239.
28. 1951 Annual Report of Medical Department Activities, 8063rd, National Archives II, Suitland, Maryland, box 240.
29. 1952 Annual Report of Medical Department Activities, 8055th, National Archives II, Suitland, Maryland, box 240.
30. 1951 Annual Report of Medical Department Activities, 8076th, National Archives II, Suitland, Maryland, box 240.
31. War Department. *Management of Battle Casualties*. Washington, DC: War Department; Technical Medical Bulletin 147 (rev); 1951.
32. 1951 Annual Report of Medical Department Activities, 8209th, National Archives II, Suitland, Maryland, box 240.
33. 1951 Annual Report of Medical Department Activities, 1st, National Archives II, Suitland, Maryland, box 239.
34. 1951 Annual Report of Medical Department Activities, 8225th, National Archives II, Suitland, Maryland, box 240.
35. 1951 Annual Report of Medical Department Activities, 8228th, Endorsement, National Archives II, Suitland, Maryland, box 241.
36. 1952 Annual Report of Medical Department Activities, 8228th, p. 6, National Archives II, Suitland, Maryland, box 241.
37. Horwitz, DG, ed. *We Will Not Be Strangers: Korean War Letters Between a MASH Surgeon and His Wife*. Urbana, Ill: University of Illinois Press; 1997.
38. 1952 Annual Report of Medical Department Activities, 8063rd, National Archives II, Suitland, Maryland, box 240.
39. 1952 Annual Report of Medical Department Activities, 8076th, National Archives II, Suitland, Maryland, box 240.
40. 1952 Annual Report of Medical Department Activities, 8209th, National Archives II, Suitland, Maryland, box 240.

41. 1952 Annual Report of Medical Department Activities, 8225th, National Archives II, Suitland, Maryland, box 240.
42. 1953 Annual Report of Medical Department Activities, 8076th, National Archives II, Suitland, Maryland, box 239.
43. 1953 Annual Report of Medical Department Activities, 8209th, National Archives II, Suitland, Maryland, box 240.
44. 1953 Annual Report of Medical Department Activities, 8225th, National Archives II, Suitland, Maryland, box 240.
45. 1953 Annual Report of Medical Department Activities, 8228th, National Archives II, Suitland, Maryland, box 241.
46. Howard JM. Introduction: historical background and development. In: Howard JM, ed. *Battle Casualties in Korea: Studies of the Surgical Research Team*. Vol 1. *The Systemic Response to Injury*. Washington, DC: Army Medical Service Graduate School, Walter Reed Army Medical Center; 1955.
47. Artz CP. Preface. In: Howard JM, ed. *Battle Casualties in Korea: Studies of the Surgical Research Team*. Vol 3. *The Battle Wound: Clinical Experiences*. Washington, DC: Army Medical Service Graduate School, Walter Reed Army Medical Center; 1956.
48. Scott R Jr, Olney JM, Howard JM. Hepatic function of the battle casualty. In: Howard JM, ed. *Battle Casualties in Korea: Studies of the Surgical Research Team*. Vol 1. *The Systemic Response to Injury*. Washington, DC: Army Medical Service Graduate School, Walter Reed Army Medical Center; 1955.
49. Sako Y, Artz CP, Howard JM, Bronwell AW, Inui FK. A survey of evacuation, resuscitation, and mortality in a forward surgical hospital. In: Howard JM, ed. *Battle Casualties in Korea: Studies of the Surgical Research Team*. Vol 3. *The Battle Wound: Clinical Experiences*. Washington, DC: Army Medical Service Graduate School, Walter Reed Army Medical Center; 1956.
50. Reister FA. *Battle Casualties and Medical Statistics: US Army Experience in the Korean War*. Washington DC: The Surgeon General, Department of the Army; 1973.
51. Artz CP. Discussion on consultants and organization of surgical service. In: *Recent Advances in Medicine and Surgery: Based on Professional Medical Experiences in Japan and Korea 1950–1953*. Vol 1. Washington, DC: Army Medical Service Graduate School, Medical Science Publication No. 4, Walter Reed Army Medical Center; 1954.
52. Van Buskirk KE. The Mobile Army Surgical Hospital. *Mil Surg*. 1953(July–December);113:27–31. National Archives II, Suitland, Maryland, box 342.
53. Leedham CL. Use of medical consultants in the Far East Command. In: *Recent Advances in Medicine and Surgery: Based on Professional Medical Experiences in Japan and Korea 1950–1953*. Vol 2. Washington, DC: Army Medical Service Graduate School, Medical Science Publication No. 4, Walter Reed Army Medical Center; 1954.

Chapter Eight

Vietnam: The Rise of Helicopter Medical Evacuation in a War Against a New Kind of Enemy

LANCE P. STEAHLY, MD

INTRODUCTION

THE VIETNAM WAR PRESENTED CHALLENGES to the Army Medical Department (AMEDD) that were unique to the conflict and terrain. The signal change in forward surgery was the widespread use of the helicopter in medical evacuation. In a sense, the soldier was brought to the surgical treatment facility rather than having forward surgery come to the soldier. These facilities were located within accessible distances by air. Hence, rapid and more definitive surgery could be rendered in reduced time compared to previous conflicts.

AN OVERVIEW OF VIETNAM

It is necessary to understand the geography and people of Vietnam to follow the Vietnam conflict's often confusing and shifting battlefronts. Only 20% or so of Vietnam is truly level land. Vietnam has three distinct areas: (1) the Mekong Delta, (2) the Chaine Annamitique (Annamite Mountains) (including the Central Highlands plateau area/mountains), and (3) the Central Lowlands.[1(pp4–5)] The Mekong Delta is well known from wartime press coverage and is the largest area, occupying the southern 40% of the country. The Delta was created by the five branches of the Mekong River. The heavy rainfall during the flood periods made combat there a challenge.[1(p4)] The Central Highlands consists of bamboo/broadleaf forests with rubber plantations and farms. The Highlands feature mountains ranging from 5,000 to 8,000 feet in elevation. The Central Lowlands features a narrow coastal strip of land. The coastal plain varies in width from 15 to 40 kilometers (km) but runs for most of the 1,400 km of the Vietnamese coast. Rice, sugar cane, and fishing villages are typically found here. Some of the larger Vietnamese cities such as Da Nang, Hue, and Cam Ranh are located along the coast in this region.[1(pp4-5)]

These geographic areas formed boundaries for the South Vietnamese military zones. The I Corps zone (northern) largely had mountains and jungles in it. The II Corps area incorporated much of the coastal plain. The III Corps zone was a mixed type of geographical constituents centered in Saigon but extending from the North Mekong Delta to the Southern Central Highlands. The IV Corps zone consisted largely of the Mekong Delta area. The climate varied with the location. The north of the country is a humid subtropical area, while the Mekong Delta is a tropical climate with distinct wet and dry seasons. In the north and in the Central Highlands, fog and low clouds were common. Vietnam generally was well described as a land of oppressive heat with temperatures in the 90s moving into the 100s. The dry season in the winter would mean heat that could range from 100 to 110 degrees Fahrenheit. In the winter, the south is dry while copious rains are abundant for the rest of the year. In the summer, the monsoon rains are epic in degree. Snakes, leeches, mosquitoes, ants, and rodents were in abundance all the time.[2(p101)]

The Vietnamese people proper mostly lived in small urban centers or in rural areas. Only 10% of the Vietnamese lived in major city centers. In the mid-1960s, ethnic Chinese made up over 85% of the population in the Mekong Delta, the river valleys, and the coastal regions. The Montagnards (mountain people) were a minority group living in the highlands, consisting of some 30 diverse tribes that played an increased role as irregular anti-Viet Cong fighting forces.[3(pp21-22)] The Montagnards were among the groups that were not trusted by the Communists.

BACKGROUND OF THE VIETNAM CONFLICT

After the French took control of Vietnam as a colony in the mid-19th century, Saigon became known as the "Paris of the Orient." In the past, most Vietnamese people lived in the delta area around Saigon. Later, the majority of the population actually lived in rural or small urban centers. The French had created rail and roads, rubber plantations, and irrigation systems that increased cultivation in the Mekong Delta. The French also had established universities at the Pasteur Institute in Saigon as a medical research institution, hospitals, and schools. The French reduced the incidence of malaria and also reduced the incidence of other tropical diseases.[1(pp1-8)]

American involvement in the Vietnam conflict followed a complicated regional history. The treaty of Hue, in 1883, effectively established Vietnam as a French colony. The French had bombarded Da Nang in 1857 and captured Saigon in 1861.[4(pp4-5)] However, despite the French military, social, and environmental successes, the nationalist spirit was raised early in the 20th century. Not surprisingly, the Vietnamese aspired to return to an independent state. Ho Chi Minh made an appearance at the Paris Peace Conference in 1919, following World War I, pushing for an independent Vietnam. The French continued their role in Vietnam after World War I until World War II and the fall of France. In World War II, the Vichy French capitulation allowed the Japanese to take over Vietnam.[5(p8)]

The Communist Ho Chi Minh formed the Viet Minh, which began military operations when Japan lost the war. Following the end of World War II, the French reasserted their colonial status in Vietnam. Starting in November 1946, the Viet Minh, under General Vo Nguyen Giap, started a war of attrition against the French and Vietnamese government. The Franco-Viet Minh War (March through May 1954) ended following the French defeat (despite American logistical and financial support) at Dien Bien Phu. The French became encircled there by the Viet Minh and could only be resupplied by air. The Americans declined to help relieve the beleaguered French. After the French defeat, the war ended and an armistice was signed in Geneva between the French and the Viet Minh in July 1954. Another agreement was also signed in July 1954, titled the "Final Declaration of the Geneva Conference," which separated North and South Vietnam at the 17th parallel. The demarcation was supposed to be temporary but it was envisioned as a compromise that would satisfy all.[4(p19)] The country north of the 17th parallel was to be controlled by the Viet Minh. Ho Chi Minh was to lead the Democratic Republic of Vietnam. The country south of the parallel (the Republic of Vietnam) was led by President Ngo Dinh Diem (until he was assassinated in 1963). The Americans effectively took over from the French starting in 1954 in an attempt to avoid more losses to the Communists in Southeast Asia.[6(p30)] In January 1955, the US Military Assistance Advisory Group–Indochina was established.[4(p21)]

The first casualties among the American advisor group occurred in 1961. US involvement increased with the Kennedy and later the Johnson administrations. General William Westmoreland assumed command of the US Military Assistance Command, Vietnam (MACV) and US Army, Republic of Vietnam (USARV) in late 1964, preceding a major troop buildup starting in 1965. In 1965, the landing of the 9th Marine Expeditionary Force at Da Nang signaled the expansion of the American involvement in Vietnam. Troop strength continued to increase through 1965, with 184,300 reported by 31 December 1965. The troop numbers peaked in 1969, with 543,300 reported as of 20 April 1969. The numbers fell to 24,200 by 31 December 1972. Only 240 were left on 30 March 1973. On 30 April 1975, "Operation Frequent Wind," the evacuation of the American Embassy in Saigon, was completed with a helicopter lifting off from the Embassy rooftop with the last 11 US Marine guards.[4(p449)]

Soldiers in Vietnam were younger than those in either Korea or World War II due to the draft excluding those who were in college or divinity school, or were fathers.[1(p111)] In World War II and the Korean War, the soldier was older because there were no college deferments, although there were occupational (war essential) deferments. Because there were so few years between the end of World War II and the beginning of the Korean War, the Selective Service System worked much the same for both mobilizations. In Vietnam, however, the Reserves (and National Guard) were never mobilized as in the other conflicts. (The Reserve component has traditionally held older members.)

Whatever their age, as Marine MAJ Curt Munson said, "the real learning took place"[2(p113)] in combat with an operational unit. Much of the flavor of combat and especially helicopter airmobile operations can be gleaned from the book *We Were Soldiers Once . . . and Young,* written by Lieutenant Colonel (LTC) (later Lieutenant General) Harold G Moore and Joseph L Galloway. The intensity of the battle and the role of the medical personnel are also characterized in *We Were Soldiers*. The demands on personnel and material could be enormous.[7(p313)]

The Tet Offensive in 1968, actually won by the Allies (which included the Republic of Vietnam and the Republic of Korea [South Korea]), was lost in the rancor of antiwar protest in the United States. In January 1968, the Viet Cong and elements of the North Vietnamese Army (NVA) initiated extensive attacks on Saigon, Da Nang, Pleiku, Nha Trang, and other cities. The Tet Offensive involved some of the most extreme fighting of the war and phases continued into September 1968 and later. Combined Allied forces successfully repulsed the enemy forces. However, the media and antiwar activists were successful in obscuring any victory aspects, while concentrating on the futility of the war. President Nixon, elected in November 1968 on an end-the-war promise, initiated peace talks while continuing operations, especially by air.[8(p307)]

The experience of the troops helped define the complexity of the political and military equation. As one example, an American soldier said in *Voices From the Vietnam War*,[2] the soldiers "were unprepared for what they would experience in combat against Communist forces in an unfamiliar land"[2(p101)] and "did not fully understand what was going on in Vietnam."[2(p101)] Or as Philip Caputo wrote in *A Rumor of War*[9] about the Vietnam War, "What had begun as an adventurous expedition had turned into an exhausting, indecisive war of attrition in which we fought for no cause other than our own survival."[9(pxiv)] Caputo had entered the Marines by joining the Platoon Officer Candidate Program, much as the fictional Mellas in Marlantes' Vietnam novel *Matterhorn*.[10] The real and the fictional Marines both experienced the Vietnam War on a most complex and personal note.

In the early years of the Vietnam War, the Army dealt largely with insurgent forces. Later, the commitment of large concentrations of regular NVA forces made the war more like a conventional one.[4(p309)] Yet, the Vietnam conflict illustrates the adage that there are no winners in a war. North Vietnam did enjoy victory in terms of eventually occupying all of Vietnam and control of the government, but they also lost many people. As recorded in the *Embers of War*,[5] the Vietnamese conflict "killed in excess of three million Vietnamese and wreaked destruction on huge portions of Vietnam, Laos, and Cambodia."[5(pxv)]

CASUALTY STATISTICS OF THE VIETNAM WAR

To get some idea of the nature of the Vietnam War, a look at casualty statistics is instructive. In that regard, the Vietnam Conflict Extract Data File of the Defense Casualty Analysis System is the official reference for casualties. For the Vietnam War, it lists "Killed in Action" (KIA) as totaling 40,934, with later additional deaths of 17,286 for a total of 58,220. (Each year the number of additional deaths is adjusted to reflect those who have subsequently died of their original wounds.) The statistics it notes for "Non-Fatal Woundings" are a total of 153,303 for the 1960 to 1974 period.[11] The *Vietnam War Almanac*[4] lists a total KIA from 1960 to 1974 for the United States of 46,370, with a US total of 153,735 wounded in action (WIA). These figures from the Almanac represent a pooling from several diverse sources.[4(p529)]

DEPLOYMENT OF MEDICAL UNITS AND EVOLUTION OF MOBILE ARMY SURGICAL HOSPITALS AND MEDICAL UNIT, SELF-CONTAINED, TRANSPORTABLE SETS

As discussed, in 1961 President John F Kennedy started measures that over the next 4 years resulted in the United States being committed to Vietnam. In 1961, the 8th Transportation Company (Fort Bragg, North Carolina) and the 57th Transportation Company (Fort Lewis, Washington), both light helicopter units, arrived in Vietnam with H-21 helicopters. Two more helicopter companies arrived in 1962.[3(pp23–24)]

In 1962, the 8th Field Hospital and the 57th Medical Detachment (Helicopter Ambulance) were the first medical units in Vietnam. The 57th Medical Detachment's UH-1 (Hueys) began to evacuate Army of the Republic of Vietnam (ARVN) troop casualties by May 1962. By November 1962, the Army had 199 aircraft of various types in support of ARVN operations.[3(p26)] In 1963, the call sign "Dust Off" was adopted by the 57th.[3(p30)] By 1964, the "dust off" helicopters, commanded by Major (MAJ) Charles Kelly, did not have the resources to answer the call for all medical evacuation missions (Figures 8-1 and 8-2). (MAJ Kelly was lost to hostile action that year.[3(pp37–38)]) The Army perfected techniques of helicopter evacuation in the period 1965 to 1970. The two original "dust off" units, were augmented by others with the start of the 1965 buildup.[3(p32)]

The flavor of Army medicine in the early years can be gained by reading a book such as the one written by Jerry Martin, MD, titled *Soldiers Saving Soldiers. Vietnam Remembered: A History of the 18th Surgical Hospital*.[12] In it he describes his experiences as a physician at the 18th Surgical Hospital during the period June 1966 to June 1967 while deployed to the Pleiku Province area. There are other books of this nature but this is especially informative because it contains a copious number of color photographs.[12]

In 1965, the 1st Air Cavalry (Airmobile), and the attached 15th Medical Battalion (Airmobile), participated in its first combat operation in the Battle of the Ia Drang Valley in western Pleiku Province. This involved regular NVA troops and insurgent Viet Cong. Ia Drang Valley is located in a remote region of the Central Highlands of Vietnam. Regular NVA soldiers were engaged in the first major fighting with American troops. Martin recalled that the 1st Air Cavalry moved a large group of helicopters to a field across the highway from his 18th Surgical Hospital (MA [Mobile Army]). Soon thereafter, this hospital began receiving wounded from the fight in the Ia Drang River Valley.[12(p62)] In the 4 days of fighting, the NVA suffered 1,800 killed and an equal number wounded, contrasted with 240 killed and 300 wounded for US forces.[13(p2)]

The importance of the airmobile medical support battalion with its air ambulance platoon (12 helicopters) was established in this 4-day battle.[14(p87)] These "dust off" helicopters evacuated casualties to the clearing stations, although they could bypass if needed and go directly to the hospitals.[14(p88)] The 23rd (Americal) Infantry Division used helicopters to evacuate wounded in their area of operation; it used ground ambulances for other activities. The 25th Infantry Division deployed to the northwest sector of South Vietnam and air evacuated to the 45th Surgical Hospital in Tay Ninh, a city in southwestern Vietnam about 90 km to the northwest of Saigon. The 45th Surgical Hospital was one of the notable forward-located hospitals and a Medical Unit, Self-Contained,

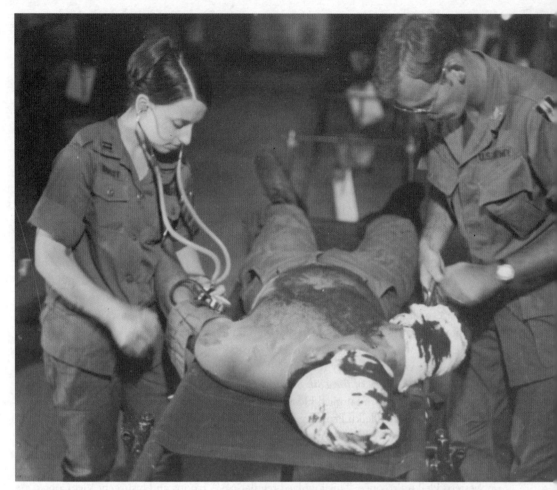

FIGURE 8-1. [Top] Male and female nurse cut the bandages from a newly admitted patient at the 2nd Surgical Hospital, Lai Khe, Vietnam, September 1969. Photograph courtesy of the Army Medical Department Center of History and Heritage, Fort Sam Houston, Texas, Image #MU-VN-B1-001.

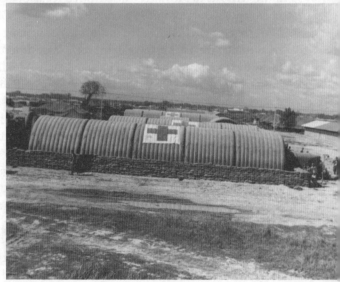

FIGURE 8-2. [Bottom] 45th Surgical Hospital Admission/Disposition Section—a five-section inflatable shelter. Photograph courtesy of the Army Medical Department Center of History and Heritage, Fort Sam Houston, Texas, Image #MU-VN-B1-002.

Transportable (MUST) unit. This hospital was a mobile shelter with expandable patient care wards, radiology, laboratory, pharmacy, dental, and kitchen areas. The 326th Medical Battalion, with an air ambulance company added, was known as an "Eagle Dust Off" unit with the 101st Airborne. The air ambulance company provided air evacuation in areas where the 101st operated, which included some of the more notorious "hot spots."[14(p89)]

A New Approach to Forward Surgery

Brigadier General (BG) Elliott C Cutler had served as the Chief Surgical Consultant for the European Theater of Operations in World War II. His war diary provides a unique view of his thoughts during that conflict.[15(pp353–356)] In World War II, while speaking of the future, Cutler wrote, "I heartily approve the system for care of the heavily damaged non-transportable in Field Hospital platoons. I would even urge an extension of this forward surgery, believing 'surgery should be brought to the soldier,' not the soldier to the surgeons."[15(p122)] However, the direction of the medical support in the Vietnam War didn't proceed exactly as Cutler envisioned. The wide use of helicopter air evacuation did, in fact, quickly bring the patient to the surgeon.

As the war progressed, military medical care in Vietnam was generally excellent. Ben Eiseman, MD, Emeritus Professor of Surgery, University of Colorado, was quoted in 1967 in his role as a naval surgical consultant as saying that if "wounded in the remote jungle or rice paddy of Vietnam, an American citizen has a better chance for quick definitive surgical care by a board-certified specialist than if he were hit on a highway near his hometown in the continental United States."[16(p237)] The Neurosurgery Consultant for USARV, LTC Robert C Leaver, Medical Corps, said that the best equipment found in United States civilian hospitals could also be found in Vietnam.[17(pp4,45,308)]

As Neel points out, the hospital mortality rate was only 2.6% for the period from January 1965 to December 1970. The rates for World War II and Korea were 4.5% for the former, while the latter was 2.5%.[18(pp50–51)] The slightly lower rate for Korea reflects the rapid evacuation characteristic also seen in Vietnam. Most of those wounded would have died before reaching treatment in the earlier conflicts. Further, the ratio of KIA to WIA in Vietnam was 1.5:6. Korea was a ratio of 1.4:1 while World War II was a ratio of 1.3:1.[18(pp50–51)]

Hospitals

MOBILE ARMY SURGICAL HOSPITAL

A development in the war was the replacement of the tents and equipment of the Mobile Army Surgical Hospital (MASH) from the Korean War with the aforementioned Medical Unit, Self-Contained, Transportable (MUST) set (1965), which was viewed as a significant improvement. The MASH was usually a 60-bed setup, which could be augmented with several MUST units. Hence, some MASH operations were converted to 200-bed combat support hospitals by such means.[10(p65)] In the Korean War, MASH units could be 60 to 100 beds and still be expanded to 200 beds.[18(p503),19(pp423–424)] MASH units were also used by US allies, such as the 9th Mobile Army Surgical Hospital of the 9th Infantry Division, Army of the Republic of Korea.[2(p178)]

THE MEDICAL UNIT, SELF-CONTAINED, TRANSPORTABLE SET

The MUST sets were conceptualized as early as 1961, but they were not demonstrated until 1965 at Fort Sam Houston, Texas, for Surgeon General Leonard D Heaton and Senator Richard Russell, Chair of the Senate Armed Services Committee. Surgeon General Heaton, writing in 1968, stated that "demand from the field for MUST equipment far exceeds availability."[20(p371)] Heaton announced plans to reequip Army units with MUST equipment within 5 years.[20(pp371-372)]

MUST units were utilized in Vietnam with differing levels of success, if one considers the limitations to a concept that seemed forward thinking at the time. The MUST unit was transportable, which was an asset not used to advantage as the facilities moved to permanent or semi-permanent locations. Still, the logistics of transportation and setting up the MUST were cumbersome. The three basic elements of a MUST could be moved by air or flatbed truck. The three components consisted of (1) the expandable surgical element, (2) the air-inflatable ward, and (3) the utility element or power package. The power element consisted of a turbine that could use a variety of fuels. The turbine's engine power packages were termed utility packs. The packs required constant maintenance, adding to the logistical worries. The gas turbine powered a generation unit that supplied electricity for the air-conditioning, heating, lighting, refrigeration, hot water, and air to keep the inflatable elements up (Figure 8-3). The surgical element was rigid walled and self-contained. The sides were expanded out in an accordion-like fashion. The air-inflatable ward was a unit with double walls to house the casualties. Extra expandable units were used to house radiography, laboratory, dental, and pharmacy facilities.[18(p65)]

The MUST unit's particular advantage was to provide controlled temperature and humidity, unlike the tents of the MASH hospital sets. However, MUST units used up to 2,400 gallons of JP4 aviation fuel each day.[8(p313)] More fuel could be needed depending on the requirements. For instance, the 2nd Surgical Hospital reported using more than 3,800 gallons of JP4 fuel per day.[4(p332)] Some units had to refuel every day to avoid running out. The requirements for fuel of all types were staggering, despite the usual ready availability of jet fuel.[8(p313)] Mortar attacks were fairly common, with the resulting shrapnel easily deflating the wards and bringing them down on their patients. Also, the wards needed concrete pads to prevent their floating after heavy rains. Especially in the monsoon season, the rains could be heavy and continuous.[8(p313)]

The mechanics of setting up the MUST units were complicated by the need for good alignment, although the MUST hospital had no organic forklifts or other lifting equipment to move the pieces. The equipment had to be borrowed from neighboring engineer or supply units that did have the requisite equipment. Large equipment wrecker trucks could be used to set up the units. Because the MUST hospital was planned to be moved in 72 hours and to be set up in less time, such infrastructure problems were significant. A more realistic timetable would be to allow many more days.[8(p313)]

The 45th Surgical Hospital is an example of a successful MUST-equipped unit. It arrived in Vietnam October 1966; on 4 and 11 November 1966, the 45th came under mortar attack and its commander was a casualty. The hospital came under several more attacks until it received its first surgical patients on 13 November. It operated as a true forward surgical hospital in 1967.[18(pp65-68)]

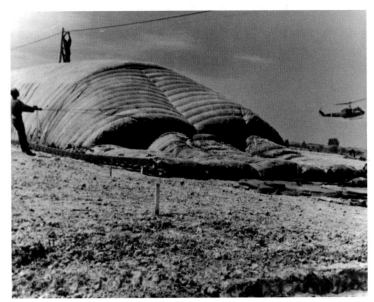

FIGURE 8-3. 45th Surgical Hospital. Inflation of the units using an air supply from the utility pack with connected valve manifold system. Note the UH-1 "Huey" helicopter in the background. Photograph courtesy of the Army Medical Department Center of History and Heritage, Fort Sam Houston, Texas, Image #MU-VN-B1-003.

Three additional MUST-equipped hospitals were set up in 1967: the 3rd, 18th, and 22nd Surgical Hospitals. The 95th Evacuation Hospital was given some MUST equipment, pending completion of its fixed facilities. Previous attempts to move the 18th and 22nd Surgical Hospitals were difficult. Neal noted that the MUST units were not used as mobile units until mid-1968, when the USARV Surgeon ruled that two MUST units were to keep their equipment and train to be mobile. The 18th and 22nd Surgical Hospitals were therefore deemed mobile MUST units. In a 1968 attack, the 3rd Surgical Hospital sustained hits in the bachelor officers' quarters, a MUST main tent, and shrapnel deflated part of the MUST. Later the 3rd Surgical Hospital sustained three separate mortar attacks in that same year, causing damage to physical structures, but only minor wounds to staff.[18(p67)]

Byerly and Pendse described their experience at the 22nd Surgical Hospital, a MUST-equipped unit in the area of an old French rubber plantation at Lai Khe, northwest of Saigon.[21] Their description spanned the period of 9 January to 30 November 1969. There were 1,963 admissions during this period, of which 92% required surgery. Of these, 73% were battle injuries, with the majority being small arms bullet injuries. More than one anatomical area was involved for 75% of these admissions. Their average of 65 minutes between wounding and admission spoke to the efficient evacuation system.[21(pp221–226)]

Kelly, writing in the journal *Neurosurgery*, described the development of a "refined system for the triage, management, and evacuation of wounded military personnel that evolved in Vietnam."[22(p939)] In Fisher's oral history project interview of Dr Steven Phillips, some of the limited experience that he had assigned to a MASH hospital toward the end of his tour in Vietnam (1968–1969) is detailed for the reader.[23] Dr Jerry Martin perhaps best summed up his experience the year he spent with the 18th Surgical Hospital. He commented that "[i]nnumerable anecdotes of narrow escapes and harrowing experiences could be described. There are multitudinous, unreported memories that could be recalled and recorded, although among them are those unpleasant and unwanted memories which are intentionally left untold."[12(p143)] He is speaking to the loss of life and suffering that are so difficult to talk about and perhaps best forgotten.

Demands on personnel and equipment could be enormous. During the 1967 Battle of Dak To, for example, the 71st Evacuation Hospital at Pleiku had to run six overloaded operating rooms while expending large amounts of medical supplies.[8(p313)] From September 1968 through August 1969, the 250- to 300-bed 67th Evacuation Hospital at Quinhon received, on average, 50 surgical admissions each day, and during large-scale combat operations, like the Tet Offensive, the surgical workload rose to as many as 200 cases per day.[24(p227)]

Adapting to Meet Changing Needs

The policy in Vietnam had called for minimal movement of hospitals (although modified somewhat in 1968 and 1969 in support of increased combat activity in certain locales). Hospitals were not moved in the support of tactical operations, as had been the case in World War II and Korea. In this conflict, the move was toward more permanent structures for hospitals.[21(pp61–63)] MAJ Allgood reviewed the use of his unit, the 24th Evacuation Hospital, as an experimental unit to try different configurations. The World War II cantonments that were parallel and unconnected could not be used in Vietnam for a number of reasons. Instead, the 24th adopted a series of interconnecting corridors. The corridor concept allowed a way to deal with the heat, humidity, rains, and dust that were everywhere. The operating room, the preoperative area, and the intensive care unit were surrounded by a 6-foot high security reinforced wall to protect against explosions. Three other permanent hospitals were built like the 24th.[25(pp12,14)]

The nature of the war and the ready availability of rotary air evacuation contributed to limited hospital movement before 1968. The movement policy was changed somewhat in 1968 and 1969. However, these moves were made in support of increased combat in certain areas. In Korea and World War II, more mobile hospitals contributed to combat units logistical and tactical military support. Aside from the brief use of MUST units, the moves were to semipermanent facilities. The fact that forward hospitals in Vietnam were, in the main, stable allowed the utilization of more advanced equipment.[18(p50)]

The number of hospitals and air ambulance units was reduced in the period between 1969 and 1970, corresponding to reduced combat operations. In 1969, a number of hospitals were deactivated (the 7th and 22nd Surgical Hospitals and the 29th and 36th Evacuation Hospitals) and three US Army Reserve units were returned to the continental United States. By 1970, more hospitals were deactivated or redeployed (8th Field, 2nd Surgical, 45th Surgical, and 12th Evacuation Hospitals).[18(p78)]

In retrospect, the MUST units were generally used as stationary structures (Figures 8-4 through 8-6). The transportability factor was a serious shortcoming of the concept. However, they could be raised more quickly than fixed structures. Hence, the MUST units could have been used as the resource for immediate treatment in a new operation area, to be later replaced as needed by more permanent structures. The lack of transportability is being addressed in current iterations of this concept.[26(p174)]

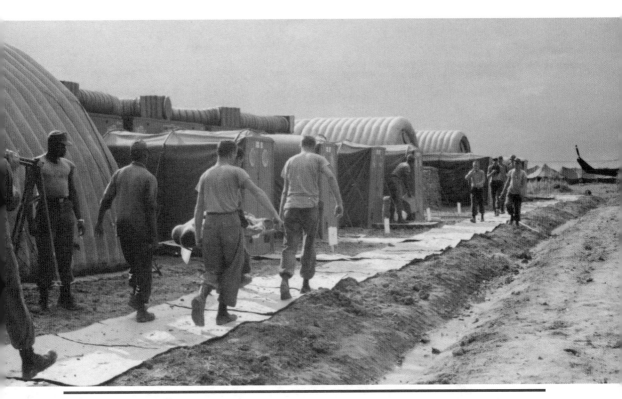

FIGURE 8-4. 45th Surgical Hospital. Patient being moved by litter toward surgery. Photograph courtesy of the Army Medical Department Center of History and Heritage, Fort Sam Houston, Texas, Image #MU-VN-B1-004.

Evacuation

Helicopter medical evacuation, employing Sikorsky helicopters, was used in a few cases by the Army in World War II (on a limited basis in India and in the Philippines[19(p9)]). This set the stage for a more aggressive use in Korea, although helicopter medical evacuations in Korea were small (17,700) compared to the much larger number in Vietnam.[19(p4)] Air ambulance evacuations by helicopters in Vietnam moved between 850,000 and 900,000 Allied military personnel and Vietnamese civilians who were sick, injured, or wounded between May 1962 and March 1973.[3(pp115–116)] In addition, the Korean air evacuation situation had enemy aircraft as a factor, which was not the case in Vietnam.[27(p18)] (By comparison, the French had 18 medical evacuation helicopters in use at the end of 1953. The French, in the period of 1950 until 1954, evacuated 5,000 casualties by helicopter.[27(p4)])

The Sikorsky H-5 was first delivered to the military in February 1945. The H-5 gained fame in medical evacuation in Korea as well as in pilot rescue.[28] The original H-5 (designated the R-5 by the military) helicopters were replaced by the more powerful H-13.[29] The Bell H-13 Sioux was the helicopter featured in the famous M*A*S*H television series. It carried two stretchers attached externally. Originally, no litter attachments were

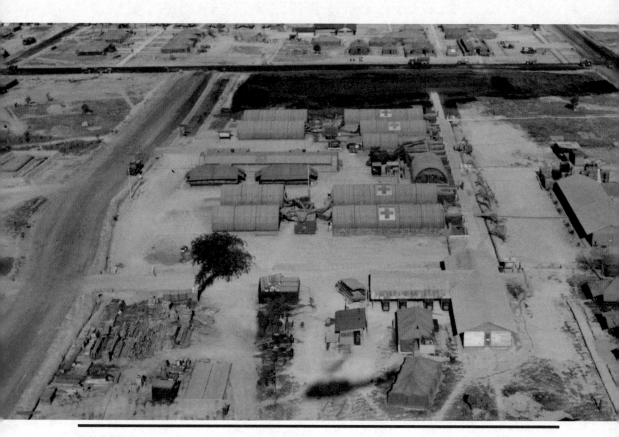

FIGURE 8-5. Improvements include sidewalks, landscaping, and painting of buildings at the 45th Surgical Hospital, as seen from the air, January 1967. Note the inflation system behind the units. Photograph courtesy of the Army Medical Department Center of History and Heritage, Fort Sam Houston, Texas, Image #MU-VN-B1-005.

available, so attachments were made for the skid rails. No medics were on board. Most of the helicopter aeromedical evacuations were done by the H-13.[3(p15)] These craft, however, were not designed for air-evacuation roles due to inadequate power and no designed litter attachments.

The original Hueys (UH-1 models A and B) lacked enough power to operate in the heat and humidity of Vietnam. The UH-1D was introduced in the early 1960s and could handle six litter cases due to its longer body. The improved gas turbine engine gave it more lifting power for that model, but it was still not enough for mountainous regions. In 1967, the newly arrived 45th Medical Company (Air Ambulance) brought the new UH-1H model, which finally solved the engine power issue. The UH-1H and the later UH-1G models were fully instrumented for night and poor weather flying and had sufficient lift to effectively use a hoist.[3(pp67–69)]

"Hueys," the UH-1 (models A to the late war H, and the H to G series with litters), were the aircraft used, with a crew of four including a pilot, copilot, medic, and crew

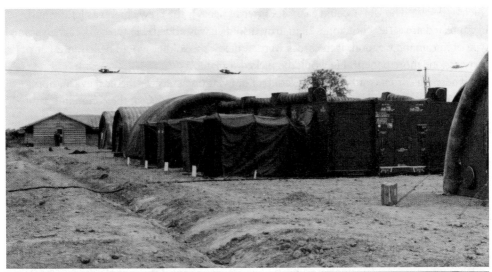

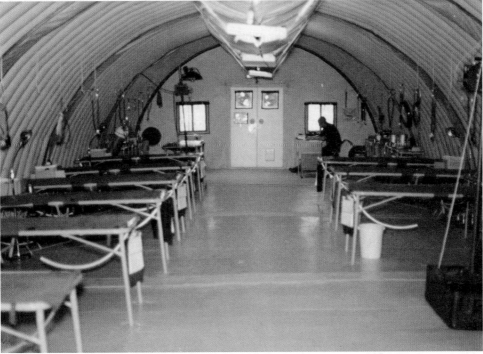

FIGURE 8-6A. [Top] MUST (Medical Unit, Self-Contained, Transportable) surgical complex. Three complete surgeries and a sterile preparation area constitute the four expandable units. Photograph courtesy of the Army Medical Department Center of History and Heritage, Fort Sam Houston, Texas, Image #MU-VN-B1-007.

FIGURE 8-6B. [Bottom] Preoperative Ward of the 45th Surgical Hospital. Beds are left undressed and are used as litter stands. Photograph courtesy of the Army Medical Department Center of History and Heritage, Fort Sam Houston, Texas, Image #MU-VN-B1-008.

chief.[4(p321),11(p66)] The UH-1 could carry six litter patients if the crew chief was left behind. In contested areas (ie, "hot zones") an armed soldier was added. He typically carried some type of automatic weapon. If the areas were "quiet," the soldier would be left in favor of carrying one more patient. He would be picked up later.[18(p75)]

There was often conflict over the control of aviation assets for medical evacuation. When the first dedicated air evacuation helicopters were introduced, the command wanted to use them for troop/supply transport activities, when available. While these differences of opinion on use continued, dedicated air evacuation assets were defined. The UH-1D was then turned over to troop transport duties when the "H" model became the standard for medical evacuation.[3(p67)]

The thick jungle made helicopter evacuation difficult. The Army used a variation of the "Jungle Canopy Platform System" as a means of extracting the wounded from the jungle below while the helicopter hovered above. The "Personal Rescue Hoist" advanced the state of performing jungle extraction.[3(pp70–71)] The hoist device was created to more effectively lift the wounded while the helicopter hovered. The hoist system was introduced in 1966, but required constant modification to the design until the end of the war.[3(p71)] The more powerful "H" model of the UH-1 made hoist operation less risky. Prior to the "H" model, the crew would be reduced to the pilot, co-pilot, and a hoist boom operator. The helicopter also carried a reduced amount of fuel to lessen weight and thus allow more lift. The hoist consisted of a winch with a cable on a boom. The cable could hold a hook and ring to which a jungle penetrator, a Stokes litter, or a rigid litter was attached. Another extractor device, the "Air Jungle Penetrator," provided seats to which casualties could be strapped—a preferred method by the crew as the device was less likely to become snared in the foliage.[18(p75)]

The evacuation helicopter was most exposed while extracting a patient in a high hover mode. Ground fire of any type was a definite risk. The extra weight of the hoist/litter mechanism added to the tension of the maneuver. When the enemy got new weapons such as the AK-47, RPD light machine gun, and the SKS carbine in 1964, these weapons and the exposed hover time caused an increase in hits on medical evacuation helicopters. The introduction of the SA-7 heat-seeking missile in 1972 could have greatly increased the loss of aeromedical evacuation assets had the war continued.[3(pp85–86)]

Patient Experience

The typical casualty could arrive at the helipad of a medical facility sometimes less than 30 minutes after helicopter pickup. The casualty was usually received within the "golden" 6-hour period after injury, often within 30 minutes.[29(pp1–2)] He would have been splinted and bandaged and the nature of the casualty's wounds would have been relayed by radio. The patient was then moved directly to the preoperative and resuscitative area to be evaluated, treated for shock, and moved to the operating room as needed.[18(p66)] The hospital receiving areas had intravenous hangers and litter racks, and adequate radiography areas. Most operating rooms and recovery areas were in air-conditioned spaces.[29(pp1–2)] This rapid evacuation changed the nature of forward surgery perhaps more than any other factor. There were, however, some cases where evacuation was delayed due to weather or heavy fighting.[30(p34)] The rapid helicopter evacuations increased the survival rate; it also brought in more seriously wounded than in past conflicts, many of whom survived.

Most surgery in military hospitals in Vietnam was performed under a general anesthetic. The usual method involved thiopental induction followed by halothane, nitrous oxide, and oxygen maintenance. Halothane was the preferred inhalational anesthetic over the explosive and flammable ether and cyclopropane.[19(p55)] The use of local anesthetics was only for minor wounds or in some rare cases where there was primary delayed closure. Spinal anesthetics were rarely used.

The experience of the 12th Evacuation Hospital is illustrative of the many different types of surgeries done. Their unit history for the period 1 January 1970 to 15 November 1970 recorded 5,418 operative procedures, of which 4,004 were classified as major procedures. The operations consisted of 753 delayed closures, 3,576 debridement procedures, 425 thoracotomies, 951 laparotomies, 379 major amputations, 189 minor amputations, 147 vascular injuries, 10 craniotomies, and 201 ocular procedures.[31]

The importance of the clearing station in the evacuation chain was well recognized. In the 1965 Ia Drang Valley campaign, the value of an airmobile medical support battalion in transporting wounded to the 1st Cavalry Division's four clearing stations was established. The personnel at the clearing station became well skilled in triage, treating shock, and administering blood.[32(pp87-88)] Yet, as pointed out by Neel, by 1967 with the reliance on helicopter evacuation, the battalion and divisional clearing stations were excluded from the evacuation chain. A surgical, field, or evacuation facility was often within the same flying distance.[18(p92)]

In a 1968 report, "Operations Report–Lessons Learned 2-68: Medical Lessons Learned," emphasis was placed on the role of the clearing station, which had a medical officer with approximately 3 years of surgical specialty training. The report pointed out that the heavy fighting in the Dak To area showed that relatively immediate professional care at the clearing station for casualties brought there by helicopter saved many who might have been lost in the evacuation over extended distances to a hospital. None of the 929 wounded in action admitted to the clearing station at Dak To died there or in subsequent evacuation. In this situation, the availability of the air evacuation helicopter made the clearing company relevant.[33(pp22-23)] In Captain (CPT) Goodrich's description of his 9 months as a battalion surgeon in 1965 to 1966, he spoke to the role of the clearing station in evacuation. Specifically, he addressed the life-saving role of immediate treatment of casualties in his facility.[34(p796)]

American forces in the Central Highlands in the period of 1968 to 1969 featured widely dispersed combat troops who were supported by "light" clearing stations. A physician and nine to 10 medics went with the units they supported. The main medical company was located at the semipermanent base camp in protected bunkers. The "light" clearing company triaged the wounded, gave care, and prepared the wounded for evacuation to the base camp. The clearing station possessed basic equipment for emergency treatment and resuscitation. This innovative use of clearing company assets fit the particular situation of that combat.[18(p92)]

The effective use of the clearing station can be seen in 1970 when the 4th Medical Battalion was in support of the 4th Infantry Division in the Cambodian incursion in May and June. Six "dust off" helicopters were available to support the clearing station. The majority of the casualties received at least initial treatment at the clearing station at the Cambodian border.[18(p92)] Because combat units were often dispersed, the "light" clearing station evolved to subdivide the assets of the unit. A doctor and seven to 10 enlisted would form the complement of the "light" clearing station. They were deployed to landing zones or fire support bases for a week to 10 days. The clearing station was to prepare the wounded for helicopter evacuation to the base camp. The base camp field operation would further triage and stabilize the wounded to be passed on to the next level of care.[18(p92)]

Helicopter Air-Evacuation System

A radio medical network aided the helicopter evacuation. An in-flight assessment was made of the casualties and then they could be directed to an appropriate facility by radio.[18(p70)] Field regulators (noncommissioned officers) at troop concentrations or at the combat point could call in the flights. Combat medics on site could also call in flights via the "dust off" network.[18(p76)] Hence, the helicopter evacuation was guided by the medical radio system and formed the nucleus of the medical regulator system to direct patients to the correct facility. Time was the critical factor more so than the distance.[18(p74)] The 44th Medical Brigade assumed management of the regulator system for all of the airspace in South Vietnam. As a rule, the telephones were unreliable, so single sideband radios were acquired.[18(p73)]

Pilots and their crews braved enormous odds. Air ambulances and crews sustained casualties equal to one-third their number. Indeed, air ambulance helicopters received more damage than even combat helicopters or gunships.[2(pp117,198)] In that regard, the exploits of Patrick Brady, a helicopter pilot, are worthy of recognition. Brady had been sent to evacuate soldiers, including wounded, surrounded by the enemy in the vicinity of Chu Lai, which he did successfully despite enemy fire. He returned to rescue more soldiers trapped in a mine-field, landing in the middle of that field to extract the wounded.[2(p65)] (In recognition of his bravery and daring, President Nixon awarded the Medal of Honor in 1969 to then-MAJ Patrick Brady, Medical Service Corps [MSC] becoming the first MSC officer to receive that award. Brady later became a major general in the Transportation Corps.[8(pp326–327)])

The Vietnam-era helicopter medical evacuation system helped to improve the civilian care system later. A civilian version of the air evacuation radio/control system, the MAST (Military Assistance to Safety in Traffic) Program, has a direct link to the experience gained in the Vietnam War.[8(p180)]

Air Evacuation to Japan/Philippines/Continental United States

At the start of the major American involvement in Vietnam, the US Air Force would evacuate patients from the Republic of Vietnam to Clark Air Force Base (AFB) in the Philippines. The evacuation could continue to Hawaii, Ryukyu Islands, or Japan proper, depending on the condition of the patient and the nature of the wounds. In 1966, air-evacuation was extended directly to the continental United States (CONUS). It could involve a direct flight to Travis AFB in California or a flight to Andrews AFB in Washington, DC, after refueling in Alaska. Soldiers could be sent to military general hospitals nearest their homes or to selected Class I hospitals (larger military facilities such

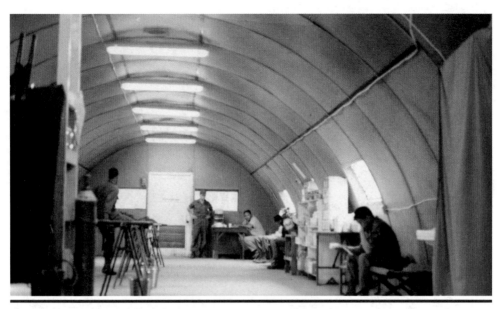

FIGURE 8-7. Emergency room before patients arrive. Photograph courtesy of the Army Medical Department Center of History and Heritage, Fort Sam Houston, Texas, Image #MU-VN-B1-009.

as Walter Reed) within more immediate proximity to their homes, if beds were available. In Japan, the Army set up the equivalent of three general hospitals to handle the evacuation load.[18(p70)]

In the early years of the conflict, all of Vietnam was designated as a combat zone so that the usual long-term treatment facilities were not in-country. The three general hospitals that were set up in Japan were to treat patients who could be returned to duty in Vietnam in 60 days, or those who were not stable enough for immediate transport to the United States. While in Japan, they would be held in a treatment facility or its medical holding company while undergoing treatment that would allow their return to Vietnam. In Vietnam, the treatment plan was to retain soldiers in a medical facility in-country if they would be able to be returned to duty in 15 to 30 days.[18(p71)]

Combat Medicine

Following Korea, the Army added a medical brigade (to command and control corps-level medical assets) headed by a brigadier general,[35(pp125–128)] while the medical command (to command and control medical assets in the larger theater such as Vietnam) was commanded by a major general.[8(p308)] In Vietnam, the 44th Medical Brigade was created to handle nondivisional medical units. An example of this asset type would be the surgical and evacuation hospitals at the field Army level.[8(p313)] The 44th was assigned to the 1st Logistical Command, rather than having it serve as a major subordinate command.[36(p39)] The position of the Surgeon, USARV and the 44th Brigade commander were made one in 1967. The US Army Medical Command, Vietnam, was established in 1970, with four surgical hospitals, three field hospitals, eight evacuation hospitals, and one convalescent

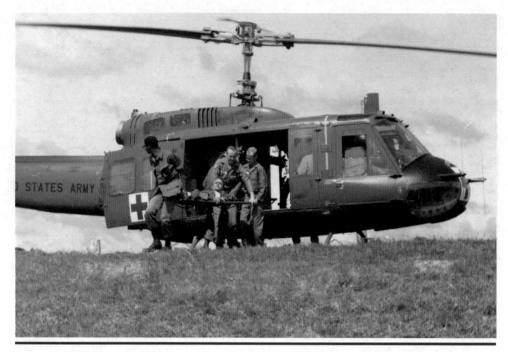

FIGURE 8-8A. UH-1 "Huey" helicopter—the workhorse of aeromedical evacuation in Vietnam. Photograph courtesy of the Army Medical Department Center of History and Heritage, Fort Sam Houston, Texas, Image #MU-VN-B1-010.

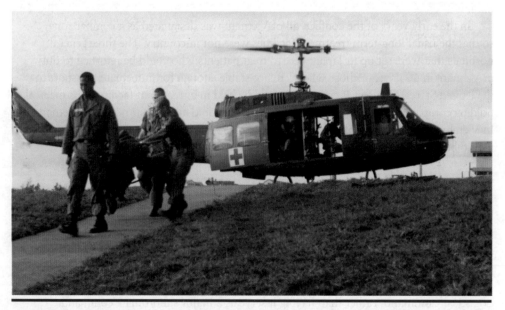

FIGURE 8-8B. Note the rotor on the helicopter is still turning while the patient is off-loaded. Photograph courtesy of the Army Medical Department Center of History and Heritage, Fort Sam Houston, Texas, Image #MU-VN-B1-011.

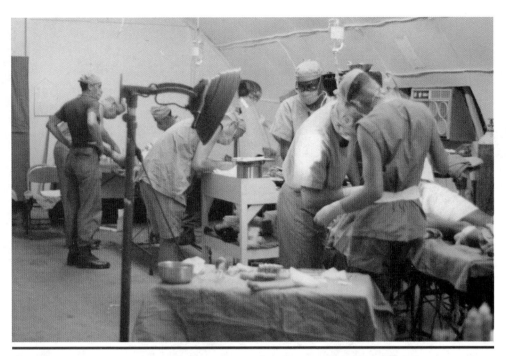

FIGURE 8-9A. Operating room scene. New surgeons acquired new skills in trauma. Debridement was a skill difficult to learn at first for the new surgeon. Photograph courtesy of the Army Medical Department Center of History and Heritage, Fort Sam Houston, Texas, Image #MU-VN-B1-013.

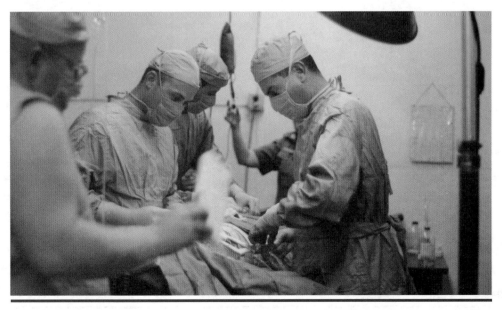

FIGURE 8-9B. Surgeons at work. Surgeons maintained a high level of care despite the turnover in staff. Photograph courtesy of the Army Medical Department Center of History and Heritage, Fort Sam Houston, Texas, Image #MU-VN-B1-014.11.

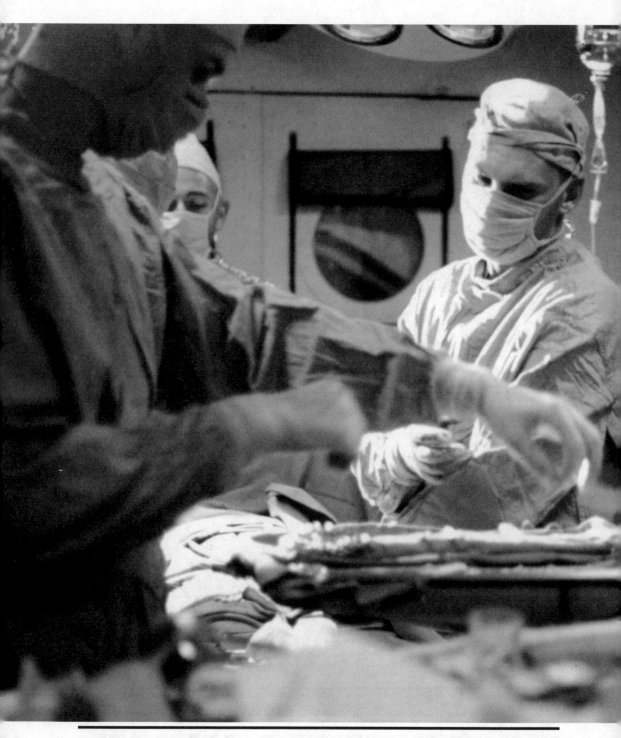

FIGURE 8-9C. Another operating room scene. The typical operating room was functional but simplistic in setup. Prompt triage brought the injured to the operating room. Photograph courtesy of the Army Medical Department Center of History and Heritage, Fort Sam Houston, Texas, Image #MU-VN-B1-015.

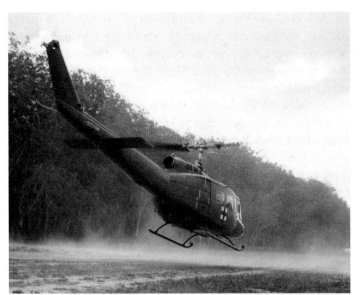

FIGURE 8-10. Helicopter landing at the 3rd Surgical Hospital at Bau Cat, Vietnam, to pick up casualties secondary to engagement with the Viet Cong, 10 miles away. The casualties were to be flown to the 1st Division Headquarters near Bien Hoa, November 1965. Photograph courtesy of the Army Medical Department Center of History and Heritage, Fort Sam Houston, Texas, Image #MU-VN-B3-CC-32318.

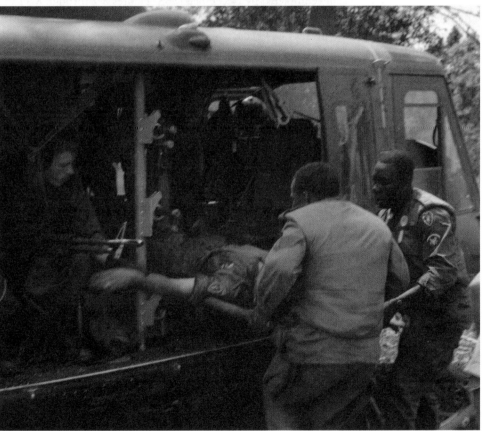

FIGURE 8-11. Loading wounded officer on UH-1 helicopter. Photograph courtesy of the Army Medical Department Center of History and Heritage, Fort Sam Houston, Texas, Image #MU-VN-B3-CC-33940.

center. The 44th Medical Brigade was released from the 1st Logistical Command. At that time the 44th Medical Brigade assumed a number of functions previously delegated to the 1st Logistical Command. It was to ensure central control that the 44th Medical Brigade was to report directly to USARV headquarters. BG (later Major General [MG]) Glenn J Collins was the first to command; MG Spurgeon Neel followed.[37(p25)]

Prior to 1965, the only Army facility in Vietnam was the 8th Field Hospital (100 beds) at Nha Trang.[36(p59)] There was a Navy medical operation in Saigon of 100 beds.[18(pp60–61)] The 3rd Field Hospital arrived in April 1965. Later that year, two evacuation and two field hospitals, along with field units, arrived. They were located near the 8th Field Hospital in Nha Trang and the 3rd Field Hospital in Saigon.[1(pp60–61)] In 1965, evacuations from Vietnam happened within 15 days of wounding. In mid-1966, patients were evacuated after 30 days due to more in-country facilities. If they could be returned to duty within that period, the soldiers were retained in Vietnam.[36(p50)] By 1967, there were six evacuation and four surgical hospitals, along with the 6th Convalescent Center[36(p61)] (at Cam Ranh Bay). More hospitals arrived in 1968, including the 312th Evacuation Hospital, the largest US Army Reserve unit in Vietnam. As of December 1968, there were 5,283 beds in country. The medical build-up was basically completed by December 1968 (Figures 8-7 through 8-11). After the Army strength fell from 331,000 in January 1970 to 119,700 at the end of 1971, there was a proportional fall in AMEDD beds, with only 1,000 beds then. US medical operations in Vietnam ended by the end of 1972.[36(p50)]

OTHER PROGRAMS SUPPORTED BY MEDICAL ASSETS

Civilian medical aid programs started in the early years of US involvement. Programs were initiated to help the people of Vietnam. Such programs included MILPHAP (Military Provincial Health Assistance Program), MEDCAP (Medical Civic Action Program), and CWCP (Civilian War Casualty Program). These programs had mixed success due to problems of civil strife, geographic isolation, and warfare.[18(pp162–163)]

The medical needs of special groups were additional duties. The Special Forces operated small hospitals to provide medical care for the Montagnards, the hill people who supported US troops.[18(p314)] They were trained by Special Forces troops in the methods of irregular warfare. The largest detractor in using these irregular troops was that due to their help, these peoples were at risk for serious retribution by the NVA and the allied Viet Cong irregulars. However, they were motivated fighters and more familiar with their terrain than the Viet Cong or NVA regulars.[18(p332)]

Initially, the enemy (NVA and Viet Cong) prisoners of war (POWs) were medically and surgically treated by both the ARVN and US Army units. The POW treatment program was turned over to the ARVN by 1969. US units continued to treat POWs in their regions until they could be transported to ARVN facilities.[18(pp69–70)]

Internists and Pediatricians

Originally, fully trained internists were assigned to surgical hospitals (and MUST units). These hospitals did not have beds for prolonged holding of the sick or wounded;

however, attached laboratory facilities were able to complete the usual surgical tests. The internists functioned as triage doctors and surgical assistants. The internists were reassigned to larger hospitals starting in 1968 so that they could function more as internal medicine physicians.[36(p41)] In 1969, 52 internists were assigned to hospitals in teams of three or four. Medical illnesses in such a tropical climate were varied and included amebiasis and other parasitic diseases, malaria, bacterial diseases, and arboviruses and other viral diseases.[36(p52)] Internists added to the improved "team" care of the wounded after surgery.[36(p50)]

The ability of internists to deal with the ever-present malaria was greatly valued because many of the wounded had malaria as an additional medical problem that had to be addressed. *Plasmodium falciparum* was the major prevalent strain. An increase in the chloroquine-resistant malaria cases presented a crisis because these new malarial cases were not prevented by the usual prophylaxis regimes. In 1965, these cases were typically found in combat troops in contact with the Viet Cong because the troops were in areas where mosquitoes were common and combat units tended to not always observe chemoprophylaxis regulations. In 1966, a major breakthrough came in the control of malaria with the introduction of a new drug. DDS (4-4-diaminodiphenylsulfone), initially recognized as an important agent in the treatment of leprosy, was also shown to be an effective agent to treat resistant strains of malaria. Internists also had to deal with infectious hepatitis and used immunoglobulin in that regard.[26(pp170–171)]

Interestingly, pediatricians were assigned to Vietnam as part of the Civilian War Casualty Program. All USARV hospitals accepted civilians on a space available basis under this program. The use of pediatricians in hospitals and the field was limited. These physicians augmented adult caregivers as needed, including duty as surgical triage doctors and surgical assistants.[36(pp43,44)] US Province Senior Advisors (civilian advisors) tried to implement programs to help the local people and to neutralize the influence of the Viet Cong. Medical care for civilians, including children, went along with programs such as Village Self-Development and Public Works.[38(pp244–245)] The Agency for International Development (AID) had sent civilian teams of physicians, nurses, and technicians to Vietnam as early as 1962.[26(p162)] Indeed, the MILPHAP was a joint venture of AID and MACV, which provided civilian physicians and nurses with a mission to improve the health of Vietnamese civilians.[26(pp162–163)]

Convalescent Facilities

The 6th Convalescent Center, located near Cam Ranh Bay, was the major convalescent center in country. It opened in 1965 upon the recommendation of Surgeon General Heaton. In its first year of operation alone, 7,500 medical and surgical patients were admitted. Later, the average admission rate was about 1,000 per month.[18(pp67–68)] Internists provided much of the staff for this center.

SURGICAL/MEDICAL CARE ADVANCES OF THE VIETNAM WAR

The hallmark of surgical care in Vietnam centered on wound debridement, wound exploration, and delayed closure. The wounds resulted in a low infection rate and no gas gangrene. Burkhalter pointed out that assignment of Regular Army (RA) medical officers (in the case of more senior surgeons from Korea and more junior surgeons from work in emergency rooms and operating rooms of Army facilities) with experience in wound management avoided having to relearn the lessons of past conflicts.[39(pp210–211)]

The level of surgical skill was high and was maintained despite surgeon rotation turnover. However, due to assignment variables, surgical specialists were often used as general surgeons. A case in point, Colonel (COL) Harold Griffiths, US Air Force Reserve, Medical Corps, was a general surgeon in Vietnam. He spoke of the situation where subspecialists were assigned to a hospital and were expected to function as general surgeons. He described the importance of trauma skills and triage in treating those injured in combat, as well as the transfer of these skills to those meeting trauma in the civilian world, especially in mass casualty situations.[40(pp228–229)]

The trauma surgery skills were increased for the surgeons involved. Because the new surgeons arriving in country had little in civilian trauma experience to prepare them, they were attached to experienced teams that could get them trained. In the larger facilities, the team approach, involving multiple disciplines operating even simultaneously, added to the overall success. Debridement (particularly fasciotomy for orthopedic surgeons) was difficult to learn, especially making wide incisions and aggressive removal of devitalized tissue.[39(p211)] Delayed closure was an emphasis in World War II and Korea.[41,42] However, a feature of the high-velocity Vietnam wound was that delayed closure could cause problems, primarily of infection and delayed healing.[39(p212)] Surgeons concluded that closure could be an elective procedure to be done when appropriate.

Every war has its own unique advances that benefit the military and civilians as well. Vietnam was no exception. Areas of advancement and interest in the war included: the military blood program, treatment of shock, treatment of metabolic and respiratory problems, body enzyme changes resulting from wounding and shock, advances in antibiotic therapy, treatment of posttraumatic renal insufficiency, burn treatment, advances in vascular surgery, and innovative advances in the use of tissue adhesives and aerosolized antibiotics.

The Vietnam Military Blood Program

In the conflict, frequent transfusion of whole blood was done with type O low-titer blood well before the injured reached a facility with cross-match capability. From 1965 forward, the push for blood was expedited because liquid (unlike frozen) whole blood had an expected life of only 21 days from donor to recipient. A source of whole blood from outside the country was an early priority. In 1965, the 8th Field Hospital did the only transfusions and they received 10 units each week from Japan. Early surges in need were met with local donor sources. As Neel points out, the whole blood program in Vietnam was supported by donors from the military, their dependents, and civilians employed at military facilities throughout the world.[32(p126)]

The arrival of the 3rd Field Hospital in 1965 allowed it to become the central blood depot for Vietnam. The 406th Mobile Medical Laboratory was given the distribution task in country.[33(pp114–115)] The continued expansion of the blood program required the establishment of the USARV Central Blood Bank in 1967. The first shipment of whole blood from the United States arrived in Japan in 1966. After that date, blood shipments came from the United States weekly to Japan and from there to the Central Blood Bank in Vietnam.[32(p122)]

In 1965, it was decided to ship only universal donor low-titer group O blood to Vietnam. More specific blood types were reserved for the Philippines and off-shore facilities. After 1965, while clearing and field hospitals were still unable to cross-match and continued to use universal O blood, the evacuation hospitals switched to more specific transfusion programs. As the Vietnam in-country facilities became more advanced, specific blood types were made available.[32(p122)]

Blood was generally to be used within 21 days. Because the blood received from out-of-country sources was 4 to 7 days old already, the effective life of the supplies was only about 2 weeks. Blood that was 21 days to 31 days old was given to the ARVN units and the civilian facilities. Originally, blood over 31 days old was destroyed, but later in the conflict, the blood was converted to plasma. It was found that the addition of the amino acid adenine could extend the useful blood life to 40 days.[32(p124)]

In 1968, fresh frozen plasma was sent to Vietnam to deal with coagulopathies following surgery and massive transfusions. Because the freezer compartments in the standard cooling units were inadequate, a freezer was adapted from one used in construction to cool steel rivets. By 1969, freezers specifically designed for fresh frozen plasma had been introduced.[32(p123)]

The Styrofoam blood box was introduced in 1965. Many authorities called Vietnam the "war of the white Styrofoam blood box." The Collins box replaced the earlier Hollinger box because it could hold 18 units of blood, was smaller in size, and retained its coolant twice as long.[32(p125)]

Extensive transfusions could also have their problems. Neel describes one case requiring 92 units of blood.[19(p56)] There could be bleeding posttransfusion, which could be controlled by fresh whole blood or fresh frozen plasma. A drop in the patient's temperature posttransfusion was a problem; blood warming technologies helped overcome this issue.

Metabolic/Respiratory Issues

The soldier became acclimated for Vietnam duty soon after arrival, but chronic dehydration was a continuing problem.[30p(3)] Research continued into the soldier's health in Vietnam from a number of approaches. The Walter Reed Army Institute of Research (WRAIR) pointed out in their studies the importance of the metabolic state of the soldier. The WRAIR Surgical Research Team also worked to investigate the care of the wounded.[29(p4)] BG Robert Hardaway described the state of surgical research in Vietnam while he was the Chief, Division of Surgery, at the WRAIR.[43(pp873–877)]

One prong of the studies of the WRAIR team (Heisterkamp et al) looked at respiratory insufficiency as a factor leading to casualty hypoxemia, shifts in serum sodium concentrations with anesthesia, and serum enzyme changes noted with wounds.[44(pp36–59)] Other facets of the Heisterkamp studies included study of serum enzymes in wounding,[44(pp1-8)] study of oxygen tensions postsurgery,[44(pp49–96)] and the effects of massive transfusions.[44(pp111–118)] Shock is an issue when the arterial blood flow is not adequate to deal with metabolic needs of tissues. Regional hypoxia results from subsequent lactic acidosis (due to anaerobic metabolism in peripheral tissues) as well as eventual end-organ failure. Shock and acidosis complicated hypoxemia (defined as a p02 less than 80%). There are many causes of shock recorded. Hypovolemic shock is due to loss of blood, plasma, and loss of fluid and electrolytes. Obstructive shock can be due to tension pneumothorax.[45(pp422–423)]

Shock

Hardaway wrote an excellent review of the history of shock and its treatment by military surgeons through the wars. He had a unique background that included handling casualties from the Japanese attack on Pearl Harbor. He pointed out that the Vietnam War was characterized by "the beginnings of serious shock research in the Army."[46(pp267–268)] Hardaway published an article describing shock lung[47(pp311–315)] (now called acute respiratory distress syndrome [ARDS]). Surgeons attributed the condition to a postulated intravascular coagulation.

Hardaway described the establishment of the first shock trauma unit at Walter Reed Army Medical Center in 1963 followed by a duplicate unit in Vietnam in 1965.[47(p268)] Hardaway's 2009 article details the Army's extensive experience in the study of shock and his own experience from Pearl Harbor to the present.[48(pp944–947)]

Prolonged shock was found to lead to DIC—disseminated intravascular coagulopathy. The WRAIR team noted sporadic DIC occurred in severe trauma, as indicated by an abnormal prothrombin time and partial thromboplastin time tests. Platelets and fibrinogen are reduced. Episodic nonlethal DIC probably occurred in the recovery from shock and trauma as postulated by Heisterkamp et al.[44(pp111–148)]

Serum Enzyme Changes in Wounds/Shock

Studies of serum enzyme changes with wounds noted that changes came about in specific enzymes such as SGOT (serum glutamic-oxaloacetic transaminase, now known as AST or aspartate aminotransferase); LDH (lactate dehydrogenase); and SGPT (serum glutamic-pyruvic transaminase, now known as ALT or alanine aminotransferase). All of these enzymes can be elevated in liver, heart, or muscle disease. Of these enzymes, the SGOT test was felt at the time to be the most accurate and sensitive test for soft tissue trauma.[44(pp49–96),49(pp272–274)]

Antibiotic Use

Antibiotic use prior to 1944 mainly featured sulfanilamide drugs. Penicillin became available in mid-1944 in significant quantities. The clinical approach in World War II for antibiotic use included having soldiers start oral sulfanilamide antibiotics when wounded; sulfa granules were sprinkled into the wound by the corpsman when first seen. As noted by Cleveland, the low rate of infection in World War II was attributed to good debridement and whole blood use, rather than the use of penicillin or sulfa.[50(p169)]

Arts et al stated in the WRAIR Research Team Report that 13 different species of bacteria were found in Korean War wound cultures.[43(p606)] Lindberg, writing in the *Annals of Surgery*, described the finding of a large proportion of cases showing both anaerobic and aerobic pathogens. Those studies found *Staphylococcus aureus, Aerobacter aerogenes, Pseudomonas,* and *Proteus* present; penicillin was not the drug of choice for these pathogens.[51(pp369–374)]

Antibiotics used in Vietnam after injury included penicillin or penicillin in combination with chloramphenicol or streptomycin.[40(p211)] The most commonly used were penicillin and streptomycin. However, it was noted that this combination was ineffective in over half of the patients evacuated in Vietnam. Mandelamine was found to be useful. Matsumoto, of the WRAIR Surgical Team, reported in 1968 that the effectiveness of penicillin was dose-related, requiring larger doses to be administered intravenously. Starting with the work of the WRAIR Surgical Research Team, surgeons learned the value of microbiological cultures to guide them in which antibiotic agents to use later. The WRAIR team also commented on the fact that wound infection was to be considered not as a response to soft tissue/bone destruction but rather to the environment and the level of foreign material in the wound. Surgeons also learned that prolonged treatment, which was often unnecessary, could lead to problems of hospital-acquired infections of another organism or further complications such as a pulmonary embolus.[40(p212)] Broad spectrum antibiotics were available only late in Vietnam.[29(p12)]

In Vietnam, the WRAIR Surgical Research Team found organisms causing morbidity and mortality included *Staphylococcus aureus, Pseudomonas aeruginosa,* and *Klebsiella* pneumonia. The most common organism in Vietnam wounds causing problems was *Staphylococcus aureus* (in 30% of wounds), followed by *Pseudomonas* (18%) and *E. coli* (17%).[29(p13)] The bacterial flora found in orthopedic wounds as reported by Heggers et al were quite instructive.[52(pp602–603)] *Serratia marcescens* had increased in wound cultures. Aggressive blood culture techniques and an attempt to provide good respiratory care to patients on ventilators were both done in an attempt to prevent *Serratia* sepsis.[29(p13)]

Despite widespread antibiotic use, the old standard of widespread debridement and delayed closure significantly helped to reduce infection.[29(p13)] The principles of debridement and delayed closure had not undergone much evolution since World War II. The 1958 *NATO Emergency War Handbook* and its 1975 revision discuss antibiotic use as a support therapy, not to replace good surgical debridement.[53] In debridement, an adequate and aggressive incision is necessary to reach the devitalized tissue. Inadequate exposure may mean missing the damaged tissue. Debridement of muscle tissue is difficult in that the surgeon may have trouble judging the soundness of muscle. Fascia should be incised to allow decompression of underlying injured tissue. The Korean War taught that muscle tissue viability can be evaluated by its consistency, ability to bleed, and contractility.[53(pp266–273)]

The incidence of gas gangrene and tetanus was almost nonexistent in Vietnam casualties. Tetanus toxoid was given as a routine to each wounded soldier. The rapid debridement of wounds and antibiotic use was in part responsible. However, it was reported that gas gangrene and tetanus were seen in Viet Cong casualties.[54(pp1445–1451)]

WRAIR had worked with the Pasteur Institute in 1964 to set up a plague research laboratory in Vietnam.[8(p315)] The plague laboratory did work to help combat an expanding problem at the start of the war. In another research area—the management of shock—the onset of shock lung/wet lung after a wound to the chest was noted. The use of diuretics was helpful in dealing with this manifestation.[29(p5)]

Posttraumatic Renal Insufficiency—Advances in Treatment

The advances in treatment of acute renal insufficiency (ARI) following trauma were significant in the Vietnam experience. The 629th Medical Detachment (Renal) was organized to deal with ARI. Of note, the 629th was a specialized intensive care operation that used hemodialysis and peritoneal dialysis to combat renal failure. It served as a referral center for renal patients of the US military and US civilians. It also treated Vietnamese civilians and military, as well as other foreign nationals in Vietnam. Once the patients were stabilized after a round of dialysis, they could be then evacuated to CONUS. Facilities in the Philippines, Japan, or Hawaii could be used en route if more immediate dialysis was needed.[37(pp465–466)]

The largest group of patients with ARI treated there were those resulting from trauma following wounding in battle. This entity was known in World War II and treated in Korea with hemodialysis. In World War II (prior to the development of the artificial kidney), the fatality rate was 90% among the wounded with ARI.[37(p466)] With early hemodialysis treatment in Korea, the fatality rate was lowered to 68% in the wounded.[37(p466)] The mortality rate in the first year of operation in Vietnam was 87% (for the posttraumatic renal failure) versus 6% for those with only medical causes. The posttraumatic cases were more complicated, demonstrating multiple organ failure and extremity wounds with attendant oligemic shock and hemorrhage.[37(pp471–473)] The rapid evacuation of the wounded by helicopter, rapid treatment, and resuscitation reduced the incidence of ARI from one in 200 woundings in Korea to one in 600 in Vietnam. Despite improvements in treatment, still two out of three soldiers died once ARI had occurred. (Of interest is that the 629th became the first Army unit to perform a successful renal transplantation in June 1969. The patient was a Vietnamese civilian. Military transplantation centers in CONUS followed this success.[37(pp475–476)])

Other Advances

Rehabilitation was quite important to the wounded soldier, especially in orthopedic injuries and amputations. The Army introduced a physical therapist to Vietnam in 1967.[30(p6)] The use of an expanded physical and occupational program in the Convalescent Center and the larger facilities added greatly to recovery of the wounded.

The use of "flak jackets" body armor greatly reduced the number of chest wounds. Hence, the proportional number of wounds of other areas was increased.[19(p55)] When worn, the flak jackets were said to be effective against three-fourths of the fragments striking the thorax. Exact figures on the wear of the jacket are not known. The primary issue was the extra heat generated and the extra weight. As in any military situation, the level of command oversight had an obvious bearing.[19(p55)]

The Vietnam War ushered in improvements in anesthesia, burn care, and the employment of plasma expanders. The usual general anesthesia was a thiopental induction followed by a mix of halothane, nitrous oxide, and oxygen. Halothane proved to be a great anesthetic in Vietnam offering safe inductions and uncomplicated recoveries.[19(p56)]

BURN TREATMENT

In the Korean War, the experience of the 46th Surgical Hospital and the experience of other facilities were coordinated with the Burn Study Ward at Brooke Army Hospital in San Antonio, Texas. The so-called "Universal Protective Dressing" was found to be helpful. A report was sent to the Surgeon for the 8th Army in Korea in July 1953, discussing the "Universal Protective Dressing," which was very effective and more comfortable for the patient. The dressing continued to be used throughout the Vietnam era.[55(p189)] Suggestions for the management of burns in the field were evolved. Suggestions for the level of response in critical care at each level of evacuation were formulated. Attention to fluid replacement in the first 24-hour period and continuing fluid replacement in the next 24 hours were outlined. The patient was to be transported on the third day to an evacuation hospital, provided fluid replacement therapy had been done. The importance of designating centers specializing in burns had been noted during the Korean War years.[55(pp189–190)]

In Vietnam, burns were often fatal if associated with enemy action (as opposed to the half that were accidental). The 70% of the deaths due to burns were associated with enemy action because of their severity and the fact that other wounds were often sustained at the same time.[19(p56)] The percentage of combat burn injuries was 5% of the total casualties in Vietnam. It is surprising that over half of the burns in Vietnam were accidental and therefore presumably preventable. Burn patients were only stabilized before evacuation to Japan. Later, over 66% of these were sent to the Burn Center at Brooke Army Medical Center in San Antonio, Texas.[19(pp56–57)] Sulfamylon ointment was started to reduce the infection rate.[19(p56)] In the specialized centers, teams of physicians and nurses were joined by occupational therapists, physical therapists, and respiratory therapists. Burn casualty management included timely triage, resuscitation, initial treatment, and air evacuation to a tertiary burn center. In the years since World War II and the Korean War, the treatment of burns greatly improved with the onset of specialized centers and the use of ancillary personnel. In the Korean War, phosphorus burns were treated with a copper sulfate solution. The solution was no longer used as it was found to be toxic in itself. Hence early debridement was deemed even more important for those burns.[19(p57)]

TISSUE ADHESIVES AND AEROSOL ANTIBIOTICS

In 1968, the WRAIR Surgical Research Team devised tissue adhesives and an aerosol antibiotic to be given by medics at the combat site. The WRAIR Team also tested a number of experimental products in Vietnam designed to aid wound healing. The aerosol antibiotic was given out to a number of tactical units and it was found to retard bacterial growth when given early on an open wound. Morbidity could be thereby reduced. Plastic polymers were used as tissue adhesives. Such adhesives could help with controlling bleeding and in facilitating tissue repair.[19(p57)] The tissue adhesives had low toxicity with fairly rapid degradation. The WRAIR Surgical Research Team found tissue adhesives valuable in surgery of the liver, lung, and kidneys, which were difficult to suture.[19(p57)] The treatment of severe liver injuries was a challenge because it involved significant transfusions and removal of large amounts of tissue. In addition, control of bleeding was a problem because it involved gaining access to relatively inaccessible spaces. As discussed, tissue adhesive use proved helpful in liver cases.

VASCULAR SURGERY

Vascular surgery started irregularly in the Korean War but it became common in Vietnam. Vascular injuries were common in both conflicts but the experience and resolve to deal with these injuries in Korea was not common. Vascular surgery techniques, operation tools, and experience rose precipitously in Vietnam. The surgery was performed by the general surgeon, the orthopedic surgeon, or the vascular surgeon, depending on personnel availability. These surgeons became quite proficient in the now commonplace vascular procedure without regard to their subspecialty. Of the wounded, 2% to 3% had arterial/venous vascular injuries. The amputation rate of limbs with vascular injury was 13%, which was the same as Korea; compared to the 49% rate of World War II, the improvement is impressive.[19(pp52–53)] In a few interesting cases, limbs were salvaged by the construction of an extra anatomic bypass, with tunneling the graft through a new route around the area. When the wound healed, a permanent graft could be done.[19(p57)] COL Norman Rich pointed out that the documentation and repair of both arteries and veins became more common in Korea and especially in Vietnam. In his article recalling the historical heritage of vascular trauma, Rich points out the value of mentorship and the legacy to be passed on of the management of arterial and venous injuries.[56]

"SIGNATURE" WOUND OF THE VIETNAM WAR

In each conflict, the nature of the combat yields a characteristic "signature wound." In the Vietnam conflict, severe wounds caused by high-velocity projectiles were common. These wounds were more severe than low-velocity projectiles from prior conflicts. As Rich discusses, the high-velocity projectile (such as the AK-47/M-16 round) produced greater tissue destruction than any other weapon used in Vietnam or other wars.[57(pp157–158)] The high-velocity projectiles caused much tissue damage, but the jungle foliage could also cause the rounds to tumble, thus increasing the wound damage, with increased cavitation effect and secondary fragments (such as pieces of fragmented bone).[19(p53),30(pp7–8)] Additional tissue damage was invariably caused by rounds that yawed or disintegrated into pieces. The high-velocity projectile wounds show characteristics of explosive nature due to the high kinetic energy of the missile. The energy exceeds the elastic limit of the injured tissue.[57(pp157–158)]

Statistical data on Army troop wounds from January 1965 to June 1970 showed more small arms deaths and injuries in Vietnam than in Korea or World War II. The numbers of "booby trap" and mine injuries were also greater in Vietnam than the other conflicts. However, there were fewer artillery, mortar, and other projective device wounds in Vietnam than in Korea or World War II.[9(p53)]

Of those injured by the various means above, 31% were returned to duty immediately.[19(pp51–52)] Of the wounded actually admitted to the hospital, approximately 42% returned to duty in Vietnam.[19(p52),29(p8)] This impressive return-to-duty rate reflected the dedication and hard work of the doctors, nurses, administrative officers, medical evacuation pilots, and medics.

Neel, in his 1973 *Medical Support of the US Army in Vietnam 1965–70*,[19] reported that multiple wounds were more commonly seen than in prior conflicts.[19(p53)] The multiple wounds in Vietnam were due to the lightweight high-velocity round, the rapid fire of automatic weapons, and the use of mines/booby traps.[30(p7)] This finding was, again, due to the extremely high velocity and kinetic energy of the wounding agent. Automatic weapons accounted for high rates of fire that was often at close range. Further, these projectiles could cause cavitation, which also resulted in external contamination and secondary fragments (such as bone) entering the wound. In the extremities there could also be nerve damage and fractures.[19(pp53–55)]

Claymore mines could cause serious wounds with the multiple steel ball projectiles. The Claymore was fielded by both sides in Vietnam (the ARVN and Viet Cong used captured mines of this type). The Claymore mine resulted in peppering with multiple fragments that often penetrated deeply. The mines could be specifically directed by positioning for a certain trajectory field. The enemy often used booby traps with significant contamination.[19(pp53–54)] In the Republic of Vietnam, mine and booby trap wounds were three times the rate of those of the Korean War or World War II.[26(p173)] The booby traps and mines caused increased injury due to the close nature of the wounding. In addition, multiple fragments with contaminants (such as dirt, fragments, and micro-organisms) made the surgery complicated. The alternatives often involved a choice of more radical surgical debridement and excision versus a more conservative approach attempting to salvage more tissue, which could result in more infection.[19(p53)]

The Vietnam conflict also saw the Viet Cong use Punji stakes. These stakes were bamboo spikes sharpened to a point at the end and smeared with animal or human fecal material, and generally placed in groups. Dr Jerry Martin, the author of *Soldiers Saving Soldiers. Vietnam Remembered: A History of the 18th Surgical Hospital* and an Army surgeon in the RVN, didn't see many of these wounds, but he did note that they required wide debridement and thorough irrigation to prevent life-threatening infections.[12(p121)]

SURGEONS GENERAL OF THE VIETNAM WAR PERIOD

Silas B Hays (1 June 1955–31 May 1959)

Hays received his medical degree from the State University of Iowa in 1928. He was commissioned in 1928 when he started his internship at Letterman General Hospital, San Francisco, California. He completed the Army Medical School and the Medical Field Service School in 1930 to 1931. Hays received 20 months of training in general surgery and urology at Walter Reed General Hospital in the period 1934 to 1937. Hays graduated from the Army Industrial College in 1940 before being assigned to the Surgeon General's Office Finance and Supply Division. In 1944, Hays was assigned to the European Theater of Operations as Chief of Supply in the Theater's Surgeon Office. In 1950, Hays was appointed as the USARMY Pacific Surgeon. In 1951, Hays became the Deputy Surgeon General. In March 1955, Hays became the Army Surgeon General.[58] Hays pursued significant construction to replace aging medical care facilities. He began a medical care program for military dependents, which greatly helped troop morale. Hays encouraged research projects and was particularly interested in the study of radioactivity effects on health.[58]

Leonard D Heaton (1 June 1959–30 September 1969)

Heaton graduated in medicine from the University of Louisville in 1922. He entered active duty in 1926. He was an intern at Letterman General Hospital. Heaton served in a variety of assignments leading up to Hawaii in 1940. At that time, Heaton became the Chief of Surgery for the hospital at Schofield Barracks. On 7 December 1941, Heaton and a colleague were strafed by Japanese planes in their car. He immediately headed to his hospital where he treated casualties. Heaton was assigned to England in 1944 where he commanded two hospitals. In 1948, Heaton was promoted to brigadier general. In 1950, he became a major general and Commander of Letterman General Hospital. In 1953, Heaton became the Commander of the Walter Reed Army Medical Center. In 1959, he became the Army Surgeon General and the first Medical Corps officer to be appointed in the rank of lieutenant general. Heaton retired in 1969 and subsequently died in 1983 at Walter Reed.[59] Heaton had many famous patients including President Eisenhower. Heaton encouraged the use of helicopters for medical evacuation and led the rapid expansion of medical services for the Vietnam War.[59]

Hal B Jennings (1 October 1969–30 September 1973)

Jennings graduated from the University of Michigan in 1941. He interned at the University of Michigan and entered active duty in 1942. Jennings served in the South Pacific until the end of the war. Jennings completed a general surgery residency at Letterman and a 2-year plastic surgery training period at Washington University. He gained certification as a plastic surgeon in 1953, and subsequently became the Chief of Plastic Surgery at Walter Reed in 1959. After assignments in Europe, Jennings deployed to Vietnam with the 1st Cavalry Division (Air Mobile). In May 1968, he became the command surgeon to the US Military Assistance Command, Vietnam. In September, he was promoted to brigadier general. In July 1969, Jennings became the Deputy Surgeon General. On 1 October 1969, he became a lieutenant general and the new Surgeon General.[60]

Richard R Taylor (1 October 1973–30 September 1977)

Taylor graduated from the University of Chicago in 1946. He completed an internal medicine residency at Letterman General Hospital, 1951 to 1953. He served in Korea from September 1953 to December 1954. In 1955, he completed a 1-year residency in pulmonary disease at Fitzsimons Army Medical Center, Aurora, Colorado. Taylor spent the years from 1956 through 1964 in a number of research and development units. In 1969, he became the Command Surgeon, US Military Assistance Command, and RVN. From 1970 to 1973, Taylor was the Commanding General, US Army Medical Research and Development Command, Washington, DC. From March to September 1973, Taylor served as the Deputy Surgeon General, and then he became the Surgeon General on 1 October 1973.[61] Taylor guided the drawdown of assets in the closing years of the Vietnam War. True to his background, he fostered research and development projects providing the template for programs in the coming decades.[61]

THE WAY FORWARD

The Army Medical Department acquitted itself well in the Vietnam War. In an excellent review of this showing from his unique perspective, COL Kenneth Swan gave the Heaton Lecture at the 7th Medical Command Medical-Surgical Conference in Germany in 1990. His talk, "Combat Casualty Care," was later published in 1992. Swan had the particular perspective of being a trauma surgeon in Vietnam (as well as Operation Desert Storm in 1991). He had the added perspective of being a professor of surgery in a major school of medicine. He attributed the success of the AMEDD in combat casualty care to six factors. Swan listed air superiority as the first point because the threat was removed of air attacks. Ground security followed. He spoke to the high density of "semimobile hospitals" that were in truth fixed. This concentration of hospitals, including evacuation hospitals, resulted in the success of the evacuation system. In allowing facilities to be less mobile, the evacuation hospital rose to the level of a university or level-1 trauma center. Fourth, he noted that a large number of trauma-trained surgeons were available and that the whole period of the Vietnam War provided an unparalleled experience to a generation of surgeons. Fifth, Swan spoke to the importance of the ready availability of whole blood, and finally, he quite correctly gave a great deal of credit to the effective use of the air evacuation ambulance.[62(pp4-10)]

BG Hardaway's 1982 Sir Henry Wellcome Prize Essay spoke to the achievements in medicine on the battlefield. He had calculated the increased losses that would have occurred in Vietnam had the medical care been the same standard of care employed in World War II or Korea.[63(pp1011-1017)] Still to be considered in the assessment of the success of medical care in Vietnam is a thought-provoking 1984 editorial by Bzik and Bellamy.[64(p230)] They speculated that Hardaway's picture of the Vietnam era care was too favorable. They noted the relative lethality of the Vietnam battlefield, while acknowledging the rapid evacuation from the battle to surgical treatment facilities. They discussed that in Vietnam the Marines had an emphasis upon forward/field resuscitation of casualties while awaiting air evacuation, which they felt had a favorable outcome. Bzik and Bellamy surmised that a more balanced approach calling for forward resuscitation and rapid evacuation might be the way to go in doctrine.[64] Clearly therein lays a challenge to incorporate such thinking for the future.

REFERENCES

1. Ognibene A, Barrett O, eds. *Internal Medicine in Vietnam.* Vol 2. *General Medicine and Infectious Disease.* Washington, DC: Office of The Surgeon General, Center of Military History; 1982.
2. Li X. Long days and endless nights: an artillery story. In: *Voices From the Vietnam War; Stories From American, Asian, and Russian Veterans.* Lexington, Ky: The University of Kentucky Press; 2010.
3. Dorland P, Nanney J. *Dust Off: Army Aeromedical Evacuation in Vietnam.* Washington, DC: Center of Military History, US Army; 2008.
4. Willbanks J. *Vietnam War Almanac. An In-Depth Guide to the Most Controversial Conflict in American History.* New York, NY: Skyhorse Publishing; 2009.
5. Logevall F. *Embers of War.* New York, NY: Random House; 2013.
6. Walker J. Indochina 1952; the Battle of Na San. *Modern War.* 2014;10(Mar-Apr):30.
7. Moore HG, Galloway JL. *We Were Soldiers Once . . . and Young: Ia Drang—The Battle That Changed the War in Vietnam.* New York, NY: Random House; 1992.
8. Ginn RVN. Medical Service Corps officers in Vietnam. In: *The United States Army Medical Service Corps.* Washington, DC: Office of The Surgeon General, Center of Military History; 1997.
9. Caputo P. *A Rumor of War.* New York, NY: Owl Books–Henry Holt and Company; 1977.
10. Marlantes K. *Matterhorn.* New York, NY: Atlantic Monthly Press; 2010.
11. Vietnam War Casualties. National Archives at http://www.archives.gov/research/military/vietnam-war/casaulty-statistics.html. Accessed 19 February 2014.
12. Martin JW. *Soldiers Saving Soldiers. Vietnam Remembered: A History of the 18th Surgical Hospital.* Morley, Mo: Acclaim Press; 2011.
13. Steinman R. *The Soldiers' Story; Vietnam in Their Own Words.* New York, NY: Fall River Press; 2011.
14. Neel S, ed. Division and brigade support. In: *Vietnam Studies: Medical Support of the US Army in Vietnam 1965–1970.* Washington, DC: Department of the Army; 1991.
15. Cutler EC. The chief consultant in surgery. In: *Activities of the Surgical Consultants.* Vol 2. In: Coates JD, ed. *Medical Department of the United States Army: Surgery in World War II.* Washington, DC: Office of The Surgeon General, Department of the Army; 1964: Chap 2.
16. Naythons M. *The Face of Mercy: A Photographic History of Medicine at War.* New York, NY: Random House; 1993.
17. Leaver RC. Neurosurgery—Vietnam 1967–1968. *USARV Med Bull.* 1968;45–49.
18. Neel S. Hospitalization and evacuation. In: *Vietnam Studies: Medical Support of the US Army in Vietnam 1965–1970.* Washington, DC: Department of the Army; 1991: Chap 4.
19. Neel S. Care of the wounded. In: *Vietnam Studies: Medical Support of the US Army in Vietnam 1965–1970.* Washington, DC: Department of the Army; 1991: Chap 3.
20. Heaton LD. From the Surgeon General. Portable Hospital (MUST). *Med Bull Eur.* 1968;25(10):371–372.
21. Byerly WG, Pendse PD. War surgery in a forward surgical hospital in Vietnam: a continuing report. *Mil Med.* 1971;136(3):221–226.
22. Kelly PJ. Vietnam, 1968–1969: a place and a year like no other. *Neurosurg.* 2003;52(4):927–939 [text]; 939–943 [discussion].
23. Fishel B. The Vietnam War and the American medical effort: and an interview with Dr Stephen J Phillips. http://collections.mdch.org/cdm/ref/collection/saac/id/21467. Accessed 17 January 2014.

24. Sebesta D. Experience as the Chief of Surgery at the 67th Evacuation Hospital, Republic of Vietnam 1968 to 1969. *Mil Med.* 1990;155(5):227.
25. Allgood GD. Contemporary hospital construction in Vietnam. *USARV Med Bulletin.* 1968;12.
26. Neel S. *Vietnam Studies: Medical Support of the US Army in Vietnam 1965–1970.* Washington, DC: Department of the Army; 1991.
27. Dorland P, Nanney J. The early years. In: *Dust-Off Army Aeromedical Evacuation in Vietnam.* Washington, DC: Center of Military History; 1991.
28. Kirkland RC. *MASH Angels: Tales of an Air-Evac Helicopter Pilot in the Korean War.* Short Hills, NJ: Burford Books; 2009.
29. Feagin JA. The soldier and his wound in Vietnam. In: *Surgery in Vietnam.* Washington, DC: Medical Department, US Army, Office of The Surgeon General, Center of Military History; 1994.
30. Dimond FC. The mobile surgical hospital in Vietnam: a lesson in flexibility. *USARV Med Bull.* 1968;3–4.
31. Harder RC. 12th Evacuation Hospital, 1 January 1970–15 November 1970. *Army Medical Department Activities Report* (RCS MED 41 [R4]). APO San Francisco 96353: Department of the Army, Headquarters 12th Evacuation Hospital (SMBL); 1970.
32. Neel S, ed. The military blood program. In: *Vietnam Studies: Medical Support of the US Army in Vietnam, 1965–1970.* Washington, DC: Department of the Army; 1970.
33. *Operations' Report Lessons Learned 2-68: Medical Lessons Learned.* Washington, DC: Department of the Army, Office of the Adjutant General; 16 April 1968: 22–23.
34. Goodrich I. Emergency medical evacuation in an infantry battalion in South Vietnam. *Mil Med.* 1967;132(10):796–798.
35. Heaton LB. Medical support in Vietnam. *Army.* 1966;16:125–128.
36. Ognibene AJ, Barrett O. Full-scale operations. In: Ognibene AJ, Barrett O'N Jr, eds. *General Medicine and Infectious Diseases.* Vol 2. In: *Medical Department, US Army, Internal Medicine in Vietnam.* Washington, DC: Department of the Army, Office of The Surgeon General, Center of Military History; 1982.
37. Neel S, ed. The medical command structure. In: *Vietnam Studies: Medical Support of the US Army in Vietnam 1965–1970.* Washington, DC: Department of the Army; 1991.
38. Boylan K. US Provincial advisors in Vietnam. *J Mil History.* 2014;78(1):244–245.
39. Burkhalter WE, ed. General thoughts on the management of orthopedic casualties lessons learned and unlearned [epilogue]. *Orthopedic Surgery in Vietnam.* Washington, DC: Office of The Surgeon General, Center of Military History; 1994.
40. Griffiths H. A general surgeon in Vietnam: lessons learned the hard way. *Mil Med.* 1990;155:228–229.
41. Treuta J. *The Principles and Practice of War Surgery.* St Louis, Mo: CV Mosby Company; 1943.
42. Heaton LD, Hughes CW, Rosegay H, Fisher GW, Feighny RE. Military surgical practices of the United States Army in Vietnam. A monograph. *Current Problems in Surgery.* Chicago, Ill: Year Book Medical Publishers, Inc; 1966.
43. Hardaway RM. Surgical research in Vietnam. *Mil Med.* 1967;132(11):873–877.
44. Heisterkamp CA III, ed. *Activities of the US Army Surgical Research Team WRAIR–Vietnam: A Technical Report for the Period 17 June 1967 to 20 January 1968.* Washington, DC: US Army Medical and Research and Development Command; 1970.
45. McPhee SJ, Papadakis MA. *Current Diagnosis and Treatment.* New York, NY: McGraw Hill Lange; 2009.

46. Hardaway RM. Wound shock: a history of its study and treatment by military surgeons. *Mil Med.* 2004;169(4):267–268.
47. Hardaway RM. Shock lung. *Int Surg.* 1973;58(5):308–310.
48. Hardway RM. One surgeon's Army experience with "wound shock" from Pearl Harbor to the present. *Mil Med.* 2009;174(9):944–947.
49. Sleeman HK, Simons RL, Heisterkamp CA. Serum enzymes in combat casualties. *Arch Surg.* 1969:(98);272–274.
50. Cleveland M. Adjunct therapy. In: *Orthopedic Surgery in the European Theater of Operations.* Part 2. *Clinical Policies and Practices.* Washington, DC: Office of The Surgeon General, Department of the Army, Government Printing Office; 1956.
51. Lindberg RB, Wetzler TF, Marshall JD, Newton A, Strawitz JG, Howard JM. Bacterial flora of battle wounds at the time of primary debridement. Study of Korean battle casualties. *Annals Surg.* 1955;141:369–374.
52. Heggers JP, Barnes ST, Robson MC, Ristroph JD, Omer GE. Microbial flora of orthopedic war wounds. US Department of Defense. *NATO Emergency War Surgical Handbook.* Washington, DC: Government Printing Office; 1958, 1975 1st Rev. *Mil Med.* 1969;134:602–603.
53. Bronwell AW, Artz CP, Sako Y. Debridement. In: *Recent Advances in Medicine and Surgery. Based on Professional Medical Experiences in Japan and Korea. 1950–5.* Vol 1. Washington, DC: US Army Medical Service Graduate School, Walter Reed General Hospital; 1954: 266–273.
54. Brown PW. Gas gangrene in a metropolitan community. *J Bone Joint Surgery.* 1974;56(A): 1445–1451.
55. Artz CP. The battle wound; clinical experiences. In: *Battle Casualties in Korea: Studies of the Surgical Research Team.* Vol 3. Washington, DC: Government Printing Office and Army Medical Service Graduate School, Walter Reed General Hospital; 1956.
56. Rich NM. Vascular trauma historical notes. *Perspect Vasc Surg Endovasc Ther.* 2011;23(1): 7–12.
57. Rich N, Johnson E, Dimond F. Wounding power of missiles used in the Republic of Vietnam. *JAMA.* 1967;199:157–168.
58. US Army Medical Department. Office of Medical History. *Surgeons General. Silas B Hays* at http://history.amedd.army.mil/surgeongenerals/S_Hays.html. Accessed 8 May 2015.
59. US Army Medical Department. Office of Medical History. *Surgeons General. Leonard D Heaton* at http://history.amedd.army.mil/surgeongenerals/L_Heaton.html. Accessed 8 May 2015.
60. US Army Medical Department. Office of Medical History. *Surgeons General. Hal B Jennings* at http://history.amedd.army.mil/surgeongenerals/H_%20JenningsJr.html. Accessed 8 May 2015.
61. US Army Medical Department. Office of Medical History. *Surgeons General. Richard R Taylor* at http://history.amedd.army.mil/surgeongenerals/R_Taylor.html. Accessed 8 May 2015.
62. Swan KG. Heaton Lecture: Combat casualty care. *J US Army Med Dept.* 1992;Sept–Oct:4–10.
63. Hardaway RM. The Sir Henry Welcome Prize Essay: Wartime treatment of shock. *Mil Med.* 1982;147:1011–1017.
64. Bzik KD, Bellamy RF. A note on combat casualty statistics [editorial]. *Mil Med.* 1984;149: 229–230.

Chapter Nine

From the Falklands to the Balkans: Toward Formal Designation of the Forward Surgical Team

CHRISTOPHER A. VANFOSSON

INTRODUCTION

THE CURRENT MANIFESTATION OF FORWARD surgical elements in the US Army evolved over several iterations of combat experience, shifting more capable surgical assets farther forward as the operating environment became less linear. Between World War I and Vietnam, the percentage of troops killed in action (KIA), defined as those who died before reaching a military hospital, hovered between 18% and 24%.[1(pp1–8)] However, the percentage of casualties who eventually died of their wounds (DOW) after reaching a military hospital improved as healthcare evolved (9% in World War I, 5% in World War II, less than 3% in Korea, and just over 3% in Vietnam).[1(pp1–8)] Advances in technology altered military tactics and equipment, while also improving medical care to the combat wounded. In Vietnam, air evacuation brought patients to military treatment facilities earlier than in the past, so that many who previously would have died on the battlefield reached a hospital. If the Vietnam DOW is statistically corrected to exclude casualties who died within 24 hours of admission to the military treatment facility, it becomes 1%.[1(pp1–8)]

As medical and military capabilities progressed, so too did the implementation of medicine on the battlefield. The meandering, linear battlefields of the two world wars and Korea gave way to the low-intensity conflicts of Vietnam and the fast-paced maneuvers of Operation Desert Storm. Tactical medicine transitioned, at first through ad hoc means, to forward surgical elements that moved closer to the battlefield. These efforts, supported by Army Medical Department studies demonstrating that 67% of all casualties listed as KIAs actually died within 10 minutes of wounding—a period in which little can be done to save the casualty—were aimed at saving the 33% of KIAs who survived the 10-minute mark.[1(p9)] It was not until the late 1990s that forward surgical teams (FSTs), seen as an innovation to the modern mechanisms of war, became formal, permanent parts of Army medical doctrine and structure.[2,3] The presence of such highly skilled and mobile teams on the battlefield today, coupled with a focus on implementing combat lifesaver training, the development and use of "blood expanders," and the advent of improved evacuation platforms reduced the DOW rate to 0.5% by the end of Desert Storm.[1(p8)] Formal inclusion of the FST into Army tactical doctrine made permanent the changes necessary to support the Army in today's nonlinear operating environment.

DEPLOYMENT OF FORWARD SURGICAL ASSETS IN THE 1980S AND 1990S

This chapter will explore four deployments of forward surgical assets in the period since the Vietnam War —the Falklands War, Operation Urgent Fury, Operation Just Cause, and Operations Desert Shield and Desert Storm—to demonstrate the evolution of the FST in the 1980s and 1990s. These deployments set the stage for the transition to the FST's formal designation as a permanent unit.

Falklands War: The 1982 British Invasion of the Falklands Islands

Although the United States was not directly involved in the Falklands War, the lessons learned from the British experience during the invasion of the Falklands Islands provided the US Army a recent reference operation for the rapid deployment of troops to island protectorates. As an indicator of possible future American military operations, the British experience demonstrated the need for medical planning prior to rapid deployments to far off lands. The sudden Argentinian invasion of the Falklands Islands, a United Kingdom-owned chain of islands 450 miles off the coast of Argentina, on 2 April 1982 triggered an unexpected deployment for the Royal Navy and its medical department. Three days later, the United Kingdom deployed its first naval units to expel Argentinian troops from the Falklands.[3,4]

The British possessed no contingency plan for combat service support for the defense of the island territory nearly 8,000 miles away. The lone staging base for the Royal Navy, at an American airfield (Wideawake Airfield) on the Ascension Islands,[3] was only halfway to the Falklands, lending little comfort to the logistics planners that rapid replenishment of combat service needs would be possible.[4(p50),5] During the Falklands campaign, air operations at Wideawake expanded from 40 flights per day to 400 flights per day and solidified Ascension Island's place in British military plans for contingent operations south of the equator in the decades to come.[3]

Although the Royal Navy was responsible for the overall operation in the Falklands, the Royal Navy Medical Department split from tradition to liaise with its counterparts in the British Army and Royal Air Force to develop a rough medical plan before the first units departed for the Falklands.[6] The SS *Uganda*, a cruise ship transporting a group of students to Gibraltar just off the southern coast of Spain, was called to military service on 2 April. Within 3 days, the *Uganda* was refitted as a hospital ship. The students were flown home to Britain while the hospital staff flew to Gibraltar to populate the new floating infirmary. Within 4 days of its call-up, the fully outfitted SS *Uganda* set forth toward the Falklands in preparation for war.[3]

By 5 April, medical planners had identified and activated the 16th Field Ambulance of the Royal Army Medical Corps, surgical teams drawn from the 16th Field Ambulance (Parachute Clearing Team) and the 2nd Field Hospital of the Royal Army Medical Corps, and the regimental medical officers already assigned as organic personnel to each of the major combat units.[6] The field surgical teams, potentially the most important asset of the group, consisted of a surgeon, an anesthetist, a resuscitation officer, four operating room technicians, a blood transfusion technician, and a clerk.[4(p57)] Their employment would place these teams as far forward as possible on the battlefield, aiming to provide surgery and resuscitation to the combat wounded within 6 hours of injury.[7]

Medical evacuation was anticipated to be difficult. Ground evacuation, the first line of evacuation from the point of injury to the regimental aid post, would be limited by the "rocky, craggy terrain."[4(p61)] It was planned that the small forward surgical elements would move forward on foot with the regimental aid posts, resuscitating patients and stabilizing them for evacuation to the next level of care. Rotary wing aircraft were the planned primary means of evacuation from the battlefield. Their use would be limited, however, by the weather and the medical commander's lack of command and control over the medical evacuation assets.[4(p57)] In anticipation of fierce fighting, and reflecting his concern over the limited evacuation capabilities once the invasion began, the British medical commander ordered the landing of the 2nd Field Hospital at Ajax Bay in the Falkland city of San Carlos.[4(pp60–62)] The 2nd Field Hospital would then serve as a staging facility for those patients who required surgery after injury. According to the plan, these patients would eventually be evacuated to the *Uganda* for stabilization before being transferred to one of three ambulance ships (the *Hecla,* the *Herald,* or the *Hydra*) for transport to Montevideo, Uruguay. From Uruguay, the Royal Air Force would fly the casualties back to Britain for convalescence.[3,4(p68)]

To compensate for the short mobilization timeline, British military leaders used the 3-week movement to the Falklands to more completely plan the operation and gather intelligence. Much of this intelligence came from Britons fleeing the Falklands after the Argentinian invasion, who provided important insight into the topography of the obscure island chain and the weaponry used by the Argentinian forces.[3] Additionally, the Royal Navy used the voyage to the Falkland battlefield to more specifically plan the medical support for the operation and to train the infantry on the essentials of combat first aid. British soldiers were trained on immediate resuscitation, treatments for shock, hemorrhage control, the use of first-aid dressings, and the proper administration of morphine as an analgesic.[3,8] In the end, this training compensated for long ground evacuation times. The patients arrived at the aid station more stable, requiring less resuscitation, and thereby allowing for an earlier evacuation to the *Uganda*.[3] In anticipation of the ensuing battle, and recognizing the possible length of the evacuation trains, soldiers on the ships also donated units of blood to the medical teams, augmenting the supply already shipped by the Royal Army Blood Supply Depot in Britain.[4(p58)]

The British invasion of the Falkland Islands, aimed at ejecting the occupying Argentinian troops, began on a wintery 8 May 1982, with troops setting forth from the inhospitable South Georgia Island east of the Falklands.[3,4(pp46–49)] Almost immediately, limitations in the medical support plan became apparent. The British troops struggled to get many of their casualties to surgery within the aimed-for 6-hour window, often because the rotary wing aircraft used for evacuation were diverted for transportation of supplies and other needs.[4(pp62–63),9] Also, at least one helicopter was shot down while extracting patients, possibly as a result of its dual use as a transport for ammunition into the fight.[4(p63)]

Regimental aid posts and field surgical teams were essential to the medical success of the mission, moving forward on foot as maneuver elements surged across the islands toward Port Stanley. Much of the ground evacuation to the regimental aid posts took an average of 2.5 hours, with patients often carried by stretcher rather than transported by ambulance. Though weather, terrain, and aircraft availability limited medical evacuations to the 2nd Field Hospital, the regimental aid posts and forward surgical units filled the gap in patient care. These patients eventually ended up at the Fitzroy and Teal Inlet.[3,4(p66)] Once it became operational on 21 May 1982, the 2nd Field Hospital, set up in a refrigerator plant at Ajax Bay near Port San Carlos, became the primary destination for evacuations.[3,10] At one point, the 2nd Field Hospital's staff performed 100 surgeries in a single 48-hour period.[10] By 9 June, when the 2nd Field Hospital ceased operations, the staff had treated 450 out of the 783 casualties treated during the Falklands War and conducted almost all of the initial surgeries needed during the campaign.[3,11] Despite the prolonged evacuation times, only three British casualties died after reaching a hospital, indicating the importance of forward surgical asset availability when medical evacuation capabilities are limited.[9]

The British medical experience in the Falklands solidified British medical doctrine and demonstrated that the medical support system could support tactical operations.[4(p68)] Only once in the deployment did the medical support system nearly crack, when the *HMS Sir Galahad* was bombed, producing 179 casualties.[7] After-action reports identified numerous shortages in planning and logistics support, such as insufficient heating, communication, paper, and potable water.[4(pp62–65),11] Some reports indicated that many casualties who died likely exsanguinated due to underuse of tourniquets.[12] Yet, with the cooperation of the three British services and the medical commander's ability and willingness to maneuver personnel on the battlefield, the adaptability and professionalism of British medical support personnel ensured that the medical needs of the Falkland Islands Campaign were met.[4(p68)]

Operation Urgent Fury: The 1983 US Invasion of Grenada

At first glance, Cold War-era national security strategies might seem focused wholly on the linear conflict that might have erupted between the United States and the Soviet Union. The battlefields of the 1980s and 1990s, however, were less linear and on a much smaller scale than military planners anticipated. The geopolitical environment was changing, and therefore, so were the potential military missions. These changes also affected the medical support structures in the US Army. The conflict in the small island country of Grenada served as a successful example of rapidly deployable American land forces in this new geopolitical environment and highlighted the need for American medical planners to develop small, rapidly deployable elements to support these missions.

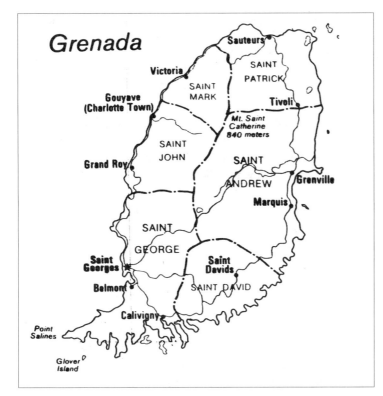

FIGURE 9-1. A map of the island of Grenada, October–November 1983. Note the location of Point Salines and Saint Georges in the southwestern portion of the nation. The medical clearing station and surgical team were established at the airstrip near Point Salines. Photograph courtesy of Colonel (Ret) Joseph P. Jackson, Jr, MD (private collection).

Maurice Bishop, a communist-leaning political player in the nation of Grenada, assumed power of the small island country in 1979. Amid Cold War concerns for the growth of communism in the Americas, Bishop's ascension to power concerned the US Department of State, which feared Bishop might move the island nation politically closer to America's Cold War nemesis, the Soviet Union.[13] These concerns appeared justified as Bishop, while claiming to be neutral, garnered Cuban support and embarked on the construction of a 10,000-foot reinforced runway. Such an airstrip concerned US officials due to the strategic location of the island nation and the potential for the Cubans or Soviets to use the strip for military purposes. The island location and the airstrip length could allow for aircraft capable of interdicting US air and sea routes, as well as serving as a collection point for Soviet arms bound for Central American communist sympathizers.[4(pp81–84),13–16] By late 1983, the airstrip was complete and Bishop had been overthrown by a more hardline Marxist regime, led by Bernard Coard and backed by the Grenadian army.[4(pp81–84),13,17] With the new airstrip complete and Coard in charge, the nation of Grenada could assume the role of a "Soviet aircraft carrier" within striking distance of the United States.[14]

Concerned that the sudden change in Grenadian leadership posed a significant threat to the 600 American students in Grenada, and with the Iranian hostage crisis in recent memory, US President Ronald Reagan ordered the Joint Chiefs of Staff on 17 October 1983 to begin planning to evacuate the students from Grenada (Figure 9-1).[18] The execution of Bishop on 19 October increased tensions even more. By 21 October, the

Organization of Eastern Caribbean States requested American assistance to ensure the stability of the government of Grenada and the safety of the students from the United States and those from other regional countries.[19(p2)] With little time for preparation, Combined Joint Task Force 120 (led by Vice Admiral Joseph Metcalf III of the US Navy's Second Fleet) commenced Operation Urgent Fury on 25 October 1983.[20] Land forces made up of "two Army Ranger battalions, some Special Forces, two 82nd Airborne Division brigades and a Marine Amphibious Unit secured all significant military objectives and successfully rescued all US citizens" within 4 days of commencement of the operation.[4(pp83–84)] While successful in accomplishing its objectives, the Task Force mission resulted in 18 service members KIA, 116 wounded in action (one of whom died of wounds later), and 28 nonbattle injuries.[21]

Planning for such a rapidly developing operation was challenging for military leaders, especially those charged with sustaining the maneuvering forces. In contrast to the British challenges in the Falklands (where distance served as the greatest challenge), American military planners struggled with the compressed timeline of the situation.[4(p84)] Most elements, such as the 82nd Airborne Division assets, operated on preexisting contingency plans.[22] Unfortunately, due to operational security considerations, many of the planning elements within the 82nd Airborne Division and the XVIII Airborne Corps were bypassed, eliminating planning elements that were well versed in rapid deployment planning scenarios.[4(pp91–92),20] The two 82nd Airborne Division brigades, who made up the bulk of the American land forces bound for Grenada, relied heavily on their preexisting rapid deployment packages to provide the appropriate amount of sustainment (including medical sustainment) for the entire operation.[4(pp93–94)]

Once mobilized for deployment, medical planners within the 82nd Airborne Division brigades began to unofficially alter their task organization to better support the mission. This was difficult, however, because some leaders within the organization were unaware of the mission destination until combat operations began.[4(p90)] The 307th Medical Battalion, 82nd Airborne Division, led by Lieutenant Colonel (LTC) Edward B Wilson, would serve as the division-level medical support for all land forces during the operation. Medical platoons organic to the Ranger elements, Special Forces teams, and the Airborne battalions would provide all medical support doctrinally organic to the unit.[4(p91),13] Fortunately, due to the division's normal tactical mission capability, 82nd Airborne Division medical assets were well suited for "maneuvering on the fly."

Based on its forced-entry mission, the airborne division is potentially separated from the larger medical support capabilities in the combat zone. The larger hospitals of the day, such as the MASH (mobile Army surgical hospital), were too large to "jump in" with the airborne medical assets during insertion operations.[20,23] The airborne medical companies were therefore augmented with small surgical teams of personnel and materiel, which would perform urgent surgeries normally provided only in a MASH or CSH (combat support hospital). Alerted on 24 October 1983, the 307th Medical Battalion sent an orthopedic surgeon (Colonel [COL] Joseph Jackson) and five medics with the 2nd Battalion, 2nd Brigade of the 82nd Airborne, which departed from Pope Air Force Base in North Carolina.[14,18,24] The team's mission was to augment the 2nd Battalion's battalion aid station and, if the battalion aid station moved off the airfield, remain at the airfield to establish a casualty collection point (CCP).[14,20] This CCP on the airfield would become the hub of patient evacuation throughout the operation.

As the invasion of Grenada commenced on 25 October, the first medical assets on the ground were the medics assigned to the Rangers, who parachuted from an altitude of 500 feet onto the airfield at 0500 hours, 12 hours before the advance elements of Charlie Company, 307th Medical Battalion (with 2nd Battalion, 2nd Brigade), arrived at Point Salines.[4(p83-84),14,20] COL Jackson and his team, however, did not jump into Grenada. Instead, they remained in the aircraft until it landed on the airfield,[25,26] reaching Point Salines at 2200 hours on 25 October. Jackson's team had no surgical capacity, bringing with them only a few items to conduct Advanced Trauma Life Support operations.[14] Furthermore, the only blood products and narcotic pain medications arrived in the Styrofoam container Jackson hand-carried onto the airfield in Point Salines.[25,26] Until the 307th could become more established, the medical support plan called for the Rangers and the other land forces to rely on Navy medical assets floating off shore. Ground commanders in the 82nd Airborne Division believed that these assets, the USS *Guam* and the USS *Saipan*, had a medical support capability equal to a 100-bed CSH or MASH.[4(p91)]

Early elements of the Rangers and the 82nd Airborne were expected to face stiff resistance upon landing in Grenada. Early intelligence indicated that Cuban workers and the Grenadian forces were organizing against the invasion.[13] Based on his understanding that the Navy could provide the medical support needed by his troops, the 82nd Airborne Division commander, Major General (MG) Edward L Trobaugh, delayed the arrival of critical combat support assets, including medical personnel, in exchange for more combat troops.[4(pp93-96)] By the morning of 26 October, MG Trobaugh and his staff learned that the Navy ships were not as capable as first thought.[4(pp97-98)] The USS *Guam* had one general surgeon and an orthopedic surgeon, as well as one operating room and eight patient beds.[14,25] The USS *Saigon* was not a fully staffed medical asset either. This misunderstanding of the capabilities available delayed the arrival of the rest of the 307th Medical Battalion (which included three physicians, a nurse anesthetist, and 14 others) until the afternoon of 26 October and the evening of 27 October.[4(pp97-98),25] Fortunately the Rangers experienced only light casualties initially, which allowed the few Army medical personnel on the ground to determine which assets were actually required in the forward areas and coordinate for shifts in deployment priority to get the needed medical assets on the ground—all while providing care to the few injured Rangers in Point Salines.[4(p99)]

Originally setting up operations in a construction shack just off of the runway at Point Salines (Figures 9-2 and 9-3), COL Jackson and his team received their first casualty at 0600 hours on 26 October (Figure 9-4). The soldier, who arrived on the hood of a dump truck, sustained gunshot wounds to bilateral sides of his chest, requiring chest tubes. Unfortunately, the medical aide bags airdropped for COL Jackson and his team contained no chest tubes. Jackson inserted a 14-gauge needle into both sides of the patient's chest before sending him off to the USS *Guam* by helicopter. Because there was no established coordination for medical evacuation, COL Jackson's team had to flag down a helicopter flying overhead. Unqualified to land on vessels at sea, the aircraft carrying this patient moved to three different naval vessels before finally locating and landing aboard the *Guam*. Fortunately, the prolonged evacuation did not negatively impact this patient's outcome.[14,24,25]

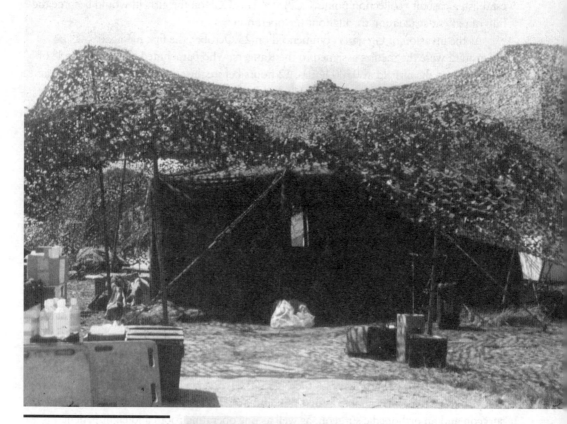

FIGURE 9-2. [Top] A view of the 307th Medical Battalion clearing station located just off of the airstrip at Point Salines, October–November 1983. Photograph courtesy of Colonel (Ret) Joseph P. Jackson, Jr, MD (private collection).

FIGURE 9-3. [Bottom] This tent, made out of a parachute, poles, and tree branches, served as the living quarters for a member of the surgical team located just off of the airstrip at Point Salines. October–November 1983. Photograph courtesy of Colonel (Ret) Joseph P. Jackson, Jr, MD (private collection).

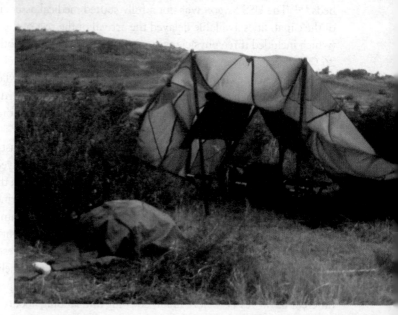

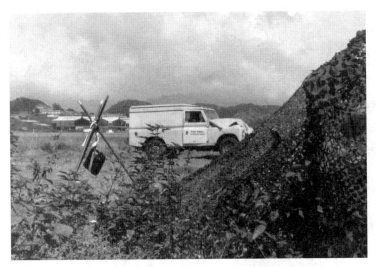

FIGURE 9-4. An "ambulance," acquired from the Grenada locals, sits outside the 307th Medical Battalion clearing station, October–November 1983. A makeshift hand washing station is also visible. Photograph courtesy of Colonel (Ret) Joseph P. Jackson, Jr, MD (private collection).

Later that day, COL Jackson's team moved the CCP from the shack to an area near the "jungle trees and out of mortar range." Continually working to improve their patient caring capacity, the team coordinated with the Rangers and Special Operations soldiers headquartered in the area to obtain much needed intravenous fluids and other medical supplies. Meanwhile, the young medic who escorted the patient to the *Guam* took time while aboard the ship to gather many badly needed medical supplies before returning to the Point Salines airfield. The throughput of medical supplies, equipment, and personnel was an apparent afterthought to the military planners, and personnel involved struggled to keep pace with operations on the ground.[24,25]

With the medical students secured by the morning of 26 October (Figure 9-5), the arrival of three medical evacuation helicopters from the 57th Medical Detachment on the morning of 27 October almost appeared unnecessary.[4(p100)] However, the arrival of the helicopters and the rest of Charlie Company, 307th Medical Battalion, on 27 October turned out to be fortunate, because the Rangers and paratroopers were poised at the time to assault the Cuban headquarters at Calivigny Barracks.[24,26] Though this objective was secured by 2100 hours,[26] two helicopters collided during the operation, and an attack helicopter inadvertently fired upon the 2nd Brigade tactical operations center, sending 45 casualties to Charlie Company, 307th Medical Battalion, in a 30-minute period.[4(p101),14,24,25] These patients, who arrived amid a violent rainstorm, were evaluated by flashlight while lying in the mud. Army chaplains, there to minister to the wounded, were asked to hold bags of intravenous fluids and assist with bandaging.[25] Nearly overwhelmed, the 307th evacuated four patients (and an accompanying physician and nurse anesthetist) by a US Air Force C-130 aircraft to the hospital at Roosevelt Roads Naval Air Station, Puerto Rico. The USS *Guam* was reserved for those casualties needing more urgent surgical care beyond the capabilities of the 307th Medical Battalion assets on the ground.[4(p101),14,24,25] The remainder of the 307th Medical Battalion would not arrive until the 6th day of the operation.[27]

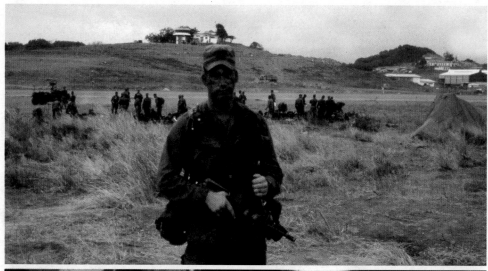

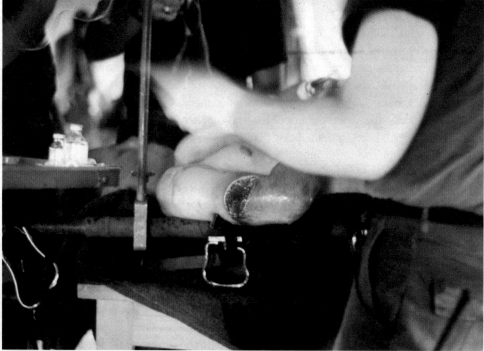

FIGURE 9-5. [Top] Rangers near the airstrip at Point Salines preparing for an air assault, October–November 1983. The Ranger in the foreground took time to show the medical team his assault camouflage. Photograph courtesy of Colonel (Rer) Joseph P. Jackson, Jr, MD (private collection).

FIGURE 9-6. [Bottom] Members of the surgical team at Point Salines clean a wound to the right arm of a soldier after he was injured by a 50-caliber round that ricocheted off of the front of a nearby weapon, October–November 1983. Photograph courtesy of Colonel (Ret) Joseph P. Jackson, Jr, MD (private collection).

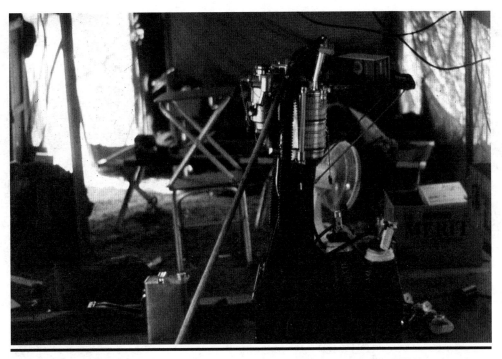

FIGURE 9-7. The interior of the surgical team's treatment tent, October–November 1983. Note the anesthesia apparatus in the foreground. Photograph courtesy of Colonel (Ret) Joseph P. Jackson, Jr, MD (private collection).

By the end of combat in Grenada (Figures 9-6 through 9-8), it became apparent to medical planners that many lessons would be learned from their experiences on the small island nation. While the medical mission was hindered significantly by the omission of medical planners from the planning stages of Urgent Fury and the absence of a senior medical commander in the Joint Task Force, the ingenuity of the medical leaders overcame most planning failures.[4(pp101–102),14,20] Perhaps the most glaring lesson was that the ground forces needed a "small, easy-to-insert surgical capability" to maneuver on the battlefield with the combat forces.[28] The experiences of COL Jackson and his team[24,25] reinforced the recommendations of medical leaders of the early 1980s, which advocated for the integration of small surgical assets into the medical plan of numerous tactical operations (real and training).[3–11] Based on British experiences in the Falklands, medical planners advocated for field surgical teams that are rapidly deployable and operational within 15 minutes.[14] Adding credence to this position, in 1984 COL Ron Bellamy published an article in *Military Medicine* that described the real concern for medical planners.[29]

Mid-1980s Evolution of Medical Planning

In his article, Bellamy identified the statistical reasons for combat deaths on the modern battlefield and found that many were preventable. The statistical significance of preventable

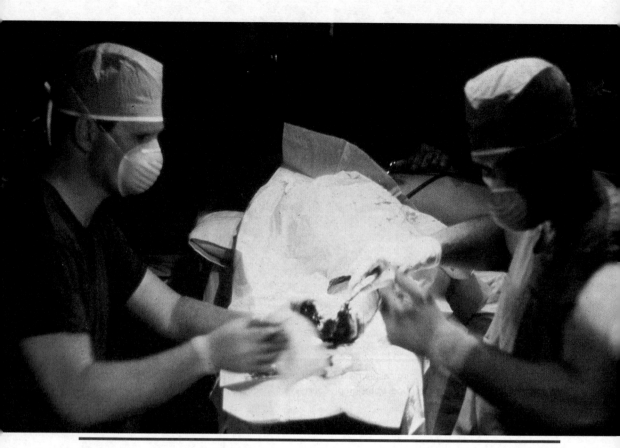

FIGURE 9-8. Surgeons cleansing a hand wound of a soldier in the makeshift operating room just off of the airstrip at Point Salines, October–November 1983. Photograph courtesy of Colonel (Ret) Joseph P. Jackson, Jr, MD (private collection).

deaths from extremity hemorrhage, tension pneumothorax, and airway obstruction caused a revolution in medical training in the Army.[29] Combat medic training was realigned, and combat lifesaver training developed, to focus on identifying and treating these conditions.[30] Medical leaders began to consider the development of small, agile surgical assets to fill the geographic void between the fast-maneuvering combat units and the large, cumbersome surgical hospitals. Also in 1984, after the Army's Medical System Program Review at the Academy of Health Sciences, 82nd Airborne Division medical planners began looking at developing such a surgical capability, modeling it after the French parachutist surgical unit or the British parachute clearing troop.[20] In efforts that were replicated by the 326th Medical Battalion, 101st Airborne Division,[27] this "surgical squad field light," a portion of the treatment platoon assigned to the headquarters and Alpha Company of the 307th Medical Battalion, was a precursor to the eventual 782nd FST.[31]

Surgical squads, such as the one assigned to the 307th Medical Battalion, became one of six modular support systems for division-level and corps-level units. The 10-person squad consisted of one general surgeon, one orthopedic surgeon, two medical-surgical nurses, two certified registered nurse anesthetists, two operating room technicians, and two licensed practical nurses. Although surgical squads were normally a corps-level asset, the Army allocated two organic surgical squads to each airborne and air assault division. The squads were meant to save lives, provide resuscitative surgery for seriously wounded or injured casualties, and preserve physical function. To accomplish their mission, the squads had to co-locate with some sort of holding capability (such as a division clearing station), usually in the brigade or division support area, for postoperative support. These assets were placed in the divisions in the mid to late 1980s, and in 1991 they were included in Army doctrine.[32]

The 44th Medical Brigade, a subordinate command of the XVIII Airborne Corps at Fort Bragg, North Carolina, also participated in the early development of a forward surgical capability. The brigade first established the 274th Medical Detachment as a test organization in 1987. COL Bruce T Miketinac, commander of the 44th Medical Brigade, carved the 274th Medical Detachment (General Surgical) from the airborne positions allocated to the 36th Clearing Company, which held the majority of the brigade's airborne positions. The 274th was given provisional status.[27,33] Colloquially referred to as the 1st FAST (Forward Airborne Surgical Team), the 274th was activated after Vietnam as a general surgery detachment.

An Army Nurse Corps officer, Captain Steve Janney, recommended that the surgical detachment add a postoperative capability and equip the team so that it could participate in airborne operations. Janney teamed with Major David Rivera, a surgeon assigned to Fort Bragg's Womack Army Community Hospital, to identify the needed changes to the 274th Medical Detachment table of organization and equipment (TO&E) to meet this new airborne, surgical, and postoperative capability.[27] From 1987 to 1989, leaders within the brigade tested personnel and equipment schemes during field training exercises. Some equipment posed a challenge for the brigade, which worked around normal Army acquisition processes to purchase and redistribute supplies to stand up the team. The draw-over anesthesia device, for example, was used by the British during the Falklands campaign but was not approved for use in the United States amid concerns about inconsistent delivery of the volatile gases used for anesthesia. The sturdy construction and size of the draw-over device, however, made it the optimal choice for use by the new surgical capability, and the unapproved piece of equipment was added to the 274th Medical Detachment TO&E. The draw-over, however, would be limited to combat use only.[27]

As designed, the team of 17 personnel was capable of loading a two-bed operating room and four-bed intensive care capability onto two Air Force pallets and into a C-130 aircraft for movement to an area of operation. The team and equipment could parachute from the same aircraft and were capable of becoming fully operational within 2 hours of exiting the aircraft.[33] LTC Alan Muench, assigned to Eisenhower Army Medical Center at Fort Gordon, Georgia, soon joined the team as a Professional Filler System (PROFIS) officer. A former Special Forces Group surgeon familiar with operating in austere environments, Muench recommended adding a communications specialist, an administrative officer, and an additional noncommissioned officer to the team.[27]

On 8 March 1989, as a demonstration of the team's capabilities, the 274th Medical Detachment parachuted into Honduras as a part of the annual Ahuas Tara 89 exercise. After securing their equipment on the drop zone near La Paz and preparing it for sling load, the surgical team moved by helicopter to Soto Cano Air Base The team was accompanied by MG James Rumbaugh, then commanding general at Walter Reed Army Medical Center, who provided instrumental support for the development of the 274th Medical Detachment while serving as the commander of Womack Army Community Hospital at Fort Bragg.[27,33,34] Tragically, Rumbaugh suffered a hard landing on the drop zone and died while being transported to Brooke Army Medical Center in San Antonio, Texas, for treatment.[33,34]

The 5th MASH, another subordinate unit of the 44th Medical Brigade, also began developing a forward surgical capability in the mid-1980s. Called the 5th FST, this team would be heavier than the 274th Medical Detachment and would not be air-droppable. Instead, it was "designed to enhance the medical capability organic to the Joint Special Operations Command." Both the 274th Medical Detachment and the 5th FST were allocated canvas tents, a small generator for operating room lights, and supplies needed for life-saving resuscitative surgery.[27] Though small surgical elements such as these were the beginning of the development of forward surgical capabilities,[27,28] it would be another decade and two significant conflicts before the American FST became a doctrinal reality.

Operation Just Cause: The 1989 US Invasion of Panama

The US invasion of Panama in 1989 did not suffer from the planning shortages that befell Operation Urgent Fury. The situation in Panama developed slowly over the course of the 1980s, leading American leaders to believe that military action in the isthmus nation might become necessary.[35] Expecting a short-notice need for agile assets on the ground, Operation Just Cause was the first time in US Army history that a forward surgical asset, though only considered provisional, was formally deployed to a theater of operations. Developed after the American experience in Grenada, and with strong consideration of Bellamy's information about preventable combat deaths, the Army's new surgical squads were in the works by 1986. By the time of the invasion of Panama, the surgical teams were trained parachutists and were important members of the invasion plan.[28]

Operation Just Cause stemmed from a long, complicated relationship between the United States, Panama, and Manuel Noriega. The United States had been involved in the security of Panama since the beginning of construction on the Panama Canal in 1904, deeming the operability of the canal to be a matter of national security.[36(p5)] In 1983, after the death of his dictator mentor, Brigadier General Omar Torrijos, Noriega took command of the Panama Defense Force and began to wield absolute power in the small nation. By 1987, the United States had become concerned about Noriega's abuse of power in Panama and his known involvement in the drug trade. On 5 February 1988, the Panamanian dictator was indicted in US federal courts on drug trafficking charges, irritating an increasingly aggressive Noriega. Concerned that his increasing hostility toward the United States, and his growing relationships with Cuba and Nicaragua, might threaten the Panama Canal (which accounted for $35 billion in cargo traffic annually) and the 35,000

Americans (including 9,500 service members) living in Panama or stationed near the Canal Zone, the Department of Defense began in 1988 to develop plans for the possible invasion of Panama.[35,36(p6),37]

Dubbed "Blue Spoon," the contingency plan called for the gradual build-up of troops in the Canal Zone (to a maximum of 13,000 troops just prior to the commencement of operations), with increasing economic and diplomatic pressure being placed on the Panamanian government in an attempt to "minimize the adverse effects of economic sanctions on the Panamanian people, while demonstrating the US resolve to secure the Canal Zone and force Noriega from power."[36(pp7–8)] As American forces moved into the Canal Zone, relations with Panama deteriorated rapidly. On 15 December 1989, the Panamanian legislative body declared war on the United States and named Noriega the "maximum leader." By 17 December 1989, violence towards Americans in Panama reached new heights, climaxing with the death of a Marine at the hands of a Panamanian soldier. President George HW Bush grew frustrated with the situation in Panama and ordered the commencement of Operation Just Cause, an escalation from "Blue Spoon."[35,36(pp27–28)]

A well-planned operation, Just Cause was led by Joint Task Force South (under the XVIII Airborne Corps) and consisted of the 193rd Separate Infantry Brigade, elements from the 82nd Airborne Division, the 7th Infantry Division (Light), the 5th Infantry Division (Mechanized), a Marine expeditionary battalion, a military police brigade, Special Forces elements, and a contingent of combat support elements.[38] Joint Task Force South was tasked to protect American lives, secure key sites and facilities, and neutralize the Panamanian Defense Force. American troops would also be expected to restore law and order while supporting the installation of a US-recognized government in Panama.[37]

Operational security remained a concern, but combat leaders had learned from the lessons of the recent past and integrated medical personnel into the operational planning, beginning in March 1989. COL Jerome Foust, commander of the 44th Medical Brigade, and four other medical planners (two of whom were Special Operators) took part in the medical planning.[27,37] Medical support was aligned under the Joint Task Force South Surgeon[39] (COL Foust) and included the organic medical assets of each maneuver unit, the 5th MASH FST, the 274th Medical Detachment, the Air Force's 24th Medical Group and 1st Aeromedical Evacuation Squadron, a portion of the 7th Medical Battalion, a portion of the 307th Medical Battalion, the 142nd Medical Battalion, and the 214th Medical Detachment.[37,38,40] The mission of the 44th Medical Brigade and its subordinates included: the provision of resuscitative surgical and postoperative care and patient holding capacity for all Joint Task Force South elements; the provision of ground and air evacuation; the provision of medical supply and resupply to all forces; the assumption of command and control for all Army and Air Force nondivisional and installation medical assets in theater (Gorgas Army Hospital and the clinics at Howard Air Force Base); and the provision of medical regulating for all patients leaving the joint operating area. Unfortunately, due to operational security, most of the leadership subordinate to COL Foust was unaware of these requirements until the units were already moving towards Panama.[37]

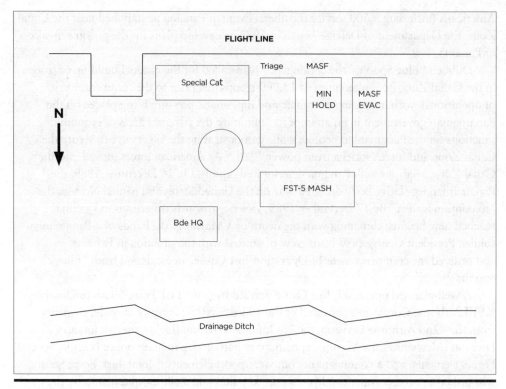

FIGURE 9-9. A diagram of the Joint Casualty Collection Point at Howard Air Force Base, Panama, early in Operation Just Cause, December 1989. Diagram courtesy of the Army Medical Department Television and Multimedia, Fort Sam Houston, TX, Video #A1701-90-0087.

The initial medical support plan (Figure 9-9) anticipated a very short operation and called for establishing a joint casualty collection point (JCCP) at Howard Air Force Base in Panama, where casualties would be triaged, treated, and evacuated as necessary. Evacuated casualties would be medically regulated to either Wilford Hall Medical Center at Lackland Air Force Base or Brooke Army Medical Center at Fort Sam Houston, both in San Antonio, soon after being surgically stabilized. Initially, Air Force leadership expressed concern that patients evacuated so soon after surgery might not fare well during transport. LTC Robert Brannon, commander of the 1st Aeromedical Evacuation Squadron (AES), intervened, however, and equipped the evacuation aircraft with the supplies and equipment necessary to care for critically ill patients, assuring Air Force leaders that his team was ready for the mission. Gorgas Army Hospital, in Panama, was not included in the plans to cover the medical needs of the operation, largely because much of the staff was made up of Panamanian local nationals.[27,38] The facility's proximity to Panamanian Defense Forces strongholds also made its use in the initial invasion a high-risk proposition.[39] The medical assets at Howard Air Force Base were the focus of the medical support for the majority of the mission (Figures 9-10 through 9-13).

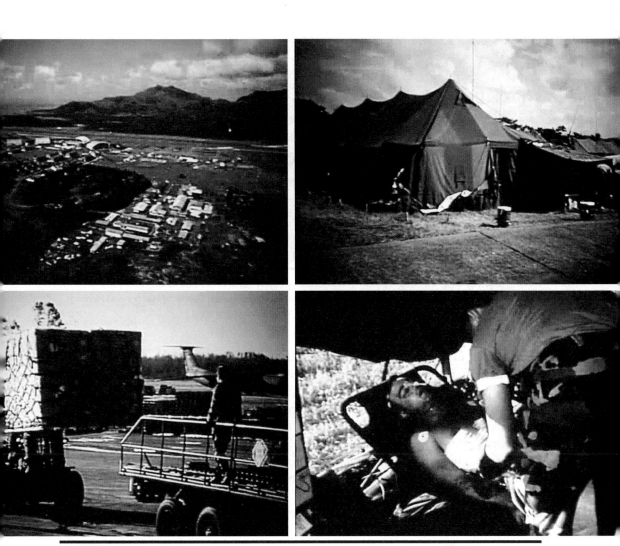

FIGURE 9-10. [Top Left] An aerial view of Howard Air Force Base, Panama. Photograph courtesy of the Army Medical Department Television and Multimedia, Fort Sam Houston, TX, Video #A1701-90-0087, 1990.

FIGURE 9-11. [Bottom Left] Airmen off-loading supplies at Howard Air Force Base, Panama. Army Medical Department Television and Multimedia, Fort Sam Houston, TX, Video #A1701-90-0087, 1990.

FIGURE 9-12. [Top Right] One of the tents used as the Joint Casualty Collection Point just off of the flight line at Howard Air Force Base, Panama. Army Medical Department Television and Multimedia, Fort Sam Houston, TX, Video #A1701-90-0087, 1990.

FIGURE 9-13. [Bottom Right] A soldier recovering from abdominal surgery at the Joint Casualty Collection Point just off of the flight line at Howard Air Force Base, Panama. Army Medical Department Television and Multimedia, Fort Sam Houston, Texas, Video #A1701-90-0087, 1990.

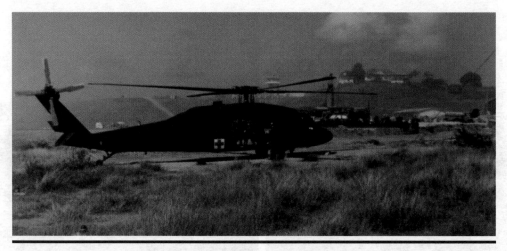

FIGURE 9-14. An Army medical evacuation helicopter sits in a field in Panama, awaiting an evacuation mission. Undated. Photograph courtesy of the Army Medical Department Center of History and Heritage, Fort Sam Houston, TX, Image #19851176-5-large.jpg.

Expecting to be in Panama until 5 January 1990, the 1st AES mobilized almost immediately after the National Command Authority ordered the invasion.[39] The first of thousands of additional troops bound for Panama,[35] the initial echelon of the 1st AES and the provisional FST from the 5th MASH flew from Pope Air Force Base, North Carolina, at approximately 2045 hours on 17 December 1989, 3 hours after being notified for mobilization. This early element of medical professionals arrived at Howard Air Force Base, Panama, and became operational at approximately 0200 on 19 December, nearly 24 hours before the invasion was scheduled to begin.[39] By 0100 hours on 20 December, Special Operations forces began attacking key Panamanian targets. Forty-five minutes later, conventional forces began movement to seize the land approaches to Panama City.[36(pp38–40),37] By 0115, the first casualties arrived at Howard Air Force Base. The first C-141, carrying approximately 40 patients and two medical attendants, lifted off for Kelly Air Force Base in San Antonio at approximately 0715 on 20 December 1989.[39]

The JCCP, located just off of the runway at Howard Air Force Base, was home to the 44th Medical Brigade tactical operations center, the 5th MASH FST, and the 1st AES. The Air Force's 24th Medical Group, normally assigned to staff the medical facilities at Howard, also provided personnel and coordinated for some power, billeting, communication, and supply requirements for the JCCP. Initially, 14 physicians (including 10 surgeons) triaged patients as they arrived at the JCCP. While the primary means of evacuation was air (Figure 9-14), the JCCP received patients from a variety of sources, including UH-1, UH-60, OH-6, HH-53, CH-47, and C-130 aircraft, as well as bus, van, pick-up truck, high-mobility multipurpose wheeled vehicle (HMMWV), and motorcycle. Some patients also walked in.[27,37]

Those patients requiring surgical intervention were taken to the tent for the 5th MASH FST for care. The patients remained at the FST for up to 4 hours before being transferred

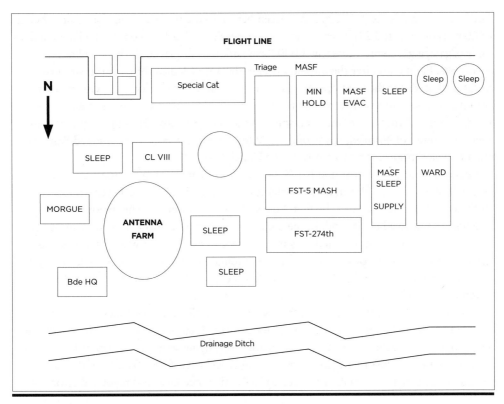

FIGURE 9-15. A diagram of the Joint Casualty Collection Point at Howard Air Force Base, Panama, late in Operation Just Cause, December 1989–January 1990. Diagram courtesy of the Army Medical Department Television and Multimedia, Fort Sam Houston, TXs, Video #A1701-90-0087.

to the nearby mobile aeromedical staging facility (MASF), manned by the 1st AES, in preparation for evacuation to Kelly Air Force Base. In the first 48 hours of the operation, the JCCP had no holding capacity, and all patients were evacuated out of theater if they could not be immediately returned to duty. Eventually, the JCCP was augmented with the 274th Medical Detachment and a clearing platoon that, combined with the MASF, provided an 80-bed holding capacity.[27,37] The 307th Medical Battalion deployed a small surgical team with the 82nd Airborne Division as well. However, while the 307th Medical Battalion treated 474 Americans and 288 Panamanians in a 23-day period, the seriously injured patients were taken to the JCCP (Figure 9-15) for treatment and evacuation rather than being treated surgically by 307th Medical Battalion personnel.[27]

By Christmas 1989, most of the Panamanian Defense Forces were neutralized, the Panama Canal remained open, and American forces secured the release of thirteen hostages held by remnant Panamanian Defense Forces.[36(pp49–53)] With Noriega's capture still outstanding, the American military focus in Panama turned to securing the new Panamanian government and providing humanitarian assistance to local nationals in need. Dubbed Operation Promote Liberty, the civil affairs mission took ownership of most Joint

Task Force South assets.[36(p65)] From 26 December to 3 January, American forces distributed 1,660 tons of food and 218 tons of medical supplies (worth $3 million) to the Panamanians while organizing a camp for nearly 5,000 local nationals displaced during combat operations. Eight days after the invasion began, the 44th Medical Brigade transitioned all surgical needs for the joint operations area to a team of professionals at Gorgas Army Hospital, whose staff was augmented by staff from a medical mission in Honduras as well as Fitzsimmons Army Community Hospital in the United States. On 3 January 1990, just after the capture of Noriega, many of the 17,000 American troops (who entered Panama just a few days prior) began to return to the United States.[36(pp63–69),37]

According to COL Foust, the JCCP medical staff treated a total of 365 patients, over half of which were Panamanian civilians or Panamanian Defense Force troops. Of these, 261 patients came in the first 2 days of the operation.[27,37] The majority of the patients (233) arrived by ground. In the 8 days they supported Just Cause, the 5th MASH FST and the 274th FST conducted 73 surgical procedures. Only 22 were categorized as "major surgeries," most of which involved abdominal or chest procedures. Specifically, the cases were categorized as: head (5, or 7%), chest (10, or 14%), abdomen (11, or 15%), extremity (35, or 48%), and multiple wounds (12, or 16%).[37]

All told, of the 26,369 American troops deployed to Panama for Operation Just Cause, 322 suffered injuries and an additional 23 were fatalities.[31,36(p65),37] Only two of these service members reached an FST prior to death,[38] one dying while in surgery at Howard Air Force Base and the other dying after arriving at Kelly Air Force Base.[39] Of the 322 American casualties, 258 were evacuated to Kelly Air Force Base and regulated to one of the two military hospitals in San Antonio. Of these casualties, 149 suffered only one injury, while approximately 90 had two or more injuries. The vast majority of all injuries (86%) were the result of penetrating injuries, and 71 casualties were injured during the nighttime airborne operation into Panama.[39,41]

As a low-intensity conflict, Operation Just Cause provided valuable insight into the future doctrine of American FSTs. The mission marked the first time an American FST parachuted into a combat zone. Unfortunately, the team's effectiveness as a medical asset on the drop zone was hindered by the need to wait for the aircraft to land before the team could access and set up its equipment.[28] Future iterations of the airborne FST would see the equipment (hardened for the airborne mission) parachuted onto the drop zone minutes prior to members of the team exiting their own aircraft.

Establishing a medical logistics train and an evacuation pathway soon after combat operations began were also important factors. The early hours of the operation resulted in the greatest workload for the medical teams. Of the 257 patients treated at the JCCP, 192 casualties were treated, stabilized, and evacuated in the first 27 hours. Furthermore, the surgical team at Howard conducted 20 major surgeries in the first 36 hours of operation.[39] Additionally, and unexpectedly, one battalion aid station reported caring for more than 140 casualties in the first 12 hours of the operation, 100 of whom were Panamanian local nationals. This early transition to humanitarian care forced upon the American medical logistics system a sudden need for obstetrics and gynecological, field sanitation, and pediatric supplies and equipment.[38,42] Such factors may not have been anticipated prior to

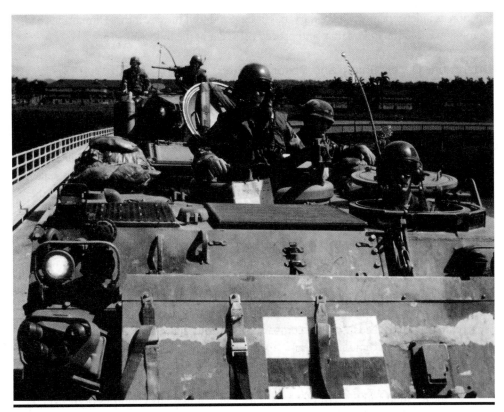

FIGURE 9-16. Medics of the 4th Battalion, 6th Infantry Regiment, 5th Infantry Division (Mechanized) crossing the Panama Canal in an M113 ambulance days after the invasion into Panama, December 1989–January 1990. Photograph courtesy of the Army Medical Department Center of History and Heritage, Fort Sam Houston, TX, Image #19851176-22-large.jpg.

Operation Just Cause, but this American experience would serve as a prelude to important considerations prior to the employment of FSTs in future operations (Figure 9-16).

Operation Just Cause served as an important step towards the formal establishment of FSTs in the US Army, validating their usefulness in a combat zone.[27,37] Vetted in the experiences of Urgent Fury and Just Cause, agility and adaptability would soon become a benchmark of forward surgical doctrine. Various Army units began to create ad hoc, locally funded and equipped surgical squads similar to the 274th Medical Detachment or the 5th MASH FST. The 25th Infantry Division developed a "light surgical unit deployable," while the 6th Infantry Division deployed an airborne-capable team to Australia in 1991 to conduct exercises with the Royal Australian Surgical Team.[27] In rapid deployment scenarios, health service support operations face numerous challenges, including operating in urban, mountainous, and jungle environments. Additionally, in operations during this period medical planners found that supply, communication, evacuation, patient accountability, and task force composition considerations were hindered by operational security considerations.[37,38] The ability of the FST to adapt to the operating environment, and to function as independently as necessary, might have reduced the effect these limitations had on mission execution in Panama, and proved prescient in the following years.

Operations Desert Shield and Desert Storm: The 1990–1991 Persian Gulf War

As the operational environment has evolved, rapid deployment of American military assets in response to a sudden tasking from the National Command Authority has become an increasingly likely occurrence. These small, low-intensity conflicts, while more frequent, have not completely replaced the large-scale wars of decades past. For the US military, the consecutive operations Desert Shield and Desert Storm served as the first large-scale conflict since the Vietnam era, resulting in more than 500,000 personnel deployed to the Middle East by the end of hostilities in March 1991.[43,44] As the conflict began, there was no immediate need for small-scale surgical assets in the deserts of the Middle East. American forces moved into the region over several months prior to the start of combat operations, allowing for the gradual buildup of medical assets in Saudi Arabia and other Arab nations in the region, which eventually peaked at 44 Army hospitals (more than 13,000 hospital beds).[43,45] The US Air Force also provided 15 hospitals (more than 1,000 beds), while the US Navy provided three fleet hospitals (approximately 1,500 beds) and two hospital ships (approximately 2,000 beds).[45] Once combat operations began, however, the need for a highly mobile surgical capability became apparent.

In the months after the fall of the Berlin Wall, the strategic equation throughout the world changed significantly. The Soviet Union fell, and with its collapse, the alliances between the Kremlin and Eastern Block nations, Cuba, and many countries of the Middle East disintegrated. The United States became the lone "super power" and began to renegotiate alliances with some former members of the Soviet Union and Warsaw Pact nations. Free of the diplomatic reins laid upon him through Iraq's patron-client relationship with the Soviet Union, Saddam Hussein grew emboldened to lay claim to the oil-based wealth of the kingdom of Kuwait in order to pay off the debt his nation accrued during the Iran-Iraq War of the 1980s.[46(pp1–2)] Hussein invaded Kuwait in the first days of August 1990. The United States, at the behest of the Saudi king, acted quickly to position troops between Iraq and Saudi Arabia, signaling America's intent to protect the oil-rich nation. The first American troops began arriving in Riyadh, Saudi Arabia, on 9 August 1990.[46(pp5–6)] Within a few short months, as tensions rose and Saddam Hussein became more resistant to international pressures to withdrawal from Kuwait, the American-led coalition grew to more than 500,000 soldiers.[43]

Months of political wrangling between the United States, the United Nations (UN), the Arab community, and Iraq proved fruitless. Hussein refused to withdraw his forces from Kuwait. The prelude to a lightning quick defeat of the Iraqi forces began on 17 January 1991.[46(p29)] Massive air strikes and missile bombardments nearly eliminated the Iraqi military command and control capabilities. The coalition achieved air supremacy and began targeting the Iraqi Scud missile architecture in an attempt to limit the missile's impact on the coalition ground forces staging in the region.[46(pp29–30)] Thirty-eight days into the air campaign, the ground assault into Kuwait and Iraq began.[46(p35)] Starting on 24 February 1991, General Norman Schwarzkopf's now infamous "left hook" sealed the Iraqi forces in Kuwait and cut off the Iraqi logistics trains coming from Baghdad, eliminating any opportunity for the Hussein regime to mount a significant resistance, while the bulk of the coalition pushed the Iraqi forces from Kuwait.[46(pp34–63)] Coalition forces achieved their objective, the liberation of Kuwait, in a little more than 4 days.

The health service support plan for operations Desert Shield and Desert Storm required the "fastest military buildup the AMEDD [Army Medical Department] had ever undertaken."[47] Concerned over the potential use of chemical weapons (Hussein was known to have used chemical weapons against Iranian soldiers during the previous decade), the Army ordered 23,493 healthcare personnel to Southwest Asia. In addition to executing other medical missions, these healthcare providers equated to 13,580 patient beds in 44 hospital units throughout the theater of operations.[48,49(pp12–13)] By the time combat operations began, 198 medical units littered the deserts of Southwest Asia.[48(p12)]

Because the Army was in the midst of a medical support reorganization, which saw many Army Forces Command medical units fielding deployable medical systems (DEPMEDS) and doctrine moving to the Medical Force 2000 concept, many of these hospital units were ill-equipped for maneuvering on the battlefield with the high-speed flow of operations.[43,47,48(pp4–5),49,50] Of the 44 Army hospitals in theater, 35 completed the transition to DEPMEDs before the operation began. The other nine hospitals (from the Reserve component) staffed host-nation facilities in Saudi Arabia and did not need to transition at that time.[51] However, hospital units lacked the equipment necessary to move the supplies and equipment needed to function. Moving a MASH, with its personnel and 1,450 tons (or 42,000 cubic feet) of supplies and equipment, required enough trucks to move 21 M1A1 Abrams main battle tanks.[48(p40)] Similarly, moving a CSH, with all of its personnel and equipment, would take approximately 7 calendar days.[48(p42)] In development since the early 1980s, the Medical Force 2000 concept did not recognize the need of FSTs beyond an augmentation capability. The goal of this concept was to move state-of-the-art surgical capabilities forward, but it did not formally call for movement of forward resuscitative capabilities outside of the hospital setting.[27] Instead, to meet the health service support challenges brought on by General Schwarzkopf's fast-paced maneuvers on the battlefield, commanders developed adjustments in the operability of these medical units.

To meet the need for speed and mobility, the two Army component command elements took varying approaches to adjusting how they employed the CSHs and MASHs, assigned as corps-level assets. Deployed in a ratio of roughly one per division, the MASH became the locus of healthcare for the maneuver units.[52] The XVIII Airborne Corps attempted to make its hospital units completely mobile. In doing so, the Corps actually reduced the surgical and bed capacity of its hospitals by half, including one MASH that had 12 beds and four operating room tables.[48(p43),52] Rather than reducing capacity, the VII Corps decided to keep its hospital units intact, moving them as complete sets when necessary. They were unable to keep up with the combat operations, however, and were forced to accept increasingly long evacuation routes as a consequence.[43,46(p43–44)] In the end, only the 159th MASH became fully operational for the VII Corps.[52]

Although it was unplanned, employment of the 5th MASH and the 274th FST (Airborne), formerly the 274th Medical Detachment, both assigned to elements of the XVIII Airborne Corps, served as the "proof of concept" for the FST of future Army medical doctrine. The 5th MASH FST, a subcomponent of the MASH (as it was designed and employed during this war), was meant to break off from the MASH and push forward in an area with the advancing maneuver units.[43,44,48,53] Once in place, the FST would function independently while the rest of the MASH moved forward (over 24–36 hours). The FST's 20 personnel and two operating room tables were designed to be operational within 2 hours.[43,44,53]

During the ground portion of Operations Desert Shield and Desert Storm, the 5th MASH was tasked with moving into Iraq as a part of the "left hook." The 5th MASH forward surgical element (FSE), a 110-person element with four operating room tables, pushed into Iraq and operated fully for 48 hours before being joined by the 5th MASH (-). The 5th MASH (-), a slightly larger portion of the MASH (but not the main body of the hospital), provided a 36-bed hospital capacity and four operating room tables. Once joined up, the 5th MASH FSE and 5th MASH (-) combined to care for injured patients for 7 days inside of Iraq. The 5th MASH FST, a subcomponent of the 5th MASH FSE, pushed even farther into Iraqi territory and operated for a week while American combat elements retrograded into Saudi Arabia, receiving much of its logistical support from other medical elements (battalion aid stations and forward support companies) in the area.[27,43,44,54]

The 274th FST (Airborne), commanded by LTC Al Muench, became the lead element of Task Force 6, a medical task force created by COL Eldon Ideus, commander of the 1st Medical Group. Supported by a platoon from the 595th Clearing Company, a platoon from the 547th Clearing Company, and the 565th Ground Ambulance Company, Task Force 6 was attached to the 24th Infantry Division (Mechanized) and provided care to elements of the lead brigade as they entered Iraq. Although 100% mobile, proximity and poor weather forced the task force to work closely with the division medical company, using the company's expandable container trucks to perform surgery after the division's first engagement. Once weather improved, Task Force 6 moved with the assaulting elements of the 24th Infantry Division, using its canvas shelters to provide cover during surgery on three separate occasions. By the time the cease-fire was announced, Task Force 6 had moved past Objective Orange near the Euphrates River and began movement east along Highway 8. Unexpectedly, the medical element's largest onslaught of casualties came after the cease-fire, when an Iraqi element unaware of the cessation of hostilities attacked the 24th Infantry Division, producing a large number of Iraqi casualties.[27]

While not the only FSTs operational during Operations Desert Shield and Desert Storm, the XVIII Airborne Corps employment of the 5th MASH FST and the 274th Medical Detachment demonstrated how the operational limitations of MASH and CSH units could be overcome. In the years following Operations Desert Shield and Desert Storm, medical planners began to evaluate future developments in combat operations, operating environments, and strategic threats.[48] For example, during a September 1991 forward surgery conference sponsored by the Army Medical Department Center and School, medical leaders from the 5th MASH, 101st Airborne Division, Special Operations Command, 44th Medical Brigade, and XVIII Airborne Corps used their combat experiences to shape forward surgical doctrine, establishing that an FST would have enough supplies to be capable of treating 10 seriously injured patients in 24 hours. Further, conference attendees agreed that after 48 hours of continuous operations, the assigned FST personnel would need to be rotated out in order to maintain the surgical capability at that location.[27] Non-Department of Defense entities, such as the General Accounting Office, made recommendations on the future of war as well.[48] Medical units needed to be lighter, more rapidly deployable, and fully mobile, many reports argued.[48,50,55] Foreseeing an operational environment that did not include air superiority, but required fast-moving or distant combat operations, medical planners recognized that "[p]roviding good medical care to wounded soldiers *where* they really need it may require [the Army] to sacrifice equipment and supplies as a cost of doing business."[55] In time, many MASH units were deactivated as a part of the Medical Reengineering Initiative, the successor concept to Medical Force 2000,[27] making room on the Army rolls for the rise of individually designated FSTs.

TRANSITION TO FORMAL FORWARD SURGICAL TEAM DESIGNATION

It would be more than a decade before the Army faced another major conflict that required the linear battlefield and fast-moving pace of combat seen in Operation Desert Storm. The downward trend of DOW rates for American forces (from 9.0% in World War I to 0.5% in Operation Desert Storm), and the ease of victory in Operation Desert Storm, gave the American military a newfound sense of strength.[1(p8)] As the 20th century came to a close with the United States as the lone "super power," the National Command Authority increasingly tasked American military personnel to enforce peace in situations throughout the world. These relatively small, low-intensity conflicts (sometimes referred to as asymmetric warfare) appeared to be the future of American military missions. Yet major combat operations, and the desire to reduce the DOW rates even further, remained at the forefront of medical operational planning. Medical planners recognized the usefulness of the FST in a variety of operational settings and knew that such environments would require "increasingly mobile and flexible trauma surgical support."[43]

Operations Restore Hope and Continue Hope: Somalia 1993

Though interested in demonstrating the capabilities of the FST, military medical planners could not justify the use of FSTs in every military operation in the 1990s. Popularized by the storied events of October 1993, commonly referred to as the "Black Hawk Down" incident, Operations Restore Hope and Continue Hope (8 December 1992–25 March 1994) were generally inconsequential to the development of FSTs in the US Army.[56,57(pp483–485)] Aimed at providing armed delivery of relief supplies to the impoverished and famine-stricken citizens of Somalia, the UN-sanctioned operations developed in phases, allowing for deliberate medical planning and positioning, rather than the urgent deployment of an agile FST. Additionally, with the involvement of some 38,000 soldiers from 23 different nations, the operations were on a larger scale than could be adequately supported by FSTs.[56]

Instead, operations Restore Hope and Continue Hope were supported by the 86th Evacuation Hospital out of Fort Campbell, Kentucky, followed by the 42nd Field Hospital (Fort Knox, Kentucky) and the 46th CSH (Fort Devens, Massachusetts) in rotation.[57(pp484–485)] The facility, which at one point reached a capacity of 104 beds, consistently cared for 40 to 50 patients in the emergency room and approximately 50 inpatients per day, well beyond the capabilities of a FST.[57(p491)] It was the 46th CSH that absorbed the brunt of the casualties when Task Force Ranger attempted to capture Somali warlord Mohamed Farrah Aidid on 3 October 1993. The 46th CSH had only 52 beds, half of the previous iterations of the hospital, and was only staffed for 32 beds. In 2 days, the 46th CSH received 60 casualties from the operation, conducted 56 operative procedures, and evacuated 55 patients to Landstuhl Army Medical Center in Germany.[57(p495)] Across the span of the operations, the 11 contingency hospitals in Somalia saw a total of 5,938 admissions and 198 strategic evacuations.[56] Certainly, the scope and length of medical coverage required in Somalia could not have been better provided by a FST.

United Nations Intervention in the Former Republic of Yugoslavia: 1992–2004

Almost simultaneously, along the Mediterranean Sea, unrest in the formerly Soviet-backed Republic of Yugoslavia splintered the nation into eight geopolitical entities. By December 1991, nearly 10,000 Balkan citizens died at the hands of their fellow countrymen and another 600,000 became refugees[57(p503)] as the various political entities jockeyed for power and the republics maneuvered for independence. By April 1992, as civil war erupted, the UN (under Security Council Resolution 749) authorized the movement of a peacekeeping contingent to the region, scattering personnel throughout the Bosnia and Croatia republics.[57(p503),58] UN Protection Forces, led by a US contingent, swelled to more than 40,000 personnel from 38 different countries by 1995.[59] Throughout this civil war, even with the UN troop presence, between 140,000 and 250,000 people were killed and 1.3 million sought refuge throughout the Balkan region by the time the Dayton Peace Accords were signed in 1995.[58]

Health service support for the initial peacekeeping contingent in Bosnia and Croatia came from Europe-based MASHs, which were charged with providing Role 3 coverage to the UN Protection Force. The 212th MASH was ordered to deploy in October 1992, landing in Zagreb, Croatia, the following month. The 60-bed hospital located at Camp Pleso, just outside of Zagreb, was ordered to provide care and a 30-day patient hold capability for the over 20,000 strong UN forces, including UN civilians in the area.[57(p505),60(pp18–20)] A joint, unified effort, the Role 3 responsibility at Zagreb rotated from the 212th MASH to the 502nd MASH (April 1993–October 1993), then to the Air Force's 48th Air Transportable Hospital (October 1993–March 1994), and finally to the Navy's Fleet Hospital 6 (March 1994–August 1994).[60(p16)] Role 2 care in theater was assigned to the European partners in the UN Protection Force.[60(pp19–23)]

FSTs were used in the early operations in Bosnia and Croatia, specifically in locations such as Kinin in the Republic of Serbian Krajina and Visoko in Bosnia and Herzegovina.[59] They were not, however, employed by American units. During the initial rotations of American medical units, the 212th and 502nd MASHs (surrounded by a large population of refugees) clung to the initial guidance for the medical rules of engagement and avoided sending medical personnel out into the various sectors of the theater.[60(p20)] It was not until the 48th Air Transportable Hospital took charge of Role 3 care that Americans began supplying medical personnel at the Role 2 locations, providing liaisons to various regions of the theater, and expanding the mission to include refugee care. During its rotation, Fleet Hospital 6 expanded the healthcare mission in theater even further, taking on the Role 4 mission (in conjunction with local hospitals) as well as much of the Role 2 mission.[60(pp20–23)]

It was not until American forces returned to Bosnia and Herzegovina in 1995, as a part of Operation Joint Endeavor, that an American FST-type unit was deployed to the Balkans. After the North Atlantic Treaty Organization (NATO) launched air strikes into the region in August 1995, representatives from the warring Serbians, Croatians, and Bosnian Muslim factions gathered at Wright Patterson Air Force Base near Dayton, Ohio. An agreement, eventually referred to as the General Framework Agreement for Peace, was signed in Paris on 14 December 1995.[58] However, medical assets would still be needed, and the 67th CSH was notified of its impending mobilization in support of Operation Joint Endeavor (20 December 1995–20 December 1996) on 11 December 1995.[57(p513)] By the time the contingent of 67th CSH personnel arrived in the Balkans in January 1996, the 212th MASH FSE was already in place near the Sava River.[57(p514)] Once the 67th CSH was in place, the 212th MASH surgical element redeployed to Germany. As stability began to spread in the region, numerous MASH and CSH units rotated to theater in support of the NATO peacekeeping mission in Bosnia and Herzegovina.[57(pp520–524),58]

As Bosnia and Herzegovina stabilized, however, ethnic Albanians in the Serbian region of Kosovo began an aggressive pursuit of independence. In 1996, the Kosovo Liberation Army began launching attacks on Serbian police forces. In response, the Serbian government began a practice of expulsion of ethnic Albanians, resulting in 1,500 dead and 400,000 Albanian refugees.[61(pp9–10)] In early April 1999, in preparation for execution of Operation Allied Force, the 67th FST deployed to Camp Able Sentry, Macedonia, in support of Task Force Falcon. At approximately the same time, a sliced portion of the 212th MASH (roughly equivalent to 1.5 FSTs) deployed to Tirana-Rinas Airport in Albania, with lead elements of NATO forces, in support of Task Force Hawk.[57(pp524–525),61] The two FSEs provided forward resuscitative surgery in their respective regions for several months. On 16 June 1999, just after Operation Joint Guardian began, the 67th FST moved to Camp Bondsteel, near Urosevac, Kosovo, where it provided resuscitative surgery until 14 July 1999, when the larger 67th Contingency Medical Force took over responsibility for the region.[57(p524)] By 2 August 1999, the 212th MASH and all Task Force Hawk units departed Albania, and Operation Allied Force had ended.[61] As Task Force Falcon settled into the 6-month rotations of personnel in and out of Kosovo in support of Operation Joint Guardian, two new medical elements entered the rotation as augmentations to the medical task forces slated for service in the theater.

Formal Establishment of the Forward Surgical Team: 1994

In January 1994, based on the rapid deployment and high mobility needs of the Army in Panama and Iraq, the Army chief of staff approved the formal establishment of the FST on the Army manning documents.[57(p526)] In March, proponents of the FST began circulating for comment draft TO&E documents for the "medical team, forward surgical" and "medical team, forward surgical (airborne)."[27] With the goal of reducing the overall DOW rate by providing early intervention and rapid evacuation, the formal fielding of the new units began in fiscal year 1997.[1] In September 1997, the first version of Field Manual 8-10-25, *Employment of the Forward Surgical Team*, was published.[27] The deployment of the 67th FST into Kenya in 1998 and the 160th FST and 250th FST into the Kosovo theater of operations in 1999 and 2000 marked the first formal deployments for the newly minted Army FST.[25,57(p526)]

A little closer to home, in mid-September 1994, elements of the XVIII Airborne Corps, the 82nd Airborne Division, and the 10th Mountain Division deployed in support of Operation Uphold Democracy.[57(p541)] Bent on protecting Americans in the small island nation and returning to power the democratically elected president, Jean Bertrand Aristide, American forces gained control of Haiti on 19 September 1994 without shots being fired.[62(pp69–79)] Members of the 274th FST were among the first medical assets to arrive on the island, establishing a surgical capability by the end of the day on 20 September 1994. Within days, portions of the 28th CSH and the 47th Field Hospital followed.[57(p543)] The relatively uneventful operation gave the military medical teams opportunity to provide humanitarian assistance to the Haitian locals and identify health requirements that could be addressed by nongovernment organizations already operating in Haiti.[62(pp130–132)]

On 31 March 1995, the American mission in Haiti was formally turned over to the UN as a nation-building mission. The 25th Infantry Division replaced the 10th Mountain Division as the senior command element on the ground and began working to establish some semblance of normality within the small island country.[62(pp136–137)] In the years that followed, the UN Mission in Haiti continued to provide humanitarian assistance to Haitian locals, and American military elements continued to be a part of that mission. Until 2000, medical personnel from all three branches of the US military rotated through Haiti on scheduled organizational rotations. FSTs, including the 555th FST out of Fort Hood, Texas, were a part of that medical rotation.[57(p548)]

On the recommendation of many government agencies, including the Government Accounting Office, FSTs were increasingly included in military and medical training scenarios, including the establishment of an FST-specific training program at Ben Taub Medical Center in Houston, Texas, in September 1998. Transformation of the Army medical force structure continued as personnel and equipment were regularly reallocated to field the 44 FSTs across the Army (active and Reserve components). In October 2001, just weeks after the terrorist attacks on the World Trade Center, the Army opened the doors to the Army Trauma Training Center at the Ryder Trauma Training Center in Miami, Florida.[27] Coupled with the realistic, combat-oriented training at their home stations, FSTs that rotated through the Army Trauma Training Center soon became hardened teams ready for the eventuality of war.

SURGEONS GENERAL DURING THE POST-VIETNAM ERA

LTG Bernhard T Mittemeyer (Falklands War and Grenada)

Lieutenant General (LTG) Bernhard Theodore Mittemeyer served as the surgeon general of the Army from 1 October 1981 to 31 January 1985.[63] Mittemeyer immigrated to the United States from Holland in 1944, when he was 14 years old. At the outset of the Korean War, the young college student was deferred from the draft so that he could attend medical school. When he eventually came on active duty, Mittemeyer volunteered for the 101st Airborne Division, in appreciation of the American unit that previously liberated his native country.[64] A urologist by training, Mittemeyer served primarily in clinical roles throughout his early career. He was then assigned as commander of the 326th Medical Battalion and division surgeon of the 101st Airborne Division in Vietnam. Later, Mittemeyer was multi-hatted as the commander, US Army Medical Command-Korea; command surgeon, UN Command/US Forces Korea/Eighth US Army; and commander, 121st Evacuation Hospital, before moving to the Office of The Surgeon General, where he served as the director of Professional Services and chief of Medical Corps Affairs. Mittemeyer served as the commanding general of Walter Reed Army Medical Center just prior to his appointment as the surgeon general.[65] During his tenure as surgeon general, the Army instituted the three-event Army Physical Fitness Test for soldiers of all ages. Prior to 1982, only soldiers under the age of 40 participated in the Army Physical Fitness Test due to concerns that rates of sudden cardiac death may rise for soldiers over 40.[57]

LTG Quinn H Becker (Mid-1980s Evolution)

LTG Quinn H. Becker served as the surgeon general of the Army from 1 February 1985 to 31 May 1988.[1] An orthopedic surgeon by training, Becker served primarily in clinical roles until he was assigned as commander of the 5th Surgical Hospital (Mobile Army) at Heidelberg, Germany. He later served as the division surgeon and commander of the 15th Medical Battalion, 1st Calvary Division (Airmobile), in Vietnam as well as surgeon of the XVIII Airborne Corps and commander of the US Army Medical Activity at Fort Bragg, North Carolina. Becker served as the surgeon, US European Command; chief surgeon, US Army Europe; and commander, 7th Medical Command, Heidelberg, Germany, just prior to his appointment as the surgeon general.[66] During LTG Becker's tenure as surgeon general, he oversaw the implementation of major quality assurance reforms in the Army Medical Department amid reports of serious problems with the medical care provided in the Army healthcare system.[67,68]

LTG Frank F Ledford, Jr (Mid-1980s Evolution)

LTG Frank Finley Ledford, Jr, served as the surgeon general of the Army from 1 June 1988 to 30 June 1992.[1] Also an orthopedic surgeon, Ledford served primarily in clinical roles until he was assigned as the surgical consultant at the Office of The Surgeon General. He later served as commander of the US Army Medical Activity, Fort Riley, Kansas, and then commander of the US Army Medical Activity, Fort Benning, Georgia. Ledford also served as the commanding general of Letterman Army Medical Center at the Presidio of San Francisco, California. Just prior to being appointed surgeon general, Ledford served as commanding general of the 7th Medical Command and surgeon of US Army Europe/Seventh Army, Heidelberg, Germany.[69] Operations Desert Shield and Desert Storm occurred during Ledford's tenure as surgeon general. Due to concerns about Saddam Hussein's propensity to use chemical weapons in combat, Army medical leaders, under Ledford's direction, undertook unprecedented training and preparation for these Operations.[70] Operations Desert Shield and Desert Storm required the first large-scale call-up of Army Reserve medical personnel since Vietnam.[4] Many of the reservists bore a significant personal cost as they sacrificed their personal medical practices, often risking bankruptcy, to serve overseas.[9] LTG Ledford also oversaw the medical operations for Operation Just Cause in 1989 and the initial operations into Yugoslavia in 1992.

LTG Alcide M LaNoue (Restore/Continue Hope, Formal Forward Surgical Team Establishment)

LTG Alcide Moodie LaNoue served as surgeon general of the Army from 8 September 1992 to 30 September 1996. The third consecutive orthopedic surgeon to be named surgeon general, LaNoue served primarily in clinical roles until his assignment as commander of the 209th General Dispensary, 97th General Hospital, US Army Europe, the first of four consecutive command positions. LaNoue next served as commander of the US Army Medical Activity, Fort Stewart, Georgia, then at the US Army Medical Activity, Fort Benning, Georgia. LaNoue then served at Eisenhower Army Medical Center, Fort Gordon, Georgia, as the commanding general. He also served as commandant of the US Army Academy of Health Sciences, deputy surgeon general at the Office of The Surgeon General, and commanding general of the US Army Health Services Command prior to his appointment as surgeon general.[71] During his tenure as surgeon general, LTG LaNoue oversaw the medical operations for operations Restore Hope and Continue Hope in Somalia. Additionally, LaNoue directed the development and maintenance of a new readiness posture in the Army Medical Department while significant downsizing occurred throughout the Army.[72]

LTG Ronald R Blanck (Yugoslavia Operations)

LTG Ronald Ray Blanck served as surgeon general of the Army from 1 October 1996 to 30 June 2000. An internist by training, LTG Blanck initially served as a battalion surgeon in Vietnam before taking on roles primarily in clinical arena until his assignment as commander of the US Army Hospital, Berlin. Subsequent positions included commander, Frankfurt Army Regional Medical Center, Frankfurt, Germany, and director of professional services and chief of Medical Corps affairs in the Office of The Surgeon General. Just prior to his appointment as surgeon general, Blanck was assigned as commander of Walter Reed Army Medical Center and Northern Regional Medical Command.[73] During his tenure as surgeon general, LTG Blanck also led the Army Medical Department through significant downsizing while balancing the need for medical personnel to support peacekeeping operations in Yugoslavia, a humanitarian mission in Haiti, and chemical/biological terrorist concerns in Japan.[74]

CONCLUSION

The evolution of forward surgery in the US military has followed an arduous path toward the reality of today's battlefield. The medical lessons learned on the battlefields of yesterday helped shape the care provided to the combat casualties today and in future conflicts. Adding FSTs to the medical formations on the battlefield provided the operational commander an element of agility and adaptability not previously known in American military history. Military operations since Vietnam provided a thorough testing ground for forward surgical doctrine. Through the continued evolution of that doctrine, the battlefield of the future may become more survivable.

REFERENCES

1. Syvertson RL. *A Computer Simulation and Analysis of the Forward Surgical Team* [thesis]. Monterey, Calif: Naval Postgraduate School; 1995. http://www.dtic.mil/cgi-bin/GetTRDoc?AD=ADA304803. Accessed 4 December 2012.
2. Stinger H, Rush R. The Army forward surgical team: update and lessons learned, 1997–2004. *Mil Med*. 2006;171(4):269–272.
3. *Falkland Island Campaign, Medical Aspects, Part 1* [videotape]. Fort Sam Houston, Tex: Army Medical Department Television and Multimedia Division; 6 April 1983. A1701-83-1604V.
4. Broyles TE. *A Comparative Analysis of the Medical Support in the Combat Operations in the Falklands Campaign and the Grenada Expedition* [thesis]. Fort Leavenworth, Kans: US Army Command and General Staff College; 1987. http://www.dtic.mil/cgi-bin/GetTRDoc?AD=ADA184721. Accessed 4 December 2012.
5. Adams V. Logistic support for the Falklands Campaign. *J Royal United Serv Inst Defense Stud*. 1984;129(3):43–49.
6. Harrison J. Naval medicine in the Falklands Conflict, April–July 1982, overall policy and operations. *Trans Med Soc London*. 1982;99-100:75-81.
7. Marsh AR. A short but distant war—the Falklands Campaign. *J R Soc Med*. 1983;76(Nov):972–982.
8. Bailey J. Training for war: Falklands 1982. *Mil Rev*. 1983;Sep:58–70. http://cgsc.contentdm.oclc.org/utils/getfile/collection/p124201coll1/id/298/filename/299.pdf. Accessed 1 March 2013.
9. Harmon JW, Llewellyn C. Lessons on the Falklands. *Med Bull US Army Eur*. 1984;41(2):11-13.
10. Mosebar RH. *Lessons Learned in Lebanon and the Falklands*. Fort Sam Houston, Tex: US Army Medical Department, Academy of Health Sciences, Directorate of Combat Development; 6 January 1987.
11. Mosebar RH. *Field Hospital in the Falkland Islands*. Fort Sam Houston, Tex: US Army Medical Department, Academy of Health Sciences, Directorate of Combat Development; 18 January 1984.
12. Jackson DS, Jowitt MD, Knight RJ. First and second line treatment in the Falklands Campaign: a retrospective view. *J R Army Med Corps*. 1984;130:79-83.
13. Cole RH. *Operation Urgent Fury: The Planning and Execution of Joint Operations in Grenada*. Washington, DC: Joint History Office, Office of the Chairman of the Joint Chiefs of Staff; 1997.
14. *Lessons Learned—Grenada* [videotape]. Fort Sam Houston, Tex: Army Medical Department Television and Multimedia Division; 4 May 1987. A1701-87-0101.
15. Wolf J. The invasion of Grenada. The American Experience website. http://www.pbs.org/wgbh/americanexperience/features/general-article/reagan-grenada/. Accessed 19 May 2013.
16. Gailey P, Weaver W Jr. Touching down in Grenada. *New York Times*. 26 March 1983. http://www.nytimes.com/1983/03/26/us/briefing-058430.html?module=Search&mabReward=relbias%3Ar, Accessed 14 July 2014.

17. Payne AJ, Sutton P, Thorndike T. *Grenada: Revolution and Invasion*. London, England: Croom Helm, Ltd; 1984.
18. Bennett RK. Grenada: anatomy of a "go" decision. *Read Dig*. 1984;(February):72–77.
19. US Department of State and Department of Defense. *Grenada: A Preliminary Report*. Washington, DC: DoS/DoD; 1983. http://www.dod.gov/pubs/foi/Reading_Room/International_Security_Affairs/153.pdf. Accessed 19 May 2013.
20. Nolan DL. Airborne tactical medical support in Grenada. *Mil Med*. 1990;156(3):104–111.
21. Bolger DP. Operation Urgent Fury and its critics. *Mil Rev*. 1986;66(7):57–69.
22. Radin RM, Bell RA. Combat service support of Urgent Fury. *Army Logistician*. 1984;16(6):16–19.
23. Walsh DP, Lammert GR, Devoll J. The effectiveness of the Advanced Trauma Life Support system in a mass casualty situation by non-trauma experienced physicians: Grenada 1983. *J Emerg Med*. 1989;7(2):175–180.
24. COL Joseph Jackson (orthopedic surgeon, 307th Medical Battalion sent an orthopedic surgeon); written communication, personal diary of his experiences during Operation Urgent Fury, October 24–17 November 1983.
25. COL Joseph Jackson (orthopedic surgeon, 307th Medical Battalion sent an orthopedic surgeon); written communication, personal notes from Operation Urgent Fury, 1984.
26. Cragg D. The US Army in Grenada. *Army*. 1983;33(12):29–31.
27. Barger LL. Developments in forward surgery during the second half of the 20th century. 2015. Unpublished manuscript, Army Medical Department Office of History and Heritage, Fort Sam Houston, Tex.
28. Stinger H, Rush R. The Army forward surgical team: update and lessons learned, 1997–2004. *Mil Med*. 2006;171(4):269–272.
29. Bellamy RF. The causes of death in conventional land warfare: implications for combat casualty research. *Mil Med*. 1984;149:55–62.
30. Hetz SP. Introduction to military medicine: a brief overview. *Surg Clin North Am*. 2006;86:675–688.
31. SGM Michael D Bivins (chief medical noncommissioned officer, XVIII Airborne Corps Surgeon's Office); email, 11 July 2013.
32. US Department of the Army. *Brigade and Division Surgeons' Handbook*. Washington, DC: Government Printing Office; 10 June 1991. Field Manual 8-10-5.
33. BG Robert D Tenhet (executive officer to the Army Surgeon General); email, 9 July 2013.
34. General James H Rumbaugh, 49, Director of Army Medical Center. *New York Times*. 10 March 1989. http://www.nytimes.com/1989/03/10/obituaries/general-james-h-rumbaugh-49-director-of-army-medical-center/. Accessed 8 December 2013.
35. Phillips RC. *Operation Just Cause: The Incursion Into Panama*. Fort McNair, Washington, DC: US Army Center for Military History; 2004.
36. Cole RH. *Operation Just Cause: The Planning and Execution of Joint Operations in Panama*. Washington, DC: Joint History Office, Office of the Chairman of the Joint Chiefs of Staff; 1995.
37. *Operation Just Cause* [videotape]. Fort Sam Houston, Tex: Army Medical Department Television and Multimedia Division; 1 March 1990. A1701-90-0087.
38. US Department of the Army. *Health Service Support Observations: Operation Just Cause*. Fort Sam Houston, Tex: Academy of Health Sciences; 1990.
39. Brannon RH. *1st Aeromedical Evacuation Squadron After Action Report, Operation Just Cause*. Howard Air Force Base, Panama: US Department of the Air Force; 1990.

40. US Army Center of Military History. XVIII Airborne Corps and Joint Task Force South Operation Just Cause list of participating units. http://www.history.army.mil/documents/panama/unitlst.htm. Accessed 1 June 2013.
41. US Army Medical Department. Medical Lessons Learned [database online]. Fort Sam Houston, Tex; AMEDD; 2010. https://mll.amedd.army.mil. Analysis of US casualties during Operation Just Cause. Observation summary 12620. Accessed 28 July 2010.
42. US Army Medical Department. Medical Lessons Learned [database online]. Fort Sam Houston, Tex; AMEDD; 2010. Demand for humanitarian aid during Just Cause. Observation summary 12613. Accessed 28 July 2010.
43. Beekley AC. United States military surgical response to modern large-scale conflicts: the ongoing evolution of a trauma system. *Surg Clin North Am*. 2006;86:689–709.
44. King BT, Jatoi I. The mobile army surgical hospital (MASH): a military and surgical legacy. *J Natl Med Assoc*. 2005;97(5):648–656.
45. *Operation Desert Shield: AMEDD Lessons Learned* [videotape]. Fort Sam Houston, Tex: Army Medical Department Television and Multimedia Division; 17 April 1991. A1701-91-0160.
46. Stewart R. *War in the Persian Gulf: Operations Desert Shield and Desert Storm, August 1990–March 1991*. Washington, DC: US Army Center for Military History; 2010. http://www.history.army.mil/html/books/070/70-117-1/CMH_70-117-1.pdf. Accessed 22 June 2013.
47. Ledford FF. From The Surgeon General of the Army: Medical support for Operation Desert Storm. *J US Army Med Dept*. 1992;(January/February):3–6. http://history.amedd.army.mil/booksdocs/AMEDDinODS/AMEDDODS1Ledford.pdf. Accessed 22 June 2013.
48. US General Accounting Office. *Operation Desert Storm: Full Army Medical Capability Not Achieved*. Washington, DC: GAO; August 1992. http://www.gao.gov/assets/160/152150.pdf. Accessed 9 October 2012.
49. US General Accounting Office. *Wartime Medical Care: Personnel Requirements Still Not Resolved*. Washington, DC: GAO; 1996. http://purl.access.gpo.gov/GPO/LPS29773. Accessed 9 October 2012.
50. Rigdon KA. *US Army Health Service Support in 2025*. Fort Leavenworth, Kans: School of Advanced Military Studies, US Army Command and General Staff College; 2004. http://www.dtic.mil/cgi-bin/GetTRDoc?AD=ADA436131. Accessed 1 December 2012.
51. *Operation Desert Shield: AMEDD Logistics Lessons Learned* [videotape]. Fort Sam Houston, Tex: Army Medical Department Television and Multimedia Division; 17 April 1991. A1701-91-0161.
52. Pattillo DA. *Portable Surgical Hospitals in the North Burma Campaign: Lessons for Providing Forward Surgical Support to Nonlinear Operations in Airland Operations* [thesis]. Fort Leavenworth, Kans: US Army Command and General Staff College; 1993. http://www.dtic.mil/cgi-bin/GetTRDoc?AD=ADA272689. Accessed 1 December 2012.
53. Steinweg KK. Mobile surgical hospital design: lessons learned from the 5th MASH surgical packages from Operation Desert Shield/Desert Storm. *Mil Med*. 1993;158:733–739.
54. Alan G Muench, MD (former commander, 274th Medical Detachment), email, 14 April 2014.
55. Kerchief KR. Combat casualty care: ready for the last war? *Mil Rev*. 1991;(April):78–83.
56. US Department of the Army. *United States Forces, Somalia After Action Report and Historical Overview: The United States Army in Somalia, 1992–1994*. Washington, DC: US Army Center for Military History; 2003. http://www.history.army.mil/html/documents/somalia/SomaliaAAR.pdf. Accessed 7 July 2013.
57. Sarnecky MT. *A Contemporary History of the US Army Nurse Corps*. Washington, DC: Borden Institute, Office of The Surgeon General of the Army; 2010. http://www.cs.amedd.army.mil/borden/Portlet.aspx?ID=099df372-1e64-4a5f-99a6-c814bd87fe6c. Accessed 7 July 2013.

58. Phillips RC. *Bosnia-Herzegovina: The US Army's Role in Peace Enforcement Operations, 1995–2004*. Washington, DC: US Army Center for Military History; nd. CMH Pub 70-97-1. http://www.history.army.mil/html/books/070/70-97-1/cmhPub_70-97-1.pdf. Accessed 9 April 2016.
59. Covey DC. The role of the orthopedic surgeon in United Nations peacekeeping operations. *J Bone Joint Surg*. 1995; 77-A(4):495–499.
60. Davis LM, Hosek SD, Tate MG, Perry M, Hepler G, Steinberg PS. *Army Medical Support for Peace Operations and Humanitarian Assistance*. Santa Monica, Calif: RAND Arroyo Center; 1996..
61. Phillips, RC. *Operation Joint Guardian: The US Army in Kosovo*. Washington, DC: US Army Center for Military History; nd. CMH Pub 70-109-1. http://www.history.army.mil/html/books/070/70-109-1/cmhPub_70-109-1.pdf. Accessed 9 April 2016.
62. Kretchik WE, Baumann RF, Fishel JT. *Invasion, Intervention, "Intervasion": A Concise History of the US Army in Operation Uphold Democracy*. Fort Leavenworth, Kans: US Army Command and General Staff College Press; 1998.
63. Army Medical Department, Office of Medical History. The surgeons general of the U.S. Army and their predecessors. http://history.amedd.army.mil/surgeons.html. Accessed 1 May 2015.
64. General Bernie Mittemeyer, a hometown hero. KCBD Television website. http://www.kcbd.com/story/19005422/general-bernie-mittemeyer-a-hometown-hero. Accessed 31 May 2015.
65. Army Medical Department, Office of Medical History. The surgeons general: Berhard T. Mittemeyer. http://history.amedd.army.mil/surgeongenerals/B_Mittemeyer.html. Accessed 1 May 2015.
66. Army Medical Department, Office of Medical History. The surgeons general: Quinn H. Becker. http://history.amedd.army.mil/surgeongenerals/Q_Becker.html. Accessed 31 May 2015.
67. Sosa I. Lieutenant General Quinn H. Becker, Surgeon General for the Army Medical Department, interviewed by Ms. Ingeborg Sosa, the Editor of the Medical Bulletin. *Medical Bulletin*. 1987:44(Feb/Mar):3-7. http://cdm15290.contentdm.oclc.org/cdm/ref/collection/p15290coll5/id/494. Accessed 31 May 2015.
68. Boffey PM. Inaction on problem doctors spurs doubts about military crackdown. *New York Times*. 21 June 1985. http://www.nytimes.com/1985/06/21/us/inaction-on-problem-doctors-spurs-doubts-about-military-crackdown.html. Accessed 31 May 2015.
69. Army Medical Department, Office of Medical History. The surgeons general: Frank F. Ledford, Jr. http://history.amedd.army.mil/surgeongenerals/F_LedfordJr.html. Accessed 1 June 2015.
70. Sosa I. The Journal interviews–LTG Frank F. Ledford, Jr., Surgeon General, United States Army. *J US Army Med Department*. 1992;Mar/Apr. http://cdm15290.contentdm.oclc.org/cdm/ref/collection/p15290coll3/id/680. Accessed 1 June 2015.
71. Army Medical Department, Office of Medical History. The surgeons general: Alcide M. LaNoue. http://history.amedd.army.mil/surgeongenerals/A_LaNoue.html. Accessed 1 June 2015.
72. Sosa I, Danford F. The Journal interviews–Lieutenant General Alcide M. LaNoue, The Surgeon General of the United States Army. *J US Army Med Department*. 1993;Sept/Oct. http://cdm15290.contentdm.oclc.org/cdm/ref/collection/p15290coll3/id/871. Accessed 1 June 2015.
73. Army Medical Department, Office of Medical History. The surgeons general: Ronald R. Blanck. http://history.amedd.army.mil/surgeongenerals/R_Blanck.html. Accessed 1 June 2015.
74. Philadelphia College of Osteopathic Medicine. Ronald R. Blanck oral history. 1997. http://digitalcommons.pcom.edu/cgi/viewcontent.cgi?article=1001&context=oral_histories. Accessed 1 June 2015.

Chapter Ten

Put to the Test: Forward Surgical Teams Challenged During the Global War on Terrorism

JASON M. SEERY, MD, and DAVID W. CANNON, SR

INTRODUCTION

THE SURPRISE ATTACKS ON THE WORLD TRADE CENTER and the Pentagon, and a third failed attack on an unknown target, by hijacked airliners on 11 September 2001 marked the beginning of a new era in the United States that will be felt around the world for decades to come. Not since the surprise attack on Pearl Harbor had there been such support by US citizens, the government, and the military for a common cause. With the onset of the Global War on Terrorism (GWOT), the capabilities of US Army surgical personnel and forward surgical teams (FSTs) would be put to the test.

> IN THE MIDST OF CHAOS, THERE IS ALSO OPPORTUNITY.
>
> Sun Tzu[1(p41)]

In 2001, Army forward surgery entered into an accelerated period of development, innovation, and overall significance. Members of US Army FSTs, their sister component surgical team equivalents from the Air Force, Navy, and the North Atlantic Treaty Organization (NATO), and the various supporting medical units, including logistical and evacuation assets, enabled the provision of life-, limb-, and eye-saving resuscitation for tens of thousands of military, civilian, and enemy patients.[2] The FSTs' ability to improve patient outcomes grew significantly over this period due to theater maturity, innovative concepts, and innovative technology. These capabilities were made possible by dedicated and passionate surgical leaders from the Medical Corps, Nurse Corps, Specialty Corps, Medical Service Corps, and Medical Enlisted Corps who chose to go beyond what was required of them. These leaders documented events, passed on lessons learned, and pushed for improvements.

They followed their hearts rather than the expected path. This chapter will tell their story, describing how, in the chaos of war, they found opportunities to improve survival chances for the soldiers who took the greatest risk. Following in the footsteps of Napoleon's famous chief surgeon and the father of modern military surgery, Baron Dominique Jean Larrey,[3] these FST leaders and team members put the desire to save the combat wounded above their own fears of injury, made great sacrifices, and devoted themselves entirely to their patients. Their service in this period is the latest example of a time-honored tradition among combat surgeons and combat surgical support staff dating from the first wars of this country.

Over the course of the GWOT, the terminology for some key elements changed. One example was the evolution of the term "echelons" of care to "levels" of care, and then to the currently used "roles" of care. The term "levels," which replaced "echelons" in 2001,[4] aligned joint assets into the level of care they were capable of providing when tactically employed. As the battlefield changed from linear to nonlinear, the term "roles" came into use about 2006 to better describe the medical unit's capabilities, rather than the level or quality of care provided.[5] This change also aligned with NATO medical terminology to ensure that all allied countries involved in the GWOT were following similar standards and "speaking the same language."[6] For the purpose of this chapter, the word "role," when used to discuss the location and capacity of a unit, will refer to "echelon," "level," and "role," unless otherwise specified, to lessen confusion.[7-9]

Another key definition that changed over the GWOT was what made up the Role 2 surgical element or team for each of the services. During this period the US Department of Defense (DoD) conventional forces Role 2 surgical team varied significantly among the services. The Army Role 2 surgical unit, the FST, is a 20-person team made up of three general surgeons, an orthopedist, two anesthetists, an emergency care registered nurse, an operating room registered nurse, a critical care registered nurse, three licensed practical nurses, three operating room technicians, four medics, and one medical administration officer. Over the past 15 years, the FST has commonly been employed in a split 10-person configuration. The FST is assigned to augment a Role 3 Army combat support hospital (CSH), but is usually forward employed attached to a Role 2 medical company. Although the FST was specifically designed to not stand alone, it can conduct limited stand-alone operations (usually while supporting Special Operations forces). While working with a Role 2 medical company, the FST has access to additional physicians and registered nurses, dental support, combat and operational stress control staff, preventive medicine staff, and limited laboratory and X-ray capabilities.[8,9] At times other nondoctrinal units have been established to fill the Role 2 surgical team position within the Army. This was usually done by forwardly deploying a section of a CSH. Known as a forward surgical element (FSE), its size ranged from 6 to over 30 staff members, based on unique mission needs.

The Air Force Role 2 surgical unit comes in three basic platforms. First is the mobile field surgical team (MFST), a five-person team made up of a surgeon, orthopedist, anesthetist, emergency medicine physician, and an operating room registered nurse or operating room technician. The MFST is the basic surgical component of the two other Air Force Role 2 surgical assets. The second is the small portable expeditionary aeromedical rapid response (SPEARR) team. This is a 10-person team made up of the MFST with the addition of a three-person critical care air transportation team (CCATT) and a two-person preventive medicine team. The CCATT consists of an intensivist physician, a critical care registered nurse, and a cardiopulmonary technician, while the preventive medicine team has a flight surgeon and public health officer. The third platform is the expeditionary medical support (EMEDS) basic, a 25-person team that includes the 10-person SPEARR team and an additional 15 staff members who provide medical or ancillary capabilities including sick-call capability, dental care, and limited laboratory and X-ray capability. The Role 2 EMEDS can be expanded with 10 extra staff and additional equipment (known as the EMEDS +10) that provide added holding capability, but no additional surgical capabilities.[8,9]

The Marine Corps Role 2 surgical unit comes in two basic platforms. First is the forward resuscitative surgical system (FRSS), an eight-person team with two surgeons, an anesthesiologist, a critical care registered nurse, two operating room technicians, and two corpsmen. Four FRSSs, along with four Role 1 shock trauma platoons and four en-route care teams, make up the larger surgical element known as the Marine surgical company. Of note, the surgeons, nurses, and enlisted corpsmen in the Marine Role 2 surgical units are Navy personnel, since the Marine Corps has no organic medical personnel.[8,9] Similar to the US Army and Air Force, the Marines created nondoctrinal appropriately sized teams to perform the Role 2 surgical team mission. One example was the surgical shock trauma platoon (SSTP), which consisted of two FRSSs and one shock trauma platoon.[10]

The Navy Role 2 surgical units also consist of two platforms, the casualty receiving and treatment ship (CRTS) and the fleet surgical team.[8,9] These teams are ship-based, as opposed to the above-mentioned land-based platforms for the Army, Air Force, and Marines.

Also of interest is how the NATO definition of the Role 2 is different than that used by the DoD. US forces use a more basic definition of Role 2 for a medical treatment facility providing greater resuscitative capability than that available from a Role 1 individual or facility. Surgical capability is not mandatory at Role 2 per US military doctrine, as opposed to the NATO definition, which states that a Role 2 facility will have the ability to provide damage control surgery. Therefore, in addition to the term "role" covering all prior definitions for the continuum of care, the term Role 2 surgical team, and at times FST, will describe the generic DoD or NATO Role 2 surgical unit, unless otherwise specifically stated.[6]

THE TWO MAJOR OPERATIONS OF THE GLOBAL WAR ON TERRORISM

Operation Enduring Freedom

Intelligence agencies identified al-Qaida, a terrorist network led by Osama bin Laden, as the group that designed and executed the 11 September 2001 attacks. Al-Qaida was a global terrorist organization, but at the time of the attacks its leader and main facilities were based in Afghanistan. Afghanistan's ruling government party at the time, the Taliban, was supportive of al-Qaida, protecting them from the United States and allied governments. After diplomatic efforts with the Taliban government leadership failed to resolve the capture of the al-Qaida attackers, military actions were implemented. Operation Enduring Freedom (OEF) commenced on 7 October 2001 in Afghanistan, marking the beginning of the GWOT. OEF's initial primary mission was to locate and capture or destroy al-Qaida equipment, members, and leadership. Intense bombing of known training and command and control areas was done by the US Navy, with Tomahawk cruise missiles, and the US Air Force, with a variety of air-delivered bombs and missiles. Various Special Operations forces were simultaneously inserted to capture or kill remaining al-Qaida members and to coordinate an anti-Taliban movement.[11,12]

Healthcare for US and coalition conventional units and Special Operations forces was initially provided by each unit's organic Role 1 and 2 medical assets, with very limited surgical capabilities.[13] Special Operations forces were the first units to deploy in the war, with their organic medical personnel, which included Special Forces medical sergeants (military occupational specialty 18D) and Special Operations combat medics (68WW1), assigned to Special Forces Groups and Ranger regiments, respectively, as well as physician and physician assistant providers. These healthcare providers had received significantly advanced training in tactical combat casualty care (TCCC) and could perform limited surgical procedures to stabilize patients or avoid preventable causes of death. These medical soldiers also had advanced training in all aspects of the military, allowing some to enter the theater by airdrop parachute-forced entry (airborne units), air-assault entry via rotary wing, or air-land entry via fixed wing aircraft. Very limited numbers of US Special Operations Command surgical elements were forward deployed.[14] These teams had various compositions of traditional trauma team members and could provide advanced surgical operations on individuals with lethal injuries. However, they could care for only a very limited amount of patients.[8,14,15] These small teams provided life-saving resuscitation and surgery for the initial Special Forces soldiers in OEF. The patients were then evacuated from Afghanistan to surgical facilities located in surrounding countries and oceans.

A US Marine medical detachment with surgical capabilities was established at Camp Rhino, approximately 190 km southwest of Kandahar, Afghanistan, on 25 November 2001. Its mission was to support the Marine Expeditionary Force, Army Ranger units, Army air assault units, Navy SEAL (sea, air, and land) units, local national forces, and enemy prisoners of war in their area of operations.[16] The detachment was made up of a standard battalion aid station and shock trauma platoon, along with an operating room section from a different element. In total, it was staffed with 32 members, including two general/trauma surgeons, two anesthesiologists, three emergency physicians, two emergency nurses, one critical care nurse, one perioperative nurse, one physician assistant, one general medical officer, one medical regulator, one independent duty corpsman, three surgical technicians, and one general duty corpsman.[8,16] The medical-surgical detachment provided initial resuscitative and surgical care to soldiers. Patients would then be evacuated to a Role 2 facility on a CRTS (the USS *Peleliu* or USS *Bataan*), located in the Arabian Sea, or to the Role 3 theater hospital in Seeb, Oman, for continuing care.

The detachment was operational on 4 December 2001 and received a total of 48 casualties over a 6-week period. The first group (and largest number) of patients arrived one day after activation. When a NATO-fired Joint Defense Attack Munitions was dropped too close to friendly forces, 21 US and 20 local national forces were injured. Due to the distance from point of injury to the medical facility, communication issues, and aircraft mechanical issues, patients arrived 5 to 6 hours after their initial injuries. Of the 41 patients, 19 US casualties were taken immediately to Seeb, while two US and 20 local nationals remained at Camp Rhino. One of the US casualties was actually killed in action, and the other was moribund on arrival and deemed expectant secondary to a massive head injury, requiring only catastrophic injury management. Of the 20 local national casualties, one required surgery for a neck injury, two required chest tubes for thorax injuries, six had open fractures, and the remainder had superficial injuries. The following day the detachment received four additional patients, but none required surgical intervention.

Ten days later, the detachment received the last group of patients during its rotation. Three US Marines were injured by an antipersonnel land mine located near Kandahar. Injuries included a hand-degloving injury to one Marine, a near complete lower-extremity traumatic amputation to a second Marine, and minor injuries to the third. The casualties arrived at Camp Rhino about 1.5 hours after their injuries. The patient with the leg injury was sent directly to Seeb, while the other two were treated at Camp Rhino. The patient with the hand injury underwent surgical debridement and washout.[16]

This medical-surgical detachment set-up, consisting of a shock trauma platoon and operating room section, along with a surgeon and anesthesiologist from the 2d Medical Battalion and personnel from a health service support detachment from the 15th Marine Expeditionary Unit, overcame many challenges early in the US war in Afghanistan. Its lessons learned helped ensure that future missions were better supported by leadership, staffing was improved, units were issued enhanced equipment and supplies, and pre-mission training was significantly enhanced.

The first US Army FSTs to deploy in the GWOT and treat surgical wounds were the 250th FST (Airborne) from Fort Lewis, Washington, and the 274th FST (Airborne) from Fort Bragg, North Carolina.[11,17] Both the 250th and 274th were among the initial set of modern FSTs officially activated in 1997. Both had the prestigious and challenging additional capability of being an airborne deployable FST, trained and equipped for early entry missions.[18] In addition, the 274th was the final version of one of the initial surgical squads developed in the late 1980s that had participated in Operation Just Cause and Operation Desert Shield/Storm. Both FSTs supported the Combined Joint Special Operations Task Force-Afghanistan (CJSOTF-A). They would successfully perform numerous doctrinal and nondoctrinal tasks and missions, setting the tone for all others to follow.

274TH FORWARD SURGICAL TEAM (AIRBORNE)

The 274th FST (Airborne) was assigned to CJSOTF-North and initially set up at Karshi and Khanabad Air Base (K2) in Uzbekistan between 14 October and 27 December 2001.[11,12] Major (MAJ) Brian S Burlingame had recently taken over as the team commander. During their deployment, in addition to saving the lives, limbs, and eyesight of numerous soldiers, Burlingame and his team created several innovative tactical solutions used as foundational methods by many follow-on units. The 86th CSH arrived at K2 on 17 October 2001, but was not fully functional until 27 December. During these months

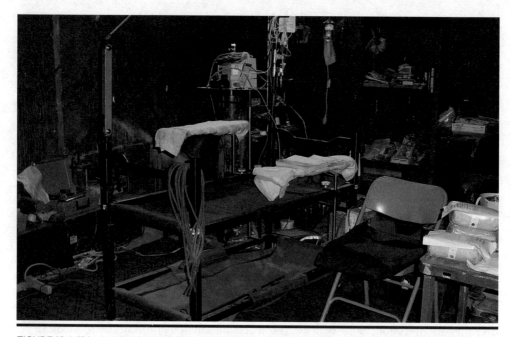

FIGURE 10-1. This area inside an abandoned building at Bagram Airfield was used for surgery by the 274th Forward Surgical Team in 2002, initially with only a litter, litter stand, and a few medical equipment set chests. This rudimentary operating room slowly became more advanced as better facilities and equipment became available in theater. Photograph courtesy of MSG John Dominguez, former operating room specialist 274th FST.

the 274th cared for over 100 patients requiring surgical evaluation and treatment. K2 was many hours from the point of injury for some patients injured in Afghanistan and not the ideal place for an FST to perform its primary mission. To stabilize patients with preventable causes of death within the "golden hour" prior to evacuation to a higher role of care, the FST needed to be closer to the actual combat.

Once the battlefield was more mature, with basic force protection and logistic channels better established, the FSTs could move farther forward. On 5 December 2001, the 274th sent a small slice of their 20-person team into southern Afghanistan to help treat US casualties injured in a friendly fire incident near Kandahar. Once there, this five-person team joined and assisted the local Marine medical-surgical detachment team at Camp Rhino taking care of both US and Afghan Militia Forces casualties. Patients were evacuated to supporting Navy ships or to the surgical facility at Seeb Air Base. The five 274th personnel accompanied the patients on two C-130 Hercules aircraft, performing in-flight surgical procedures on some casualties. Two days later, the 274th was again asked to send a five-person surgical team into Afghanistan. This time the five-person team set up at Bagram Airfield and supported ongoing combat operations in eastern Afghanistan (Figure 10-1). This move placed surgical assets much closer to the point of injury and improved the potential of survival and salvage. The remaining 15 team members and equipment stayed operational at K2 until the 86th CSH became functional and assumed surgical care for that area of responsibility.

On 27 December 2001, the 274th FST main element left K2 and joined their colleagues in Bagram. The 274th FST would stay at this location until the end of their deployment on 8 May 2002, caring for over 130 casualties. A few days earlier, on 24 December, a British Role 3 unit, the 34th Field Hospital Troop, set up at Bagram approximately 300 meters from the 274th FST forward echelon, and quickly established a mass casualty incident plan. On 20 January 2002, the 34th and 274th had their first opportunity to work together, caring for US Marines injured in a CH-53 (Sea Hawk) helicopter crash. On 28 January, a US Army CH-47 (Chinook) helicopter from the 101st (Airborne) Division crashed during a night mission with 26 personnel on board. Fortunately, no one died on impact, but 16 sustained injuries. Two other CH-47s on the mission collected the 26 passengers and patients and transported them to Bagram, approximately 1 hour away. Unit medics provided en route care. Seven patients went directly to the 34th Field Hospital Troop. The 274th FST provided care for 12 of the patients with assistance from medical staff from the 10th (Mountain) Division. Three patients were later transferred to the 34th Field Hospital for continuing care. Patients requiring further treatment went on to the 86th CSH in Uzbekistan. In the end, all of the patients from this mass causality incident survived their wounds. The 34th Field Hospital and the 274th FST would again work together during the care of multiple patients from a US Air Force C-130 Hercules crash on 13 February.[19]

The 274th and 34th experienced their largest number of casualties during Operation Anaconda. Operation Anaconda, the largest and longest US military operation since the Vietnam War, began on 1 March 2002 and was staged out of Bagram Airfield. It also occurred at the highest altitude ever recorded for combat engagement by US forces.[11,12,20] The operation involved multinational forces, including the Afghan Militia Forces, with the aim of destroying the largest stronghold of Taliban and al-Qaida terrorists residing in the Shah-e-Kot Mountains in southeastern Afghanistan. The enemy was well entrenched and trained, and American and coalition forces met strong resistance. During the second day of the mission, the 274th cared for 50 casualties, performing five minor and eleven major surgeries with the collaboration of British and Spanish field hospitals in the area. The next day only three casualties arrived at the FST's location. On mission day four, a CH-47 was shot down by enemy fire along with a search and rescue helicopter that went out to assist their colleagues. Eleven of the survivors had injuries requiring care at the FST, with six undergoing surgery.

By the end of Operation Anaconda, 119 soldiers had been seen at the 274th FST, with 32 major and minor surgical procedures performed. In total, the 274th provided trauma care to over 200 casualties and performed 103 surgeries.[11,12] Without the FST's presence during the initial invasion, many soldiers would have died. The staff's collaboration with an allied force medical unit was unique at the time, but such collaboration would become common as the conflict in Afghanistan, and then Iraq, evolved. The FST's personnel recognized the benefits of collaborating and worked through protocol and equipment differences. Their documentation of this partnership helped others who found themselves in similar situations over the years. The 274th's professionalism and willingness to perform surgery in a high-risk and immature theater set a high standard for all who followed.

250TH FORWARD SURGICAL TEAM (AIRBORNE)

Providing an equally important mission and high level of care in the southern region of Afghanistan was the 250th FST (Airborne). It was assigned to CJSOTF-South and initially set up at Seeb Air Base, from 20 October 2001 to 24 December 2001.[17] Lieutenant Colonel (LTC) Clifford Porter led the 250th during this important initial deployment. He and his unit overcame numerous obstacles and worked alongside many joint and allied colleagues, ensuring the unit successfully provided the necessary surgical and resuscitative support to the combat and support personnel in southern Afghanistan. While in Oman, they cohabitated with an EMEDS unit from the US Air Force 320th Expeditionary Medical Group.[17,21]

Within 24 hours of arriving at Seeb Air Base, the FST and EMEDS unit were ready to receive patients. The combined units had four trauma/resuscitation beds; eight emergency/acute beds; seven intensive care beds with ventilators; 10 medical/surgical beds; a laboratory; digital radiography, angiography, and computed tomography (CT); and four fully functional operating tables.[17] This joint facility took care of casualties from southwestern Afghanistan and areas near the Pakistani border. Similar to the situation with the 274th FST (Airborne), the location was many hours from the point of injury and not the ideal proximity for an FST to best perform its primary mission. Evacuation times from point of injury to the surgical facility could be as long as 6 to 12 hours.[21] Soldiers with preventable causes of death requiring surgery might not make it to this location in time. Fortunately, combat forces were able to quickly secure the area around Kandahar.

Once the area was secured, with basic force protection and logistic channels established, the 250th relocated. The team set up in a more forward position at Kandahar International Airfield on 25 December 2001 and remained there until 2 April 2002. These early teams would learn how to cope with the desert cold, snow and winds (Figure 10-2). On arrival, they briefly integrated with a Marine shock trauma platoon from the 26th Marine Expeditionary Unit. The team was fortunate to also spend a short period of time in late February 2002 with the forward support medical company from the 3rd Brigade of the 101st Airborne (Air Assault) Division.[17] Because the US Army FST is not designed to operate for long periods without Role 1 or 2 medical assistance, as well as other logistical and administrative support, these partnerships were welcomed while they lasted. The 250th spent its remaining time at Kandahar functioning independently without the doctrinal support of a battalion aid station, forward support medical company (also known as "Charlie Med" and now referred to as a brigade support medical company), or area support medical company.[7-9,22-26]

Evacuation times from Role 2 to Role 3 early in OEF were far from the approximately 1-hour evacuation period for combat casualties of the mature theater during the Vietnam War.[11,12,27] While patients were seen by their Role 1 providers to address their injuries and some of the preventable causes of death within minutes to hours, the surgical facilities in K2 and Seeb Air Base were hours away for many casualties, so patients were held longer prior to evacuation to definitive care. During this period (October 2001 to May 2002, when the 274th FST was the primary medical treatment facility for combat casualties in

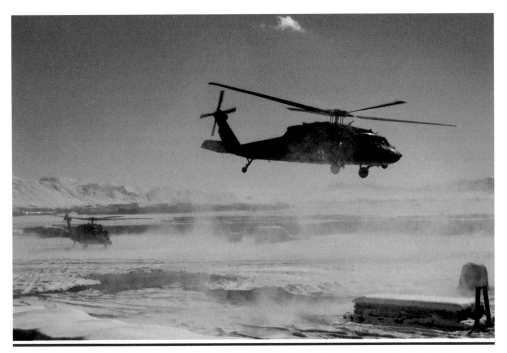

FIGURE 10-2. A Blackhawk helicopter takes off on a MEDEVAC mission at Forward Operating Base Orgun-E in the Afghanistan winter, 2011. The 250th and 274th Airborne Forward Operating Teams (FSTs) were the first US Department of Defense surgical teams to carry out combat trauma resuscitation and surgery in Afghanistan. Their personnel learned to work in extreme cold, strong winds, rain, and snow. The 1980th and 947th FSTs replaced the 250th and 274th in spring 2002, and were the first to experience the opposite extremes of high temperatures, sand storms, and very dry conditions. Photograph courtesy of LTC Dean Felldabaum, former commander of the 2nd FST.

Afghanistan), these facilities were not in an ideal geographical location to provide life-saving surgical intervention to the approximately 10% of casualties with surgically correctable torso injuries, the 9% with significant extremity vascular injuries, and all patients needing advanced resuscitation management or care from other lethal injuries.[11,12,27] However, these early OEF prolonged evacuation times to Role 3 facilities were comparable to the 3- to 4-hour evacuation times that the Soviets experienced during the occupation of Afghanistan in the 1980s.[28]

Once the 250th was established at Kandahar and the 274th at Bagram, evacuation times from point of injury dropped to a maximum of approximately 3 hours, significantly improving the chances of a soldier's life or limbs being saved.[21] During this deployment, the 250th cared for 50 surgical patients, conducted 68 surgical procedures, and established a surgical resuscitative care facility that served as the model in terms of the types of injuries and treatments provided by FSTs in Afghanistan for a brigade-sized unit.[29] Like the 274th, the 250th proved that a small group of highly motivated and properly trained and equipped medical providers could save the lives, limbs, and eyesight of patients no matter where they were called to duty.

1980TH AND 102ND FORWARD SURGICAL TEAMS

As combat continued, President George W Bush made it clear that the conflict would be much different from previous wars and that it would last for many years, and possibly decades. The US Army Reserves would become very active in supporting the GWOT. The 1980th FST from Fresno, California,[30,31] was activated in February 2002 and arrived in Kandahar that April to conduct a handover of surgical coverage from the 250th FST (Airborne). A few days later 1980th personnel found themselves saving the lives of six Canadian soldiers injured by a 500-pound laser-guided bomb, secondary to a friendly fire mishap from a US Air National Guard F16 aircraft.[32] By the end of their 6-month activation, the 1980th FST had cared for over 70 cases of combat trauma, including gunshot wounds and blast injuries, to all regions of the body in adult and pediatric patients.[33]

In August 2002, the 1980th passed on their experiences and trauma responsibilities to the 102nd FST, another forward surgical team from Fort Lewis, Washington, commanded by LTC Robert Handy.[34] The 102nd FST deployed for 7 months, from August 2002 until March 2003. Their primary mission was to provide damage control resuscitative surgery in support of combat actions by the 101st and 82nd Airborne Divisions, Special Operations forces, and Afghanistan militia forces. The vast majority of the casualties were trauma related and consisted of a mix of US soldiers, Afghan militia and civilians, and coalition forces. The FST performed 112 surgeries on 90 patients during this time period.[34]

947TH AND 909TH FORWARD SURGICAL TEAMS

The 947th FST, a Reserve medical unit from West Hartford, Connecticut, was notified on 11 March 2002 that it would mobilize and deploy to Afghanistan in support of OEF. LTC Robert W McAllister and his team arrived at Bagram Airfield on 28 April and began proceedings to relieve the 274th FST (Airborne).[30] Under the CJSOTF-A's command and control, the 947th FST would continue the hard work of the previous FST. However, in May 2002, the team was unable to save the life of an American Special Forces soldier who had been injured many hours from their location.

The FST commander, LTC McAllister, coordinated with CJSOTF-A and explained that an FST could function even closer to the point of injury to provide high-quality life-saving resuscitation and surgery to injured soldiers if other support measures were taken by higher elements. The Alpha echelon of the FST jumped forward to Camp Harrison in Orgun-E to be closer to the current area of enemy engagement. The Bravo echelon stayed at Bagram and received additional support from members of the 405th CSH (Reserve) stationed in Kuwait.

In July 2002, the 339th CSH (Reserve) was established (see below for more details), providing a more robust theater Role 3 facility. This allowed the 947th Bravo echelon to move forward to Orgun-E and reunite with the rest of its team. When not seeing patients, 947th FST members assisted with other camp activities, including working with local national police forces and supporting various requests by the local US civil affairs units. The unit cared for, and saved, numerous combat trauma patients in its area of responsibility, and was well respected by its CJSOTF-A leadership. On 28 October 2002, the team left the theater and was replaced by another Reserve unit, the 909th FST, from Fort Sheridan,

Illinois, commanded by Colonel (COL) Dirk Wassner.[35,36] With a little over half of the US Army's FSTs in the Reserve, teams such as the 1980th, 947th, and 909th would be key in the success of forward resuscitation and surgery on the modern battlefield.

The 1980th and 947th FSTs also represented other "firsts" in this war. They were the first US FSTs to perform combat trauma management in the sweltering heat of an Afghanistan summer. Their ability to overcome the environmental conditions, combined with other logistical, communication, and evacuation challenges, set a new standard. They also continued to build the FST's strong reputation; their combatant colleagues and leaders soon came to consider the FST as the new "gold standard" of casualty care on the battlefield.

555TH FORWARD SURGICAL TEAM

The last of the initial FSTs during the early period of OEF was the 555th FST from Fort Hood, Texas. Commanded by MAJ Young Choi, the unit was deployed to Kuwait from 21 November 2001 to 31 March 2002 in support of US military stationed in Kuwait. The FST primarily supported the 1st Cavalry Division. The team worked out of the Kuwait Armed Forces Hospital, where they evaluated and treated US service members, including trauma evaluations and a few surgeries. During their deployment, the 555th FST was tasked with sending a small surgical element to Kandahar to support a temporary mission gap. The care provided by the 555th FST was not on the same scale as that of the 274th or 250th FSTs, but it demonstrated a different capability of a modern US Role 2 surgical team, working with an allied nation and deploying a split element to a different country thousands of miles away for a special support mission. This deployment would also help the 555th prepare for an unexpected deployment one year later.[37]

339TH COMBAT SUPPORT HOSPITAL

Department of Army doctrine for the employment of the various levels of military medical treatment is based on Army Techniques Publication 4-02.5, *Combat Casualty Care*.[38] FSTs are normally employed in brigade combat teams on the basis of one per maneuver brigade. They are usually attached to a CSH for general support. When operationally employed, FSTs are attached to medical companies. An FST may also be a part of a medical task force in support of Special Operations forces.[22,24,38,39] CSHs are normally assigned to a medical brigade (support). CSHs were first deployed to Afghanistan and Iraq under the Medical Force 2000-designed table of organization and equipment (TOE) and consisted of two modules: a hospital unit base and a hospital unit surgical. Later deployments were under the Medical Reengineering Initiative design (corps CSH), consisting of a hospital company A (84-bed) and a hospital company B (164-bed). Hospital company A was capable of providing an early entry hospitalization element of 44 beds and a follow-on hospitalization augmentation element of 40 beds. Many of the CSHs conducted split-based operations utilizing the 84-bed and 164-bed hospital facilities to provide healthcare support in separate locations. Other CSHs conducted operations in more than two locations, using a variety of deployment manning documents, requests for forces, and requests for augmentation to add additional personnel needed to operate multiple locations. As both theaters matured, it became increasingly common for CSHs to operate in fixed facilities and to utilize theater-provided equipment. If the CSH was within 1 hour of the point of injury, then taking a patient to an FST is usually not required because the patients can get advanced surgical care within the "golden hour" at the CSH.

The 339th Reserve CSH, from Pittsburgh, Pennsylvania, was alerted on 23 April 2002 that it would be the first US military hospital deployed within the borders of Afghanistan. On 24 June 2002, LTC James C Post and his CSH arrived in theater and established the first Role 3 facility within the country's borders at Bagram Airfield. They set up their 44-bed CSH element 4 days after arrival and were fully ready to accept patients on 1 July, 4 days ahead of schedule.[40,41] Due to their proximity to the combat operations, the CSH would receive numerous patients directly from the point of injury. On 2 July the first patients arrived. They included four Afghani children injured by crossfire between US military and opposition forces. The proximity of CSHs to the point of injury remained the same for over a decade, up to the writing of this chapter, allowing CSHs in various regions to be the initial recipients of numerous casualties and the FSTs to be located even further forward.

The 339th medical staff performed trauma evaluation on 531 patients and treated hundreds of others for sick call and other disease and nonbattle injuries. Patients included 337 US military troops, 26 troops from allied countries, 15 US civilians, 10 enemy prisoners of war, and 140 local nationals (90 adults and 50 children). The team performed 518 life-saving or stabilizing surgeries and procedures over a 5-month period.[40] The 339th CSH set up the first military CT scanner in theater and introduced many other technologically advanced pieces of medical equipment.[40]

48TH COMBAT SUPPORT HOSPITAL

On 6 December 2002, 6 months after its arrival in theater, the 339th CSH was replaced by the 48th CSH.[11,30] The 48th, commanded by COL Alan L Beitler, had been reactivated less than 2 years before, on 16 October 2000, and was the US Army's first multicomponent CSH. The 48th CSH was designed to function as a 44-bed hospital; however, as with most other medical and surgical units during the GWOT, it was employed in a different manner. The 48th CSH was set up as a 28-bed hospital with 12 intensive care unit and 16 intermediate care ward beds, not using the remaining 16 intermediate care ward beds. The staff consisted of two general surgeons, one vascular surgeon, one orthopedic surgeon, two oral maxillofacial surgeons, two anesthesiologists, two anesthetists, one emergency medicine physician, two family medicine physicians, one internal medicine physician, one pediatrician, one radiologist, one physician assistant, sixteen registered nurses, and numerous licensed practical nurses, technicians, and medics. Patients were seen in a sick call area for routine issues or in the emergency treatment section for urgent medical, surgical, and psychiatric needs. There were two operating rooms arranged to perform three procedures simultaneously.

During their 6-month deployment, from 6 December 2002 to 7 June 2003, staff of the 48th saw 10,679 patients, including US forces, allied forces, Afghan militia forces, Afghan civilians, and enemy combatants, performing 358 surgical procedures on 168 casualties. The CSH also received all of the patients from the two FSTs that were functioning as smaller, split elements. Combined, the FSTs treated 91 casualties prior to sending them

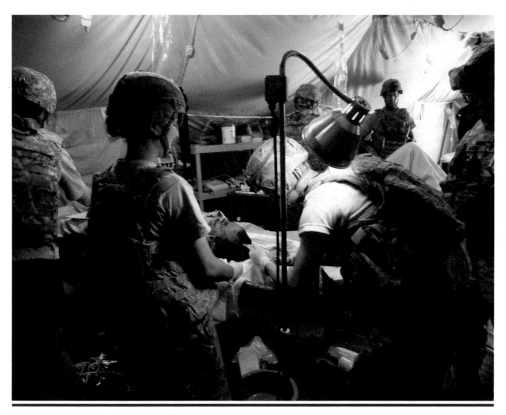

FIGURE 10-3. Far forward surgery holds risks for the providers. Here a forward surgical team at Camp Pannonia, Afghanistan, cares for a soldier during an offensive in which the compound came under direct and indirect attack. Team members continued to provide care while wearing their protective gear. Photograph courtesy of MAJ Christopher Vanfosson, critical care nurse, 541st FST.

to the 48th CSH. Patients were sent from the CSH to either Landstuhl Regional Medical Center in Germany, their host allied nation hospital, the Afghan military hospital in Kabul, or local civilian Afghan hospitals, based on the type of patient. US soldiers were transferred to Germany via the Air Force CCATT.[13,42]

ROLE 2 AND ROLE 3 EXPANSION

The FST and CSH elements continued to expand their coverage over the next decade. As of late 2014, there were four regional commands (RCs) in Afghanistan. There was a NATO Role 3 facility at Mazar-i-Sharif in RC-North, an Army/Air Force Role 3 at Bagram in RC-East, a Navy Role 3 in Kandahar in RC-South, and another Army Role 3 split between various locations in RC-West. Numerous Army, Navy, and Air Force Role 2 surgical and resuscitative units were located within each RC under the command and control of the Task Force Medical Brigade or CJSOTF-A. Most functioned as split, 10-person elements, but some were full teams. All have faced tactical, operational, administrative, security, logistical, training, communication, information technology, and other challenges

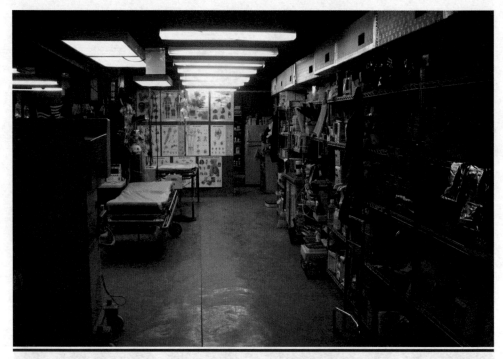

FIGURE 10-4. An image of the split forward surgical team facility at Forward Operating Base Orgun-E, Afghanistan, in 2010. Surgical capability at Orgun-E was initially established in 2002. Note the significant difference from conditions in Figure 10-1, including powerful overhead lighting, walls of supplies, dedicated office space, refrigerator, and fluoroscopy machine. Not visible are oxygen lines providing flow to the facility from a large oxygen generator located outside. Photograph courtesy of LTC George Johnson, former certified registered nurse anesthetist, 541st FST.

over the last 13 years (Figure 10-3). They evolved from split-based operations and working in tents to being mostly in fixed, semipermanent facilities. Most were located within a 45-minute patient evacuation area, had reliable electricity, good communication equipment, and numerous morale opportunities. Their staff significantly contributed to the current 95% survival rate from combat trauma, and have also been key in reducing the 10% died of wounds rate from truncal bleeding amenable to surgical correction.[27,43–46] These medical units have become a necessity for the combatant commanders and are well respected and supported by combat leaders.

However, most notable is the recognition of the importance of TCCC as the gold standard for combat medic training, which has brought about a revolution in casualty care through enhanced prehospital medical care. These enhancements emphasize hemorrhage control from extremity wounds by nonmedical personnel, either in support of combat medics or in their absence, and life-saving interventions such as application of tourniquets, maintaining airway and breathing, and control of shock at the point of injury. The combat casualty care experience of the 75th Ranger Regiment in Iraq and Afghanistan demonstrated how key life-saving interventions on the battlefield can be delivered by nonmedical

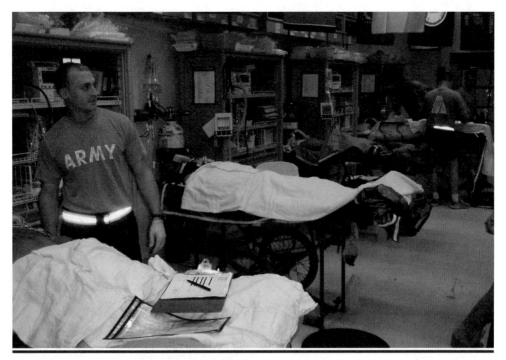

FIGURE 10-5. Image of the new facility at Jalalabad, Afghanistan, after its opening in 2008. Providers of the 772nd Forward Surgical Team (Air Assault) and their patients enjoyed the enhanced amenities of this fixed facility, which are similar to those in a US hospital. Photograph courtesy of LTC Kyle Remick, former commander of the 772nd FST.

personnel or by combat medics. Both the Ranger Regiment and the Canadian armed forces identified their all-combatant TCCC training programs as key elements in their unprecedented success in reducing preventable death on the battlefield.[47,48]

FST leaders have developed new tactics, techniques, and procedures to address the austere environment they work in, as well as the changing enemy methods of attack. This has resulted in doctrinal and logistical changes that will be discussed later in this chapter. FSTs have been involved in many projects to support the Special Forces community, civil affairs community, Department of State, other US government agencies, and many nongovernment agencies. These include training local national military medical staff, working with local national civilian and military medical facilities, and other "winning the hearts and minds" types of projects.

As the war in Afghanistan evolved, medical assets grew from the first two FSTs to, at times, over 20 locations with established FST elements. All US services, as well as many NATO allies, have contributed to trauma care via their various versions of Role 2 surgical units and forward deployed Role 3 hospitals (Figures 10-4 and 10-5). On 1 January 2015, the conflict's name changed from OEF to Operation Freedom's Sentinel as the US mission focuses more on training, advising, and assisting the Afghan security forces to take over protection of their own government, lands, and people.[49] As the war draws to an

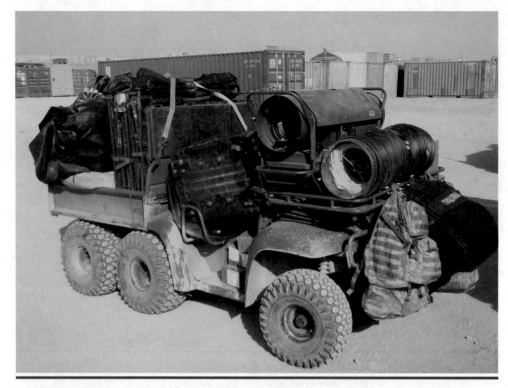

FIGURE 10-6. Early set-up (2007) of a non-doctrinal wheeled vehicle configured for forward surgical team (FST) missions in support of Special Operations forces. The vehicle would be transported via a rotary-wing aircraft to a far forward location. Photograph courtesy of LTC Kyle Remick, former commander of the 772nd FST.

end, the units are supporting more and more Special Operations forces as the number of conventional forces declines (Figure 10-6). As local national forces take over responsibility, these surgical units are closing down some areas while performing missions in new areas. Increasingly they are performing temporary missions outside of their large forward operating bases for short periods of time in support of Special Operations forces or for coverage in times and areas of need to conventional forces. FSTs have developed their own mobile mission concepts, using rotary wing aircraft to rapidly move a 6- to 10-person slice element around the battlefield. The passion and creativity of team members is impressive and will surely lead to even better care in the future (Figure 10-7).

Operation Iraqi Freedom

Due to increasing concerns about the potential Iraqi use of weapons of mass destruction (WMDs), the United Nations Security Council passed Resolution 1441 in 2002.[50] This resolution called for the country of Iraq to fully work with and support UN weapons inspection teams. Despite the UN resolution, Saddam Hussein and his staff failed to support the full disclosure of certain facilities and documents thought to provide evidence of

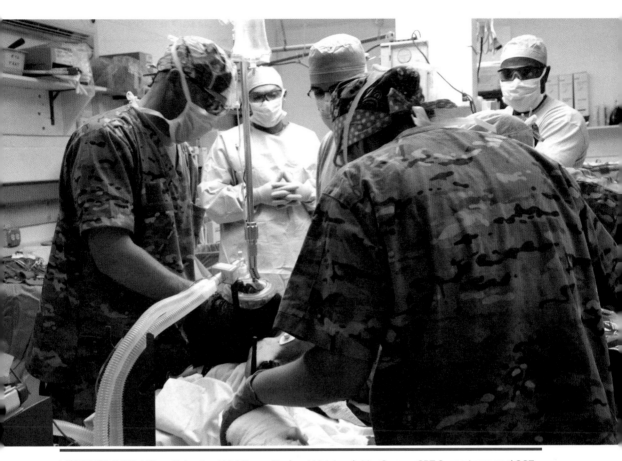

FIGURE 10-7. MAJ Cleve Sylvester, MAJ Tyson Becker, MAJ Jacob MacGregor, CPT Suzan Laux, and SGT Keith Shackelford operate on an Afghan National Police officer at their facility in Farah, Afghanistan, in 2014. Many forward surgical team members have deployed multiple times over the years. US Navy photograph by Chief Hospital Corpsman Josh Ives/Released.

a WMD program. Due to the concerns that Iraq was developing WMDs, or could easily acquire them from another source, and intelligence sources indicating Saddam was supporting terrorist organizations, an invasion of Iraq was planned. On 20 March 2003, conventional forces entered Iraq and started the official ground war known as Operation Iraqi Freedom (OIF). This war would be supported by 40 different countries with different languages, combat trauma protocols, and skill levels, and occur simultaneously with OEF, creating unique challenges throughout the DoD and especially for the medical units.[51] Combat maneuver units were under the command of US Central Command and operationally controlled by US Army V Corps. Just under 300,000 soldiers took part in the initial invasion. Of these, 248,000 were US troops split among elements of the 3rd Infantry Division, 4th Infantry Division, 82nd Airborne Division, 101st Airborne Division, 1st Marine Expeditionary Forces, and various Special Operations units.

TABLE 10-1. **UNITS PARTICIPATING IN INITIAL PHASES OF OPERATION IRAQI FREEDOM**

Unit	Home Base
1st FST (Reserve)	Brooklyn, NY
2nd Armored Calvary Regiment FST (Airborne)	Fort Bragg, NC
126th FST	Fort Hood, TX
160th FST	Miesau, Germany
240th FST	Fort Stewart, GA
250th FST (Airborne)	Fort Lewis, WA
274th FST (Airborne)	Fort Bragg, NC
555th FST	Fort Hood, TX
624th FST (Reserve)	Erie, PA
628th FST (Reserve)	San Antonio, TX
745th FST	Fort Bliss, TX
782nd FST (Airborne)	Fort Bragg, NC
801st FST (Air Assault)	Fort Campbell, KY
912th FST (Reserve)	Cranston, RI
915th FST (Reserve)	Vancouver, WA
932nd FST (Reserve)	Indianapolis, IN
934th FST (Reserve)	Salt Lake City, UT
936th FST (Reserve)	Paducah, KY
945th FST (Reserve)	Minneapolis, MN
1st Medical BN-FRSS Alpha	Camp Pendleton, CA
1st Medical BN-FRSS Bravo	Camp Pendleton, CA
1st Medical BN-FRSS Charlie	Camp Pendleton, CA
2nd Medical BN-FRSS Alpha	Camp Lejeune, NC
2nd Medical BN-FRSS Bravo	Camp Lejeune, NC
2nd Medical BN-FRSS Charlie	Camp Lejeune, NC

BN: battalion
FRSS: forward resuscitative surgical system
FST: forward surgical team

As in OEF, FSTs, as well as FRSSs, were deployed in support of combatant commanders.[52] In total, nineteen FSTs and six Marine FRSSs participated in the initial phases of OIF. These units are listed in Table 10-1.[52–54]

Various Army, Navy, and Air Force Special Operations surgical assets were in place to support Special Operations forces already coordinating the invasion and subsequent overthrow of the Baath party, securing any potential WMDs, and disrupting any terrorist cells. One of these units would become the newly designed Air Force Role 2 surgical unit known as the Special Operations surgical team, which was usually accompanied with a Special Operations critical care evacuation team. Various NATO and allied forces also had Role 2 surgical and Role 3 facilities that took care of combat injured soldiers.[55,56]

The conventional surgical units accompanied their assigned combat units as they moved north from Kuwait or as they moved south after being air deployed in the north. Some of the members on the 274th FST (Airborne), 250th FST (Airborne), and 555th FST

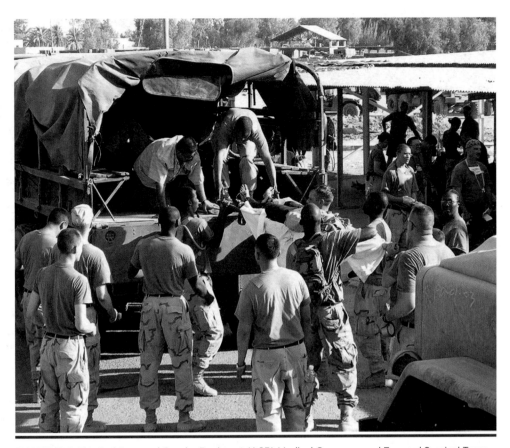

FIGURE 10-8. The 2nd Armored Cavalry Regiment (ACR) Medical Company and Forward Surgical Team accept patients at Camp Muleskinner via CASEVAC after the 19 August 2003 bombing of the UN headquarters at the Canal Hotel in Baghdad, Iraq. The bombing caused at last 22 deaths and over 100 casualties. The 2nd ACR was the closest medical/surgical facility in the area, located approximately 6 miles southeast of the incident, and received many patients. Photograph courtesy of COL Kim Smith, former perioperative nurse, 2nd ACR FST.

had memories of serving in Afghanistan during the early phases of OEF still fresh in their minds. These units would again be initial deployers and help lead the way with their lessons learned.[17,57] During the initial invasion phase and the early period of the follow-on security and stabilization phase, most of these units remained in theater. While some FSTs stayed as little as a few months, most stayed 12 months, with a few extended to 15 months. Over this time, FST personnel would care for thousands of friendly military, local civilian, and enemy combatant patients, resulting in hundreds of surgeries performed. The FSTs would set up and tear down their facilities multiple times using various configurations, including their organic tents as well as abandoned buildings. The 2nd Armored Cavalry Regiment FST (Airborne) acquired an expandable surgical shelter like the ones used at CSHs, which remained set up on the back of a 5-ton truck. The unit was able to keep up with the

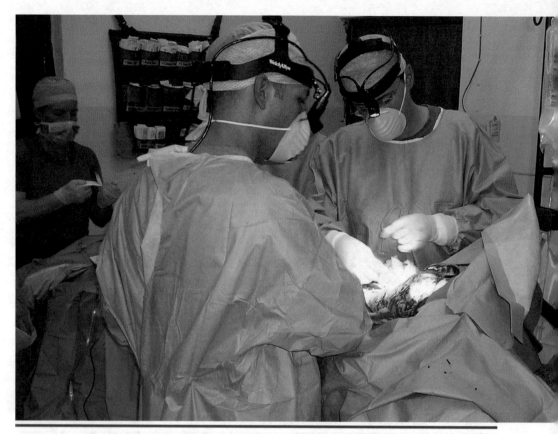

FIGURE 10-9. LTC Thomas McCorey, LTC Alexander Stojadinovic, and MAJ Kim Smith perform surgery on victim of the UN headquarters bombing. The 2nd Armored Cavalry Regiment Medical Company and Forward Surgical Team occupied the Al Rasheed Military Hospital in the southeastern area of Baghdad early after the initial phase of the invasion of Iraq. Photograph courtesy of COL Kim Smith, former perioperative nurse, 2nd ACR FST.

cavalry's quick advancements and could rapidly be ready to conduct surgery without setting up all the tents or much equipment.

Coordination for unit movement and patient transfers was complex due to the vast number of medical units on the battlefield; however, the resourceful and passionate FSTs, medical companies, various surgeons' cells, and MEDEVAC units were able to function fairly well. As the mission converted from the first to the second phase after 1 May 2003, the unit movements slowly stabilized and the type of patients and types of injuries changed (Figures 10-8 and 10-9).

Injury patterns early on were as expected for a ground war with dismounted and mounted troops taking on a force with conventional weapons. The majority were gunshot wounds, blast injuries, and burns. Due to the protection of armored vehicles and body armor, many injuries were to the limbs. Vehicle armor and individual body armor would significantly improve in quality and increase in quantity early on in this theater. The enemy's method of attack would also change to reliance on improvised explosive devices (IEDs) and indirect fire, with much less gunfire. The combination of improved armor and change in the enemy's tactics caused a shift in injury patterns to more isolated extremity wounds or polytrauma including the extremities. Role 2 surgical teams were flexible and able to continuously provide the care needed to save many soldiers.

FORWARD RESUSCITATIVE SURGICAL SYSTEMS

Other innovations being introduced at the time included the new Navy and Marine Corps surgical unit, recently added to address injured service members in this type of conflict. Like the Army, the Navy and Marines had been working with various small and mobile surgical platforms to meet the needs of their new combat missions to prevent the problems that occurred during Operation Desert Shield/Storm. With news of the upcoming potential war in Iraq and ongoing war in Afghanistan, the Navy Bureau of Medicine and Surgery solidified its plans and created the FRSS. The Marine FRSS was a new surgical unit that had only been in prototype development prior to January 2003. It was designed to augment medical units already in the Marine inventory, including the battalion aid station and shock trauma platoon, or to boost capability on a Naval vessel when increased surgical capability was required. Like the FST, the FRSS could be moved by its own ground tactical vehicles, via military aircraft, swing-loaded under a rotary wing, or (unique to the Navy) it could also be moved on air-cushion vehicles. The unit was manned by eight personnel, including a general surgeon, orthopedic surgeon, anesthesiologist, critical care registered nurse, independent duty corpsman, two operating room technicians, and one general duty field medical technician. The team could be augmented with additional critical care or emergency care nurses to assist with the transport of critical patients. There were two prototype FRSSs, one stationed on the east coast and one on the west coast. These units would become official FRSSs after January 2003.

Between February and March 2003, four additional FRSSs were rapidly assembled and prepared for deployment to OIF under the leadership of Captain HR Bohman and Commander Robert Hincks.[58] In April and May, four additional Reserve FRSSs were stood up from the 4th Medical Battalion so they could relieve their active duty colleagues that summer. The six primary units moved with the 1st Medical Expeditionary Force along the eastern side of southern Iraq toward Baghdad. During a bad sandstorm, one of the teams had vehicle problems and lost the ability to move its equipment. The personnel were reassigned to a different FRSS so their skills could still be used. This consolidated team traveled with the combat service support element in support of the 1st Medical Expeditionary Force. The remaining four teams moved far forward of their two parent surgical companies. After bounding forward, they would set up surgical capabilities and then meld in with the full surgical company once it arrived. During the period from 22 March to 1 May 2003, the FRSSs treated 34 Marines and 62 wounded Iraqi soldiers and civilians, performing 151 surgical procedures, with a zero died of wounds rate.[53,59] The FRSSs performed 14% of all surgeries while functioning as jump elements and assisted in many other surgeries when they cohabitated with the surgical company. FRSS staff performed in an exemplary manner while providing care to their fellow Marines.

212TH MOBILE ARMY SURGICAL HOSPITAL

Another key combat surgical team that contributed to the initial phases of the war was the 212th Mobile Army Surgical Hospital (MASH). Commanded by LTC Ken Canestrini and based out of Miesau, Germany, the 212th was the Army's only remaining MASH. The 212th MASH initially co-located with the 86th CSH at Camp Udairi, in Kuwait, prior to the war. Once the invasion began, the unit of 160 soldiers, including 9 physicians and surgeons, 29 nurses, and a mixture of pharmacy and operating room technicians, laboratory and radiology technicians, medics, licensed practical nurses, nutritionist, administrators, logisticians, computer and communication specialists, laundry and motor pool staff, and others moved north. Over a 3-day convoy, they encountered combat action as they moved toward Objective Rams and set up at the logistics support area (LSA) Bushmaster near An Najaf. Personnel were able to rapidly assemble tents and surgical shelters to provide an emergency medical treatment area, three operating room tables, and 36 recovery beds divided into three 12-bed areas.[60,61]

During the early phases of OEF and OIF, Role 2 surgical unit members had to conduct many other duties, such as field sanitation and area security, in addition to their jobs as medical care providers. While not pleasant and often time consuming and disruptive to work-rest cycles, these duties were necessary to ensure that the unit functioned and was secure. The 212th MASH, as did their sister surgical units, would also experience something they never saw in the United States or Europe, massive sand storms. Personnel had to ensure that their equipment was not damaged and then decontaminate as best they could to provide the cleanest facility possible.[60,61]

After a few weeks of operations at LSA Bushmaster, the team moved farther north, to LSA Dogwood, located just south of Baghdad. There they conducted capabilities assessments of area Iraqi medical clinics and hospitals. The 212th returned to Germany in June 2003. Of the 701 patients treated during the deployment, 132 orthopedic procedures were performed on 74 patients, while an additional 33 patients required abdominal, thoracic, or neck explorations. This was the final combat mission for the 212th MASH because it was converted to a CSH in 2006. The team members demonstrated one last time that the MASH, designed after World War II, was still a capable surgical unit.[60,61]

COMBAT SUPPORT HOSPITALS

In addition to the 212th MASH, three combat support hospitals deployed into Iraq during the initial phase of OIF. The 21st CSH from Fort Hood, Texas; the 28th CSH from Fort Bragg, North Carolina; and the 86th CSH from Fort Campbell, Kentucky, all crossed the border and entered Iraq, while the 47th CSH from Fort Lewis, Washington, and 10th CSH from Fort Carson, Colorado, provided medical care and support from Kuwait.[61-64] As with their Role 2 surgical colleagues, these Role 3 units would care for initial wounded due to the nonlinear aspect of the war after phase one was competed. They would also receive all casualties from the numerous Role 2 facilities. These casualties' injuries were caused by direct and indirect contact with the enemy, IEDs, helicopter crashes, suicide bombings, and nonbattle trauma. Casualty evacuation rarely occurred with only single patients. Many of their patients arrived in groups or as part of a true mass casualty incident, such as the attack on the United Nations headquarters building in Baghdad on 19 August 2003.[65]

From January to July 2003, the 86th CSH was deployed in support of preparations for and during the invasion of Iraq.[60,66] After its initial staging in Kuwait, the 86th was split into multiple elements once OIF began. These elements included a 44-bed hospital at Tallil Air Base near An Nasiriyah and two FSEs in the V Corps headquarters area. An additional 84-bed primary element remained in Kuwait to provide medical care to support elements that remained in Kuwait, and to receive initial patients from the invasion phase from various FSTs, FRSSs, and the 212th MASH.[60,61]

The 28th CSH supported the 3rd and 101st Infantry Divisions' area of responsibility during the initial ground invasion.[63] Personnel established a 44-bed hospital while en route to Baghdad. Once the city was in the control of US and allied forces, the 28th CSH split and established two facilities. The main element was a large facility in the "Green Zone" just east of Baghdad International Airport. A second, smaller hospital was established in Tikrit. While many medical-surgical facilities came under attack during the war, the 28th's location in the Green Zone made it a target of opportunity, and the area was shot at routinely with rockets and artillery. While no CSH members died of wounds during this rotation, a few years later, in 2006, the 28th CSH would return to this location and lose a team member to indirect fire.[67]

The 21st CSH convoyed from Kuwait to sites in northern Iraq.[64] The unit had the furthest convoy from its starting point in Kuwait of all the initial CSHs that moved into theater. Their 3-day drive ended about 100 miles north of Baghdad, where they established a 44-bed hospital at the airfield in Balad. The 21st would establish two sites, known as "Bear North," located in Mosul, and "Bear South," located in Balad. The Bear South site was expanded to a larger 164-bed facility, while Bear North was enlarged to the 84-bed configuration. These sites became very busy as the war transitioned. Two periods of significant patient inflow were during the Battle of Mosul and the Battle of Fallujah.[68,69]

The 47th CSH, from Fort Lewis, Washington, also played an important role in the initial phases of the invasion, but its primary mission was to provide hospital support in Kuwait.[70,71] The unit would provide combat support and combat service support, and treat DoD civilians who ran the massive logistical and support mission for the troops who advanced across the border into Iraq. Support personnel in Kuwait were often victims of job-related injuries and accidents while working with heavy and dangerous military equipment and supplies. The 47th also received combat trauma cases from Role 2 surgical teams during the initial invasion phase until the various other Role 3 facilities were established during phase two of the war. The unit's efforts provided care for numerous battle and nonbattle injuries and served as a safety net for the military service members conducting the fighting to the north.

The 10th CSH, from Fort Carson, Colorado, had prepared to accompany and support the 4th Infantry Division as it moved through Turkey into northern Iraq, but was not able to conduct this mission when the Turkish Parliament denied the US and British forces use of its ground or air space for the invasion.[72] After the mission was scrapped, the 10th CSH was notified that it would go to Kuwait and advance north into the area it had previously been tasked to support. However, upon arrival in Kuwait, the mission changed again. The

10th CSH established itself there to provide support for local military and associated civilians, and prepared to receive patients from Iraq, if needed. At one point, team members were told they might move to northern Iraq for a humanitarian mission, but again they were selected to stay and provide care in Kuwait. After approximately 4 months, the 10th CSH returned to Colorado and prepared for a return mission to Iraq in 2005. While the unit never entered the combat zone, it was prepared to do so, and it did provide essential care to support personnel in Kuwait.[68,72]

AIRBORNE INSERTION OF FORWARD SURGICAL TEAMS

Of the initial modern FSTs stood up in 1997, five were designated as airborne capable: the 782nd FST (Airborne) within the 82nd Airborne Division at Fort Bragg, North Carolina; the 274th FST (Airborne) and 2nd Armored Cavalry FST (Airborne) within the 44th Medical Brigade, also at Fort Bragg; the 250th FST (Airborne) within the 62nd Medical Brigade at Fort Lewis, Washington; and the 67th FST (Airborne) within the 30th Medical Brigade in Germany. Other FSTs would also receive the prestigious airborne designation and the challenging mission capability during the GWOT era (see Chapter 11 for details). The mission of airborne FSTs was to jump into combat along with their combat arms colleagues. Personnel would then assemble to provide advanced trauma care alongside their fellow medical company paratroopers. Approximately 1 to 4 hours after the jump, with the area secured, the FST's Alpha echelon could set up for more advanced resuscitation and surgery, functioning separately for 6 to 48 hours while awaiting reconstitution with the Bravo echelon once the airfield was repaired and aircraft could air-land the second wave of soldiers.[73,74]

The 250th FST (Airborne) was the first conventional modern US Army FST to execute this mission during the initial invasion of Iraq in 2003. The team was led by LTC Harry Stinger, a long-time leader in the FST community, especially in the airborne FST units. In 1996 he had been the commander of the 82nd Airborne Surgical Squad, which was converted to an official FST, the 782nd FST (Airborne), in 1997. While with the 782nd, Stinger and his unit supported the Defense Readiness Brigade mission, now known as the Global Response Force mission. He led the development of many administrative, logistical, training, and operational concepts used by airborne FSTs today. The 250th FST (Airborne) thus had the most knowledgeable airborne FST commander, along with other highly trained and qualified surgical soldiers in the Alpha and Bravo echelons.

FSTs usually train with their local brigade combat teams for the Global Response Force mission. This facilitates development of standard operating procedures and supports unity as a combined Role 2 medical-surgical trauma team. Unfortunately, in 2003 the 250th FST (Airborne) had limited information on the mission and associated details. Its mission, originally for a possible airborne assault, was changed first to an air-land mission and later back to an airborne assault mission. Also, the 250th would support an infantry brigade that it had never trained with, one on the other side of the world. Team members joined the 173rd Airborne Infantry Brigade in Vicenza, Italy, only 5 days before the mission, without taking part in the initial medical planning. Because the 173rd did not have a dedicated FST stationed with it, its members were not familiar with the integration concepts of FSTs, which were not part of their airborne medical standard operating procedures. Fortunately LTC Stinger had years of experience with airborne FSTs and was able to coordinate with the 173rd brigade surgeon, MAJ Richard Malish, and other organic medical staff on how to best employ their assets. These leaders had to make hard decisions on short notice that could have a huge impact on soldiers' outcomes a few days later.

LTC Stinger and MAJ Malish developed plans on who would jump versus be air-landed.[75] Due to limited space on the initial heavy drop aircraft, the vehicles carrying the FST's equipment and supplies replaced two previously loaded vehicles from the medical support company. The 173rd Brigade Medical Company would now be short their patient-hold capability for the initial phases of the mission. It is not uncommon for some vehicles to be bumped during training, so airborne FSTs know that two vehicles' worth of equipment is the minimum they must bring to provide advanced resuscitative and surgical care to up to 10 severely initial injured patients. It is also not uncommon for the number of FST jump personnel to be changed to nine or even eight from the planned ten.

The 250th FST (Airborne) experienced this situation when its members executed their airborne forced entry mission into Iraq on 26 March 2003. The exact makeup of the Alpha echelon is mission dependent, based on many factors. The following members of the 250th made this first, and to date only, jump of a modern FST into combat: LTC Harry Stinger (general surgeon and 250th FST commander), MAJ John Devine (orthopedic surgeon), MAJ Brad West (nurse anesthetist), CPT Glen Carlsson (emergency room registered nurse), Sergeant First Class (SFC) Robert Novak (licensed practical nurse and FST detachment sergeant), SFC Luke Fullerton (healthcare specialist), Staff Sergeant (SSG) Robert Burns (healthcare specialist), SSG Abel Tavarez (operating room specialist), and Specialist (SPC) William Goldsworth (operating room specialist). (See previous chapters for information about early surgical squads and detachments that air-landed into Operation Just Cause and air-dropped during World War II.[76,77])

The team heavy rigged and jumped two M998 highly mobile military wheeled vehicles (HMMWVs) loaded with a single deployable rapid assembly shelter; one 5-kw diesel generator; multiple medical equipment sets with enough equipment and supplies to set up and care for approximately 10 surgical patients; and 20 units of packed red blood cells.[78,79] Blood products were acquired from DoD resources in Europe. The team also requested nonstandard fresh frozen plasma (FFP) and platelets, but these were not provided. Of note, later in both theaters FFP was provided to all FSTs, but, due to their short shelf life, platelets are still not available. The packed red blood cells the team acquired were packed in two standard commercial Styrofoam coolers with ice, with one cooler placed in the front of each vehicle.[80] The issued blood refrigerators were not loaded because they took up valuable space in the back of the HMMWVs. The Bravo echelon carried the remainder of the unit's military and medical personnel, equipment, and supplies.

Over 950 paratroopers exited the airplanes that night and jumped not only into the pitch darkness over Iraq, but also into history.[79] Not since the British Army's 1st Surgical Team, led by Lieutenant Charles Rob, parachuted into Souk-el-Arba, Tunisia, in World War II had a similar event occurred.[81] The jump made by the 250th FST (Airborne) is considered the first of its type by a US military conventional surgical unit (see Chapter 9

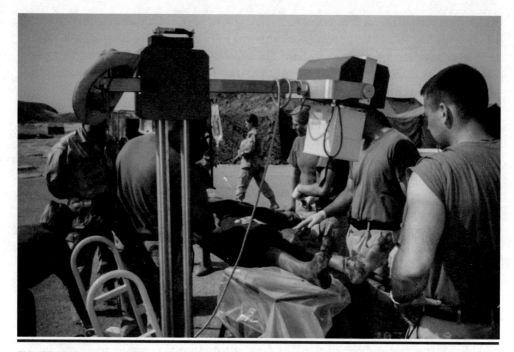

FIGURE 10-10. Members of the 173rd Infantry Brigade (Airborne) Medical Company and the 250th Forward Surgical Team (Airborne) care for patients on the airfield they occupied in Northern Iraq in March 2003. These paratroopers were trained to perform triage, resuscitation, medical management, and surgery with minimal assets after jumping into a combat zone. The unit would later have better tents and facilities as the battlefield matured. Here they are evaluating a patient in an outside care area with a portable x-ray machine. Photograph courtesy of COL Richard Malish, former brigade surgeon, 173rd Infantry Brigade.

for further details). Fortunately, the 250th's patient load was much less than what Dr Rob experienced. A total of 18 patients were injured on the drop zone and treated by the 173rd Medical Company and 250th FST (Airborne). Injuries ranged from mild jump injuries to a possible leg fracture. Luckily, there were no life-threatening injuries due to jump complications or initial combat action.

Contributing factors to this success included an intense pre-mission parachute-training regimen, a large drop zone that was free of obstacles, favorable wind conditions, soft terrain secondary to recent rainfall, and no enemy contact. The FST Alpha echelon helped with the evaluation and management of many of the initially injured soldiers, including minor extremity injuries, a soldier with bilateral dislocated shoulders, and a jumper with a presumed tibia-fibula fracture (later diagnosed as a grade III sprain).[78,82] After the initial air insertion, the team linked up with the Bravo echelon to establish the full FST (Figure 10-10).

Members of the 250th supported numerous medical and surgical needs of US and allied personnel, civilians, and enemy prisoners of war in their area of responsibility. They also assisted other unique support missions during their deployment. These included medical civil affairs mission support, in which they worked with the local surgical community to help with numerous projects. The 250th provided much needed support to the local population and showed the Iraqis in this area what the Americans could provide. The surgical staff was able to coordinate with the American College of Surgeons to provide valuable training material for the local national surgeons to use. They also worked with the Air Force EMEDS unit at Kirkuk Military Airfield on a few occasions.

By the end of their 1-year deployment, 250th staff had performed 59 surgeries on 48 patients (including US troops, allied troops, and enemy prisoners of war). An additional 16 patients with nonoperative trauma were treated. The patients had an average revised trauma score of 7.0 +/- 2. Approximately 25% of injuries were nonbattle related, 35% were blast injuries, and 40% were gunshot injuries. These various mechanisms caused torso injuries in 21% of patients, head and neck injuries in 28%, and extremity injuries in 51%. Four patients died in the FST's triage area or facility, including three from nonsurvivable head injuries and one secondary to exsanguination from a superficial femoral artery and vein injury.[17,83]

Overall, the unit had a very successful mission and provided high-quality care to the soldiers in its area of responsibility. In addition, it validated that the airborne FST concept could be executed, from loading the proper equipment, jumping the equipment and surgical team out of a plane, and set-up on the drop zone, to providing care prior to the main body's arrival. The 250th's lessons learned have been passed on to other airborne FST members via various publications and word of mouth. Their actions were recognized with the Bronze Star, Combat Parachutist Badge, and Arrow Head Device.[77,78,82]

TRANSITION FROM MANEUVER BRIGADES TO AREA SUPPORT MISSION

Once the linear battlefield was no longer present, the management of various support elements in theater became complex for a period of time. Coalition forces were spread throughout the country, and small pockets of friendly forces and anticoalition groups were mixed in between. Units might live and work next to other units that could not support their administrative and logistical needs due to differences in branch of service or chains of command. This was also true for the FSTs.[52]

The FSTs at this time were attached to maneuver brigades, except for three unique FSTs that were direct reporting units permanently assigned to a regiment or division. These were the 2nd Armored Cavalry Regiment FST (Airborne), 801st FST (Air Assault), and 782nd FST (Airborne), which always fell under the 2nd Armored Cavalry Regiment, 101st Airborne Division (Air Assault), and 82nd Airborne Division, respectively, even in garrison.

The location of surgical assets was determined by the combatant commander, based on recommendations of his or her medical staff, which did not always take into account the needs of the entire theater of operations. To solve the problem, administration, tactical, and operation control of FSTs was transferred from brigade combat teams to a medical task force. This change allowed for one governing body to oversee the placement of Role 2 surgical assets and Role 3 assets to best meet the need of the theater commander's mission, regardless of which combat and support units moved in and out of the region.

As the mission transitioned to counterinsurgency operations, the entire system was able to manage the needs of a mobile and difficult adversary. FSTs were placed in areas that better met the needs of a region, instead of the unit they were first assigned to. Future FSTs would come into theater under this arrangement but, by virtue of location, would still support the combat unit in their area of operations. Some units were able to collaborate with local facilities and providers (Figure 10-11). Some FSTs augmented the CSH in their area and could rapidly move to an area that required additional support for both conventional and Special Operations soldiers. This change had an impact on the garrison management of the three direct reporting FSTs.

Between late 2004 and 2006, these three units were deactivated and then reactivated under new command. First, the 2nd Armored Cavalry Regiment FST (Airborne) left the 2nd Armored Cavalry Regiment in 2004 and became the 759th FST (Airborne), under the 44th Medical Brigade, while under the command of LTC Richard Ellison.[84,85] Next, in 2005, the 801st FST (Air Assault) left the 101st Airborne Division and became the 772nd FST (Air Assault), also under the 44th Medical Brigade, while under the command of LTC Kirby Gross. Lastly, in 2006, the 782nd FST (Airborne) left the 82nd Airborne Division and became the 541st FST (Airborne), again under the 44th Medical Brigade, while under the command of LTC Shawn Nessen. The 772nd stayed at Fort Campbell, Kentucky, and the 541st and 759th stayed at Fort Bragg, North Carolina, continuing the traditions of their former units while also setting new standards and developing proud reputations for their new designations.[84,86,87]

THEATER CLOSURE

Beginning 1 September 2010, OIF officially ended and became the new mission known as Operation New Dawn. The focus of this operation was to finalize the training of the Iraqi military and police forces, finalize other stabilization efforts, and transition the future assistance of the Iraqi government and people to the Department of State. The US Army XVIII Airborne Corps performed command and control duties of US Forces-Iraq during the final phases in 2011. One of the main focuses of the deputy corps commander, Lieutenant General (LTG) Frank Helmick, was the maintenance of the advanced surgical capability that the United States and allied countries had become accustomed to.[88,89] Plans were developed to ensure that this would be possible. The medical task force coordinated with their assigned FSTs to create a method of coverage and evacuation.

There were three basic types of facility closures involving FSTs. They included (1) smaller outpost or station closures, (2) large operating base closures, and (3) medical-surgical unit transitions of authority from DoD to the Department of State. The FSTs were often already functioning in their 10-person split capacity, but would need to function with even less personnel and equipment for a short period just prior to leaving their sites. Instrumental in these closures was the 912th FST.

Commanded by COL Timothy Counihan, 912th personnel knew that high-quality surgical care could be provided by four to six skilled members for short periods of time, based on their experience from early OEF deployments and knowledge of published and unpublished sources. However, due to operational needs during the closure of Contingency

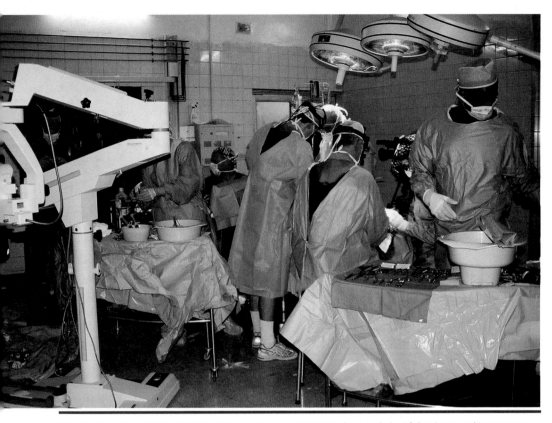

FIGURE 10-11. Partnership training and care became commonplace early in Afghanistan and Iraq as part of winning the hearts and minds of local citizens. Here a local national patient receives surgical care from members of the 2nd Armored Cavalry Regiment Forward Surgical Team and a local surgeon. These collaborations included local providers conducting joint medial training with US and allied staff. Photograph courtesy of COL Kim Smith, former perioperative nurse, 2nd ACR FST.

Operating Station (COS) Gary Owen, 912th team members had to limit their final "jump" team to four members. This jump team would remain as the only real trauma management asset for damage control resuscitation and surgery for the final 2 days that COS Gary Owen was open. The jump team ensured that all 1,200 soldiers leaving the area during those last few days would have combat surgical coverage, and departed by rotary wing only 4 hours before the final American soldiers left.[88]

The next closure was slightly different from COS Gary Owen. Through careful planning and availability of assets (including nearby fixed and rotary wing service), the split 912th was able to function as a complete 10-person team for the closure of the much larger Camp Adder. The team provided coverage until 18 hours prior to the final ground convoy departure time. This gave them 6 hours to tear down their facility, pack it, palletize their equipment, and deliver it to the convoy area. They then moved to the airfield and were transported by C-17 Globemaster aircraft.[88]

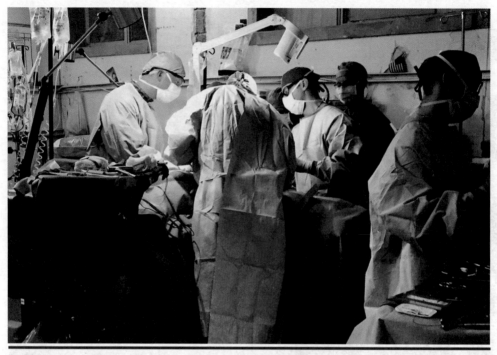

FIGURE 10-12. MAJ Ronald Kembro and MAJ Timothy Placket of the 772nd Forward Surgical Team (Air Assault) perform surgery at a newly established location in Iraq in 2015 in support of Operation Inherent Resolve. While the facility is brick and mortar, the team is using standard field equipment. The return to Iraq is a new beginning in a traditional immature theater of support, which is developing at this time. Photograph courtesy of MAJ Timothy Placket, trauma surgeon, 772nd FST.

The other half of the 912th split FST was responsible for the transition of medical coverage to a new Department of State medical unit at Contingency Operating Base (COB) Basrah. The United States had taken over responsibility of this area in 2009 from British medical units that had been there for most of OIF. The 912th FST provided training and mentorship to the new Department of State medical-surgical staff. The old and new team collaborated for a short period of time and provided capabilities and capacity similar to a 20-person FST. Once the final US convoy was beyond the area of coverage and closer to the combat support hospital in Kuwait, the 912th broke down its equipment and supplies and the team members said their final good-byes. They left Basrah in the hands of the Department of State team and flew via rotary wing to Kuwait.[88]

Leaving bases like Gary Owen, Adder, and Basrah is much different than moving to a new site, as some units had done earlier in the war. Instead of having a large amount of support locally to move somewhere that may or may not be mature, FSTs that close or transition bases are leaving an area with minimal support and possibly heading home (Figure 10-12). The positive and negative emotional impact of these missions can adversely affect a team if not managed well. The 912th did an exemplary job of maintaining high morale, staying as long as they operationally could to provide coverage, and remaining focused on their core mission: to be far forward, possibly in harm's way, to stabilize casualties for further transport along the continuum of care, with the final destination being home with friends and family.[88]

US ARMY SURGEONS GENERAL CONTRIBUTIONS TO THE SUCCESS OF THE FORWARD SURGICAL TEAM

The significance of the FST was clear to the Army surgeons general since their initial inception in the late 1980s. Lieutenant generals Ledford, LaNoue, and Blanck had the vision to realize that the old field and general hospital and MASH systems were dated and needed to be replaced. Their collaboration with subordinate units' recommendations and surgical subject matter experts, along with analysis of lessons learned from various US and NATO units in the 1980s and 1990s, led to development of a sound platform and mission for future FSTs.[90] During the GWOT, four Army surgeon generals maintained strong support for the FST community.

Just prior to the GWOT, LTG James B Peake became the 40th US Army surgeon general.[91] As a general/thoracic surgeon, he truly appreciated that the FST was the Army's premier medical-surgical unit of the future. His vision and timing were paramount to the success of FSTs for the next 15-plus years. Before becoming surgeon general, LTG Peake was the Army Medical Department (AMEDD) Center and School commander from 1996 to 2000.[92] While there, he ensured that a new dedicated FST field manual and Army Training and Evaluation Program-Mission Training Plans were published in 1997 and 1999, respectively, to help guide FSTs to the highest level of combat medical readiness.[23,93] He also played an essential role in establishing the Joint Trauma Training Center at Ben Taub Medical Center in Houston, Texas, and the FST Commanders Course at Fort Sam Houston, Texas.[94,95] After becoming surgeon general, Peake was the senior Army medical officer as the wars in Afghanistan and Iraq began. During this time, LTG Peake successfully finalized the new training partnership with the Ryder Trauma Center in Miami, Florida, to establish the Army Trauma Training Center (ATTC), initiated the Joint Trauma Theater Registry, and supported the increased number of active and Reserve FSTs to meet the needs of a war being fought in multiple theaters.[96–99]

In 2004, LTG Kevin C Kiley succeeded LTG Peake.[91] He too was an advocate of the FST, starting before he became the 41st Army surgeon general. As the AMEDD Center and School commander from 2000 to 2002, LTG Kiley helped update the FST field manual in 2003, which improved guidance in the new types of battlefield engagement.[24,100] He also worked with LTG Peake in the approval of the Joint Trauma Theater Registry and the ATTC.[96–98] Once he became surgeon general, Kiley supported the transformation of all FSTs into medical brigade assets, as well as decreased deployment time for certain FST and CSH providers to help prevent surgical skills degradation. LTG Kiley was also instrumental in the establishment of the formal Joint Trauma System (JTS) in 2006,[98] and he pushed for all deploying FST personnel to attend predeployment trauma training at the ATTC for clinical validation.[101]

In 2007, LTG Eric B Schoomaker became the 42nd Army surgeon general.[102] Like his predecessor, Schoomaker understood that the FST was the most essential element to saving lives on the current battlefield and worked hard to ensure their success. Under his leadership, the old Army Training and Evaluation Program-Mission Training Plans system was converted to the newer Combined Arms Training Strategy System, giving teams a clearer and more complete training program to use throughout their Army Force Generation Cycle.[103,104] In 2009, he finalized a policy started by LTG Kiley to ensure that all medical and surgical units attended their appropriate predeployment trauma training.[105] LTG Schoomaker also ensured that four FSTs would be assigned to support the Homeland Security Defense Chemical Biological Radiation Nuclear Response Force mission. Near the end of his tenure, he supported a force design update for the FST to meet the needs of the next decade and future conflicts. His contributions to the FST community provided them with the proper manning, equipment, and training to save the maximum amount of lives on the battlefield.

Most recently, LTG Patricia D Horoho has maintained strong support for the Role 2 surgical team after becoming the 43rd Army surgeon general in 2011.[106] She supported the radical redesign of the FST into the new forward resuscitative surgical team, and continued to ensure that funding and personnel were available for an optimal clinical training experience at the ATTC as well as the Combat Extremity Surgery Course. In 2013, a new Army training publication replaced the previous FST field manual.[107] This new document consolidated the past medical company, FST, and CSH manuals into one brief publication.

INJURED AND FALLEN FORWARD SURGICAL PROVIDERS

Performing surgery far forward is a challenging mission for many reasons. Providers often do not have all the equipment and supplies they are accustomed to in stateside practice or at a CSH. Resupply, communication, Internet connectivity, and basic electricity are also challenges. Often the living conditions and basic morale, welfare, and recreation options are much more limited than at the larger bases. Also, the forward setting is a much more dangerous place to work. Because there is more manual labor involved, FST members are known to have more disease and non-battle injury conditions than colleagues working elsewhere. Even more dangerous is that personnel are physically closer to the conflict, both during initial ground or air assaults and later, as the FST occupies more austere forward operating bases and combat outposts closer to the enemy.

Many FST members have sustained combat wounds while deployed. At the time of this writing, injured FST personnel notably include members of the 915th FST (Reserve), 274th and 250th airborne FSTs, and, most recently, the 628th FST (Reserve).[84,108-112] In addition, four medical personnel—from the 782nd FST (Airborne), 1st FST (Reserve), 274th FST (Airborne), and the 848th FST (Reserve)—have died during combat while deployed with an FST.[113-116] Personnel assigned to CSHs endured combat injuries and some fatalities too.

On the evening of 3 July 2003, the members of the 915th FST, from Vancouver, Washington, were set up in Balad, Iraq, finishing up work and relaxing for the night. Without warning, a volley of mortars came into their compound, and one round hit their facility. Of the team's 20 members, 14 sustained some level of injury from the blast, and many of them required medical treatment and surgery. The injured received evaluation, resuscitation, and surgery at the 21st CSH and the newly arrived 1st FST, from Fort Trotten, New York, which were both located nearby at Balad. Fortunately, all team members survived their injuries.[108,110]

On 20 March 2004, US forces came under attack from insurgents in Fallujah, Iraq. This coordinated attack included the use of rockets fired from a distance at the US military compound. One of the rockets detonated near the location of MAJ Mark D Taylor, MD. Mark was a Professional Filler System (PROFIS) surgeon in the 782nd FST (Airborne) out of Fort Bragg, North Carolina. His fellow FST members were unaware of his location and, needing his assistance as other casualties arrived, frantically asked for someone to find him. Then a casualty arrived whom they recognized. It was Mark. His good friend, Womack Army Medical Center colleague, and fellow PROFIS surgeon on the 782nd, MAJ Sean Montgomery quickly realized that Mark's injuries were too severe to survive. MAJ Taylor, who was 41, became the first FST member killed in action. He has been recognized in numerous ways. At Fort Bragg, a street and a simulation training center, the Taylor-Sandri Medical Training Center, were named after him, as was a trauma lecture series at the Gary Wratten Army Surgical Symposium.[113]

The second FST member to die in combat was another surgeon, MAJ John P Pryor, DO. Previously a trauma surgeon at the University of Pennsylvania Medical Center, MAJ Pryor joined the Army Reserves in 2004 and deployed to the medical facility at Abu Ghraib in 2006. For his second deployment, he wanted an even more challenging assignment and volunteered to deploy with the 1st FST from Fort Trotten, New York. He was killed at age 42 on the morning of 25 December 2008 during a mortar attack on his compound in Mosul, Iraq. John was highly respected in the civilian and military medical community, and his loss had a significant impact on many. He, too, was recognized and remembered in numerous ways, including in articles and stories in the American College of Surgeons' *Journal of Trauma* and the *General Surgery News*. He also had a memorial lecture series named after him. On 4 February 2015, the John P Pryor Shock-Trauma and Resuscitation (STAR) Unit at Pennsylvania Presbyterian Medical Center opened. The unit was named in Pryor's honor by his former mentor, US Naval Reserves Commander C William Schwab.[114]

The third FST member to die in combat was SSG Ronald J Spino, the senior licensed practical nurse for the 274th FST (Airborne) from Fort Bragg, North Carolina. Ron started his 1-year deployment in Iraq and then moved with his unit to Afghanistan to provide much needed surgical support in Bala Murghab. This northwestern region of Afghanistan near the Turkmenistan boarder was underdeveloped and a challenging location with minimal assets. The team performed well and maintained its morale. With only 1 month to go on his deployment, SSG Spino was shot and killed on 29 December 2009 by an Afghan National Army soldier while both were on a helicopter landing zone. (Additional tragedy happened a few weeks later, in January 2010, when the site was hit by indirect fire as the 274th was conducting a site handover to the 250th FST from Fort Lewis, Washington. Multiple team members from both units sustained significant injuries, including the operating room nurse from the 274th and both the senior surgeon and orthopedic surgeon from the 250th. Fortunately, there were no lethal injuries.) SSG Spino was 45 years old. He was recognized and remembered like his fallen comrades. A large commemorative plaque hangs in the 274th FST (Airborne) team house at Fort Bragg.[111,115] In addition, the main training room at the Army Trauma Training Center in Miami, Florida, has been dedicated in his honor, reminding all deploying FST members of the risks and challenges that await them.[115]

The fourth FST member to die to date in combat was another Army Reservist, CPT Joshua M. McClimans, RN. After a 2005 tour to Iraq in 2005 with the 256th CSH, CPT McClimans was the critical care nurse for the 848th FST, from Twinsburg, Ohio, while the unit was deployed to FOB Salerno. On 22 April 2011, FOB Salerno received indirect fire attacks. At 30 years old, Joshua was fatally injured by one of the munitions that entered the FOB and detonated. Joshua's grandmother, the mayor of his hometown of Jamestown, Pennsylvania, ensured that he was honored for his service and actions.[116]

The most recent injuries sustained to FSEs by combat action occurred during the 7 August 2012 attack on FOB Shank, which was attacked by insurgents early that morning. The attack involved a vehicle-borne IED with approximately 3,000 pounds of explosives. The explosion caused a large breach, approximately 75 feet long, in the base's thick outer wall. The attack killed four individuals on the base and injured another 28, including one of the surgeons assigned to the 648th FST.[84]

All of these FST members volunteered to take on the challenges of combat trauma so they could share their knowledge, skills, passion, and empathy with the combatant soldiers. None truly believed they would one day become one of the many patients seen at their surgical facility. None actually thought they too would die in combat rather than return home in the manner they had planned. The four fallen soldiers, the other providers with injuries, and fellow FST members who have deployed since 2001 are part of a unique family of eclectic medical staff dedicated to saving lives beyond what many noncombat medical providers can comprehend.

LTC Robert Blease, SSG Ronald Spino's commander at the 274th FST (Airborne), served at the ATTC after their deployment. He ensured that SSG Spino's spirit and memory would live on as all deploying Army FSTs saw his name and story during their predeployment trauma training in Miami. The training center named after Spino also includes a "wall for our fallen FST heroes" with the photos, names, and units of the four who gave their lives while trying to save lives. The wall is pointed out on the first day of training to ensure that all students take their training seriously and understand the risk they are volunteering to take.

The US Role 2 surgical teams described in this chapter faced the challenges of forward deployment and did everything they could to improve the lives and outcomes of their fellow soldiers on the battlefield. Afterward they shared their lessons learned and worked toward process improvement back in garrison. Amid the chaos of war, they found opportunities to improve their patients' outcomes and the trauma system as a whole. This is an accomplishment of which each and every one of them is right to be proud.

TOPICS AND ISSUES AFFECTING FORWARD SURGICAL CARE

Military Working Dogs Cared for by the Forward Surgical Team

During this era, a new type of patient started showing up at the doors of the FST. FSTs were well trained and prepared to take care of US soldiers, NATO soldiers, enemy prisoners of war, and local nationals; however, when military working dogs (MWDs) began to arrive, providers had to adjust their medical-surgical knowledge and skills to help these new "soldiers." Typically, veterinarian medical detachments are co-located or near Role 3 facilities, a distance from the outposts where most of the animals worked and were injured (Figure 10-13). A significant number of these animals would not have survived if they were sent on the long journey to Role 3 facilities, so they were taken to the area Role 2 or FST instead.

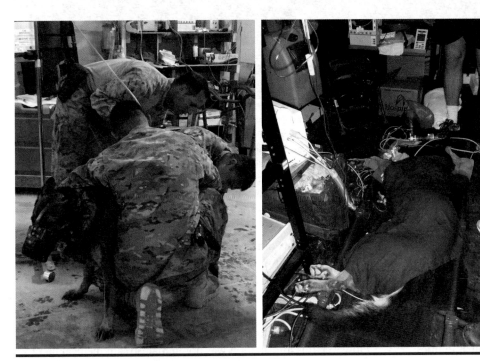

[Left] FIGURE 10-13. A canine is cared for at the 772nd Forward Surgical Team (Air Assault) during Operation Inherent Resolve after receiving multiple lacerations from concertina wire. Military working dogs are considered soldiers and receive care within the Department of Defense (DoD) system. Often they receive initial care by forward surgical teams because they are further forward than the DoD veterinarian assets. Photograph courtesy of MAJ Tmothy Plackett, former trauma surgeon, 772nd FST.

[Right] FIGURE 10-14. A NATO military working dog being cared for in the postoperative setting. This explosive ordnance disposal canine was cared for by a conventional forward surgical team supporting NATO in Regional Command–North, Afghanistan. The canine became hyperthermic after surgery. Medical management was coordinated for via cell phone with US veterinarians stationed in Bagram. Photograph courtesy of MAJ Christopher Vanfosson, former critical care nurse, 541st FST.

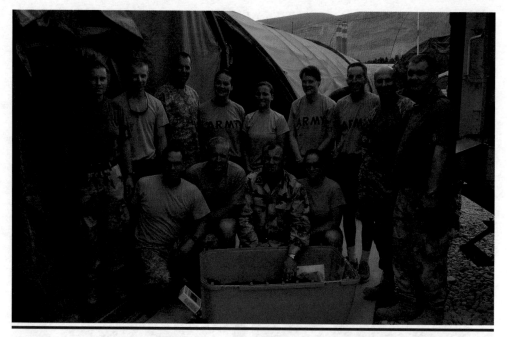

FIGURE 10-15. Trauma care not only saves the patient, but also strengthens partnerships. While most partnership building during the war was between allied countries and local nationals as part of the counterinsurgency doctrine, many times it also occurred within allied personnel. Thousands of coalition patients have been cared for at US Role 2 and 3 facilities. Here the collaboration at a multinational camp can be seen, as multiple combined and joint conventional and Special Operations units arrange for a military working dog to be transported to Bagram for further care.

Although veterinary clinical medicine officers had been assigned to deployed veterinary units since 2005 to ensure high-level care for MWDs in theater,[117] and MWD management has been detailed in military veterinarian and Special Operations doctrine for many years, veterinary trauma management was sparsely documented in the peer-reviewed literature.[118] During the GWOT era, Dr Wesley M Taylor, MAJ Janice L Baker, and a few others began publishing detailed articles addressing gaps and lessons learned in managing MWDs with combat injuries.[117,119–122] However, this information was not in mainstream medical literature or presented to the surgical staff members on FSTs. Additionally, MWD management was not part of the FST's mission essential task list and few team members ever imagined they would one day be looking at an MWD lying on a stretcher with combat injuries and in extremis. As the dogs arrived, individuals from various FSTs began documenting their experiences treating the dogs so that lessons learned could be passed on.

One of the first places where this care was documented and distributed in the conventional military medical community was in "First to Cut: Trauma Lessons Learned in the Combat Zone,"[123] a collection of case scenarios from OIF and OEF sponsored by the US Army Institute of Surgical Research (ISR) and edited by COL Lorne Blackbourne. Chapter 14, titled "Military Unique," described an MWD with a gunshot wound to the abdomen and laid out a basic pathway to manage these types of patients. After reading this case scenario or hearing about MWDs as FST patients, some units asked for additional predeployment training from their local conventional or Special Operations veterinarian units.

This training proved valuable. One FST, the 541st from Fort Bragg, was provided a canine surgery standard operating procedure by the veterinarians prior to deployment, and later performed multiple urgent and emergent procedures and surgeries on NATO MWDs in their area of responsibility. One patient was an explosive ordinance MWD with an acute gastric dilatation volvulus that was extremely sick on presentation. The dog had just arrived in-country and was lethargic and tachycardic, with significant abdominal distension. Asked to help, the FST first contacted NATO veterinarians at the Role 3, approximately 2 to 3 hours away by rotary wing, but these veterinarians did not have surgical training. The 541st then contacted US veterinarians in Bagram, and performed the surgery via phone consultation. The veterinarians in Bagram provided advice on a different way to perform a gastropexy that was slightly different from the technique used in a human patient, and later they provided postoperative advice when the dog became hyperthermic and needed intervention (Figure 10-14). Otherwise, the case was similar to human laparotomy and foregut surgery, and a few questions were answered by the canine surgery standard operating procedure. After the surgery, the MWD patient was transported to Bagram and had a full recovery (Figure 10-15). He had in-country convalescence and was ready to go out on missions with his handler a few weeks later.

The 541st documented this case in a peer-reviewed journal with collaboration from the US veterinarians in Bagram,[124] which sparked interest and controversy within the veterinarian and surgical community. The final consensus was that in certain situations, initial stabilization of MWDs with resuscitation and surgery, if indicated, could be performed by a nonveterinary surgeon if the dog could not be sent to a veterinarian in a timely manner.

The 541st also provided initial care to two NATO search-and-rescue MWDs that were severely lacerated after becoming entangled in concertina wire. These interventions saved not only the MWDs' lives and limbs, but also thousands of dollars in transportation costs and unnecessary risk to an aviation crew, while strengthening relationships with NATO allies.

A clinical practice guideline titled "Canine Resuscitation" was approved and published on 15 April 2011 by the Joint Theater Trauma System under the ISR.[125] As part of the annual review process, the clinical practice guideline was updated on 19 March 2012 and renamed "Clinical Management of Military Working Dogs."[126] All medical providers deploying to the Central Command area of responsibility are expected to be familiar with this guideline and all clinical practice guidelines, and the topic is covered at the ATTC, Navy Trauma Training Center, Centers for the Sustainment of Trauma and Readiness, and Joint Forces Combat Trauma Management Course, as part of the mandatory predeployment trauma training. Various other military units have also adapted doctrine for MWDs; for example, the US Army Special Operations Command has a canine TCCC guideline for its medical staff,[127] providing basic information to Role 1 and Role 2 providers. Additionally, it is recommended that units train in advance with their local military veterinarian center and MWD handlers as part of their routine annual training to ensure the best possible patient outcomes.

Unexploded Ordnance Embedded in Patients

FST members deployed to OEF and OIF often found themselves in unexpected situations, for instance, how to manage a patient with embedded unexploded ordnance (UXO). Also referred to as retained or impaled UXO in the literature, embedded UXO occurs very rarely. Cases of embedded UXO have involved rocket-propelled grenades (RPGs), large-caliber explosive bullets, mortar rounds, and grenades such as M79 and M203 rounds. Patients with embedded UXO usually have significant blunt injury but no true blast injury.

Most medical providers know to check for any type of ammunition and ordnance patients may have in their pockets, known as "loose" UXO, before the patient is brought into a treatment facility, especially when treating unknown local patients or known enemy patients. Loose UXO is equally or more dangerous than embedded UXO because it may be missed, and it could detonate if dropped or stepped on during patient transport or care. However, few providers were trained to handle the mental, emotional, logistical, or clinical aspects of caring for a soldier with embedded UXO.

In 1999, "Removal of Unexploded Ordnance From Patients: A 50-Year Military Experience and Current Recommendations," by LTC Brian Lein, LTC John Holcomb, CPT Scott Brill, COL Steven Hetz, and MAJ Thomas McCrorey, was published in *Military Medicine*.[128] The authors found cases of 36 patients with retained UXO dating from World War II, either in the global literature or identified by verbal communication with living military physicians. Four of these patients were noted to be moribund upon arrival and died before surgery could be provided. The remaining 32 patients all survived the removal of the UXO, with no injuries sustained by the medical or explosive ordnance disposal (EOD) staff who took care of them. In these 36 cases, 4 injuries were located in the head or neck, 14 in the extremities, and 17 in the trunk; the remaining injury had no clearly documented location. This landmark article also laid out a basic plan for safely performing surgery on these patients with minimal risk to the surgical team.

This article was the only available guidance on the subject until the more widely distributed *Emergency War Surgery–Third United States Revision* handbook was published in 2004.[8] However, neither the article nor the handbook were required predeployment reading, and embedded UXO was not covered in any of the official predeployment training early in the wars. Although official guidance has evolved slightly since these two sources were published, they included a number of basic principles that have endured: notify the local command and the EOD team immediately, evacuate all nonessential personnel from the area, and require essential medical personnel to don individual body armor or EOD blast gear (if they have trained with it). Another recommendation is to avoid using the main care facility because valuable equipment could be lost if the UXO explodes. Instead, move the patient to a pre-designated safe area to ensure force protection and crowd control, and utilize a predetermined and prepackaged set of essential equipment and supplies that have no effect on munitions. These strict policies and procedures were created to ensure provider safety and best patient outcome.

Because fuses are armed and triggered by different methods (impact, electromagnetic, laser, rotational/centrifugal forces, acceleration, etc), these two documents recommend caution to avoid inadvertently arming or detonating the device by rotating the UXO or the patient, avoiding contact with electrical tools or monitoring equipment, avoiding metal-to-metal contact, and always gently moving the patient, thus avoiding sudden movements or impact to the device. Oxygen can safely be provided to the patient, but the oxygen canisters or oxygen generator should not be near the patient to prevent a secondary explosion if the primary UXO detonates.

Most patients with this type of injury will require general anesthesia. Totally intravenous anesthesia (TIVA) should be used instead of inhaled gases, which are contraindicated. If necessary, TIVA can be provided from a distance with an extension tube, allowing the anesthesia provider to remain in a safe location behind sandbags or a blast wall. If general anesthesia is not required, a spinal or regional block can be used. Other points to consider: radiography use is safe, but ultrasound, CT scans, and other studies should be avoided. The device should be removed en bloc, if possible; amputation should be considered if other methods fail. Once the UXO is removed, the patient should be rapidly transported to the main operating room to receive the highest level of surgical and resuscitative care.[9,128–134]

In any situation requiring triage, providers must do the most good for the most patients, so a casualty with embedded UXO should be the last individual to receive care. Also, the patient should be triaged as expectant if their injuries are too severe or the risk of UXO removal is too high (eg, in cases of embedded chemical and biological UXO).

Units should practice UXO management in garrison. Every part of managing a patient with embedded UXO will go better if it is planned for and practiced ahead of time. The set-up of an ancillary surgical site, creation of a blast wall and sandbagging, and the "do's" and "don'ts" of embedded UXO treatment cannot be safely or effectively done if performed strictly on the fly.

At the time of this writing, there have been five known cases of embedded UXO in combat casualties during the GWOT. Three occurred in OEF and are published and well known; however, very little has been published about embedded UXO in OIF and Operation New Dawn (OND). The two known OIF/OND cases will be formally documented here. One of these, the first known case of a soldier surviving embedded UXO during the GWOT, occurred in Iraq in the spring of 2005.[135,136] An RPG went through the door of an HMMWV and penetrated the thorax of a soldier, entering through the open side of his body armor. The soldier was treated in the field and transferred to the 86th CSH, where he underwent surgery. Unfortunately, he was nearly moribund on arrival and died. The device was removed and taken to the large surgical equipment sterilizer until the EOD team was able to remove it.

This case of embedded UXO was not well documented. Individual interviews of 86th CSH staff members indicate that the grenade entered the soldier's thorax in the axillary area and began exiting the anterior chest. It was also stated that the presence of embedded UXO was not clear until the patient was in the operating room, where he was immediately transferred because he was in extremis in the emergency room, before the x-ray had been developed and read. Many standard steps to ensure the safety of the medical providers and equipment were probably not taken, apparently due to the initial lack of knowledge of the embedded UXO. Because of limited documentation in this case, it is unclear whether the explosive part of the RPG was in the soldier's chest, or whether only remnants of the tail section and warhead detonator were embedded.

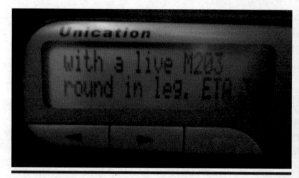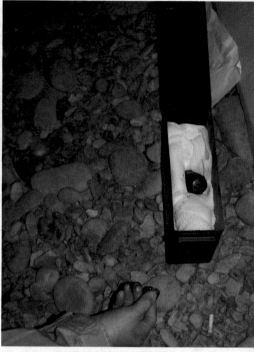

FIGURE 10-16. (a) An image from a pager used at the surgical facility in Tikrit, Iraq, in 2007, detailing information about an inbound patient with a live M203 round embedded in his leg. (b) The removed and still live M203 was placed in an ammunition can lined with medical gauze to create a soft packing. It was removed from the facility and disposed of by the local explosive ordnance disposal team. This was one of the earliest cased of an embedded unexploded ordnance in Iraq War and the first ever documented case of a live M203 round being embedded in a live patient. Photographs courtesy of MAJ John Chovanes, former trauma surgeon, 325th Combat Support Hospital.

The best-documented and most well-known UXO case occurred in OEF and involved a 23-year-old active duty male soldier, Private (PVT) Channing Moss, in 2006.[87,129,137–139] An RPG entered PVT Moss's left side, with the tip lodged in his right hip. The extensive surgery performed on Moss by the 759th FST (Airborne) in Orgun-E, under the supervision of MAJ John S Oh, was videotaped. MAJ Oh and three enlisted medical providers, along with their EOD support personnel, performed this dangerous life-saving surgery. The surgery began with an initial incision at the right anterior hip around the tip of the RPG. Next, a standard trauma laparotomy incision was made. With the assistance of the EOD experts, the grenade was stabilized and the tail section extending out of Moss's left side was safely cut off. The remaining components of the grenade were then advanced forward from left to right, following the projectile's original path, and out the initial right hip incision. The UXO was removed and handed safely off to the EOD team. Additional surgery and resuscitation was performed to stabilize the patient and transport him to Role 3 for further management. Moss survived his wounds after undergoing numerous additional operations at Landstuhl Regional Medical Center, Walter Reed Army Medical Center, and Dwight D Eisenhower Army Medical Center.[137,138]

Numerous news interviews, textbooks, journal articles, and blogs mention this unique case, primarily because of the videotaped surgery. While the cameraman was not an essential member of the surgical team, his presence was not a violation of guidelines. Clinical evaluation and consultation with EOD personnel early on revealed that the warhead was no longer connected to the sustainer motor. The casing for the base of the warhead detonator was seen on x-ray and possibly intact, but it was mechanical and did not have combustibles in it. Lastly, it was assumed that the rocket propellant in the sustainer motor was completed consumed. Due to this proper initial evaluation and consultation, the UXO was assumed to be stable and therefore fairly safe for removal and video documentation. This case and its detailed documentation spurred additional publications discussing these situations and providing guidance on how to properly address them.

A third known case occurred during OIF in 2007. A US Marine was injured and transported to the 325th CSH in Tikrit. The patient was stable, so hospital staff had time to prepare for the situation, setting up an ancillary surgical site and developing a safe plan for the UXO removal (Figure 10-16). MAJ John Chovanes, a trauma surgeon; CPT Michael Hawkins, CRNA; an unknown medic; and an unknown Navy EOD team member donned their personal protective gear and performed the procedure without complications.[140–144] The embedded 40-mm round was disposed of, and the patient was eventually transported to Landstuhl Regional Medical Center and then on to the United States. Fortunately for the patient, Dr Chovanes had discussed this exact scenario with his trauma surgery colleague, MAJ John Pryor, before he deployed (see the preceding discussion of Dr Pryor's death a year later as the second surgeon killed in action at an FST facility during the GWOT). This is the first documented case of an M203 round being embedded in a patient. While 18 of the 36 cases reported in Lein et al's article involved the M79 grenade launcher round, its replacement weapon, the M203, had not been seen previously in embedded UXO cases.

In 2008, *War Surgery in Afghanistan and Iraq*, edited by COL Shawn Nessen, COL (Ret) Dave E. Lounsbury, and COL Stephen P Hetz, was published, soon followed by "First to Cut" in 2009 (see discussion above).[123,129] Both publications included case scenarios of embedded rocket-propelled grenades in soldiers and described what the team did to address them. These scenarios reinforced the procedures recommended by Lein et al's paper, with some additional recommendations, which assisted the providers in managing the next two cases of embedded UXO.

At times UXO may be embedded so deeply that it is not recognized until the patient is inside a treatment facility, as with the first case discussed, and also the fourth reported case. This case occurred in 2010 at the Craig Joint Theater Hospital in Bagram. An Afghan National Army soldier presented with an embedded high-explosive incendiary 14.5-mm (.57 caliber) bullet from a Russian-made machine gun[145] that had not exploded on impact. The soldier had been involved in an IED attack and was brought to the facility as a standard trauma patient. It is unclear if the round was a component of the initial IED or from secondary gunfire during an ambush after the initial blast. The patient underwent a standard trauma evaluation, initial adjuncts, and radiology studies including a CT scan. He was then taken to the operating room for surgery. At this time, a second, more thorough, evaluation of the CT scan revealed something odd embedded in the patient's scalp. When the radiologist, Air Force LTC Anthony Terreri, realized what the CT was showing, he immediately notified Air Force MAJ John K Bini, the 455th Expeditionary Medical Group trauma director.

The operating room was then cleared of all nonessential personnel while essential personnel removed the UXO from the patient. After removal, the high-explosive incendiary bullet was passed on to EOD staff for proper disposal. Remaining surgeries were completed on the patient, and he survived the injury.[77] This case highlights how UXO can be embedded so deeply it can threaten medical staff and equipment inside a medical facility, and also how proper planning and quick thinking can lead to a successful resolution.

The fifth known incident of embedded UXO occurred in 2012 when an undetonated RPG injured Marine Lance Corporal (CPL) Winder Perez.[146–148] The RPG tip became lodged in Perez's leg, pelvis, and lower abdomen, creating life-threatening wounds. As often occurs in a combat zone, communication and coordination among responders was difficult. The medical evacuation (MEDEVAC) crew initially believed they were picking up a local national girl with a leg injury, but soon realized their patient was a US service member with an embedded UXO device. As in all such situations, the medics, ground MEDEVAC teams, air MEDEVAC teams, and surgical staff had to decide whether to take on this dangerous challenge.

While the literature provides guidance on the safest ways to manage these situations, it also states that sometimes the risk can be too high and the patient should be categorized as expectant. However, in this case, the pilot, copilot, crew chief, and flight medic collectively agreed to not leave the patient to die, but to take on the risk of injury and death, and the destruction of their UH-60 Blackhawk, if the round were to detonate during transport. Their decision resulted in Perez arriving at FOB Edinburgh alive.

Once there, he was evaluated by Navy nurse Lieutenant Commander (Lt Cmdr) James Gennari and his surgical staff from the Marine Corps 2nd Supply Battalion, Surgical Company, Bravo. Initial surgery was performed at an offsite location per published recommendations and the battalion's internal protocol. The RPG was removed without injury to the surgical staff or damage to any equipment. The grenade was given to EOD staff, and the surgical team was able to provide additional damage control surgical and resuscitative procedures to stabilize Perez. He was then safely transported to Role 3 for further management of his wounds.

The 1999 article written by Lein et al, the case scenarios in *War Surgery in Afghanistan and Iraq* and "First to Cut" books, descriptions in the *Emergency War Surgery Handbook* and the Defense Medical Training Institute's *Combat Casualty Care Course Handbook*,[25,26] a few other journal articles, and local standard operating procedures provide guidelines that are not part of mandatory military training but were sought out by the surgeons and surgical staff and used extensively during deployment training rotations of FSTs at the ATTC. In all known GWOT embedded UXO cases, the surgical team had some preexisting knowledge of these potential situations and possibly a basic plan for who would perform the surgery, what procedure to perform, where they would perform it, why they would choose to do so, how they would function as a team, and how they would interact with other groups such as EOD staff to ensure that the patient and the surgical team survived the procedure. Some teams had more standardized plans and had practiced these scenarios in garrison.

Because of these embedded UXO cases and the lack of training on the topic, the Joint Theater Trauma System branch of the ISR published the "Unexploded Ordnance Management" clinical practice guideline in 2012. Once this guideline became official, the proper medical management of both loose and embedded UXO became part of mandatory predeployment training. As the GWOT/Overseas Contingency Operations continues to transition, these situations will likely continue. With the additional preparation from mandatory provider training, most soldiers will survive and medical staff may be able to maintain their 100% success rate of avoiding embedded UXO detonation in surgery.

Advances In Concepts, Technologies, and Care

TACTICAL COMBAT CASUALTY CARE

US Army FSTs, and similar small surgical units, were designed to address the need for proximity and mobility of forward surgical assets, as noted in Chapter 9. One important factor in patient treatment at these facilities is the condition of the patient upon arrival, which largely depends on the quality of care rendered between the point of injury and the surgical facility. COL Ronald F Bellamy's landmark 1984 paper, "The Causes of Death in Conventional Land Warfare: Implications for Combat Casualty Care Research," published in *Military Medicine*, reviewed historical data and used complex analysis to demonstrate that a significant number of casualties' lives could be saved if proper emphasis was placed on field medical care.[27] In 1995, Bellamy presented a refined version of this data in the first chapter of the Borden Institute's *Anesthesia and Perioperative Care of the Combat Casualty*, noting that of those killed in action, 44% died from exsanguination, 31% from central nervous system injuries, and 13% from combined injuries. Additionally, 5% died of wounds due to central nervous system injury, 4% from multiple organ failure/sepsis, and 3% from shock. Twenty percent of those casualties who exsanguinated on the battlefield died as a result of bleeding from an artery in an extremity (femoral and brachial injuries were the most common locations) that could have been controlled by prompt first aid such as application of a pressure dressing or a tourniquet.[43]

COL Bellamy advocated for increased numbers of medically trained individuals, improved medical training for initial responders, and improved adjuncts at the point of injury to stabilize patients. This recommendation led to better training of combat medics, including instruction on emergency cricothyrotomy, improved resuscitation, simpler and more secure intravenous access, and evacuation of trapped air for the management of pneumothorax. Bellamy also strongly advocated for better hemorrhage control. He believed that better point-of-injury management, coupled with faster evacuation times, might save at least 26% of these causalities: those with surgically correctable torso injury, extremity exsanguination, and blast injuries.[27,149,150] Bellamy went on to state that, "To save lives, there is no substitute for prompt and effective surgery. Either the casualty must be evacuated to surgical facilities or the surgical facilities must be brought to the casualty. With helicopter evacuation of questionable feasibility, surgical care in Army 21 [the 21st century Army] will be possible only if the facilities go with the soldier. That is not possible with the large and cumbersome hospitals of today, but the answer found forty years ago—small surgical/shock teams attached to unit level medical assets—might still be applicable."[149(p410)]

In the 1990s, US Army Rangers and Navy SEALs developed what became known as TCCC, taking point-of-injury care to the next level.[151,152] TCCC standards have been codified by the DoD Committee on Tactical Combat Casualty Care (CoTCCC). These techniques and practices have significantly increased the number of wounded soldiers to arrive at the forward treatment facilities. An important consequence of this improvement, however, is that on average the casualties were arriving with more severe injuries. Patients who previously would have been killed in action (ie, died before arrival at a surgical facility) were being saved.

Proximity became more important. Combat surgeons needed to be closer to the point of injury to ensure that more of these soldiers, now surviving to reach Role 2 with central nervous system injuries, torso hemorrhage, and airway and chest wall or lung injuries, could be stabilized beyond the capabilities of the line medic. The modern FSTs provide initial surgical care of lethal head and torso injuries, as well as continuation of care rendered at the point of injury for airway, extremity, and some chest injuries. Once stabilized, patients can be transported to higher levels of care. The significant success of forward surgery is the continuing historically high survival rates, despite the increasing severity of patients' condition on arrival.

HEMOSTASIS

FSTs have embraced or helped develop numerous technology advances since the GWOT's beginning. Improved body and vehicle armor have provided enhanced soldier protection compared to previous combat engagements. Many blast injuries that historically would have caused lethal central nervous system, torso, or extremity injuries are now more survivable. Solders are living after the immediate blast, but with significant extremity injuries with involvement of one to all four limbs. While use of extremity tourniquets had been taught to every soldier for decades, only medics and combat lifesavers were issued tourniquets or had the components, cravats and dowels, to actually apply them. However, even when available, the classic strap tourniquet or the cravat and dowel tourniquets never worked as well as desired.

During the GWOT, new commercial tourniquets became available, and in 2005 they began appearing in various medical units' medical equipment sets as well as soldiers' individual first aid kits.[153–155] The most commonly used extremity tourniquet was the combat application tourniquet (CAT), followed by the Special Operations forces tactical tourniquet (SOFT-T). With the availability of these new tourniquets, soldiers with previously lethal extremity injuries were now arriving alive in larger numbers to Role 2 facilities.[155–158] Combat surgeons had to quickly develop new protocols to meet the challenges of these very sick combat trauma patients.

Once extremity tourniquets became mainstream and liberally applied, extremity exsanguination was no longer the most common cause of preventable death from a nonsurgical source of bleeding. Instead, pelvic bleeding in the inguinal area from distal iliac and proximal femoral vessels became a leading cause of lethal bleeding. Military providers were very aware of this problem, especially those familiar with the death of CPL James Smith, killed in action in Somalia in 1993.[159] Smith died of a gunshot wound and groin hemorrhage that was too proximal for a tourniquet application. The US Army Institute of Surgical Research recognized and addressed this issue in 2008 by developing the Combat Ready Clamp (CRoC), which can apply pressure to areas of the body where traditional tourniquets cannot be used.

TCCC management of junctional hemorrhage now includes training materials for three commercially available pelvic binders: the Pelvic Binder (Pelvic Binder Inc, Dallas, TX); the T-POD (Bio Cybermetrics International, La verne, CA); and the SAM Sling (SAM Medical Products, Wilsonville, OR). Additionally, two other types of junctional tourniquets may also serve as pelvic binders, the SAM Junctional Splint (SAM Medical Products) and the Junctional Emergency Treatment Tool (JETT; Chinook Medical Gear, Durango, CO).[160–162]

In addition to tourniquets, new hemostatic agents for external hemorrhage control were developed. Products such as QuickClot Combat Gauze (Z-Medica, Wallingford, CT, Celox Hemostatic (Chinook Medical Gear), and Chito Gauze (Tricol Biomedical, Portland, OR), to name the primary ones, filled the aid bags of medics and the traumatic cavity wounds of patients.[163,164] Not all products developed for the military are still used, due to various problems.

Combat Gauze became a frequently used and favorite supply of military medical providers. Beyond its traditional use to control significant soft-tissue bleeding, combat surgeons were known to pack it into liver injuries, retroperitoneal hematomas, and complex paraspinal injuries instead of using the traditional nonimpregnated plain gauze. When used in this manner, Combat Gauze is removed during a second surgery at the Role 3 facility.

The success of these hemostatic agents prompted additional research and testing so that third-generation products are used currently, with ongoing research into future products. These will possibly have different chemical agents and structural enhancements of current designs.

DAMAGE CONTROL RESUSCITATION AND BLOOD PRODUCTS

Early in the war, military physicians and surgeons began using a new technique known as damage control resuscitation.[165,166] This type of resuscitation was an attempt to limit excessive administration of intravenous fluids, to prevent their acute side effects and later sequelae, while focusing on the positive aspects of giving blood products. Also as part of this concept, combat providers were taught to be comfortable with permissive hypotension (a systolic blood pressure of 90) instead of the higher values normally taught.

In addition to reduced overall volume of transfusion, damage control resuscitation emphasized early blood replacement. FST and CSH personnel began following protocols to give 1:1 ratios of packed red blood cells (PRBCs) to plasma or 1:1:1 ratios of PRBCs to plasma to platelets, based on availability of each product at their location. Traditionally, FSTs stocked PRBCs only, but for most of the GWOT they also had fresh frozen plasma. CSHs also stocked platelets. Following these ratios, instead of those used in garrison and civilian trauma centers, resulted in increased survival rates. Of note, although FSTs did not have prepackaged platelets, they had the ability to acquire platelets via fresh whole blood.

Fresh whole blood transfusion for combat casualties was not new to the combat surgeon. The technique had been developed during World War I and was the primary type of transfusion throughout the world until the 1960s. The DoD continued to use fresh whole blood transfusion into the GWOT. Although no longer approved by the Food and Drug Administration for primary use in the United States, the technique is authorized for combat use due to logistical needs, and it has been found to be a better resuscitation product than component therapy. FSTs collaborated with their medical company colleagues to help develop robust fresh whole blood collecting systems.[167] Many soldiers are alive today due to the generosity of their fellow soldiers who lined up to donate warm fresh whole blood at a moment's notice. Currently, the US military is looking into the use of freeze-dried plasma and liquid plasma to allow for easier delivery of a resuscitation colloid at the point of injury, in transport, and at the FST facility.

Additionally, since 2001 air MEDEVAC units have slowly increased their use of blood product transfusion.[152] En-route transfusion in these "vampire" missions, commonplace since 2012,[168] have helped improve patient condition on arrival at the FST for further resuscitation and surgery. Lastly, component blood therapy, as well as fresh whole blood, is currently being considered by the CoTCCC as the primary resuscitative fluid at point of injury for future missions. Overall, damage control resuscitation was practiced throughout the second half of the GWOT and has shown significant improvements in initial and long-term outcomes.

HEMOSTATIC PHARMACOLOGICS

Hemostatic pharmacologics were also widely used at the FST and CSH during this period. Starting around 2003, recombinant Factor VIIa was being used to help address noncompressible bleeding in some trauma patients.[169,170] While British military surgical personnel were the first to use the product, the United States followed shortly after.[171] Initial findings demonstrated that recombinant Factor VIIa decreased bleeding; however, data on long-term outcomes showed a concerning increase in deep vein thrombosis and pulmonary embolism. Due to the nature of combat casualty care along the continuum of care, it has been difficult to determine whether the use of recombinant Factor VIIa offered a true benefit or a risk.[172]

Tranexamic acid, an antifibrinolytic, is the current standard of care for individuals deemed to require damage control resuscitation with massive blood transfusion (defined as 10 units of PRBCs within the first 24 hours of care).[163] Its benefits were proven in two major studies published in 2012, CRASH 2 (Clinical Randomization of an Antifibrinolytic in Significant Hemorrhage)[173] and MATTERs (the Military Application of Tranexamic Acid in Trauma Emergency Resuscitation study).[174] Both showed that tranexamic acid decreased coagulopathy and improved outcomes, leading to the CoTCCC recommendation for its use. The earlier it is administered, the better the outcomes for severe combat casualties. In August 2011, the CoTCCC recommended that TCCC guidelines include tranexamic acid and make it available for advanced level field medics to ensure that it would be in the patient's system and have effects as soon as possible.[175] It quickly replaced recombinant Factor VIIa, and new protocols were implemented.[176,177]

HYPOTHERMIA

Hypothermia management is another area in which FSTs have had a positive impact on patient outcome. All FSTs, from mobile to semipermanent facilities, have environmental control units to help ensure that trauma patients stay warm. In addition to wool or cotton blankets, these units also carried a variety of space blankets or other advanced passive and active products.[178] Patients arriving at the FST's facility have the remainder of their clothes removed, but stay warm in the operating room and recovery sections due to increased ambient air temperatures and quick placement of a space blanket or active warming device such as a Bair Hugger (3M, St Paul, MN). When patients are prepared for transport, FSTs are trained to package them using products such as the Hypothermia Prevention and Management Kit (HPMK [North American Rescue, Greer, SC]), or Blizzard Survival blankets (Blizzard Survival, Bethesda, Gwynedd, UK).[179] The HPMK is the most widely used. This device fits the patient like a sleeping bag, has access areas for lines and patient care, and has an oxygen-activated warming pad.

PAIN MANAGEMENT

Other advances in managing combat trauma pain had an impact on combat surgeons. Early on, soldiers received morphine for almost all combat injury pain. While usually effective, morphine had numerous shortcomings. It required intramuscular, intravenous, or intraosseous access; could cause additional blood pressure decreases in patients with hypotension; had to be administered by medics or higher-level providers; and was subject to abuse or theft. Intramuscular administration caused delayed effects, which could lead to accidental overdosing. Morphine's effects can also cause challenges with evaluation, resuscitation, and respiration.

In response to these problems, a new, tiered strategy for managing pain was developed. The system began (for mild to moderate pain) with administration of the combat pill pack, which contained 1,300 mg of acetaminophen and 15 mg of meloxicam for pain control, as well as 400 mg of moxifloxacin for initial antibiotic control of mild injuries. After taking these medications, soldiers could continue performing combat operations or await routine transport. Moderate to severe pain was managed with a lozenge of 800 µg of oral transmucosal fentanyl if the patient was not in hypovolemic shock, unconscious, suffering from a severe head injury, or in respiratory distress before arrival at a surgical facility. A second lozenge was authorized if the patient was hemodynamically stable and still having pain. The lozenge, commonly referred to as a fentanyl lollipop, could be taped to the patient's index finger to ensure it was not dropped or misplaced; also, if the patient went into shock, developed respiratory problems, or became unconscious, it would fall out of the mouth. Ideally the patient should be sitting up when the lozenge is administered.

Ketamine, a dissociative anesthetic medication, was added to the TCCC guidelines as a recommended alternative to morphine in 2012.[180] In October 2013, TCCC guidelines were changed to make ketamine the primary medication for patients with moderate to severe pain. Ketamine worked reliably by multiple routes (intramuscular, intranasal, intravenous, and intraosseous). Morphine could still be used, in moderation, as an adjunct in certain situations.[181] As the guidelines changed, the type of pain management the arriving patients had received in the field might be unclear, especially if treatment documentation cards were missing or incomplete. If it wasn't known whether the patient had received ketamine, neurological evaluations would be inconclusive. This problem led to improvements in care documentation (see the section on patient medical records, below).

Additionally, many patients received TIVA or regional blocks, based on their condition and injuries. Patients with isolated limb injuries often left theater surgical facilities with catheter-directed pain pumps. These devices provided excellent pain management control without the side effects of oral or parenteral narcotics, and numerous soldiers made positive comments about them.

RADIOGRAPHY, BLOOD COLLECTION, AND ANESTHESIA EQUIPMENT

Throughout the war, FSTs received numerous intratheater equipment upgrades. Some locations had fluoroscopy for vascular and orthopedic repairs, and some received their own radiography machines if they were not co-located with a medical company. All received equipment to perform fresh whole blood drives if they were not co-located with a medical company. Many had improved operating room lighting, civilian-style patient beds, and operating room tables instead of the traditional litter-based systems. The standard draw-over system used for providing anesthetic gases at the FST was difficult to use and maintain. Eventually, many FST sites received field-style Drager (Louisville, KY) Narkomed or Fabius anesthesia machines to provide better quality general anesthesia.

DAMAGE CONTROL SURGERY

In addition to damage control resuscitation, FSTs routinely employed damage control surgery. Damage control surgery was usually performed in the best interest of a cold, acidotic, and coagulopathic patient, but it was also used at times to stabilize a patient while surgeons treated another patient, or to meet a MEDEVAC opportunity that might not be available later due to missions or weather. After damage control surgery, numerous patients were left with packed abdomens, with bowel in discontinuity, or with vascular shunts to temporize their potentially lethal injuries. Soft-tissue wounds and laparatomy incisions were commonly left open, with follow-on surgery provided by a Role 3 facility. Improvised open-abdomen dressings were initially used, but many surgeons ended up using the preferred vacuum-assisted closure abdominal dressing system to control fluid losses.

MEDICAL EVACUATION

During the wars in Afghanistan and Iraq, most patients were transported by air MEDEVAC (primarily US, British, and German assets). On occasion patients who were injured on base, or near base, especially in large urban areas, were transported by ground. The primary aircraft supporting US medical transport was the UH-60 Blackhawk. The United Kingdom initially used the CH-125 Sea King, but switched from this aging aircraft to the CH-47 Chinook about 2006. German MEDEVACs initially used the CH-53 Stallion and then, starting in 2013, the NH-90. Ground transport occurred via many different ambulances. US field ambulances included the M113, M996, M997, various versions of the MRAP (mine-resistant ambush protected), or CASEVAC (casualty evacuation) vehicles.

At first MEDEVAC flights took a long time (as noted in the discussion of OEF above), but they were slowly reduced to under an hour.

In 2009, Secretary of Defense Robert Gates mandated that a surgical unit and affiliated air medical support be available within 60 minutes for all conventional forces, so that patients had a better chance of being seen with in the "golden hour" of trauma.[182] This requirement applied to Role 2 surgical teams and CSH FSEs, as well as their supporting air evacuation units, throughout both theaters. Previous 2-hour evacuation times rapidly dropped to under 45 minutes for most flights due to the assets dedicated to meet the secretary of defense's policy. By reducing evacuation times, surgical stabilization, via damage control resuscitation and surgery, could more rapidly be provided.

As the war evolved, patients also began to get better care before being picked up by MEDEVAC, and while en route to the FST. TCCC became the theater standard and helped ensure that the latest in concepts and equipment were pushed out to the front lines. However, the air and ground evacuation units had more patients to manage as the conflict continued. Some casualties in very critical condition would have died in the absence of advanced body armor or TCCC concepts. Air MEDEVAC units had to increase their ability to manage these critical patients better than they had in the past. Teams began adjusting their protocols, for example, by giving blood products while en route to surgical units. Known now as "vampire" missions, MEDEVACs with blood transfusions began early in OEF and became very common.[183,184]

The combination of improved body armor, better point-of-injury care, and faster MEDEVACs with better en-route care meant that the FSTs had more patients arriving in extremis than in the past, often with devastating injuries that would have caused death before the casualties reached surgical care in all previous wars. FSTs were now saving patients with catastrophic injuries who might be difficult to keep stable for further transport. Some FST sites were enhanced with additional critical care equipment and staff to provide limited extended care times to further stabilize the patients.

Additionally, early on in the war many patients who survived their initial surgery at the FST were packaged and ready to be medically evacuated to the Role 3 with ongoing challenges. While many patients had numerous injuries and adjuncts to address these injuries, sometimes junior flight medics were asked to care for patients with complex injuries they had no experience with. Only stabilized patients were transported. However, these patients might have a head injury; an open abdomen; missing limbs; an external pelvic or limb fixator; nasogastric tubes; multiple chest tubes, peripheral intravenous lines, central venous catheters, or intraosseous lines with numerous drips and blood products running into each; or any combination of these injuries.

MEDEVAC crews and combat surgical teams knew that some patients were beyond the scope of most flight medics' skill set. To ensure patients' best chance for survival, two major changes occurred. The first was a paradigm shift for the US Army: the recognition that within a trauma care system, the best medical staff to care for especially complex patients are in-flight critical care nurses. US civilian air rescue and some allied countries' military had this capability. However, the US Army previously did not. The AMEDD Center and School rapidly developed a program to train new en-route critical care nurses: the

Joint En-route Care Course, which provided the additional unique skills that already highly qualified nurses needed to help keep patients stabilized during air transport to Role 3.[185] These providers, who had extensive backgrounds in managing patients in a hospital-based intensive care unit, received additional flight and patient transport training. They helped increase the number of patients who arrived to the Role 3 warmer, in better physiological condition, and more stable overall.

In tandem with the deployment of en-route critical care nurses, the flight paramedic program was created to produce and maintain flight paramedics with more advanced training than earlier flight medics received.[162,186] Both en-route critical care nurses and the new flight paramedics provided improved transport care to patients, improving the level of care provided from point of injury to the FST, as well as from the FST to the CSH.[187] In response, FSTs began creating better ways to address mass casualty incidents via planning, patient flow, and clinical management.[188] For example, it was shown that in certain circumstances, with motivation and training, a two-surgeon FST could run two operating room tables.[189]

The new US air MEDEVAC model slightly resembled the German and British MEDEVAC platforms also used in Afghanistan at that time. The German CH-53 Stallion and NH-90 aircraft were usually staffed by a four-person medical team consisting of an emergency care physician, anesthesiologist or anesthetist, and two paramedics. Good outcomes with this platform were reported for movement from Role 2 to Role 3.[190] The United Kingdom deployed a unique MEDEVAC concept known as the medical emergency response team, or MERT, midway through the war. Initially stood up in 2006 by LTC Andy Griffiths, a British anesthesiologist, MERTs have saved many patients who would have otherwise died en route.[191,192] MERTs used CH-47 Chinook rotary wing aircraft staffed with a four-person medical team made up of an anesthesiologist or emergency care physician, an emergency care nurse, and two paramedics. Initially the team was an integral part of the hospital staff and rotated on shifts, performing on the MERT as an additional duty. Now the medical team is specifically selected, trained, and equipped for this role and is dedicated to it for the deployment.

The advanced level of care in larger aircraft provided by MERTs has been shown to improve the patient's condition on arrival to a surgical unit through advanced procedural skill sets, ability to transfuse blood products, and, most importantly, the decision-making expertise of a highly skilled and trained team. The MERT concept is now integral to future United Kingdom operational medicine. The United States has shown interest in the advanced provider concept used by the German and British, but has not committed to taking a larger aircraft with more equipment and providers with a higher level of training to the point of injury.

Institute of Surgical Research and the Joint Trauma System

The US Army Institute of Surgical Research (ISR), located at Joint Base San Antonio–Fort Sam Houston, Texas, has a long and proud history of supporting the medical and surgical needs of combat surgeons via extensive research efforts. During the GWOT, ISR staff worked to get information and products to Role 2 and 3 surgical teams on the battlefield and to their colleagues at the Role 4 hospitals in Germany and the continental United States. In 2005, the Battlefield Health and Trauma Research Institute was formed. This new consortium co-located all combat casualty care research leaders within the DoD at the ISR for enhanced collaboration. The ISR also ensured that the latest discoveries in initial burn management were rapidly provided to Role 2 surgical units.[193]

A few years into the war, the DoD recognized the need for better management of the vast amounts of trauma data pouring in, which could be used to analyze patient outcomes and effect process improvements.[194] This led to the creation of the JTS in 2004. Efforts were focused on three areas for the much needed feedback to the field: data acquisition, automation, and analysis. The JTS evolved to provide unequalled shared knowledge and impacts on patient outcomes. Also created in 2004 was a subordinate unit, the Joint Theater Trauma System (JTTS). This element, which resided in the Central Command area of responsibility, was established to ensure the JTS was actively engaged in combat trauma, primarily by establishing the Joint Theater Trauma Registry (JTTR) to improve collection of patient management and outcomes data for near-term and future analysis. Role 2 and 3 surgical units were provided a very detailed form to fill out on each patient, designed to collect specific information in a simple and concise manner using TCCC cards and after-action reports. The information is then input via Medical Communications for Combat Casualty Care (MC4) handheld devices.

JTS staff have conducted very successful data acquisition, provided data analysis, coordinated for performance improvement, and developed and conducted education and training programs that far exceeded anything done in the past. Performance improvement came in the form of clinical practice guidelines based on the data collected and the education and training led by the weekly Combat Casualty Care Conferences held by the JTS and ISR. While the JTS was originally stood up to meet the needs of the Role 2 and Role 3 trauma teams within the Central Command area of responsibility, its value has been recognized and addresses all roles of care and will likely be the model for all combatant command areas and theaters in the future.

Patient Medical Records

Another first during this period was the use of electronic medical records for documenting and tracking patient care. Early on, all documentation was done on standard field casualty care forms, followed by notes handwritten on hospital-based forms such as the Standard Form 600. At times patient data was written directly on the patient's skin or on strips of silk tape with a permanent marker. Research-oriented surgeons and nurses at many of the initial FSTs collected data on their patients. These local databases were used for early OEF and OIF analysis and publications until a better system was established by the DoD via the JTS. To improve individual patient care, the DoD procured a new electronic patient care system for the field. The system, called the Medical Communications for Combat Casualty Care, or MC4, provided an array of useful patient care software products. Deployed in 2003, MC4 was used in Afghanistan, Iraq, Kuwait, and Qatar.[195] It used a semi-ruggedized laptop as its primary hardware and could communicate to various servers via a satellite dish.

In addition to tracking and logistical software, the DoD's Armed Forces Health Longitudinal Technology Application (AHLTA) software program for soldiers' electronic medical records could be used in a special "theater" version known as AHLTA-T. Using AHLTA-T would ensure that all patient encounters could be entered into a permanent electronic medical record. As the patient moved from Role 2 to Role 3 to Role 4 care at Landstuhl Regional Medical Center in Germany to a continental DoD medical treatment facility, all records could be seen due to daily system-wide updates. This system provided a better trail of patients' care, incorporating quality assurance for medical documentation accuracy and accountability.[196]

One of the final challenges to battlefield patient records was at the point of injury. At the beginning of the war, medics were issued DD Form 1380, a standard field medical card dated December 1991. Although the card had areas to document many of the basics needed for initial patient care, it needed improvement. Because 87% of casualties die in the prehospital setting, analysis of the reasons for each death, via proper documentation, was strongly sought after.[46]

With the change in basic point of injury care being rapidly advanced by the CoTCCC, committee members also pushed for an improved field medical card.[195] They wanted a card that followed their three-phase system of care under fire, tactical field care, and tactical evacuation care and that was easier and faster to fill out. The CoTCCC developed the TCCC Casualty Card in 2007, based on a casualty card developed by US Army Rangers a few years earlier. The TCCC Casualty Card was initially printed as a DA Form 7656 and became the standard format for documenting prehospital care by all US Army providers.[197]

Even with an improved card, a 2011 study revealed that only 14% of casualties had care documented upon arrival at a Role 2 or Role 3 surgical unit.[198(pp44–47)] Part of this problem was due to a lack of enforcement and poor understanding of the importance of point-of-injury documentation. Another problem was that the new TCCC Casualty Card was an Army form, so many Air Force, Marines, and Navy units could not easily acquire it or use it.[199]

Two things were done to address the underutilization of the new card. First, the CoTCCC had the DA 7656 converted to a DD form in 2014. It was again called DD 1380, but the nomenclature was changed from "field medical card" to "TCCC Card." Second, an innovative initiative to inspire young medics, physician assistants, and physicians at Role 1 to increase compliance and accountability was developed. Individual soldiers and medical units received recognition and awards for having the highest card turn-in rates. Both of these changes have significantly increased point-of-injury care documentation, resulting in better follow-on care at FSTs and valuable data for analysis of the 87% who die in the prehospital setting.

Forward Surgical Team Training and Readiness

Various FSEs within the US military train using a similar format of individual and collective military and medical training. Army FSTs prepare for mission readiness and combat deployments via a number of standard and nonstandard training techniques. The Army technique will be discussed here, with major differences in the Air Force, Navy, and some

NATO units noted when appropriate. Please refer to the referenced documents for additional details and specific facts.

INDIVIDUAL AND COLLECTIVE, COMMON MILITARY, AND MILITARY MEDICAL TRAINING

Throughout the late 1980s and 1990s, the early surgical squads and detachments, which had no official doctrinal instructions, followed medical training formats that their sister medical companies were using and created additional training on their own to fill recognized medical-to-surgical gaps. Field Manual (FM) 8-10-5, *Brigade and Division Surgeons' Handbook: Tactics, Techniques and Procedures* (published 10 June 1991) briefly mentioned the structure and employment of surgical elements, but included no formal guidance on training.[200] When they could, team members performed surgery at their local military treatment facility with staff surgeons.

Once the modern FST was established in 1997, the Department of the Army provided detailed guidance on how to lead, employ, and train an FST in numerous doctrinal materials. These included basic Army references such as FM 25-100 and FM 25-101, *Training the Forces* and *Battle Focused Training*, respectively, and FST-specific references such as FM 8-10-25, *Employment of Forward Surgical Teams: Tactics, Techniques and Procedures* (30 September 1997), and Army Training Evaluation Program (ARTEP) 8-518-10-MTP, *Mission Training Plan for the Forward Surgical Team and Forward Surgical Team (Airborne)*, dated 9 February 1999.[22,93,201,202] The basic Army publications provided FST leadership and their reporting commands with the same structure that the entire Army used to ensure high-quality training for unit readiness. However, the specifics came from the new FST field manual and ARTEP, which clearly stated the duties and responsibilities of individual team members and sections, and also the units' capabilities and capacities to perform specific tactics, techniques, and procedures.

Individual military tasks, known at the beginning of the war as Common Task Training or CTT, and now referred to as Army Warrior Tasks or AWTs, were found in manuals such as the Soldier Training Publication-Soldier's Manual of Common Tasks (STP-SMCT).[203–205] These manuals listed tasks for the four different enlisted levels needed to perform soldier basic skills properly in a combat environment. Officers were expected to know up to skill level four to be equal to their sergeant first class and higher colleagues in each of these skills. Specific individual military occupational skills for enlisted soldiers were found in various editions of the Soldier Training Publication-Soldier's Manual and Trainer's Guide (STP-SM-TG).[206–208] These manuals listed the specific skills essential to performing duties as a healthcare specialist (91W, later 68W), licensed practical nurse (91C, then 68WM6 and 68C), or operating room specialist (91D, then 68D).

Likewise, officers had specific tasks they were expected to know at the company and field grade level, in addition to the soldier common tasks. These tasks, conditions, and standards were found in the military qualification standards level I, II, and III manuals for precommissioning, lieutenants and captains, and majors and lieutenant colonels.[209–211] Lastly, a publication for individual medical officer training was the *Military Qualifications Standards II for Medical Areas of Concentration*,[212,213] which covered specific medical tasks for field medical providers.

These manuals also included information about where each task is first learned and how often it needed to be repeated as part of the training cycle. The manuals were guides for setting up routine scheduled training and evaluating individual performance levels. They also often had information on the collective tasks and group training, including situational training exercises, field training exercises, culminating training events, certifying exercises, and validation exercises. The ATEP manual was the primary guide for unit collective training. FSTs also accompanied their supported units during rotations at the National Training Center at Fort Irwin, California, or the Joint Readiness Training Center at Fort Polk, Louisiana, for complex training events.

Military doctrinal manuals were updated over the years to keep up with the changes in battlefields, equipment, and overall goals. In the early 2000s, FM 25-100 became FM 7-0, *Training the Forces*; FM 25-101 became FM 7-1, *Battle Focused Training*; and FM 8-10-25 became FM 4-02.25, *Employment of Forward Surgical Teams: Tactics, Techniques and Procedures*.[24,214–216] In 2011 the Army chief of staff began a complete remodeling of the Army doctrine system.[217] Fundamental principles are now found under Army doctrine publications, while detailed information on fundamentals is found in the Army doctrine reference publications, and remaining FMs contain tactics and procedures only. Previously used FMs were replaced by Army techniques publications (ATPs). The FST field manuals were superseded by a new Army techniques publication, ATP 4-02.5 *Casualty Care*, in May 2013.[107] The original 1999 ATEP manual for the FST was modernized and eventually evolved into the newer combined arms training strategy.[103,218] Similar to the previous ATEP manual, units would use the combined arms training strategy as a guide for developing mission-essential task lists and supporting routine individual and collective training. Both the standard Army manuals and the combined arms training strategy were now electronic and more easily updated.

MEDICAL PROFICIENCY TRAINING/BORROWED MILITARY MANPOWER

An addition to task training, medical soldiers and officers had to perform their jobs in a clinical setting to maintain their overall skill set. Individuals who were professional fillers (PROFIS) to the FST performed their regular hospital jobs throughout the year and trained with their assigned FST for 2 weeks out of the year. Organic FST personnel worked at the hospital under the medical proficiency training program and the borrowed military manpower program.

The medical proficiency training program provided soldiers with an opportunity for uninterrupted work at their local or partnered medical treatment facility, usually in a 30-day rotation annually in which soldiers worked in various parts of the hospital correlating with their individual military occupational specialty. The borrowed military manpower program was used to ensure that all medical personnel with non-Medical Command assignments assisted with the hospital's patient load while staying clinically active to ensure skill retention. Although the program varied between stations and units, FST nurses generally worked 4 days a week at the local medical treatment facility and spent the other day training at the FST facility. The senior nurse might work 2 to 3 days at either facility, while surgeons spent a few days per week at the medical treatment facility in clinics and the oper-

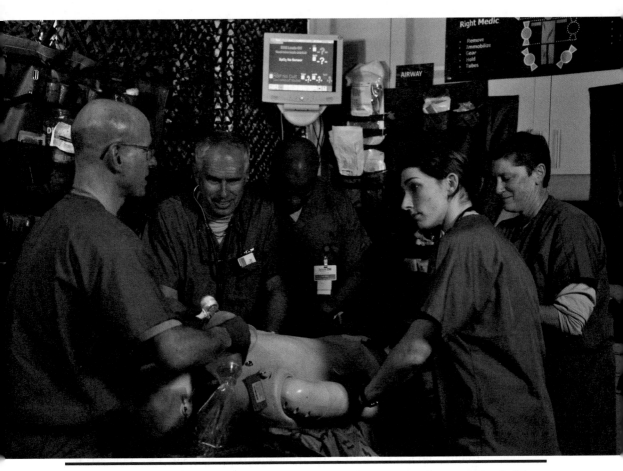

FIGURE 10-17. LTC Michael Yaffe, COL Colleen Klohen, and others from the 402nd Forward Surgical Team (Reserve) practice their roles during initial patient assessment and treatment prior to working together as a team on live patients. By knowing their specific tasks, working on a common lexicon, and gaining motor memory, forward surgical teams are able to cut their primary and secondary survey times by up to 50% while decreasing miscommunication and increasing provider and patient safety. Photograph courtesy of the US Army Recruiting Command.

ating room. Surgeons also participated in academic programs and had "on-call" duty at the hospital a few times every month. Enlisted personnel primarily participated in the medical proficiency training program because of other military obligations, although many units attempted to have their soldiers work in the local medical treatment facility more routinely, as well as having all personnel perform surgery as a team, in preparation for deployment (Figure 10-17).

PREDEPLOYMENT TRAUMA TRAINING

Throughout the majority of the GWOT, most FSTs attended what is now called predeployment trauma training. This was done near the end of the unit's training phase of the armed forces generation training cycle prior to transition into the mission/available phase.[103,104,218,219] Army Role 2 surgical units trained at the ATTC, while Navy and Air Force Role 2 surgical units trained at the US Navy Trauma Training Center and the Centers for the Sustainment of Trauma and Readiness Skills (C-STARS). These programs were originally established due to DoD Inspector General and General Accounting Office reports after Operations Desert Shield and Desert Storm, which found that many deployed medical providers were not clinically active at an acceptable readiness level, and most were not specifically trained in trauma assessment and resuscitation, trauma surgery, or trauma critical care. Those trained in trauma often did not perform these duties on a routine basis.[220–226]

In 1996, Congress passed legislation as part of the National Defense Authorization Act requiring the DoD to create military-civilian partnerships to provide opportunities for DoD personnel to sustain an acceptable level of trauma skills.[94,227] The act established a DoD group of subject matter experts, which became known as the Combat Trauma Surgical Committee, to consider the trauma personnel, equipment, and training needs of the military to meet future deployment readiness requirements and address past failures.[228] Many preexisting programs brought military trauma providers into civilian hospitals, but they were not universally available, had no standardized curriculum, and lacked consistent funding.[94]

In 1997, the Navy established a pilot program through the Naval Medical Center in Portsmouth, Virginia, and Eastern Virginia Medical School. Training was conducted at Sentara Norfolk General Hospital. The military also established a partnership with Ben Taub General Hospital in Houston, Texas, to provide a training center for all DoD Role 2 surgical teams. This program, finalized in 1998, became known as the Joint Trauma Training Center.[229] The 30-day training rotations alternated between Army and Air Force teams.[230] The program trained numerous military medical providers for 2 years prior to its closure.[231–233] Based on the overall positive feedback from rotating surgical team members, the Combat Trauma Surgical Committee sought alternative training sites that could accommodate a larger volume of rotating teams, provide an even better clinical experience, and resolve administrative issues.[234]

In 2001, the Air Force established the first of three current programs under C-STARS with Baltimore Shock Trauma. Focused on Air Force Role 2 and 3 team members, the program developed an excellent reputation.[235,236] The second C-STARS was set up with the University of Cincinnati in August 2001, focused on training for critical care air transport teams. A third program was established at St Louis University in December 2002, focused on training Reserve unit Role 2 and 3 team members.[237]

With recommendations from military personnel who trained at the Ryder Trauma Center, the ATTC was established in August 2001. This program became the model for austere resuscitation and surgery refresher training and team roles development.[238,239] The 2nd FST from Fort Carson, Colorado, was the first official team to rotate through in January 2002. Since then, numerous FSTs have participated in over 130 rotations; more than 3,000 students have attended the course (Figure 10-18).

In July of 2002, the US Navy formalized its training program in collaboration with the University of Southern California School of Medicine, providing training for Navy forward and fleet surgical units.[240–242]

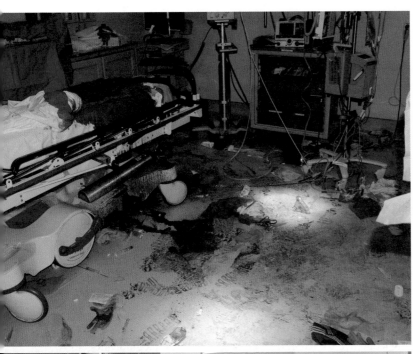

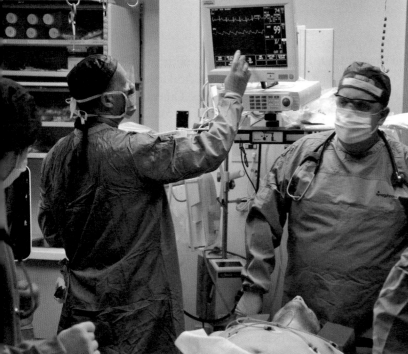

FIGURE 10-18. (a) A civilian trauma resuscitation unit bay after a patient was cared for with an emergency thoracotomy and went on to survive his surgery. High-volume Level 1 civilian trauma centers like those at the Ryder Trauma Center in Miami, the Shock Trauma Center in Baltimore, and the Los Angeles County Medical Center provided predeployment trauma training for Role 2 and some Role 3 surgical teams. Their high volume of trauma, world-renowned staff, and dedicated personnel ensured all trauma team members had the best training prior to deploying. (b) Army Trauma Training Center senior nurse instructor LTC William White works with forward surgical team members at the Ryder Trauma Center during their 6 days of clinical rotations. All three trauma training centers worked with embedded military trauma experts along with the host facilities staff to hone the skills of rotating military personnel. Photographs courtesy of the US Army Recruiting Command.

All three programs focused on basic and advanced trauma knowledge, skills refreshers, and combat-unique trauma considerations based on injury patterns, equipment, and supplies available. There were also varying levels of interprofessional team development at the training centers. While all three programs were conceptualized prior to the GWOT to ensure prewar readiness, they were well-placed to meet the ongoing need for predeployment trauma training throughout the conflict. They are considered centers of excellence staffed with subject matter experts in the areas of operational medicine, resuscitation, and surgery. In addition to didactic lectures and labs, and hands-on real life trauma training for skills sustainment, the combat trauma-specific curriculum ranged from blast and high-power rifle physics to large total body surface area burns to management of severe injuries with limited resources. Unique surgical training far in advance of residency or fellowship training included performing external fixator placement for long bone and pelvic fractures, lateral canthotomy and cantholysis for retrobulbar hematomas, and craniotomy for damage control neurosurgery.[243-247]

Various articles and numerous testimonials by surgeons have stated the significant value of being initially taught or refreshed on the most current patient care guidelines, and receiving training with their dedicated team.[245,248-253] Midway through the war, each service surgeon general made attending these courses mandatory for a certain percentage of each deploying team,[105,254,255] ensuring that personnel had the funding and opportunity for refreshing their skills and knowledge, were current on combat clinical trauma guidelines, and could work together as a team to excel in patient care.

ADDITIONAL AND OPTIONAL FORWARD SURGICAL TEAM TRAINING

Some FST members and teams attended additional training opportunities, including other Army predeployment trauma training courses for Role 2 medical units or Role 3 surgical units, as well as many other optional military medical courses. Other predeployment trauma training courses included the military transition team, brigade combat team trauma training, tactical combat medical care with a focus on Role 1 and 2 medical team providers, and the Joint Forces Combat Trauma Management Course for Role 3 CSHs. Many FST personnel attended these courses to enhance their knowledge of the overall continuum of care on the modern battlefield, gaining a better understanding of the capabilities and standards at sending and receiving units that work with the FST.

Another course attended by some FST members was the Emergency War Surgery Course sponsored by the Defense Medical Readiness Training Institute, mostly attended by Air Force and Navy surgical team members. The course provided Army FST staff another chance to receive the latest information on combat casualty management in a formal setting. As with the mandatory predeployment trauma training courses, the curriculum has changed over the years, but remained focused on current standards of cared based on TCCC and the clinical practice guidelines.

Because many combat injuries involve the extremities, and are often severe and different from those seen in civilian trauma centers, additional training was needed in this field. A preexisting Extremity War Surgery Course (created in the mid-1990s) evolved into the Combat Extremity Surgery Course in 2004. This course focuses on the initial combat trauma management of extremities, including completion amputation, proper debridement, fasciotomies, vascular shunting, and placement of external fixators to the long bones and pelvis. The course's focus audience is general surgeons and orthopedic surgeons preparing to deploy. It provides foundational knowledge of the current ways to address these injuries to help improve limb salvage or expedite patient care and transfer to the next medical treatment facility. The course is embedded into the Army Trauma Training Course, so that all deploying Army Role 2 surgical teams gain this knowledge, and is also taught multiple times a year at off-sites for others to attend.

When it became evident that some patients being transported from the forward medical and surgical facilities to the next higher level of care were having complications en route, the Army addressed this in two main ways. One was to provide improved training and hands-on experience back in garrison to all flight medics, including a new flight paramedic course. The second step was assigning advanced skilled providers to assist with MEDEVAC of complex patients. These providers were usually emergency care and critical care nurses, aeromedical physician assistants, and flight surgeons. The military developed the Joint En-route Care Course to train flight medics, licensed practical nurses, registered nurses, physician assistants, and physicians, with a focus on having nurses and flight surgeons better prepared to assist with transport care.[256]

The ISR Burn Center offered courses throughout the GWOT to help give Role 1 through Role 4 providers a better understanding of current concepts for treating burns and polytrauma in theater. One Burn Center course was the Management of Burn and Multiple Trauma Casualty Course, which provided didactic training and hands-on experience with burn and polytrauma patients at Brooke Army Medical Center/San Antonio Military Medical Center. Students at the course could see how proper management at the point of injury, and throughout the continuum of care, had resulted in improved outcomes.

Other courses attended less often by FST members include the Field Management of Chemical and Biological Casualties or the more advanced Medical Management of Chemical and Biological Casualties, provided by the US Army Medical Research Institute of Chemical Defense and US Army Medical Research Institute of Infectious Diseases. These courses covered general and specific chemical and biological concerns in the battlefield or stateside due to attacks or accidents. Those who wanted to further their understanding of trauma management in a radiation-exposed patient could also take the Medical Effects of Ionizing Radiation Course taught by the Armed Forces Radiobiology Research Institute. Another course some personnel reported attending was the Infection Control in the Deployed Environment Course held at San Antonio Military Medical Center. As in other units, a specified number of FST members needed to be Field Sanitation Course graduates. Additionally, operating room specialists and executive officers needed to complete the Combat Lifesaver Course.

The FST TO&E also formally assigned the position of FST Chief to the 61J general surgeon or 61M orthopedic surgeon who was organic to the team. The AMEDD Center and School's Department of Healthcare Operations developed the FST Commanders

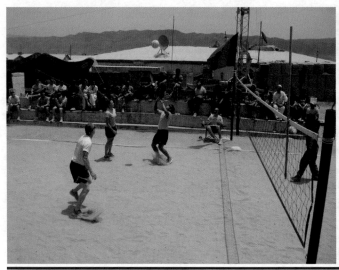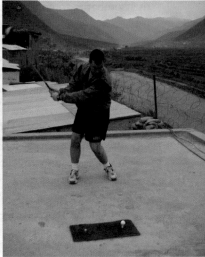

FIGURE 10-19. Exercise, entertainment, and group development are not just for the movies. Soldiers in combat zones need to stay fit and also deal with the realities of life and death. Here a friendly game of volleyball provides all of these and more. Photograph courtesy of LTC Dean Fellabaum, former commander, 2nd FST.

FIGURE 10-20. Sometimes forward surgical team members find it necessary to "recharge their batteries" by adding a little color (green fake grass) and familiar activities, like this member of the 160th FST shown in Naray, Afghanistan. Photograph courtesy of LTC Dean Fellabaum, surgeon, 160th FST.

Course in 1998 after a need for the training was noted by a surgeon, LTC Steve Swann, with the support of another surgical leader, LTC Brian Allgood, and the AMEDD Center and School's commanding general, MG James Peake.[257] LTC Allgood was a former commander of the 82nd Airborne Surgical Squad in the early 1990s and the first commander of the official modern 274th FST (Airborne) in 1997.[77,95] COL Allgood is one of the few physicians who paid the ultimate sacrifice during this era when he died in a helicopter crash in Iraq on 20 January 2007.[258]

First conducted in July 1999,[259] the FST Commanders Course provides surgeons, nurses, and others who took on the role of FST commander with appropriate administrative, intelligence/security, training/operations, logistical, information technology, budgeting, legal, and other related knowledge needed by successful commanders. The week-long course is conducted in a small group with lectures provided by subject matter experts and former FST commanders. The FST Commanders Course is held at the same time as the Brigade Surgeons Course and Division Surgeons Course, so universally useful lectures are held jointly, and students of all three courses can interact, network, and better understand how their roles interact in garrison and while deployed. When FSTs assigned to brigade combat teams were realigned to be exclusively under medical brigades, this interaction became even more important because past interactions at the home station were significantly reduced. FSTs worked with the brigade combat teams' medical staff and units during some contingency missions and many deployments, so getting an understanding of various unit's capabilities, gaps, and standard operating procedures made mission success easier (Figures 10-19 and 10-20).

Other Missions and Changes During Time of War

In addition to the theater and garrison transformations mentioned above, the Medical Command and Forces Command changed FST locations and numbers in other ways. Additional Role 2 surgical teams were established after the GWOT began in September 2001. As the battlefield changes, FSTs now perform more Special Operations forces support missions. FSTs have also worked with local national medical facilities while deployed to both Iraq and Afghanistan. And at the time of this writing, the US Army FST is preparing to be transformed into the forward resuscitative surgical team (FRST), with many changes in personnel. US Army Special Operations Command is working on acquiring up to three of its own FRSTs by fiscal year 2017.

Another major change during the GWOT was the airborne status of various units. Due to the ever-changing nature of the conflict, the Army alternated the number of FSTs that could perform their duties as part of an air-deployable joint forced entry package. A brief description follows, with more details on these changes noted in the next chapter.

The 8th FST was one of the original surgical teams that existed before the official designation of the FST in 1997. It was activated in 1986 at Schofield Barracks, Hawaii, as the 8th Medical Detachment (Forward Surgical) to support the Role 2 surgical needs of the Pacific Command. While the team members were stationed in Hawaii, they participated in OIF twice and OEF twice. In 2010, the unit relocated to Fort Richardson, Alaska, and was designated an airborne unit. While deployed in 2014, the unit was notified that it would lose its newly assigned airborne status upon its return to Alaska as part of a Department of the Army realignment of assets.[260]

The 240th FST was activated in 1997 at Fort Stewart, Georgia. The unit had two successful deployments to Iraq while based at Fort Stewart. In 2009, the 240th was relocated to Fort Bragg, North Carolina, and was designated an airborne FST. The unit deployed to OEF twice, supported the Northern Command Defense Chemical Biological Radiological Nuclear Response Force mission, and supported the XVIII Airborne Corps' Global Response Force mission multiple times. The 240th FST lost its Airborne designation as part of the same realignment in 2014.[261,262]

The 67th FST was another of the original surgical teams in existence before the FST's official designation. The 67th Medical Detachment (Forward Surgical), as it was known, was stationed in Vicenza, Italy, since its activation in 1993. This European Command FST would be one of three in Europe, including the 160th FST activated in 1999, and the 130th FST.[261] The 67th was an airborne unit that could support the 173rd Infantry Brigade, also stationed in Vicenza. In 1994, they both relocated to Giebelstadt, Germany. The 67th FST participated in numerous support missions throughout Europe and Africa, including Bosnia, Kenya, Macedonia, Kosovo, Nigeria, and the Republic of Georgia, making them one of the most highly utilized FSTs in the DoD.[263]

In 2002, the team was disappointed when it lost its prestigious airborne status. In 2005 it deployed to OIF, and on its return in 2006, relocated to Wurzburg, Germany. The 67th relocated again in 2007 to Miesau, Germany, and regained its designation as airborne. Since that move, it participated in OEF twice, supported the XVIII Airborne Corps' Global Response Force mission, and again provided support within the Africa Command area of responsibility in Tanzania and other locations. The 67th FST again lost its airborne status in 2013. This FST has been to more places, in garrison and on support missions, than any of its peers, and has changed its mission profile multiple times. Throughout this period the 67th maintained a strong reputation as a team much in demand for assignments and deployments.[264]

The number of US Army FSTs increased during the GWOT. At the time of this writing, there were 16 FSTs on active duty and 22 FSTs in the US Army Reserves. The Air Force and Navy/Marines have also increased the number of their Role 2 surgical teams, or developed new ones, in both the conventional and Special Operations communities. However, there have also been deactivations. In addition to those previously mentioned, other deactivated units include the 130th FST, which was part of European Command, stationed in Camp Darby, Italy, until 2009. However, the unit never deployed, and it probably was never stood up due to transformations going on at the time. Another deactivated unit was the 127th FST, stationed in Yongson, Korea, which was stood up in 1997 and maintained readiness for its enduring potential mission of providing Role 2 surgical care in the event of a conflict in the region.[265]

While the GWOT was the primary focus of FSTs during this era, they supported other missions outside of the Central Command area of responsibility. Some units were assigned to support DoD conventional and Special Operations forces combat units, while other missions supported disaster relief and humanitarian assistance missions. Units still rotated to various partner countries to support European Command medical needs, while others supported missions in many countries throughout the Southern, African, and Pacific Commands areas of responsibility. Additional mission assignments included the Northern Command Defense Chemical Biological Radiological Nuclear Response Force mission, the Forces Command Global Response Force mission, and presidential support missions. More information on these topics will be presented in the following chapter.

REFERENCES

1. Sun Tzu. *A Arte da Guerra—The Art of War—Sun Tzu*. Madrid, Edad; 2007.
2. US Army Institute of Surgical Research. Department of Defense Trauma Registry. Joint Base San Antonio, Tex: Joint Trauma System; 2014. http://usaisr.amedd.army.mil/10_jts.html/. Accessed March 23, 2017.
3. Richardson RG. *Larrey: Surgeon to Napoleon's Imperial Guard*. 1st ed. London, England: John Murray Publishers Ltd; 1974.
4. US Department of Defense. *Health Service Support*. Washington, DC: DoD; 2001. Joint Publication 4-02.
5. US Department of Defense. *Health Service Support*. Washington, DC: DoD; 2006. Joint Publication 4-02.

6. North Atlantic Treaty Organization. *Allied Joint Medical Support Doctrine*. Brussels, Belgium: NATO Standardization Agency; 2006. Allied Joint Publication 4.10(A).
7. Bowen TE, Bellamy RF. *Emergency War Surgery Handbook*. 2nd US rev. Washington, DC: Borden Institute; 1988.
8. Burris DG, Dougherty PJ, Elliot DC, et al, eds. *Emergency War Surgery Handbook*. 3rd US rev. Washington, DC: Borden Institute; 2004.
9. Cubano MA, Lenhart MK, Bailey JA, et al, eds. *Emergency War Surgery Handbook*. 4th US rev. Fort Sam Houston, Tex: Borden Institute; 2013.
10. Chambers LW, Green DJ, Gillingham BL, et al. The experience of the US Marine Corps' Surgical Shock Trauma Platoon with 417 operative combat casualties during a 12-month period of Operation Iraqi Freedom. *J Trauma*. 2006 Jun;60(6):1155–1161.
11. Peoples GE, Gerlinger T, Craig R, Burlingame B. The 274th Forward Surgical Team experience during Operation Enduring Freedom. *Mil Med*. 2005;170(6):451–459.
12. Peoples GE, Gerlinger T, Craig R, Burlingame B. Combat casualties in Afghanistan cared for by a single forward surgical team during the initial phases of Operation Enduring Freedom. *Mil Med*. 2005;170(6):462–468.
13. Beitler AL, Wortman, GW, Hofmann LJ, et al. Operation Enduring Freedom: the 48th Combat Support Hospital in Afghanistan. *Mil Med*. 2006;171(3):189–193.
14. Schoenfeld AJ. The combat experience of military surgical assets in Iraq and Afghanistan: a historical review. *Am J Surg*. 2012;204(3):377–383.
15. Manifold C. *Air Force Medical Service Concept of Operations for the Mobile Field Surgical Team*. Bolling Air Force Base, Washington, DC: Office of the Air Force Surgeon General; 10 September 1999.
16. Bilski TR, Baker B, Grove JR, et al. Battlefield casualties treated at Camp Rhino, Afghanistan: lessons learned. *J Trauma*. 2003;54:814–822.
17. Rush RM, Stockmaster NR, Stinger HK, et al. Supporting the Global War on Terror: a tale of two campaigns featuring the 250th Forward Surgical Team (Airborne). *Am J Surg*. 2005;189(5):564–570; discussion 570.
18. Stinger H, Rush R. The Army forward surgical team: update and lessons learned, 1997–2004. *Mil Med*. 2006;171(4):269–272.
19. Vassallo DJ, Gerlinger T, Maholtz P, Burlingame B, Shepherd AFI. Combined UK/US field hospital management of a major incident arising from a Chinook helicopter crash in Afghanistan, 28 Jan 2002. *J R Army Med Corps*. 2003;149:47–52.
20. Midla, GS. Lessons learned: Operation Anaconda. *Mil Med*. 2004;169(10):810–813.
21. Pratt JW, Rush RM Jr. The military surgeon and the war on terrorism: a Zollinger legacy. *Am J Surg*. 2003;186(3):292–295.
22. US Department of the Army. *The Medical Company: Tactics, Techniques, and Procedures*. Washington, DC: DA; 2002. Field Manual 4-02.6.
23. US Department of the Army. *Employment of Forward Surgical Teams: Tactics, Techniques, and Procedures*. Washington, DC: DA; 1997. Field Manual 8-10-25.
24. US Department of the Army. *Employment of Forward Surgical Teams: Tactics, Techniques, and Procedures*. Washington, DC: DA; 2003. Field Manual 4-02-25.
25. Defense Medical Readiness Training Institute. *Combat Casualty Care Course Handbook*. 2nd ed. Fort Sam Houston, Tex: Defense Medical Readiness Training Institute; 1999.
26. Defense Medical Readiness Training Institute. *Combat Casualty Care Course Handbook*. 3rd ed. Fort Sam Houston, Tex: Defense Medical Readiness Training Institute; 2002.
27. Bellamy RF. The causes of death in conventional land warfare: implications for combat casualty care research. *Mil Med*. 1984;149(2):55–62.
28. Grau LW, Jorgenson WA. Handling the wounded in a counter-guerrilla war: the Soviet/Russian experience in Afghanistan and Chechnya. *Army Med Dept J*. 1998;Jan/Feb:2–10.

29. Place RJ, Rush RM Jr, Arrington ED. Forward surgical team (FST) workload in a Special Operations environment: the 250th FST in Operation Enduring Freedom. *Curr Surg.* 2003;60(4):418–422.
30. CPT Peter V Arnold, CRNA (former certified registered nurse anesthetist and commander, 947th Forward Surgical Team, West Hartford, Conn); email about unit history, September 2014.
31. Kozaryn LD. Active or reserve, there's no difference—they must depend on each other. American Forces Press Service; 18 June 2002. http://www.defense.gov/news/newsarticle.aspx?id=43741. Accessed 24 March 2015.
32. Friscolanti M. *Friendly Fire: The Untold Story of the US Bombing That Killed Four Canadian Soldiers in Afghanistan.* Somerset, NJ: John Wiley & Sons; 2005: Chap 7.
33. American Association of Nurse Anesthetists. Recognition of Captain David J Kolodji, CRNA. 19 June 2003. http://www.aana.com/aboutus/inservicesofourcountry/Pages/Captain-David-J-Kolodji-CRNA-MSN.aspx. Accessed 31 December 2014.
34. Beekley AC, Watts DM. Combat trauma experience with the United States Army 102nd forward surgical team in Afghanistan. *Am J Surg.* 2004;187(4):652–654.
35. Wronski R. Call to duty could place area medics at front line. *Chicago Tribune.* 29 September 2002. http://articles.chicagotribune.com/2002-09-29/news/0209290269_1_medics-reservists-active-duty. Accessed 15 October 2014.
36. CPT Rainier J Abordo, RN (registered nurse and commander, 909th FST, Operation Enduring Freedom, Afghanistan); personal communications about unit history, August–September 2014.
37. MAJ William Vanasse, RN (former emergency care nurse for the 555th FST, Operation Iraqi Freedom, and 759th FST, Operation Enduring Freedom); personal communication, February 2014.
38. US Department of the Army. *Combat Casualty Care.* Washington, DC: DA; 10 May 2013. Army Techniques Publication 4-02.5.
39. US Department of the Army. *Operational Terms and Graphics.* Washington, DC: DA; 2004. Field Manual 1-02 (Supersedes Field Manual 101-5-1).
40. COL Donna N Hershey, RN (registered nurse and chief of clinical operations, 807th Medical Command [Deployed Support], Salt Lake City, Utah, and former registered nurse, 339th Combat Support Hospital, Operation Enduring Freedom, Afghanistan); email, August–September 2014.
41. SPC Anthony Fantasia, EMT (former 68W Healthcare Specialist [Combat Medic], 339th Combat Support Hospital, Operation Enduring Freedom, Afghanistan); email, June 2013.
42. COL Alan L. Beitler, MD (surgical oncologist, Keller Army Community Hospital, West Point, NY, and former commander, 48th Combat Support Hospital, Operation Enduring Freedom, Afghanistan); personal communication and emails, September 2010, May and August 2013, October 2014.
43. Bellamy RF. Combat trauma overview. In: Zajtchuk R, Grande CM, eds. *Anesthesia and Perioperative Care of the Combat Casualty.* In: Zajtchuk R, Bellamy RF, eds. *Textbooks of Military Medicine.* Washington, DC: Borden Institute; 1995: Chap 1.
44. Simmons JW, White CE, Eastridge BJ, et al. Impact of improved combat casualty care on combat wounded undergoing exploratory laparotomy and massive transfusion. *J Trauma.* 2011;71(1):S82–S86.
45. Eastridge, BJ, Stansbury LG, Stinger H, Blackbourne L, Holcomb JB. Forward surgical teams provide comparable outcomes to combat support hospitals during support and stabilization operations on the battlefield. *J Trauma.* 2009;66:S48–S50.
46. Eastridge BJ, Mabry RL, Seguin P, et al. Death on the battlefield (2001–2011): implications for the future of combat casualty care. *J Trauma Acute Care.* 2012;73(6 Suppl 5):S431–S437.
47. Kotwal RS, Montgomery HR, Kotwal BM, et al. Eliminating preventable death on the battlefield. *Arch Surg.* 2011;146(12):1350–1358.

48. Savage E, Forestier C, Withers N, Tien H, Pannell D. Tactical combat casualty care in the Canadian Forces: lessons learned from the Afghan war. *Can J Surg*, 2011;54:S118–123.
49. Torreon S. *US Periods of War and Dates of Recent Conflicts*. Washington, DC: Congressional Research Service; 27 February 2015. RS21405.
50. President Bush: Monday "moment of truth" for world on Iraq [press release]. Washington, DC: White House Office of the Press Secretary; 16 March 2003. http://georgewbush-whitehouse.archives.gov/news/releases/2003/03/ images/20030316-3_azores1-515h.html. Accessed 24 March 2015.
51. Operation Iraqi Freedom–coalition members [press release]. Washington, DC: White House Office of the Press Secretary; 27 March 2003. http://georgewbush-whitehouse.archives.gov/news/releases/2003/03/ 20030327-10.html. Accessed 12 April 2014.
52. Beekley AC. United States military surgical response to modern large-scale conflicts: the ongoing evolution of a trauma system. *Surg Clin N Amer*. 2006;86(3):689–709.
53. Stevens R. The forward resuscitative surgical system. *NRA News*. August 2004;34–35.
54. Fontenot G, Degen EJ, Tohn D. *On Point: The United States Army in Operation Iraqi Freedom*. Charleston, SC: CreateSpace Independent Publishing Platform; 2013: Chap 3.
55. Lt Col Daniel Crawford, RN (senior officer-in-charge, Air Force Special Operations Surgical Team); personal communication, January 2015.
56. Ervin MD. Air Force special operations command special operations surgical team (SOST) CONOPS. *JSOM*. 2008;8(2):68–75.
57. Patel TH, Wenner KA, Price SA, et al. A US Army forward surgical team's experiences in Operation Iraqi Freedom. *J Trauma*. 2004;57(2):201–207.
58. CDR Robert Hincks, MD (former commander, 2nd Medical Battalion Forward Resuscitative Surgical System); email, February 2015.
59. Chambers LW, Rhee P, Baker BC, et al. Initial experience of US Marine Corps forward resuscitative surgical system during Operation Iraqi Freedom. *Arch Surg*. 2005;140:26–32.
60. Liewer S. Army's last MASH unit stretched to its limits in Iraq. *Stars and Stripes*. 10 April 2003. http://www.stripes.com/news/army-s-last-mash-unit-stretched-to-its-limits-in-iraq-1.4194. Accessed 24 March 2015.
61. Marble S. *Skilled and Resolute: A History of the 12th Evacuation Hospital and the 212th Mobile Army Surgical Hospital, 1917–2006*. Fort Sam Houston, TX: Borden Institute, 2013; Chap 6.
62. 86th Combat Support Hospital official unit history. Fort Campbell website. http://www.campbell.army.mil/units/Eagle Medics/Pages/History.aspx. Accessed 25 January 2015.
63. 28th Combat Support Hospital official unit history. Fort Bragg website. http://www.bragg.army.mil/units/44thmedbde /28thCSH/Pages/default.aspx. Accessed 15 January 2015.
64. 21st Combat Support Hospital official unit history. Fort Hood website. http://www.hood.army.mil/1stMed/units.aspx. Accessed 10 May 2014.
65. COL Kim Smith, RN (former senior nurse for the 2nd ACR FST, Operation Iraqi Freedom); emails, January–November 2014.
66. LTC (R) Ronald M Cashion, RN (former certified registered nurse anesthetist, 86th Combat Support Hospital, Fort Campbell, Ky, and Operation Iraqi Freedom, Iraq); emails, July–August 2014.
67. MAJ Christopher Vanfosson, RN (former senior nurse 541st FST and ward nurse 28th CSH); personal communications, January–December 2014.
68. Doganis D. Life and death in the war zone [transcript]. *NOVA*. PBS television. 2 March 2004. http://www.pbs.org/wgbh/nova/military/life-and-death-in-war-zone.html. Accessed 24 March 2015.
69. Bruckart J. Operation Iraqi Freedom—21st CSH. FEViper.com. http://www.feviper.com/iraq.htm. Accessed 24 March 2015.

70. Sawyer D. Soldiers treated in desert hospital. ABC News website. 27 March 2003. http://abcnews.go.com/Primetime/story?id=125266. Accessed 24 March 2015.
71. Army docs treats wounded in desert tent. ABC News website. 11 April 2003. http://abcnews.go.com/Primetime/story?id=131983. Accessed 24 March 2015.
72. Doganis D. The producer's story: into Kuwait and Iraq with two combat support hospitals. KLRN San Antonio television website. February 2004. http://www.pbs.org/wgbh/nova/combat-docs/producer.html. Accessed 15 January 2015.
73. US Department of Defense. *Joint Forcible Entry Operations*. Washington, DC: US Department of Defense; 2008. Joint Publication 3-18.
74. 82nd Airborne Division. *82nd Airborne Division Airborne Standing Operating Procedures Edition VIII*. Fayetteville, NC: US Department of the Army; 2011.
75. COL Richard G Malish, MD (commander, Southern Command Clinic, Miami, Fla, and former 173rd Brigade Surgeon, Operation Iraqi Freedom, Afghanistan); emails, January 2015.
76. Yarbrough JC. *173rd Airborne Brigade: Sky Soldiers*. 3rd ed. New York, NY: Turner Publishing; 2006: Chap 6.
77. US Department of the Army. *Announcement is Made of the Following Award: Bronze Star Combat Parachutist Badge and Arrow Head Device*. Washington, DC: DA; 24 May 2004. Permanent orders 145-19.
78. COL(R) Harry K Stinger, MD (trauma critical care surgeon and former commander of the 250th Forward Surgical Team (Airborne), Fort Lewis, Wash, and Operation Iraqi Freedom, Iraq); telephone and email communications, May–August 2014.
79. COL (Ret) Harry Stinger, MD (former commander of the 82nd Surgical Squad, 782nd FST and 250th FST); personal communications, December 2014–January 2015.
80. Stinger HK. College plays pivotal role in Operation Iraqi Freedom. *Bull Am Coll Surg*. 2004;89(3):8–15.
81. Rob C. Some experiences with a parachute surgical unit. *J R Army Med Corps*. 1944;165.
82. COL Richard G Malish, MD (commander, Southern Command Clinic, Miami, Fla, and former 173rd Brigade Surgeon, Operation Iraqi Freedom, Afghanistan); personal communications, August–September 2014.
83. Malish R, DeVine JG. Delayed drop zone evacuation: execution of the medical plan for an airborne operation into northern Iraq. *Mil Med*. 2006;171(3):224–227.
84. COL (Ret) Richard Ellison, MD (former commander and senior surgeon for 2nd ACR FST and 759th FST in Operation Iraqi Freedom, PROFIS surgeon to the 648th FST); personal communications, January 2014–February 2015.
85. LTC (R) Thomas McCorey, MD (former commander and senior surgeon for the 2nd ACR FST, Operation Iraqi Freedom); personal communications, 2003–2004; emails, 2013.
86. COL Kirby Gross, MD (former commander and senior surgeon for the 801st FST and 772nd FST, Operation Iraqi Freedom); personal communication, February 2015.
87. COL Shawn Nessen, MD (former commander and senior surgeon for the 782nd FST and 541st FST, Operation Enduring Freedom); personal communications, January–December 2014.
88. Counihan TC, Danielson PD. The 912th Forward Surgical Team in Operation New Dawn: employment of the forward surgical team during troop withdrawal under combat conditions. *Mil Med*. 2012;177:1267–1271.
89. LTC John Detro, PA (former commander of the 240th FST, in support of the DCRF and GRF missions; senior physician assistant on 2nd ACR Medical Company for Operation Iraqi Freedom and deputy command surgeon for XVIII Corps); personal communications, January–December 2014.
90. Thomas RW. *Ensuring Good Medicine in Bad Places: Utilization of Forward Surgical Teams on the Battlefield*. Carlisle, Penn: US Army War College; 15 March 2006.
91. LTG (Ret) James B Peak. Official Department of Defense resume. https://www.gomo.army.mil/Ext/Portal/Officer/Resumes.aspx?Ltr=P&Type=Retired. Accessed 22 November 2015.

92. Cannon DW, McCollum J. Army Medical Department lessons learned program marks 25th anniversary. *Mil Med.* 2011;176(11):1212–1214.
93. US Department of the Army. *Army Training Evaluation Program: Mission Training Plan for the Forward Surgical Team and Forward Surgical Team (Airborne).* Washington, DC: DA; 9 February 1999. ARTEP-8-518-10-MTP.
94. Gebicke ME. *Wartime Medical Care: DOD Is Addressing Capability Shortfalls, But Challenges Remain.* Washington, DC: General Accounting Office; September 1996. GAO/NSIAD-96-224. http://www.gao.gov/products/NSIAD-96-224. Accessed 24 March 2015.
95. COL (Ret) Harry Warren, MD (former commander of the 82nd Surgical Squad, initial commander for the 101st Surgical Squad and 2nd ACR FST); personal communications, October–December 2014.
96. US Government. *Medical Training Agreement.* Memorandum of Agreement Between the United States of America and the Public Health Trust of Miami-Dade County, Florida, 6 November 2015.
97. US Army Medical Command. *Trauma Center Training Agreement.* Memorandum of Agreement By and Between the United States Army Medical Command and the School of Medicine, University of Miami, Miami, Florida, 7 June 2002.
98. Bailey J, Spott MA, Costanzo GP, Dunne JR, Dorlac W, Eastridge B. *Joint Trauma System: Development, Conceptual Framework, and Optimal Elements.* Fort Sam Houston, Tex: US Department of Defense, US Army Institute for Surgical Research; 2012.
99. MG (Ret) Kevin C Kiley. Official Department of Defense resume. https://www.gomo.army.mil/Ext/Portal/Officer/Resumes.aspx?Ltr=K&Type=Retired. Accessed 22 November 2015.
100. Neidinger AA. *Envision-Design-Train: A Pictorial History of the US Army Medical Department Center & School From 1920 to 2010.* Washington, DC: Borden Institute; 2012.
101. Kiley KK. *Memorandum for Record, Subject: Army Medical Department (AMEDD) Pre-Deployment Trauma Training.* Fort Sam Houston, TX: US Army Medical Command; 18 December 2006.
102. LTG (Ret) Eric B Schoomaker. Official Department of Defense resume. https://www.gomo.army.mil/Ext/Portal/Officer/Resumes.aspx?Ltr=S&Type=Retired. Accessed 22 November 2015.
103. US Department of the Army. *Combined Arms Training Strategy: Medical Team, Forward Surgical (Airborne).* Washington, DC: DA; 2010.
104. US Department of the Army. *Army Force Generation.* Washington, DC: DA; 2011. Army Regulation 525-29.
105. Robinson AM Jr. *Pre-Deployment Trauma Training Matrix (PDTTM) for Deploying Navy Medical Department Personnel.* Washington, DC: Department of the Navy; 9 August 2010. http://www.med.navy.mil/policy-guidance/Documents/2010-012.pdf. Accessed 24 March 2015.
106. LTG Patricia D Horoho. Official Department of Defense resume. https://www.gomo.army.mil/Ext/Portal/Officer/Resumes.aspx?Ltr=H&Type=Active. Accessed 22 November 2015.
107. US Department of the Army. *Casualty Care.* Washington, DC: DA; 2013. Army Techniques Publication 4-02.5.
108. CPT Gary E Bilendy, RN (commander, 915th FST); personal communications and emails about 915th FST unit history, September–August 2013.
109. 1LT Beau D McNeff, MS (executive officer, 915th FST); personal communications and emails about 915th FST unit history, September–August 2013.
110. Boivin J. No safe haven: Army surgical team injured in mortar attack. *Nursing Spectrum Career Management Magazine* [serial online]. September 2003. Available at: http://community.nursingspectrum.com/MagazineArticles/article.cfm?AID=10388. Accessed October 21, 2005.
111. LTC (Ret) Robert Blease (former commander and orthopedic surgeon, 274th FST, Operation Iraqi Freedom and Operation Enduring Freedom; orthopedic instructor at the Army Trauma Training Center); personal communications, January–December 2014.

112. LTC John Williams (former PROFIS surgeon, 250th FST, Operation Enduring Freedom); personal communication, November 2012.
113. Honor the fallen–Army Maj Mark D. Taylor. 2004. *Military Times*. http://projects.militarytimes.com/valor/army-maj-mark-d-taylor/257108. Accessed 24 March 2015.
114. Honor the fallen–Army Maj John P. Pryor. 2008. *Military Times*. http://projects.militarytimes.com/valor/army-maj-john-p-pryor/3880374. Accessed 24 March 2015.
115. Honor the fallen–Army Staff Sgt Ronald J Spino. 2009. *Military Times*. http://projects.militarytimes.com/valor/army-staff-sgt-ronald-j-spino/4441954. Accessed 24 March 2015.
116. Honor the fallen–Army Capt Joshua M. McClimans. 2011. *Military Times*. http://projects.militarytimes.com/valor/army-capt-joshua-m-mcclimans/6348288. Accessed 24 March 2015.
117. Baker JL, Truesdale CA, Schlanser JR. Overview of combat trauma in military working dogs in Iraq and Afghanistan. *Army Med Dep J*. 2009:33–37.
118. Jennings PB Jr. Initial management of injuries in military working dogs in a combat environment. *Mil Med*. 1983;148(10):808–811.
119. Baker JL, Havas KA, Miller LA, Lacy WA, Schlanser J. Gunshot wounds in military working dogs in Operation Enduring Freedom and Operation Iraqi Freedom: 29 cases (2003–2009). *J Vet Emerg Crit Care* (San Antonio). 2013;23(1):47–52.
120. Taylor WM. Canine tactical field care. Part one—the physical examination and medical assessment. *J Spec Oper Med*. 2008;8(3):54-60.
121. Taylor WM. Canine tactical field care. Part two—massive hemorrhage control and physiologic stabilization of the volume depleted, shock-affected, or heatstroke-affected canine. *J Spec Oper Med*. 2009;9(2):13–21.
122. Taylor WM. Canine tactical field care. Part three—thoracic and abdominal trauma. *J Spec Oper Med*. 2010;10(1):50–58.
123. Blackbourne LH, Cancio L, Holcomb J, Craig B, et al, eds. *First to Cut: Trauma Lessons Learned in the Combat Zone*. Fort Sam Houston, Tex: US Army Institute of Surgical Research; 2009.
124. Beitler AL, Jeanette JP, McGraw AL, et al. Emergency canine surgery in a deployed forward surgical team: a case report. *Mil Med*. 2011;176(4):477–480.
125. US Army Institute of Surgical Research. *Canine Resuscitation–Joint Theater Trauma System Clinical Practice Guidelines*. Joint Base San Antonio, Tex: Joint Trauma System; 2011.
126. US Army Institute of Surgical Research. *Clinical Management of Military Working Dogs–Joint Theater Trauma System Clinical Practice Guidelines*. Joint Base San Antonio, Tex: Joint Trauma System; 2012.
127. US Special Operations Command. Tactical trauma protocols, tactical medical emergency protocols, and canine tactical combat casualty care (C-TCCC) for special operations advanced tactical practitioners. *J Spec Ops*. 2012; Supplement:229–237.
128. Lein B, Holcomb J, Brill S, et al. Removal of unexploded ordnance from patients: a 50-year military experience and current recommendations. *Mil Med*. 1999;164(3):163–165.
129. Nessen SC, Lounsbury DE, Hetz SP. Removal of unexploded ordnance. In: *War Surgery in Afghanistan and Iraq: A Series of Cases, 2003–2007*. Washington, DC: Borden Institute; 2008: 373–376.
130. Plurad DS. Blast injury. *Mil Med*. 2011;176(3):276–282.
131. Oh JS. Removal of unexploded ordnance. *J Trauma*. 2007;62(2):S21.
132. Auerbach PS. Combat and casualty care. In: *Wilderness Medicine*. 6th ed. Philadelphia, Penn: Elsevier; 2012: 507–522.
133. US Army Institute of Surgical Research. *Unexploded Ordnance Management–Joint Theater Trauma System Clinical Practice Guidelines*. Joint Base San Antonio, Tex: Joint Trauma System; 2012.
134. US Army Medical Department. *Forward Surgical Team Handbook: Guide to Lessons Learned and Recommended Practices for Deployment Operations*. Joint Base San Antonio, Tex: AMEDD Center & School, Lessons Learned Division; 2011.

135. Matt W Ruemmler, CRNA (certified registered nurse anesthetist, 86th Combat Support Hospital, Fort Campbell, Ky, and former registered nurse, 86th Combat Support Hospital, Operation Iraqi Freedom, Iraq); personal and email communications, July–August 2014.
136. COL Karen L Wright, RN (registered nurse, 86th Combat Support Hospital, Operation Iraqi Freedom, Iraq); personal and email communications, August 2014.
137. Paparella A, LaFaille R. Channing Moss and the men who saved him: where are they now? ABC News website. 26 May 2011. http://abcnews.go.com/2020/channing-moss-men-saved-now/story?id=13684826. Accessed 24 March 2015.
138. SPC Channing J Moss; personal communications, August–September 2008.
139. LTC John Oh, MD (trauma critical care surgeon, Walter Reed National Military Medical Consortium, and former staff surgeon, 759th FST, Operation Enduring Freedom, Afghanistan); emails, March–April 2014.
140. Frangou C. Physicians in harm's way bring precious lessons home: Iraq experience likely to change US trauma care forever. *PRN*. 2008;34(5).
141. Scott A. Bedside to battlefield: trends in critical care nursing-blast injury. *Advance News*. October 2009. http://nursing.advancedweb.com/Editorial/Content/PrintFriendly.aspx?CC=189253. Accessed 19 July 2014.
142. Hawkins MR. The military experience. *JEMS*. 2008;(suppl):16–18.
143. The glidescope ranger—a unique case study. *Verathon*. http://verathon.com/content-pages/glidescope-ranger-case-study. Accessed 24 March 2015.
144. CPT Michael R. Hawkins, CRNA (certified registered nurse anesthetist, 405th Combat Support Hospital, West Hartford, Conn, and former certified registered nurse anesthetist, 325th Combat Support Hospital, Operation Iraqi Freedom, Iraq); telephone and email communications, May 2014.
145. Williams R. Medical staff removes UXO from patient at Bagram Airfield. 2 April 2010. Defense Video & Imagery Distribution System. http://www.dvidshub.net/news/47581/medical-staff-removes-uxo-patient-bagram-airfield. Accessed 24 March 2015.
146. Barker R, Schroeder D. MEDEVAC crew reacts to dangerous call. 30 May 2012. Defense Video & Imagery Distribution System. http://www.dvidshub.net/news/89156/medevac-crew-reacts-dangerous-call. Accessed 24 March 2015.
147. Fantz A. "You have an RPG in your leg." 8 June 2012. CNN website. http://security.blogs.cnn.com/2012/06/08/you-have-an-rpg-in-your-leg/. Accessed 24 March 2015.
148. Masterson J. Navy nurse pulls rocket round out of Marine's leg. 21 April 2012. Allnurses.com. http://allnurses.com/nursing-news/navy-nurse-pulls-700604.html. Accessed 24 March 2015.
149. Bellamy RF. Contrasts in combat casualty care. *Mil Med*. 1985;150:405–410.
150. Bellamy RF. Letter to the editor. *Mil Med*. 1986;151:63–64.
151. Butler FK, Hagmann J, Butler EG. Tactical combat casualty care in special operations. *Mil Med*. 1996;161(suppl):3–16.
152. US Army Institute of Surgical Research. *Department of Defense Tactical Combat Casualty Care Guidelines*. Joint Base San Antonio, Tex: Joint Trauma System; 28 October 2014.
153. Walters TJ, Wenke JC, Kauvar DS, McManus JG, Holcomb JB, Baer DG. Effectiveness of self-applied tourniquets in human volunteers. *Prehosp Emerg Care*. 2005;9:416–422.
154. Holcomb JB, McMullin NR, Pearse L, et al. Causes of death in US special operations forces in the Global War on Terrorism. *Ann Surg*. 2007;245:986–991.
155. Kragh JF Jr, Walters TJ, Westmoreland T, et al. Tragedy into drama: an American history of tourniquet use in the current war. *J Spec Oper Med*. 2013;13:5–25.
156. Kragh JF Jr, Walters TJ, Baer DG, et al. Survival with emergency tourniquet use to stop bleeding in major limb trauma. *Ann Surg*. 2009;249:1–7.
157. Kragh JF Jr, Littrel ML, Jones JA, et al. Battle casualty survival with emergency tourniquet use to stop limb bleeding. *J Emerg Med*. 2011;41:590–597.
158. Kragh JF Jr, Beebe EF, O'Neill ML, et al. Performance improvement in emergency tourniquet use during the Baghdad surge. *Am J Emerg Med*. 2013;31:873–875.

159. Hanley R. The Somalia Mission: relatives recount dreams of 2 killed in Somalia. 7 October 1993. *The New York Times* website. http://www.nytimes.com/1993/10/07/world/the-somalia-mission-relatives-recount-dreams-of-2-killed-in-somalia.html. Accessed 24 March 2015.

160. Blackbourne LH, Mabry R, Sebesta J, Holcomb JB. Joseph Lister, noncompressible arterial hemorrhage, and the next generation of "tourniquets." *US Army Med Dep J*. 2008;Jan–Mar:56–59.

161. Kragh J, Murphy C, Dubick M, Baer D, Johnson J, Backbourne L. New tourniquet device concepts for battlefield hemorrhage control. *US Army Med Dept J*. 2011;Apr–Jun:38–48.

162. Butler F. Changes to the TCCC guidelines: pelvic binders and comprehensive review. milSuite.mil. https://www.milsuite.mil/book/docs/DOC-350292. Accessed March 23, 2017.

163. Bennett B, Littlejohn L. Review of new topical hemostatic dressings for combat casualty care. *Mil Med*. 2014;179(5):497–514.

164. Cox ED, Schreiber MA, McManus J, Wade CE, Holcomb JB. New hemostatic agents in the combat setting. *Transfusion*. 2009;49:248S–255S.

165. US Army Institute of Surgical Research. *Damage Control Resuscitation at Level IIb/III Treatment Facilities–Joint Theater Trauma System Clinical Practice Guidelines*. Joint Base San Antonio, Tex: Joint Trauma System; 2013.

166. Fox CJ, Gillespie DL, Cox ED, et al. Damage control resuscitation for vascular surgery in a combat support hospital. *J Trauma*. 2008;65(1):1–9.

167. Nessen SC, Eastridge BJ, Cronk B, et al. Fresh whole blood use by forward surgical teams in Afghanistan is associated with improved survival compared to component therapy without platelets. *Transfusion*. 2013;53(suppl):107S–113S.

168. Barker R. MEDEVAC crews in Afghanistan increase en-route patient care. 4 January 2013. US Army website. http://www.army.mil/article/93788/. Accessed 24 March 2015.

169. Williams DJ, Thomas GO, Pambakian S, Parker PJ. First military use of activated Factor VII in an APC-III pelvic fracture. *Injury*. 2005;36(3):395–399.

170. Parker PJ, Adams SA, Williams D, Shepherd A. Forward surgery on Operation Telic. *J R Army Med Corps*. 2005;151(3):186–191.

171. Perkins JG, Schreiber MA, Holcomb JB. Early versus late recombinant factor VIIa in combat trauma patients requiring massive transfusion. *J Trauma*. 2007;62(5):1095–1099.

172. Wade CE, Eastridge BJ, Jones JA, et al. Use of recombinant factor VIIa in US military casualties for a five-year period. *J Trauma*. 2010:69(2):352–359.

173. Perel P, Al-Shahi Salman R, Kawahara T, et al. CRASH 2 (Clinical Randomisation of an Antifibrinolytic in Significant Haemorrhage) intracranial bleeding study: the effect of tranexamic acid in traumatic brain injury—a nested randomised, placebo-controlled trial. *Health Technol Assess*. 2012 Dec;16:1-54.

174. Morrison JJ, Dubose JJ, Rasmussen TE, Midwinter MJ. Military Application of Tranexamic Acid in Trauma Emergency Resuscitation (MATTERs) study. *Arch Surg*. 2012;147(2):113–119.

175. US Army Institute of Surgical Research. *Department of Defense Tactical Combat Casualty Care Guidelines*. Joint Base San Antonio, Tex: Committee on Tactical Combat Casualty Care; 8 August 2011.

176. CRASH-2 trial collaborators. Effects of tranexamic acid on death, vascular occlusive events, and blood transfusion in trauma patients with significant hemorrhage (CRASH-2): a randomized, placebo-controlled trial. *Lancet*. 2010;376(9734):23–32.

177. Morrison JJ, Bubose JJ, Rasmussen TE, Midwinter MJ. Military application of tranexamic acid in trauma emergency resuscitation (MATTERs) study. *Arch Surg*. 2012;147(2):113–119.

178. Blackbourne LH, Grathwohl KW, Barras P, Eastridge B. Maximizing patient thermoregulation in US Army forward surgical teams. *Army Med Dep J*. 2008;Jan–Mar:60–66.

179. Allen PB, Salyer SW, Dubick MA, Holcomb JB, Blackbourne LH. Preventing hypothermia: comparison of current devices used by the US Army in an in vitro warmed fluid model. *J Trauma*. 2010;69suppl(1):S154–S161.

180. US Army Institute of Surgical Research. *Department of Defense Tactical Combat Casualty Care Guidelines*. Joint Base San Antonio, Tex: Joint Trauma System; 30 August 2013.
181. US Army Institute of Surgical Research. *Department of Defense Tactical Combat Casualty Care Guidelines*. Joint Base San Antonio, Tex: Joint Trauma System; 28 October 2013.
182. Shanker T. Gates seeks to improve battlefield trauma care in Afghanistan. 27 January 2009. *The New York Times* website. http://www.nytimes.com/2009/01/28/washington/28military.html. Accessed 24 March 2015.
183. Place R, West B, Bentley R. In-flight transfusion of packed red blood cells on a combat search and rescue mission: a case report from Operation Enduring Freedom. *Mil Med*. 2004;124(3):181–183.
184. Malsby R, Quesada J, Powell-Dunford N, et al. Prehospital blood product transfusion by US Army MEDEVAC during combat operations in Afghanistan: a process improvement initiative. *Mil Med*. 2013;178(7):785–791.
185. Nagra M. Optimizing wartime en route nursing care in Operation Iraqi Freedom. *US Army Med Dep J*. 2011;Oct–Dec:51–56.
186. Kheirabadi BS, Terrazas IB, Hanson MA, Kragh JF, Dubick MA, Blackbourne LH. In vivo assessment of the Combat Ready Clamp to control junctional hemorrhage in swine. *J Trauma Acute Care Surg*. 2013;74(5):1260–1265.
187. Mabry R, Apodaca A. Penrod J, Orman J, Gerhardt R, Dorlac W. Impact of critical care-trained flight paramedics on casualty survival during helicopter evacuation in the current war in Afghanistan. *J Trauma Acute Care Surg*. 2012;73(2 Suppl 1):S32–S37.
188. Ran Y, Hadad E, Daher S. Triage and air evacuation strategy for mass casualty events: a model based on combat experience. *Mil Med*. 2011;176:647–651.
189. Vanfosson CA, Seery JM. Simultaneous surgeries in a split forward surgical team: a case study. *Mil Med*. 2011;176:1447–1449.
190. Willy C, Hauer T, Huschitt N, Palm H. Surgical use: experiences of German military surgeons in Afghanistan. *Langenbecks Arch Surg*. 2011;396(4):507–522.
191. Capt Steven Bree (surgeon, Royal Navy, British liaison officer for deployment medicine to the United States); personal communication, February 2015.
192. Apodaca A, Morrison J, Spott M, et al. Improvements in the hemodynamic stability of combat casualties during en route care. *Shock*. 2013;40(1):5–10.
193. Lairet KF, Lairet JR, King BT, Renz EM, Blackbourne LH. Prehospital burn management in a combat zone. *Prehosp Emerg Care*. 2012;16(2):273–276.
194. Acosta JA, Hatzigeorgiou C, Smith LS. Developing a trauma registry in a forward deployed military hospital: preliminary report. *J Trauma*. 2006;61(2):256–260.
195. *Medical Communications for Combat Casualty Care (MC4): Managing Critical Medical Information*. Fairfax, VA: General Dynamics Information Technology; 1 November 2013. http://www.gdit.com/globalassets/health/5795_mc4.pdf. Accessed 24 March 2015.
196. Smith LE. The deployed electronic medical record. *US Army Med Dep J*. 2008;Oct–Dec:63–67.
197. Kotwal RS, Montgomery HR, Mechler KK. A prehospital trauma registry for tactical combat casualty care. *Army Med Dept J*. 2011;Apr–Jun:15–17.
198. Caravalho J. *Dismounted Complex Blast Injury: Report of the Army Dismounted Complex Blast Injury Task Force: Report*. Fort Sam Houston, TX: DCBI Task Force; 18 June 2011. http://armymedicine.mil/Documents/DCBI-Task-Force-Report-Redacted-Final.pdf. Accessed 24 March 2015.
199. Eastridge BJ, Mabry R, Blackbourne LH, Butler FK. We don't know what we don't know: prehospital data in combat casualty care. *Army Med Dept J*. 2011;Apr–Jun:11–14.
200. US Department of the Army. *Brigade and Division Surgeons' Handbook: Tactics, Techniques and Procedures*. Washington, DC: DA; 1991. Field Manual 8-10-5.
201. US Department of the Army. *Training the Forces*. Washington, DC: DA; 1988. Field Manual 25-100.

202. US Department of the Army. *Battle Focused Training*. Washington, DC: DA; 1990. Field Manual 25-101.
203. US Department of the Army. *Soldier's Manual of Common Tasks: Skill Level 1*. Washington, DC: DA; October 1990. STP-21-1-SMCT.
204. US Department of the Army. *Soldier's Manual of Common Tasks: Skill Level 1*. Washington, DC: DA; October 1994. STP-21-1-SMCT.
205. US Department of the Army. *Soldier's Manual of Common Tasks: Skill Level 2–4*. Washington, DC: DA; October 1992. STP-21-24-SMCT.
206. US Department of the Army. *Soldier's Manual and Trainer's Guide: MOS 68W Health Care Specialist–Skill Levels 1/2/3*. Washington, DC: DA; May 2013. STP-8-68W13-SM-TG.
207. US Department of the Army. *Soldier's Manual and Trainer's Guide: MOS 91WM6 Practical Nurse-Skill Levels 1/2/3/4/5*. Washington, DC: DA; May 2003. STP-8-91WM6-SM-TG.
208. US Department of the Army. *Soldier's Manual and Trainer's Guide: MOS 91D Operating Room Specialist-Skill Levels 1/2/3/4*. Washington, DC: DA; July 2003. STP-8-91D14-SM-TG.
209. US Department of the Army. *Military Qualification Standards I: Manual of Common Tasks for Precommissioning Requirements*. Washington, DC: DA; 1990. STP-21-I-MSQ.
210. US Department of the Army. *Military Qualification Standards II: Manual of Common Tasks for Lieutenants and Captains*. Washington, DC: DA; 1991. STP-21-II-MSQ.
211. US Department of the Army. *Military Qualification Standards III, Manual of Common Tasks for Majors and Lieutenant Colonels* [draft]. Washington, DC: DA; 1992. STP-21-III-MSQ.
212. US Department of the Army. *Military Qualification Standards II Medical (60, 61, 62), Dental (63), Veterinary (64), Army Medical Specialist (65), Army Nurse (66), and Medical Service (68 only) Corps Company Grade Officer's Manual*. Washington, DC: DA; 1988. STP 8-II-MQS.
213. US Department of the Army. *Military Qualification Standards II Medical (60, 61, 62), Dental (63), Veterinary (64), Army Medical Specialist (65), Army Nurse (66), and Medical Service (68 only) Corps Company Grade Officer's Manual*. Washington, DC: DA; 1993. STP 8-II-MQS.
214. Steele WM, Walters RP. Training and developing Army leaders. *Mil Review*. 2001:Jul–Aug:2–9.
215. US Department of the Army. *Training the Forces*. Washington, DC: DA; 2002. Field Manual 7-0.
216. US Department of the Army. *Battle Focused Training*. Washington, DC: DA; 2003. Field Manual 7-1.
217. Jakola B. Army doctrine leaders forecast future technology, leadership needs. 26 February 2010. US Army website. http://www.army.mil/article/35088/Army_doctrine_leaders_forecast_future_technology__leadership_needs/. Accessed 24 March 2015.
218. US Department of the Army. *Combined Arms Training Strategy: Medical Team, Forward Surgical*. Washington, DC: DA; 2010.
219. US Department of the Army. *Training Units and Developing Leaders for Full Spectrum Operations*. Washington, DC: DA; 2011. Field Manual 7-0.
220. Davis R. *Operation Desert Storm: Full Army Medical Capability Not Achieved*. Washington, DC: General Accounting Office; February 1992. GAO-92-8.
221. Conahan F. *Operation Desert Storm: Full Army Medical Capability Not Achieved*. Washington, DC: General Accounting Office; August 1992. GAO/NSIAD-92-175. http://www.gao.gov/products/NSIAD-92-175. Accessed 24 March 2015.
222. Conahan F. *Medical Readiness Training: Limited Participation by Army Medical Personnel*. Washington, DC: General Accounting Office; June 1993. GAO/NSIAD-93-205. http://www.gao.gov/products/NSIAD-93-205. Accessed 24 March 2015.
223. Gebicke ME. *Operation Desert Storm: Improvements Required in the Navy's Wartime Medical Care Program*. Washington, DC: General Accounting Office; July 1993. GAO/NSIAD-93-189. http://www.gao.gov/products/NSIAD-93-189. Accessed 24 March 2015.
224. Conahan F. *Operation Desert Storm: Problems With Air Force Medical Readiness*. Washington, DC: General Accounting Office; December 1993. GAO/NSIAD-94-58. http://www.gao.gov/products/NSIAD-94-58. Accessed 22 April 2014.

225. Gebicke ME. *Wartime Medical Care. Aligning Sound Requirements With New Combat Care Approaches Is Key to Restructuring Force.* Washington, DC: General Accounting Office; March 1995. GAO/T-NSIAD-95-129. http://www.gao.gov/products/153872. Accessed 24 March 2015.
226. Brittin KA. *Medical Mobilization: Planning and Execution, Inspection Report.* Washington, DC: Defense Inspector General; 1993. 93-INS-13.
227. P Law No. 104-106. The National Defense Authorization Act for Fiscal Year 1996. 10 February 1996.
228. Martin ED. *Combat Trauma Surgery Report From the Assistant Secretary of Defense.* Washington, DC: Defense Health Agency; 13 May 1997. http://www.health.mil/policies/combat-trauma-surgery. Accessed 10 March 2014.
229. Gebicke ME. *Medical Readiness: Efforts Are Underway for DOD Training in Civilian Trauma Centers.* Washington, DC: General Accounting Office; April 1998. GAO/NSIAD-98-75. http://www.gao.gov/products/NSIAD-98-75. Accessed 24 March 2015.
230. Bruce S, Bridges E, Holcomb J. Preparing to respond joint trauma training center and USAF nursing warskills simulation laboratory. *Crit Care Nurse Clin N Am.* 2003;15:149–162.
231. Place RJ, Porter CA, Azarow K, Beitler AL. Trauma experience comparison of Army forward surgical team surgeons at Ben Taub Hospital and Madigan Army Medical Center. *Curr Surg.* 2001;58(1):90–93.
232. Schreiber MA, Holcomb JB, Conaway CW, Campbell KD, Wall M, Mattox KL. Military trauma training performed in a civilian trauma center. *J Surg Res.* 2002;104(1):8–14.
233. Holcomb JB, Dumire RD, Crommett JW, et al. Evaluation of trauma team performance using an advanced human patient simulator for resuscitation training. *J Trauma.* 2002;52(6):1078–1085.
234. Conaway CW, Campbell KD. *Report of Combat Trauma Surgical Training at Ben Taub General Hospital.* San Antonio, TX: Brook Army Medical Center; 1999. http://oai.dtic.mil/oai/oai?verb=getRecord&metadataPrefix=html&identifier=ADA420310. Accessed 24 March 2015.
235. Lt Col Raymond Fang, MD (director of the Air Force Baltimore, Md, C-STAR program); personal communications, August 2014–February 2015.
236. Col Stacy Shackleford, MD (trauma surgeon, Air Force Baltimore, Md, C-STAR program); personal communications, August 2014–February 2015.
237. Thorson CM, Dubose JJ, Rhee P, et al. Military trauma training at civilian centers: a decade of advancements. *J Trauma Acute Care Surg.* 2012;73(6):S483–S489.
238. COL (Ret) Thomas Knuth, MD (first director of the US Army Trauma Training Center); personal communication, November 2014.
239. Dr Nicholas Namias, MD (chief of trauma at the Ryder Trauma Center, Army Trauma Training Center); personal communication, November 2014.
240. CDR Jef Ricks, MD (emergency care physician, US Navy Trauma Training Center); personal communication, September 2014.
241. CDR Daniel Grabo, MD (trauma surgeon, US Navy Trauma Training Center); personal communication, January 2015.
242. CDR Patricia Hansen, RN (director, Navy Trauma Training Center); personal communications, January–August 2014.
243. Benfield RJ, Mamczak CN, Vo KT, et al. Initial predictors associated with outcome in injured multiple traumatic limb amputations: a Kandahar-based combat hospital experience. *Injury.* 2012;43:1753–1758.
244. Possley DR, Burns TC, Stinner DJ, et al. Temporary external fixation is safe in a combat environment. *J Trauma.* 2010;69:S135–S139.
245. Bell RS, Mossop CM, Dirks MS, et al. Early decompensated craniectomy for severe penetrating and closed head injury during wartime. *Neurosurg Focus.* 2010;28(5):1–6.

246. McHenry T, Simmons S, Alitz C, Holcomb J. Forward surgical stabilization of penetrating lower extremity fractures: circular casting versus external fixation. *Mil Med.* 2001;166(9):791–795.
247. Cho RI, Bakken HE, Reynolds ME, Schlifka BA, Powers DB. Concomitant cranial and ocular combat injuries during Operation Iraqi Freedom. *J Trauma.* 2009;67(3):516–520.
248. Christine E. *Maintaining Military Medical Skills During Peacetime: Outlining and Assessing a New Approach.* Santa Monica, CA: National Defense Research Institute and RAND Health; 2008.
249. Pereira B, Ryan ML, Ogilvie MP, et al. Predeployment mass casualty and clinical trauma training for US Army forward surgical teams. *J Craniofac Surg.* 2010;21:982–986.
250. Schulman CI, Graygo J, Wilson K, Robinson D, Garcia G, Augenstein J. Training forward surgical team: do military-civilian collaborations work? *Army Med Dept J.* 2010;Oct–Dec:17–21.
251. King DR, Patel MB, Feinstein AJ, Earle SA, Topp RF, Proctor KG. Simulation training for a mass casualty incident: two-year experience at the Army Trauma Training Center. *J Trauma.* 2006;61(4):943–948.
252. Schulman CI, Garcia GD, Wyckoff MM, Duncan RC, Withum KF, Graygo J. Mobile learning module improves knowledge of medical shock for forward surgical team members. *Mil Med.* 2012;177:1316–1321.
253. McCunn M, York GB, Hirshon JM, Jenkins DH, Scalea TM. Trauma readiness training for military deployment: a comparison between a US trauma center and an Air Force theater hospital in Balad, Iraq. *Mil Med.* 2011;176:769–775.
254. Office of The Surgeon General. *HQDA EXORD 096-09, Mandatory Pre-Deployment Trauma Training (PDTT) for Specified Medical Personnel.* All Army Activities (ALARACT) Memorandum; 3 February 2009.
255. Headquarters, US Air Force. *Unit Level Management of Medical Readiness Programs.* Washington, DC: USAF; 14 April 2008. Air Force Instruction 41-106.
256. Morrison JJ, Oh J, DuBose JJ, et al. En-route care capability from point of injury impacts mortality after severe wartime injury. *Ann Surg.* 2013;257(2):330–334.
257. Carol Hobaugh, PhD (former contributor to the initial Forward Surgical Team Commanders Course); personal communications, January–February 2014.
258. Honor the fallen–Army COL Brian D Allgood. 2007. *Military Times.* http://projects.militarytimes.com/valor/army-col-brian-d-allgood/2507125. Accessed 24 March 2015.
259. Hobaugh C. Army Medical Department Center and School Forward Surgical Team Commanders Course information paper. Unpublished paper in possession of author.
260. MAJ Michael Fisher, CRNA (commander, 8th FST, Operation Enduring Freedom); personal communications about unit history, August 2014.
261. CPT Bryan Malone, MS (executive officer, 240th FST, Afghanistan); personal communications about unit history, August–September 2014.
262. SSG E Rios, LPN (former licensed practical nurse, 240th FST); personal communications, January–February 2015.
263. MAJ Gustavo E Moreno, RN (commander and emergency room nurse, 160th FST); email about 160th FST unit history, April–May 2014.
264. LTC Colin A Meghoo (commander and surgeon, 67th FST); email about 67th FST unit history, February–June 2014.
265. Capt Cheuk Y Hong, MD (former member of the 127th and 135th FSTs); personal communication, September 2014.

Chapter Eleven

Homeland Defense, Contingency Operations, and Future Directions

DAVID C. LYNN and JASON M. SEERY

INTRODUCTION

AS DISCUSSED IN THE PREVIOUS CHAPTER, the post-9/11 Global War on Terrorism represented a significant era for military medicine in general, and military surgery in particular. As in other times of armed conflict, significant advancements were made: the concepts of damage control surgery and damage control resuscitation, the application of tourniquets and hemostatic agents, improvements in mechanical protection, and the institution of casualty tracking systems and data collection all helped reduce battlefield mortality to historically low levels, while the "modular" concept of forward surgery brought surgical assets closer than ever to the point of injury.[1-14]

The accomplishments of surgeons, nurses, physician assistants, medics, and other medical officers and enlisted personnel treating life-threatening injuries in Iraq and Afghanistan over this period were nothing short of heroic. Also during this timeframe, the armed services were engaged in the tasks of homeland defense, responses to severe weather and natural disasters, support of allied militaries, and the posture of readiness to support any new potential theater of operation—all the while maintaining a steady deployment cycle in support of Operation Enduring Freedom, Operation Iraqi Freedom, and Operation New Dawn. This resulted in an unprecedented operational tempo for the US military's medical personnel.

This chapter will discuss the US military's surgical contributions with respect to the Global Response Force (GRF) mission, homeland defense, responses by US Northern Command (USNORTHCOM) to natural and manmade disasters, terrorist threats including the Defense CBRN (Chemical, Biological, Radiological, and Nuclear) Response Force (DCRF) mission, readiness to support contingency operations other than Iraq and Afghanistan, and other missions. Force design updates and future directions for military surgical assets will also be discussed.

HOMELAND DEFENSE AND CONTINGENCY OPERATIONS

Operation Noble Eagle

Immediately after the 9/11 attacks on New York and the Pentagon, thousands of National Guard and Reserve personnel were mobilized to perform security missions at military installations, airports, power plants, bridges, ports, and other potential terrorist targets. As military assets were used for homeland defense and to support federal, state, and local agencies, Operation Noble Eagle rapidly expanded to include search and rescue, engineering operations, forensics, medical support, and various other missions.[15–17]

Numerous federal entities were mobilized, including USNS *Comfort*, battalion aid stations, volunteer-run first aid stations, Veterans Administration hospitals, and aid stations operated by the Federal Emergency Management Agency (FEMA). The 344th Combat Support Hospital (CSH), a Reserve unit, provided personnel, logistical support, and supplies to Jacobi Hospital in the Bronx. The unit also loaned everything from cots to weapons to other military units and fire departments. Unfortunately, Jacobi Hospital, like many others in the New York area, was waiting for patients that would never arrive. According to Dr. Sheldon Teperman, director of Jacobi's trauma center:

> We cleared out patients, we cleared out the emergency room, we set up teams of trauma doctors and emergency medicine doctors that were volunteers that came from all over the campus and then we waited, and no one came, because as everybody knows now, close to 3,000 people died at Ground Zero, and almost nobody was pulled out of that rubble.[18]

Instead, medical care focused on combat stress and the treatment (long- and short-term) of respiratory illness secondary to exposure. Individuals at Ground Zero were exposed to falling debris, fire, smoke, toxic chemicals, dust (including pulverized asbestos), and various biohazards. Mental trauma, stress, and fatigue also took a toll on rescue workers, many of whom labored for extended periods of time.

In her book *Attack on the Pentagon: The Medical Response to 9/11*, Condon-Rall describes in vivid detail the harrowing events of that day, and the heroic efforts of numerous military and civilian personnel in Washington, DC.[19] While 126 lives were tragically lost, the outcomes could have been much worse.

Before the attack, portions of the Pentagon building had been modernized with blast-resistant windows, steel-reinforced weight-bearing columns, and penetrant-resistant outer walls. The Anthony DiLorenzo Tricare Health Clinic routinely prepared for emergencies and always had two five-person teams (each with a physician, a registered nurse, and three medics) on standby. These teams systematically prepared for emergencies in conjunction with the Air Force Flight Clinic, the Navy Dental Clinic, the Washington Headquarters Services, the Arlington County Fire Department, the Federal Bureau of Investigation, FEMA, the Defense Protective Service, and the Department of Defense (DoD) law enforcement organization for the Pentagon (now the Pentagon Police Department). Condon-Rall describes how Major (MAJ) Lorrie Brown (DiLorenzo clinic chief nurse), Captain (CPT) Jennifer

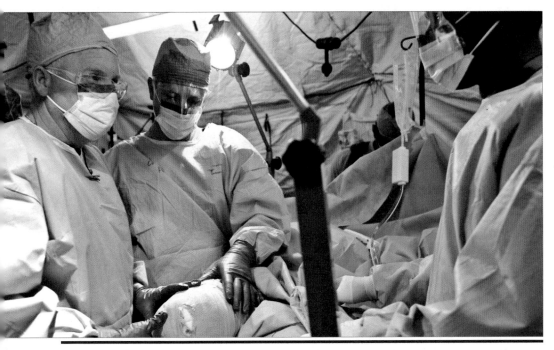

FIGURE 11-1. US Army medical providers with the 240th Forward Surgical Team at Fort Bragg, NC, complete a simulated leg amputation during a joint service field exercise, 15 October 2012, at the Joint Readiness Training Center at Fort Polk, LA. (US Air Force photo by Tech Sgt Joselito Aribuabo/Released)

Glidewell (acute care nurse), and Sergeant (SGT) Matthew Rosenburg (medic) immediately took action following the attack by organizing casualty collection points, conducting triage, providing point of injury care, and coordinating evacuation.

> With their emergency bags already packed, and only the length of the hallway to run, the teams, according to Major Brown, had all of the triage areas operational by 0943, 5 minutes after the plane hit the Pentagon.[19(p10)]

In the end, 125 patients were evacuated to 12 different surrounding military and civilian hospitals. The preparation, decisive action, and teamwork of those who responded that day has since served as an emergency preparedness model for healthcare systems and providers.

The Global Response Force Mission

The GRF mission, formally referred to as the Division Readiness Brigade (DRB) mission, includes military assets on 24/7 standby, ready to deploy anywhere in the world within hours of notification. The capabilities of these assets, if called, include forcible entry and seizure of a defended airfield, followed by the buildup of combat power to support follow-on military operations.[20–22] GRF is a joint military operation led by the Army's XVIII Airborne Corps. The Army's airborne forward surgical teams (FSTs) continuously

TABLE 11-1. **ROLES OF MILITARY MEDICAL CARE**

Role 1		Point of injury (self-aid, buddy aid, and combat lifesaver)
	Army/USMC:	Battalion Aid Station
	USMC:	Shock Trauma Platoon
Role 2	Army:	Medical Company
		Forward Surgical Team
	Air Force:	Mobile Field Surgical Team
		Small Portable Expeditionary Aeromedical Rapid Response
		Expeditionary Medical Support (EMEDS, Basic or +10)
	Navy:	Casualty Receiving and Treatment Ship (CRTS)
		Aircraft Carrier Battle Group
	USMC:	Surgical Company
		Forward Resuscitative Surgical System
		En Route Care Team
	NATO:	Any facility that provides damage control surgery
Role 3	Army:	Combat Support Hospital
	Air Force:	EMEDS +25
		Air Force Theater Hospital
	Navy:	Expeditionary Medical Facility
		Hospital Ship
Role 4		CONUS-based hospital or other "safe haven"

Adapted from: *Emergency War Surgery*. Fourth US Revision. Fort Sam Houston, TX: Borden Institute; 2013.
USMC: United States Marine Corps
CONUS: Continental United States

TABLE 11-2. **US ARMY AIRBORNE FORWARD SURGICAL TEAMS AND THEIR LOCATIONS**

2nd ACR FST	Fort Bragg, NC (airborne 1997 to 2004, when unit deactivated)
8th FST	Joint Base Elmendorf Richardson, AK (airborne 2011 to 2013)
67th FST	Miesau, Germany (airborne 2007 to 2013)
240th FST	Fort Bragg, NC (airborne 2009 to 2014)
250th FST	Joint Base Lewis-McChord, WA (airborne 1997 to 2009)
274th FST	Fort Bragg, NC (airborne 1997 to present)
541st FST	Fort Bragg, NC (airborne 2006 to present; formerly the 782nd FST)
759th FST	Fort Bragg, NC (airborne 2004 to present; formerly the 2nd ACR FST)
782nd FST	Fort Bragg (airborne 1997 to 2006, when unit deactivated)

ACR: Armored Cavalry Regiment
FST: Forward Surgical Team

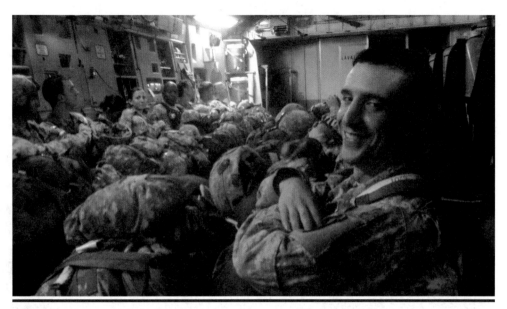

FIGURE 11-2. Team members from forward surgical teams at Fort Bragg, NC, aboard a C-17 aircraft, about to complete a nighttime combat parachute jump, 18 October 2011. Fort Bragg FSTs regularly conduct airborne training operations with the 82nd Airborne Division's brigade combat teams on the Global Response Force mission. On the right is MAJ William Vanasse, Chief Nurse, 759th FST. (Photo by MAJ David Lynn)

train with the 82nd Airborne Division's brigade combat teams and are prepared to support this enduring mission (Figure 11-1).[23,24] The FSTs are organized to conduct both airborne (parachute) and air-land insertions.[25,26] Capabilities for this mission are trained on a regular basis through the Joint Operations Access Exercise,[27,28] and FSTs are routinely co-located with their brigade support medical company counterparts to evaluate, treat, and evacuate casualties (Table 11-1).[29–32]

The concept of the airborne surgical team was developed by a British vascular surgeon, Dr Charles Rob, during World War II. As a result of Rob's work, the Royal Army Medical Corps conducted two combat jumps into North Africa, validating the ability of airborne surgical assets to decrease combat deaths.[33] In the 1990s, the first US Army airborne FSTs were established: the 782nd and 274th Medical Detachments and the 2nd Armored Calvary Regiment FST at Fort Bragg, North Carolina, as well as the 250th Medical Detachment at Fort Lewis, Washington.[34] In 2015, three Army FSTs retained the airborne designation (Table 11-2). These highly mobile, well-trained, and disciplined surgical units can be deployed anywhere in the world on short notice. They are designed to parachute into combat, allowing for the early treatment of casualties (Figure 11-2). During an airfield seizure operation, a team parachutes part of its personnel and equipment (Alpha echelon), then air-lands the other portion of the team (Bravo echelon). Alpha echelon equipment is heavy-dropped (parachuted) in one to two military vehicles, while Bravo echelon equipment and personnel is air-landed approximately 12 to 24 hours later. Thus, these

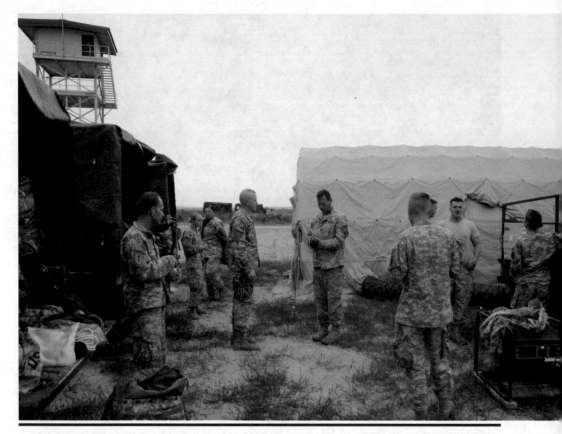

FIGURE 11-3. Team members from Fort Bragg's airborne forward surgical teams set up their Bravo echelon next to their Alpha echelon on the tactical air field after a night mass tactical jump as part of a Joint Operational Access Exercise, August 2009. Note the small 5-kw non-military generator used to provide power for the Alpha echelon shortly after parachuting onto the landing zone, enabling advanced resuscitation and surgical capabilities. (Photo by MAJ David Lynn)

units enhance the brigade medical team's ability to perform advanced trauma resuscitation during the initial phases of a mission, and conduct surgical interventions approximately 30 to 45 minutes after their heavy-dropped or air-landed equipment is recovered. Army FSTs employed in this manner are capable of performing approximately 30 life-saving surgeries over the course of 72 hours before reconstitution is required.

The personnel and equipment makeup of the Alpha and Bravo echelons, as well as their method of employment, are variable and flexible. During the 250th FST's combat jump into Northern Iraq, the Alpha echelon included one general surgeon, one orthopedic surgeon, one certified nurse anesthetist, one emergency medicine nurse, three combat medical specialists, and two operating room technicians.[35] Once on the ground and operational, the FST may stand alone, but capabilities are greatly enhanced when the team is combined with its brigade support medical company (or "Charlie Med") Role 2 counterparts.[31] Surgical and medical capabilities may be established in a cleared building (preferred if available). If a building is unavailable, the medical teams will set up their respective tents (generally best if co-located and interconnected) to begin advanced resuscitation and surgical intervention. After the runway is cleared and the air-land option is available, the Bravo echelons of the medical units arrive and augment their Alpha counterparts.[24]

An FST vastly improves its capacity by quick assembly and establishment of a footprint within the medical company area, which is composed of an administrative section, treatment platoon, patient holding squad, and ambulance platoon.[30] By combining personnel, this robust "Role 2-plus" medical team can greatly increase capability while improving the quality of care; it has ambulance support for patient evacuation to awaiting ground or air assets. This crucial integration increases the speed of care, improves patient flow and tracking, and enables medical resupply operations, as well as providing radiographic and laboratory capabilities. It also allows for damage control surgery and resuscitation to occur beyond the 30 patients in a 72-hour period limit. This method of forward surgical employment is validated on a regular basis through participation in Joint Operations Access Exercises, which include one brigade combat team from the 82nd Airborne Division, members of the US Air Force, various international partners, and multiple other enablers, including one airborne FST (Figure 11-3). Over 1,000 paratroopers conduct static-line jumps, projecting combat power into a hostile environment, and units conduct various follow-on missions over the ensuing weeks as they would in a GRF mission.

As was demonstrated after Hurricane Katrina in 2005 and the Haiti earthquake in 2010, military medical assets that stand ready on this short notice mission may be utilized for a wide variety of operations other than war.

US Northern Command and Homeland Defense

After the terrorist attacks on 11 September 2001, USNORTHCOM was created to deter, prevent, and defeat threats and aggression aimed at the United States, its territories, and its interests. This marked the first time a single military commander was charged with protecting the US homeland since the days of George Washington. Activated on 1 October 2002, USNORTHCOM's mission now includes defense support for civilian authorities. When approved by the president or secretary of defense, it may direct military resources (Army, Navy, Air Force, Marine Corps, or Coast Guard) to support federal, state, and local entities. Its area of responsibility includes all air, land, and sea approaches to North America, encompassing the continental United States, Alaska, Canada, Mexico, and the surrounding water areas out to approximately 500 nautical miles.[36]

USNORTHCOM's assigned missions for military medical units include the Joint Task Force Civil Support Defense CBRN (Chemical, Biological, Radiological, and Nuclear) Response Force (DCRF), formerly known as the CBRNE Consequence Management Response Force. DCRF assets were increased to improve its ability to assist the federal response more rapidly and reduce the impact of a homeland CBRN incident, providing critical life-saving capability. Including over 5,200 service members, DCRF is structured in two force packages that are prepared to deploy at 24 and 48 hours, respectively. The medical task force portion of the force is currently composed of Role 3 assets (three Air Force expeditionary medical support [EMEDS] units) and Role 2 assets (four FSTs and four area

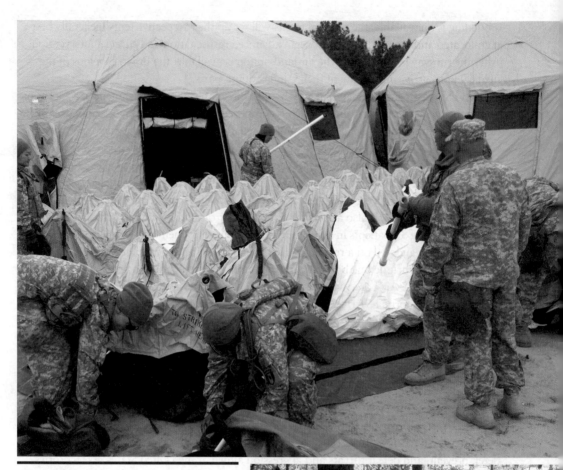

FIGURE 11-4. [Top] Members of the 759th Forward Surgical Team set their tents up adjoining the 550th Area Support Medical Company just north of Normandy Drop Zone, Fort Bragg, NC, 17 January 2012. Teams conducted a 5-day unit-level field training exercise in preparation for assuming the Defense (Chemical, Biological, Radiological, Nuclear) Response Force Mission. (Photo by MAJ David Lynn)

FIGURE 11-5. [Bottom] Fort Bragg Forward Surgical Team (FST) commanders attend the Medical Management of Chemical and Biological Casualties course at Aberdeen Proving Ground and Fort Detrick, MD, in preparation for the Defense CBRN (Chemical, Biological, Radiological, Nuclear) Response Force mission, 25 October 2011. Left to right: MAJ David Lynn, 759th FST; MAJ Jason Seery, 541st FST, and MAJ John Detro, 240th FST. (Photo by MAJ David Lynn)

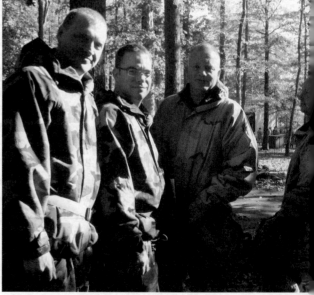

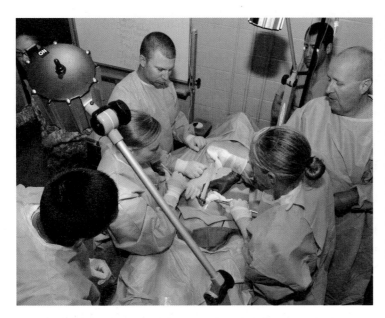

FIGURE 11-6. US Army MAJ Kelly Blair (right), commander of the 250th Forward Surgical Team, 62nd Medical Brigade, Joint Base Lewis-McChord, WA, instructs soldiers as they perform mock surgery on the Chloe Surgical Simulator during the Vibrant Response exercise at Camp Atterbury, IN, 2 August 2012. (US Army photo by SGT Mark Cloutier/Released)

support medical companies [ASMCs]), in addition to medical logistics, preventive medicine and ground ambulance units, combat and operational stress control, and veterinary services. FSTs and ASMCs are geographically "paired" for employment at or near an incident site, providing a relatively rapid, robust medical-surgical element (Figure 11-4).[37,38]

Preparation for medical units assigned to the DCRF mission consists of both individual and collective unit-level training with a renewed emphasis on CBRN threats, as well as a focus on legal aspects of military employment within the United States. All individuals are required to take courses related to antiterrorism, FEMA, and the defense support of civil authorities, as well as the Posse Comitatus Act, in order to ensure that soldiers and leaders understand their roles and limitations as they interact with civilians. CBRN training is variable and may be limited due to new restrictions on centralized funding, and is often at the discretion of unit commanders. The US Army Medical Research Institute of Chemical Defense and US Army Medical Research Institute of Infectious Diseases host numerous useful courses. These include Medical Management of Chemical and Biological Casualties, designed for nurses and providers; Field Management of Chemical and Biological Casualties, for medics and enlisted personnel; and Hospital Management of Chemical, Biological, Radiological, Nuclear, and Explosive Incidents, geared toward senior leaders and medical planners (Figure 11-5). The Armed Forces Radiobiology Research Institute hosts Medical Effects of Ionizing Radiation, a valuable course that can be tailored for physicians and nurses or medics and first responders.

Unit-level training includes medical and surgical treatment of all casualties, including pediatric and geriatric patients, animals, and CBRN victims. Training also includes the use of personalized protective equipment and specialized CBRN equipment needed for hasty decontamination and detection. These skills should be reinforced and validated regularly during field training exercises, preferably with regional ASMC units. Training culminates in the annual Operation Vibrant Response exercise, in which units respond to a simulated large-scale CBRE incident (Figure 11-6).

To date, USNORTHCOM has not had to respond to a large-scale threat calling for military support. The Robert T Stafford Disaster Relief and Emergency Assistance Act (Public Law 100-707), signed into law in 1988, authorized the federal government to help state and local governments alleviate the suffering and damage caused by disasters. USNORTHCOM has frequently been called upon to respond to requests from civil authorities in these situations, and on at least two occasions the response included provision of the military's unique medical and surgical assets.[36]

Hurricane Katrina

Hurricane Katrina first made landfall as a Category 1 hurricane on 25 August 2005 in Florida, where it caused approximately $2 billion in damage and killed 14 people. Katrina then crossed the Gulf of Mexico, making landfall again on 29 August as a Category 3 hurricane, inundating New Orleans and inflicting widespread damage as levees protecting the city failed, killing more than 1,800.

At the request of civilian authorities, USNORTHCOM forces deployed to the region under the direction of Joint Task Force Katrina commander Lieutenant General Russel Honoré.[36] More than 22,000 personnel from every branch of the US military participated in the effort, which included health and medical support; search and rescue; security; evacuation; recovery of deceased persons; debris removal; restoration of infrastructure; logistics including distribution of food, water, and ice; temporary shelter; and long-range communications.[39] The first medical unit to arrive was the 782nd FST (Airborne) under the command of MAJ (P) Shawn Nessen.[40]

The 782nd FST was assigned to the 82nd Airborne Division and supported the DRB mission. As part of the DRB mission, the team represented one of the world's few surgical assets ready to deploy at a moment's notice. The 782nd left Fort Bragg and was on site in New Orleans within 18 hours of notification (Figure 11-7). At the direction of the Medical Task Force Commander, the FST set up in the baggage claim area of the New Orleans airport and was ready to receive surgical patients within 1 hour (Figure 11-8). The 782nd maintained operations until the 14th CSH from Fort Benning, Georgia, arrived and set up almost 2 weeks later. Unfortunately, by the time either of these units was activated and operational, most people in need of medical attention had already been evacuated from the city. With few civilian patients, focus shifted to support of the 82nd Airborne Division and other military units.

When Hurricane Rita threatened the city in late September that same year, the 14th CSH was disassembled, moved, and reassembled inside the convention center in downtown New Orleans, closer to the remaining civilian population in need of assistance. The 14th CSH, an 84-bed hospital, included an emergency room, operating room, computed tomography and radiograph capability, and dental and specialty clinics. The 14th CSH continued to provide support for both military and civilian populations until being replaced by the 21st CSH from Fort Hood, Texas, on 10 October. Operations were eventually taken

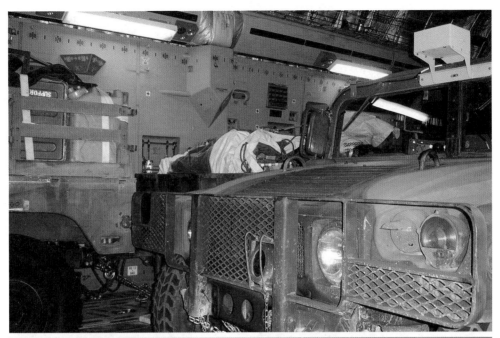

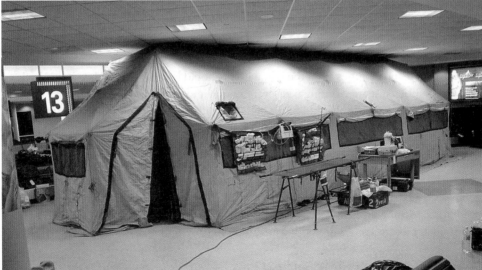

FIGURE 11-7. [Top] The 782nd Airborne Forward Surgical Team was the first Department of Defense medical asset to arrive and be ready to accept patients due to the organic mobility designed into the unit and it being on the Global Response Force Mission. Prepacked vehicles were loaded on C-17 aircraft at Pope Air Base and arrived at New Orleans Airport shortly after. (Photo by COL Shawn Nessen)

FIGURE 11-8. [Bottom] MAJ(P) Nessen team's set up next to baggage claim area 13 in a secure and powered location. Taking advantage of the enclosed facility, triage, initial trauma assessment, and resuscitation were conducted adjacent to the erected tent, saving it to be allocated as an operating room with two tables. (Photo by SFC Leonel Cubias) over by New Orleans Charity Hospital on 14 November, bringing US military medical operations to a close.[39]

Although the care of surgical patients during this time was minimal, the operation was still important for two reasons: (1) it again validated the FST as a rapidly deployable unit within the United States, and (2) it yielded powerful lessons learned for future incidents. The fact that the 782nd FST was able to reach New Orleans with all necessary personnel and equipment within 18 hours of alert speaks to the military's truly unique lift capability, as well as the FST's training, motivation, and state of readiness. While limited in the number of surgical patients that can be treated, few other military or civilian assets exist that can be employed with such expediency. It also validated the DRB/GRF medical support mission: both the need for highly trained units (including medical and surgical units) on 24/7 standby, and the possible employment of these units for missions other than overseas combat operations.

Lessons learned reinforced the known challenges regarding timeliness of employment.[41,42] Even if the decision was made to deploy surgical assets immediately, and these elements are on standby, surgical units will arrive well beyond the "golden hour" for treatment. Even after the team's arrival, obstacles exist to informing those in need about the availability and location of medical assets. Patients with life-threatening injuries from the initial event may already have died of wounds, survived without intervention, or received care elsewhere. If any surrounding infrastructure exists, as it did in the suburbs of New Orleans (and in the greater New York area during Operation Noble Eagle), patients generally find their way via ambulance or personal means to existing hospitals and medical facilities. Unless units are pre-positioned, expectations regarding the treatment of patients with life-threatening injuries from the initial event should be tempered. While individuals with new injuries sustained during post-event search and rescue missions, recovery operations, or other actions would be treated during the "golden hour" timeframe, these casualties are historically far fewer in number. Focus instead shifts toward true civilian support, an important lesson that should not be forgotten by units that currently support DCRF and other contingency missions. Surrounding hospitals may be staffed with surgeons, nurses, and technicians who have been awake and working for days, and facilities may be running low on medical supplies. Military medical units may be employed to reinforce existing medical systems with personnel and Class VIII medical supplies, while other military assets assist with food, water, fuel, security, and logistical support.[43]

Operation Lifeline and Task Force 212

In the early morning hours of Saturday, 8 October 2005, the Kashmir area of Pakistan suffered a 7.6-magnitude earthquake with its epicenter near the densely populated city of Muzaffarabad.[44] The event would claim the lives of over 86,000 and displace over 4 million. Within 48 hours, various US military assets began to mobilize, including the 212th Mobile Army Surgical Hospital (MASH), based in Miesau, Germany. The 212th was supported and augmented by the 160th FST and 123rd Main Support Battalion, also stationed in Germany, and the 240th FST from Fort Stewart, Georgia.[45,46] The first elements of Task Force 212 left Ramstein Air Base, Germany, and arrived in Pakistan on 17 October 2005.

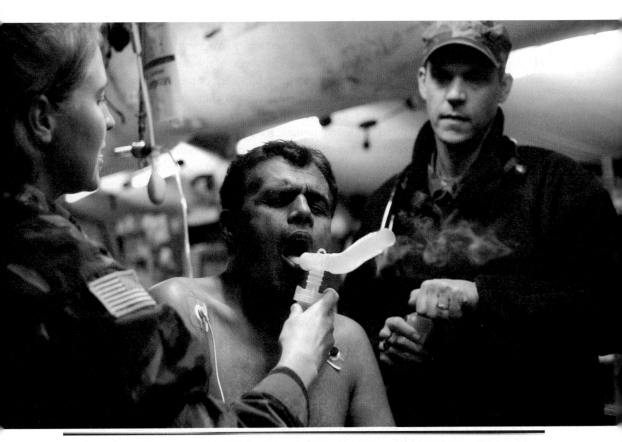

FIGURE 11-9. US Army 2LT Kristy Bischoff (left) and MAJ Tom Knisely treat a patient at the 212th Mobile Army Surgical Hospital at Muzaffarabad, Pakistan, during Operation Lifeline on 5 January 2006. Operation Lifeline was a Pakistani-led relief operation designed to aid victims of the devastating earthquake that struck this region on 8 October 2005. (US Air Force photo by Airman 1st Class Barry Loo/Released)

Medical efforts began in earnest around 29 October as part of what would be dubbed Operation Lifeline: transportation, engineering, medical, and logistical support provided by more than 1,200 troops.[46–49] Task Force 212 faced unique logistical challenges due to the region affected. Harsh weather (snow), difficult terrain, and lack of security (because of nearby Taliban forces) were constant concerns, particularly for the 240th FST, which was located several miles away from the main body at higher elevation.[44] Unlike after Hurricane Katrina, Pakistani patients walked for miles to be seen. By the end of the operation, the 212th MASH treated over 32,000 host nation patients, performed 484 surgical operations (mostly for orthopedic or extremity wounds), and provided over 13,000 vaccinations (Figure 11-9).[50] The 212th was the last active MASH in the Army prior to its conversion to a CSH, and after the operation, the US State Department purchased all $4.6 million of its equipment and donated the entire hospital to the Pakistani military.[48] The 212th MASH's sign now resides at the Army Medical Department (AMEDD) museum at Fort Sam Houston, Texas.

Operation Unified Response

On the morning of 12 January 2010, a catastrophic 7.0-magnitude earthquake struck Haiti. The epicenter was approximately 10 to 15 miles west of the capital, Port-au-Prince, and it eventually killed over 200,000 people, injuring hundreds of thousands more and displacing over one million individuals. The quake destroyed Haiti's main port and caused major damage to its infrastructure. Later that night, the president of Haiti declared a national state of emergency and requested humanitarian assistance and disaster relief aid. Military aid from the United States was coordinated through US Southern Command (USSOUTHCOM). The USCG Cutter *Forward* arrived off the coast the next morning, on January 13th. Military personnel established a liaison team with the Haitian Coast Guard to conduct damage assessments, establish command and control, and begin providing humanitarian assistance. Shortly thereafter, two USCG C-130 aircraft arrived to help the most seriously wounded and evacuate injured American citizens. During the course of the day, an Air Force South assessment team landed in Port-au-Prince to survey the airport, while elements of the First Special Operations Wing arrived to reopen Port-au-Prince International Airport. US Navy P-3 aircraft from the Cooperative Security Location of Comalapa, El Salvador, conducted aerial reconnaissance of the area. DoD officials ordered the aircraft carrier USS *Carl Vinson* and the USS *Bataan* Amphibious Readiness Group (with the 22nd Marine Expeditionary Unit embarked) to make best speed to Haiti. The first US urban search and rescue team, a 72-member unit from Fairfax County, Virginia, arrived in Haiti before 24 hours had elapsed. On January 14, four more USCG cutters and the USS *Higgins* arrived offshore. An engineering assessment team determined the pier and wharf at Port-au-Prince port too badly damaged to allow for ship-borne efforts to make land, making them effectively inoperable. On January 15, key personnel from USNORTHCOM, the XVIII Airborne Corps, and the 82nd Airborne Division arrived along with the USS *Carl Vinson*. Additional medical assets were dispatched, and the Joint Task Force Bravo (JTF-B) Medical Element (stationed in Honduras) and the USS *Bataan* arrived on January 18, followed by the USNS *Comfort* on January 20 and the 24th EMEDS on January 24. Military units were augmented by Red Cross translators and support personnel, DoD assets, and civilian physicians, nurses, and medical students from across the United States. By the end of January, JTF-Haiti controlled over 22,000 military personnel both on the ground and offshore, 1,100 of which were medical.[36,49–51]

A worldwide outpouring of support led to the arrival in Haiti of additional military units, civilian personnel, and nongovernmental organizations (NGO) from multiple nations. Numerous field hospitals were established by entities from Argentina, Canada, China, Colombia, Cuba, France, Israel, Italy, Jordan, Mexico, Russia, Spain, Sri Lanka, Turkey, and other nations. Coordination of these assets became the main focus of the military leadership. From a medical standpoint, the three main tasks now became: (1) working with engineers to find out which Haitian hospitals were standing, safe, and functional; (2) distributing medical assets across the disaster area; and (3) informing the populace about the location of various assets. In all, six Haitian hospitals remained operational, and another nine were partially operational. While coordinated through the US State Department, these efforts relied heavily on the expertise of medical planners from USSOUTH-

COM, led by Captain Miguel Cubano (a general surgeon and the first naval officer to hold this command), and the XVIII Airborne Corps surgeon cell, led by Colonel (COL) Richard Ellison (a general surgeon by training and former commander of the 759th FST).[52]

Unlike the situations encountered during Operation Noble Eagle or Hurricane Katrina, what little surrounding infrastructure that existed before the earthquake was decimated. Thirteen of Haiti's 15 government ministry buildings were completely destroyed. Nearly half of all buildings sustained significant damage in Port-au-Prince and surrounding villages. The airport control tower was rendered inoperable, and more than half the seaport was left in ruins. In contrast to previous humanitarian operations, medical units found no shortage of patients. Due to the sheer volume of patients, as well as the potential for ongoing injuries due to aftershocks, the initial units to arrive became rapidly overwhelmed. Potentially dangerous situations were encountered when medical units set up without proper security in place.[53]

Once again the US military was able to utilize its unique capabilities to employ its medical assets for circumstances other than combat operations. However, the scale of these operations was unprecedented, and never before did a noncombat operation rely so heavily on military leaders and medical planners. The effort required international and interagency coordination and communication, not only among medical counterparts, but also among engineering, logistical, and security personnel, as well as various governing bodies.[54] By the end of February, DoD personnel were directly responsible for treating nearly 10,000 patients and performing over 1,000 surgeries, as well as evacuating approximately 189 Haitian citizens in need of higher levels of care to US facilities via military aircraft. Seventy thousand prescriptions were filled, and countless additional lives were saved by preventive medicine units that worked energetically to thwart the spread of communicable diseases among the displaced.

Other Foreign Operations

US military medical and surgical assets continue to have a presence throughout the world, providing both humanitarian relief and strategic support. To serve as an academic resource, the Center for Disaster and Humanitarian Assistance Medicine was chartered in 1999 at the Uniformed Services University of Health Sciences in Bethesda, Maryland, through congressional funding. According to the Center's director, COL Charles Beadling, "Healthcare is a bridge that permits non-threatening interactions between parties that otherwise would not communicate," contributing to regional stability and global security.[55] In fact, current DoD directives place priority on security, stability, transition, and reconstruction operations equal to combat operations.[56] Most of these initiatives and projects fall into the category of primary care and preventive medicine, although surgical units play a support role. One example includes the US Africa Command's Natural Fire exercise. Although the exercise is largely an academic endeavor involving forces from Uganda, Chad, Kenya, Tanzania, Rwanda, and Burundi, US forces also provide medical care at rural clinics (Figure 11-10). In 2009, the 629th FST, from Columbus, Ohio, along with the 7225th Medical Support Unit, saw approximately 700 patients a day at the Pajimo Clinic in rural Uganda (Figure 11-11).[57,58] Numerous surgical units in Iraq and Afghanistan have also

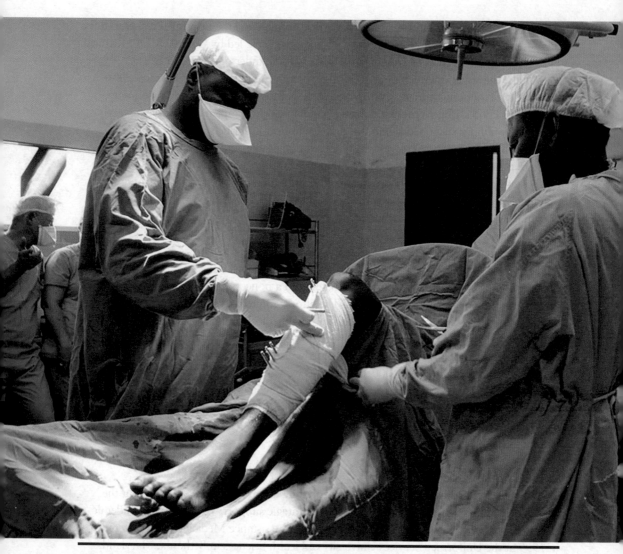

FIGURE 11-10. A joint team of Chadian and US military medical professionals work together during a surgery 14 April 2015, at the Military Teaching Hospital in N'Djamena, Chad. They performed a procedure on a Chadian soldier who sustained a gunshot wound that fractured his right femur and left tibia. The US and Chadian medical teams were working together as part of a joint exercise called Medical Readiness and Training Exercise, known as MEDRETE 15-3. The exercise was a joint effort between the Chadian government, US Army Africa, the Army Reserve Medical Command, and the 7th Civil Support Command. MEDRETE 15-3 served as an opportunity for US and Chadian forces to hone and strengthen their lifesaving skills as well as reinforcing the partnership between the countries. (US Army Africa photo by SSG Andrea Merritt)

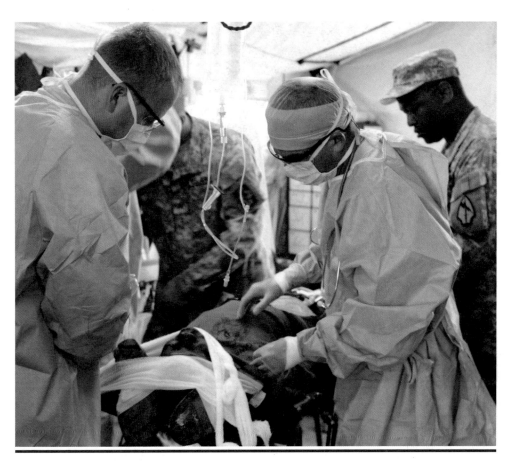

FIGURE 11-11. MAJ Scott Armen, a surgeon from Gainesville, FL, and other soldiers of the Columbus, OH, 629th Forward Surgical Team, examine a Ugandan soldier hit in the head by a steel beam. 1LT Matthew Boyer (not shown), a nurse, was the medical officer-in-charge at the site, and having no neck braces, improvised and stabilized the injured man's neck with a pair of boots. The Ugandan soldier was quickly flown by helicopter to a hospital in Kampala, 200 miles south. (US Army photo by MAJ Corey Schultz/Released)

conducted humanitarian relief projects, as well as providing training for host nation's civilian and military medical assets.[59,60]

USSOUTHCOM's JTF-B, established in August 1984 at Soto Cano Air Base, Honduras, conducts joint operations to enhance security and stability in Central America. Its personnel have ranged from 500 to 2,000 over the last 20 years and currently number about 600. The JTF-B has a medical element with an organic seven-person mobile surgical team (MST) manned with a mixture of Air Force and Army medical staff. The MST works with other Army, Navy, and Air Force medical personnel (dental, pharmacy, laboratory, veterinary services for military working dogs, preventive medicine, physical therapy, radiology, medical maintenance, medical supply, emergency medical technicians, aviation medicine, and patient administration).[61]

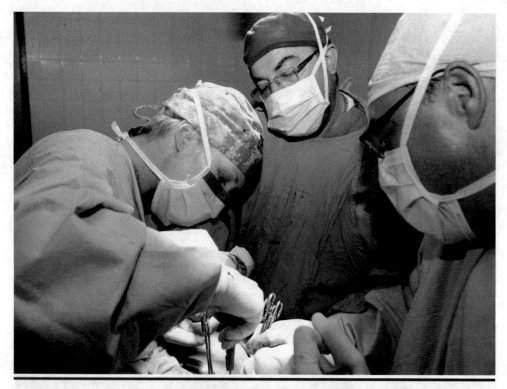

FIGURE 11-12. US Army MAJ Lisa Coviello, Joint Task Force Bravo Medical Element general surgeon, performs a gallbladder removal with Dr Jose Mejia and Dr Guillermo Saenz, Honduran general surgeons, 12 July 2011, at a community hospital in Comayagua, Honduras. (US Air Force photo by Tech Sgt Matthew McGovern/Released)

While its primary mission is to support the service members of JTF-B, the unit's medical element has a secondary mission to remain "field ready" for any emergency requiring medical or surgical support. Personnel conduct quarterly medical readiness exercises to prepare for this mission. In an effort to support the local community and build international goodwill, the forward surgical element assists local surgeons with operative cases in nearby villages twice a week (Figure 11-12). The JTF-B also provides air assets and resuscitative surgical care in response to local trauma cases.[61–64] Personnel were dispatched to Peru in 2007 under the command of Lieutenant Colonel (LTC) Esmeraldo Zarzabal in response to a severe earthquake, arriving approximately 20 hours after notification (Figure 11-13).[64–67]

As mentioned earlier, the JTF-B medical element deployed to Haiti in support of Operation Unified Response in 2010 under the command of Colonel (COL) Marie Dominguez with 23 personnel: the MST an emergency medical team and a 20-cot holding capability. It was one of the first surgical units to have "boots on the ground" (Figure 11-14). JTF-B personnel conducted inpatient and surgical operations for 20 days, working hand-in-hand with counterparts from the Haitian Coast Guard, the Mexican Navy

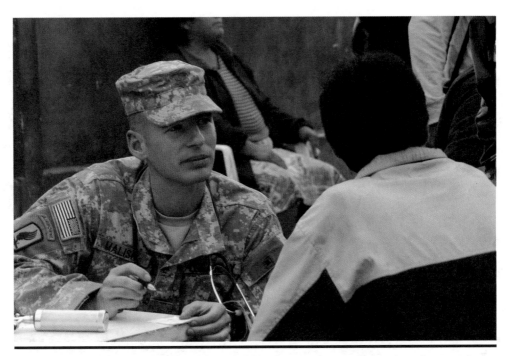

FIGURE 11-13. Army MAJ Richard Malish, a physician from Soto Cano Air Base, Honduras, listens as a patient describes his condition during the Joint Task Force-Bravo medical humanitarian relief mission 17–21 August 2007. Members from the JTF-Bravo deployed to provide medical care to the citizens of Pisco, Peru, following the 8.0-magnitude earthquake that devastated the region on 15 August. In addition to the medical assets sent, the mobile field surgical team, led by COL Rob Rush, was deployed too. (US Air Force photo by Senior Airman Shaun Emery)

and civil service, the Columbian Army and Navy, the Sri Lankan infantry, and other US military units. This unique multinational team saw over 2,000 patients, conducted 64 surgical procedures, and evacuated over 400 patients to the USS *Comfort*, Sacre Coeur Hospital, Italian and Russian military hospitals, NGO facilities, and medical facilities in the Dominican Republic.[62–64]

Perhaps the US military's most notable medical and surgical humanitarian efforts are the biennial missions conducted by the Navy ships *Comfort* and *Mercy*. Both Role 3 facilities include 1,000 beds and 12 operating rooms, with 80 to 100 intensive care unit bed capabilities. During odd years, USNS *Comfort* embarks from Norfolk, Virginia, and conducts Operation Continuing Promise, spending several months at various ports in the Caribbean and South America. Similarly, the USNS *Mercy* conducts Operation Pacific Partnership on even years, traveling to places such as Vietnam, Cambodia, and Indonesia. Utilizing various partnerships, on-site NGOs and local physicians identify potential surgical cases. The first day at port typically includes an evaluation day, when patients are examined, decisions are made based on complexity and time constraints, and cases are scheduled for the upcoming 5 days; more complex cases will be "front loaded" to maximize the ability for follow up. Patients are issued numbered tickets, and barges ferry patients to and from the ship. Gen-

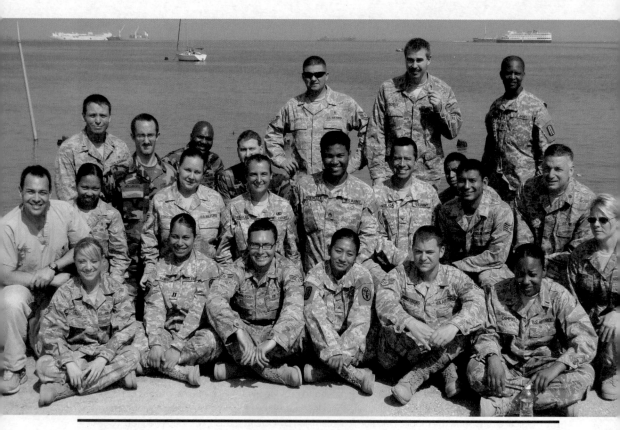

FIGURE 11-14. Members of Joint Task Force-Bravo Medical Element, led by COL Marie Dominguez, completed a 28-day deployment to Haiti 14 February 2010 in support of Joint Task Force Haiti and relief efforts stemming from a 7.0-magnitude earthquake that struck the country a few weeks prior on 12 January. (US Army photo by CPT Isabel Ramirez/Released)

eral surgeons, orthopedic surgeons, otolaryngologists, urologists, and other specialists then perform hundreds of procedures ranging from the simple to the complex. Civil engineers concurrently perform various projects ashore, while outdoor medicine clinics see patients numbering in the thousands.[68–70]

These noncombat surgical support missions are vital in enhancing US national security strategy, using "soft power" as a means of influence. They also provide challenging and unexpected situations that keep various forward surgical elements prepared and ready to execute their mission at a moment's notice. The experience and skills sustainment obtained during these missions are difficult to replicate in training, and benefit not only team members, but also future patients who will be treated by these units.

Other Forward Surgical Elements

Operational security limits the amount that can be written about many covert operations and units. However, military surgeons, anesthesiologists, nurse anesthetists, surgical technicians, nurses, and medics continually support the president and vice president of the United States and other high-level dignitaries, both in the United States and overseas. Army, Navy, and Air Force surgeons and their teams are also embedded with Special Operations Forces units across the globe, providing surgical and resuscitative care to the nation's most lethal and versatile fighting forces.[71]

FUTURE DIRECTIONS

After many years of garrison and combat experience, the keys to a successful forward surgical element are now known. These include highly motivated surgical personnel who are skilled in their profession and understand the unique needs and structure of a surgical team; durable and mobile medical equipment for performing damage control resuscitation and damage control surgery; reliable military field communication and information technology equipment to support the team's administrative, logistical, and operational needs; high-quality, consistent training that is team-oriented and patient-focused; and proper tactical employment.

The wars in Iraq and Afghanistan have validated the capabilities of smaller forward surgical units.[72] While small size undeniably places a greater strain and more training requirements on deployed personnel, data have shown that mortality rates of patients treated at Role 2 facilities are nearly identical to those at Role 3 elements, even when these small surgical teams were "split" and deployed to two different locations.[13] This data has driven much of the thought process behind the Army FST Force Design Update: current concepts for teams in the future would be composed of two mirrored "halves" that can be employed together or separately depending on mission requirements. Each half would include one orthopedic surgeon and one general surgeon. These halves could be divided even further, with a "resuscitative" unit that includes an emergency medicine provider, as well as an "operative" unit. The resuscitative unit would have the ability to "jump" forward on occasion and provide care nearer to the point of injury, as well as conducting preoperative and postoperative care when attached to the rest of the team.[73]

Ideal equipment for the forward surgical element includes items that are small, light, and durable, and have multiple functions. Much of the equipment needed is also electrical, and needs a long battery life and dual-voltage capability so it can be used in areas where only 220 voltage is available. With the establishment of the modern Army FST in 1997, units were fielded with standardized equipment that was agreed on by a working group of subject matter experts. The large amount of attention and funding this endeavor received ensured that the best equipment was provided. However, with time the missions that FSTs perform changed from those originally conceived: the length of time patients were held at the FST, the length of time the FST was supported by a towable generator for electrical power, and the length of time an FST was deployed (at times up to 15 months) all increased. In addition, there was a new expectation for Internet capability to complete reports, track patients, and maintain electronic medical records. At the same time, technology has rapidly advanced and patient outcome expectations have increased.

The AMEDD Center and School Capabilities Development Integration Directorate and the US Army Medical Materiel Agency, an AMEDD Research and Materiel Command agency, have endeavored to ensure that the proper tools are in the hands of the forward surgical elements working to save the life, limbs, and eyesight of those with combat injuries. During their triennial meetings, staff of these agencies query numerous subject matter experts and develop working groups to discuss the need for additions, deletions, or modifications to the FST medical equipment and supplies. Recently, a working group was able to capture useful data collected by the AMEDD Center and School Lessons Learned Division during FST postdeployment out-briefs. Dedicated individuals such as MAJ (R) David Cannon and others have consolidated this valuable feedback and published it in the "Forward Surgical Team Handbook: Guide to Lessons Learned and Recommended Practices for Deployment Operations." The working group has used this reference, along with feedback from the MilBook website, to make numerous recommendations, including the most recent changes. Ensuring that all equipment is dual voltage, acquiring newer technology for providing anesthesia and airway management (such as the formal addition of video-assisted laryngeal scopes to the standard equipment), and improved surgical lights are just a few of the many improvements made to the basic issue equipment and supplies.

Modern forward surgery also relies on dependable field equipment to transport its personnel and equipment, to power its facility, and to house its life-saving medical equipment. Recent improvements include replacing some Army FST High Mobility Multipurpose Wheeled Vehicles (HMMWVs) with Light Medium Tactical Vehicles, which have more space and power to transport the team and its equipment. Vehicles are fielded with modern, secure communication and global positioning satellite devices that enable them to move more freely and securely on the battlefield. The original 5-kw generators are now augmented with 18- to 20-kw generators that have onboard 5-ton environmental control units to ensure that patients will stay warm or cool, based on the medical and tactical situation. There have also been improvements in tents and related items. However, equipment unique to the GRF and DCRF missions has not been provided by the Department of the Army Headquarters, and it is left to local units to purchase such equipment, currently creating variability among units and occasional shortcomings. These issues are being aggressively addressed by the XVIII Airborne Corps and US Army North, respectively.[33]

Training for forward surgical units while in garrison remains a challenge. Newly assigned Army FST chiefs (aka "commanders") are expected to attend the FST Commanders Course taught by the AMEDD Command and Staff Branch at Fort Sam Houston, Texas. This is to ensure that Army Medical Corps and Nurse Corps officers appointed to this special assignment are equipped with foundational knowledge in the areas of administration, personnel, legal issues, security, tactics/operations, training, planning, logistics, maintenance, communication, information technology, and budgeting.

Today's forward surgical units perform weekly military and medical training during "Sergeant's Time," guided by their unit mission-essential task list and the supporting soldier training publications, including the *Soldier's Manual and Trainer's Guide* and *Soldier's Manual of Common Tasks* for various military occupational specialties. These individual and collective training tasks are reinforced at numerous situational training exercises and field training exercises. Individual team members participate in patient care at their local military treatment facility as part of the Borrowed Military Manpower program, in which they serve as part of the clinical schedule on a routine basis to ensure skills sustainment. In addition, medical proficiency training is provided as soldiers are relieved from their normal FST military duties for a period of time (30 days, for example) and work exclusively in their local military treatment facility. All deploying FSTs, and some FSTs assuming the DCRF or GRF mission, are also required to attend the US Army Trauma Training Center (ATTC) at Ryder Trauma Center in Miami, Florida. This 2-week, team-training, trauma-focused event has been the premier predeployment trauma training exercise within the DoD since 2001. The ATTC training curriculum is based on Advanced Trauma Life Support principles, the Team Strategies and Tools to Enhance Performance and Patient Safety (TeamSTEPPS) program, combat-specific instruction based on the most recent US Army Institute of Surgical Research Clinical Practice Guidelines, and Tactical Combat Casualty Care Guidelines. Once teams complete the training at ATTC, they usually conduct a culminating training event at their home station, where their reporting unit certifies or validates that they are ready to deploy or assume a special mission.

As the focus shifts from combat operations to homeland defense, surgical teams still need to be prepared to care for critically injured patients.[74] Command teams will continue to balance the requirements for individual training, soldier development, collective military training, and time spent engaging in actual patient care. Coordination with local military and civilian hospitals will therefore become even more important.[75-77] Currently, there exists a high degree of variability among surgical units and their opportunities for such training. Some military treatment facilities struggle to meet required personnel needs, and individuals from surgical units are "tasked" to meet these shortfalls, making collective team training difficult. Other units' garrison requirements make any hospital training minimal to nonexistent.[78] Airborne units have the additional challenge of added individual and sustainment training because parachutists are required to conduct one or more jumps every 3 months.[23] While the validity of this airborne requirement has been challenged, no other option exists for providing surgical support to paratroopers during the initial phases of a forced entry mission. According to COL Shawn Nessen, former commander of the 782nd FST and current Deputy Commander for Clinical Services of the 212th CSH, "As long as there is a need for airborne operations, there exists a need for airborne forward surgical teams."[40]

Future forward surgical elements supporting DCRF, GRF, humanitarian assistance, disaster relief, and other missions will be successful only if the unit is properly staffed, equipped, trained, and employed. To ensure the best patient outcomes, operational and medical commanders must fully understand an FST's abilities, requirements, and limitations. It is up to the subject matter experts to keep their commands informed regarding the units' capabilities and readiness level, and the responsibilities of the commands to take the advice of the highly specialized leaders of these units. Instructors of the Basic Officer Leadership Course, Captains Career Course, Brigade Healthcare Provider Course, Division Surgeons Course, and similar courses must ensure that thorough discussion of forward surgery is provided. Simply stating that the FST is a Role 2 asset that can work with a medical company or augment a CSH at the Role 3 level is insufficient. Recent curriculum changes at the Brigade Healthcare Provider and Division Surgeons courses added a 1-hour lecture on FST capabilities, tactics, and other vital information to ensure that future staff advisors and medical unit commanders are able to properly support and employ forward surgical units. Subject matter experts must continue to work with and educate the brigade combat team and division leadership to ensure that lessons learned, especially during Operation Enduring Freedom and Operation Iraqi Freedom, are not forgotten.

CLOSING

This chapter is by no means comprehensive. Without a doubt units from all branches of service, many of which are also on 24/7 standby, have also accomplished great tasks and touched many lives. Highlighted here were only some of the units and events that demonstrated FST capability and important lessons for the future, as well as emphasizing the training, manning, and equipment needs for the next, unknown mission. Their efforts have saved lives, provided comfort and a sense of safety to Americans and others in need abroad, strengthened international relations, and proved to the DoD leadership that the Role 2 surgical team is flexible, adaptable, extremely capable, and a very valuable asset.

ACKNOWLEDGMENTS

Mr James P Brown; Dr Dominic Storto, MD, FACS; COL James D Frizzi, MD, FACS; COL Richard Ellison, MD, FACS; COL Shawn Nessen, DO, FACS; LTC John V Salter; LTC Francis Cannizzo, MD, FACS; LTC John F Detro, PA-C; MAJ Paul Brewer, MD; MAJ Rebecca Lesemann; CPT Chris Parker; Dr Miguel Coello; and Dr Ricardo Aviles.

REFERENCES

1. Nessen SC, Cronk DR, Edens J, et al. US Army two-surgeon teams operating in remote Afghanistan—an evaluation of split-based forward surgical team operations. *J Trauma*. 2009;66:S37–S47.
2. Holcomb JB. Damage control resuscitation. *J Trauma*. 2007;62:S36–S37.
3. Holcomb JB, Jenkins D, Rhee P, et al. Damage control resuscitation: directly addressing the early coagulopathy of trauma. *J Trauma*. 2007;62:307–310.
4. Holcomb JB, Stansbury LG, Champion HR, et al. Understanding combat casualty care statistics. *J Trauma*. 2006;60:397–401.
5. Clarke JR, Trooskin SZ, Doshi PJ, et al. Time to laparotomy for intra-abdominal bleeding from trauma does affect survival for delays up to 90 minutes. *J Trauma*. 2002;52:420–425.
6. Borgman MA, Spinella PC, Perkins JG, et al. The ratio of blood products transfused affects mortality in patients receiving massive transfusion at a combat support hospital. *J Trauma*. 2007;63:805–813.
7. Cinat ME, Wallace WC, Nastanski F, et al. Improved survival following massive blood transfusion in patients who have undergone trauma. *Arch Surg*. 1999;134:964–968.
8. Shackford SR, Mackersie RC, Hoyt DB, et al. Impact of trauma systems on the outcome of severely injured patients. *Arch Surg*. 1987;122:523–527.

9. Schreiber MA, Zink K, Underwood S, et al. A comparison between patients treated at a combat support hospital in Iraq and a level I trauma center in the United States. *J Trauma.* 2008;64:S118–S122.
10. Nessen SC, Eastridge BJ, Cronk D, et al. Fresh whole blood use by forward surgical teams in Afghanistan is associated with improved survival compared to component therapy without platelets. *Transfusion.* 2013;53(Suppl1):107S–113S.
11. Kragh JF Jr, Walters TJ, Baer DG, et al. Survival with emergency tourniquet use to stop bleeding in major limb trauma. *Ann Surg.* 2009;249(1):1–7.
12. Cox ED, Schreiber MA, McManus J, et al. New hemostatic agents in the combat setting. *Transfusion.* 2009;49:248S–255S.
13. Eastridge BJ, Stansbury LG, Stinger H, et al. Forward surgical teams provide comparable outcomes to combat support hospitals during support and stabilization operations on the battlefield. *J Trauma.* 2009;66:S48–S50.
14. Remick KN, Dickerson JA, Nessen SC, et al. Transforming US Army trauma care: an evidence-based review of the trauma literature. *US Army Med J.* 2010;Jul–Sep:4–21.
15. *Operation Noble Eagle, Center for Army Lessons Learned Initial Impressions Report (IIR).* Leavenworth, Kans: TRW, Inc; 15 May 2002.
16. US Department of Defense Deployment Health Clinical Center. Operation Noble Eagle–World Trade Center. http://www.pdhealth.mil/deployments/noble_eagle_wtc/background.asp. Accessed 7 December 2015.
17. US Army Reserve Command. *The Role of the Army Reserve in the 11 September Attacks: New York City Office of the Army Reserve.* Fort McPherson, Ga: US Army Reserve Command; 2003.
18. Drexel K. Jacobi Medical Center honors lives lost on 9/11. 5 September 2011. http://nycxml.twcnews.com/content/news/health_and_medicine/146443/jacobi-medical-center-honors-lives-lost-on-9-11/. Accessed 18 August 2012.
19. Condon-Rall ME. *Attack on the Pentagon: The Medical Response to 9/11.* Washington, DC: Borden Institute; 2011.
20. Mattis JN. Quoted in: Helmick FG. Joint forcible entry. Powerpoint presented at: US Army Infantry Warfighter Forum; 15 September 2010; Fort Benning, Ga. http://www.benning.army.mil/iwc/2010/Downloads/LTGHelmick.ppt. Accessed 18 August 2012.
21. US Department of the Army. *Army Force Generation.* Washington, DC: US Department of the Army; 2011. Army Regulation 525-29.
22. US Department of Defense. *Joint Forcible Entry Operations.* Washington, DC: US Department of Defense; 2008. Joint Publication 3-18.
23. US Department of the Army. *82nd Airborne Division Airborne Standing Operating Procedures Edition VIII.* Fayetteville, NC: US Department of the Army; 2011.
24. Bender B. Airfield seizure combat health support. *Army Logistician.* 2004:10–13.
25. US Department of the Army. *Employment of Forward Surgical Teams; Tactics, Techniques, and Procedures.* Washington, DC: US Department of the Army; 1997. Field Manual 8-10-25.
26. US Department of the Army. *Employment of Forward Surgical Teams; Tactics, Techniques, and Procedures.* Washington, DC: US Department of the Army; 2003. Field Manual 4-02-25.
27. US Department of the Army. *Airborne Operations.* Washington, DC: US Department of the Army; 1990. Field Manual 90-26.
28. Kuhn DA, Alfano A. Paratroopers get back to the basics with JOAX. US Army website. 22 February 2011. http://www.army.mil/article/52366/paratroopers-get-back-to-basics-with-joax. Accessed 7 December 2015.

29. Stinger HK, Rush R. The Army forward surgical team: lessons learned, 1997–2004. *Mil Med.* 2006;171(4):269–272.
30. US Department of the Army. *The Medical Company.* Washington, DC: US Department of the Army; 2002. Field Manual 4-02.6.
31. Lynn DC, Lesemann RK, Detro JF, and Seery JM. Employment of the "Role 2-plus": lessons learned in a time of high OPTEMPO [operational tempo]. *Mil Med.* 2014;179:1412-8.
32. US Department of Defense. *Emergency War Surgery*, Fourth United States Revision. Fort Sam Houston, Tex: Borden Institute; 2013.
33. Rob C. Some experiences with a parachute surgical unit. *J Royal Army Med Corps.* 1944;165.
34. COL(R) Harry Warren, MD (former chief of orthopedics at Womack Army Medical Center, commander of the 82nd surgical squad, and initial commander of the 101st surgical squad and 2nd Armored Calvary Regiment FST); personal interviews, October–November 2014.
35. Rush RM, Stockmaster NR, Stinger HK, et al. Supporting the "Global War on Terror": a tale of two campaigns featuring the 250th Forward Surgical Team (Airborne). *Am J Surg.* 2004;189:564–570.
36. US Northern Command Office of History. *A Short History of United States Northern Command as of 31 December 2012.* Colorado Springs, Colo: Peterson Air Force Base, US Northern Command Office of History; 2013.
37. US Department of Defense Joint Task Force Civil Support. *Commander Joint Task Force-Civil Support (CJTFCS) Operational Plan (OPLAN) 3500-11.* Fort Eustis, Va; JTFCS; 30 September 2011.
38. Mathis JW. *Joint Task Force Civil Support Defense CBRN Response Force (DCRF) Employment Concept*, Version 3.0. Fort Eustis, Va; JTFCS; 1 June 2013.
39. Wombell JA. *Army Support During the Hurricane Katrina Disaster.* Fort Levanworth, Kans: US Army Combined Arms Center Studies Institute Press; 2012.
40. COL Shawn C. Nessen, DO, FACS (Deputy Commander for Clinical Services, Landstuhl Regional Medical Center, Germany, and former Commander, 782nd Forward Surgical Team, Fort Bragg, NC); telephone interview, 29 May 2013.
41. Kochems A. Military support to civilian authorities: an assessment of the response to Hurricane Katrina. The Heritage Foundation website. 28 November 2005. http://www.heritage.org/research/reports/2005/11/military-support-to-civilian-authorities-an-assessment-of-the-response-to-hurricane-katrina. Accessed 7 December 2015.
42. US Government Accountability Office. *Hurricane Katrina: Better Plans and Exercises Needed to Guide the Military's Response to Catastrophic Natural Disasters.* Washington, DC: US Government Accountability Office; May 2006.
43. James P Brown (Plans and Mobilization Specialist, Womack Army Medical Center, Ft. Bragg, NC; former Noncommissioned Officer in Charge, Plans and Operations, 43rd Aeromedical Evacuation Squadron, Pope AFB; former Theater Aero Medical Evacuation Planner, Forward, Task Force Tarawa, Operation Iraqi Freedom, Iraq; and former Assistant Noncommissioned Officer in Charge, Mobile Aero Medical Staging Facility, Camp Rhino and Khandahar, Operation Enduring Freedom, Afghanistan); personal interview, 30 May 2013.
44. US Geological Survey. Magnitude 7.6–Pakistan. 2005 October. http://earthquake.usgs.gov/earthquakes/eqinthenews/2005/usdyae. Accessed 7 December 2015.
45. US Department of Defense. 240th Forward Surgical Team, Fort Stewart, Georgia. http://www.defense.gov/News/NewsArticle.aspx?ID=18045. Accessed 19 October 2013.

46. COL James D Frizzi, MD, FACS (Chief, Department of Surgery, Dwight D Eisenhower Army Medical Center, Fort Gordon, GA, and general surgeon formerly assigned to 240th Forward Surgical Team during Operation Lifeline, Pakistan); personal interview, 19 October 2013.
47. Montgomery N. 212th MASH unit treats stoic Pakistanis. *Stars and Stripes*. 3 November 2005. http://www.stripes.com/news/212th-mash-unit-treats-stoic-pakistanis-1.40552. Accessed 7 December 2015.
48. Army News Service. Soldiers honored for Pakistan earthquake relief. 13 October 2006. http://www.army.mil/article/324/Soldiers_honored_for_Pakistan_earthquake_relief. Accessed 7 December 2015.
49. Wiseman P. Mission to quake-ravaged Kashmir is farewell for MASH. *USA Today*. http://usatoday30.usatoday.com/news/world/2006-02-15-mash-farewell_x.htm. 15 February 2006. Accessed 7 December 2015.
50. Defense Procurement and Acquisition Agency. Emergency acquisitions. http://www.acq.osd.mil/dpap/ccap/cc/jcchb/Files/Topical/Emergency_Acquisitions/resources/Pakistan_Relief_Ops_2010.pdf. Accessed 19 October 2013.
51. Fraser DM. *Posture Statement of General Douglas M Fraser, US Air Force, Commander, US Southern Command, Before the 112th Congress, Senate Armed Services Committee*. 6 March 2012. https://www.dtic.mil/DTICOnline/downloadPdf.search?collectionId=tr&docId=ADA. Accessed 5 May 2016.
52. COL Richard W Ellison, MD, FACS (Former Chief, Department of Surgery, Womack Army Medical Center, Fort Bragg, NC; former surgeon, XVIII Airborne Corps during Operation Unified Response, Haiti; and former Commander, 759th Forward Surgical Team, Fort Bragg, NC); personal interview, 28 May 2013.
53. Auerbach PS, Norris RL, Mennon AS, et al. Civil–military collaboration in the initial medical response to the earthquake in Haiti. *N Engl J Med*. 2010;362:e32.
54. Pueschel M. Civil–military medical response to Haiti earthquake may be viewed as model for disaster relief. http://intlhealth.dhhq.health.mil/newsID135.mil.aspx. US Department of Defense Force Health Protection & Readiness website. Accessed 7 December 2015.
55. Beadling CW. Director's statement. US Department of Defense Center for Disaster and Humanitarian Assistance Medicine website. http://www.cdham.org/directors-statement. Accessed 29 July 2013.
56. US Department of Defense. *Military Support for Stability, Security, Transition, and Reconstruction (SSTR) Operations*. Washington, DC: US Department of Defense; 16 September 2009. US Department of Defense Instruction 3000.05.
57. Miller B. Partnership building takes center stage at Natural Fire 2011. US Africa Command website. http://www.africom.mil/Newsroom/Article/8583/partnership-building-takes-center-stage-at-natural. Accessed 7 December 2015.
58. Schultz C. Natural Fire 10 medical clinic a success. *Warrior-Citizen*. 2010;55:1.
59. Woll M, Brisson P. Humanitarian care by a forward surgical team in Afghanistan. *Mil Med*. 2013;178(4):385–388.
60. Lynn DC, De Lorenzo RA. Advising and assisting an Iraqi Army medical clinic: observations of a US military support mission. *Mil Med*. 2011;176(9):998–1002.
61. US Southern Command. Joint Task Force-Bravo. http://www.jtfb.southcom.mil/. Accessed 7 December 2015.
62. CPT Chris Parker (Director, Medical Operations, Joint Task Force-Bravo, Soto Cano Air Base, Republic of Honduras); telephone interview, 28 June 2013.

63. Dr Dominic LP Storto, DO (former general surgeon, Womack Army Medical Center, Fort Bragg, NC, and former general surgeon assigned to Joint Task Force-Bravo, Soto Cano Air Base, Republic of Honduras); telephone interview, 29 June 2013.
64. CPT Ricardo Aviles, MD (Medical Officer, Medical Element, Joint Task Force-Bravo, Soto Cano Air Base, Republic of Honduras); email, 3 July 2013.
65. Miguel A Coello, MD (Medical Officer, Medical Element, Joint Task Force-Bravo, Soto Cano Air Base, Republic of Honduras); email, 4 July 2013.
66. Malish R, Oliver DE, Rush RM, et al. Potential roles for military-specific response to natural disasters—analysis of the rapid deployment of a mobile surgical team to the 2007 Peruvian earthquake. *Prehospital Disast Med.* 2009;24(1):3–8.
67. Sigmon MJ. *External After Action Review–Medical Element (MEDEL) Response to 15 August 2007 Earthquake in Pisco, Peru.* Soto Cano Air Base, Honduras: Headquarters, Medical Element, Joint Task Force–Bravo; 24 August 2007.
68. LTC Francis Cannizzo Jr, MD, PhD, FACS (Co A, 405th Combat Surgical Hospital; Medical/Surgical Lead, Kuwait University Health Network; International Consultant, Surgical Oncology, Kuwait Cancer Control Center; Adjunct Professor of Surgery and International Medicine, University of Toronto; and surgeon assigned to USNS *Mercy*, Operation Pacific Partnership); telephone interview, 5 June 2013.
69. Kremer V. USNS *Comfort* to support Continuing Promise. American Forces Press Service. 18 March 2011. http://www.defense.gov/News/NewsArticle.aspx?ID=63210. Accessed 29 July 2013.
70. Miles D. USNS *Mercy* heads home from pacific partnership mission. American Forces Press Service. 13 September 2012. http://www.defense.gov/news/newsarticle.aspx?id=117839. Accessed 29 July 2013.
71. Remick KN. The surgical resuscitation team: surgical trauma support for US Army Special Operations Forces. *J Spec Ops Med.* 2009;9:4.
72. Vanfosson CA, Seery JM. Simultaneous surgeries in a split forward surgical team: a case study. *Mil Med.* 2011;176(12):1447.
73. *Medical Team, Forward Resuscitative and Surgical (FRST), Force Design Update (FDU).* Fort Sam Houston, Tex: Army Medical Department; 2013.
74. Peleg K, Jaffe DH. Are injuries from terror and war similar? A comparison study of civilians and soldiers. *Ann Surg.* 2010;252:363–369.
75. Pereira BMT, Ryan ML, Olgilve MP. Predeployment mass casualty and clinical trauma training for US Army forward surgical teams. *J Craniofac Surg.* 2010;21:982–986.
76. Thorson CM, Dubose JJ, Rhee P, et al. Military trauma training at civilian centers: a decade of advancements. *J Trauma Acute Care Surg.* 2012;73:S483–S489.
77. Sohn VY, Miller JP, Koeller CA, et al. From the combat medic to the forward surgical team: the Madigan model for improving trauma readiness of brigade combat teams fighting the Global War on Terror. *J Surg Res.* 2007;138:25–31.
78. MAJ Paul A. Brewer, MD (Commander and orthopedic surgeon, 758th Forward Surgical Team, Joint Base Lewis-McChord, WA, and Operation Enduring Freedom, Afghanistan); personal interview, 29 July 2013.

Acronyms and Abbreviations

AAJT	Abdominal Aortic Junctional Tourniquet
AAT	Abdominal Aortic Tourniquet
ABN	Airborne
ACR	Armored Cavalry Regiment
ADP	Army doctrine publication
ADRP	Army doctrine reference publication
AEF	Army Expeditionary Forces
AES	aeromedical evacuation squadron
AFB	Air Force Base
AF-SOCCET	Air Force Special Operations Critical Care Evacuation Team
AF-SOST	Air Force Special Operations Surgical Team
AID	Agency for International Development
ALT	alanine aminotransferase
AMEDD	Army Medical Department
AMF	Afghan Militia Forces
ANA	Afghan National Army
ARDS	acute respiratory distress syndrome
ARFORGEN	Armed Forces Generation
ARI	acute renal insufficiency
ARTEP	Army Training Evaluation Program
ASC	advanced surgical center
ASMC	area support medical company
AST	aspartate aminotransferase
ATP	Army techniques publication
ATTC	Army Trauma Training Center
AWT	Army Warrior Tasks
BAMC	Brooke Army Medical Center
BAS	battalion aid station
BCT	brigade combat team
BCT3	Brigade Combat Team Trauma Training
BEF	British Expeditionary Force
BG	brigadier general
BMM	borrowed military manpower

BSMC	brigade support medical company
CAT	combat application tourniquet
CATS	Combined Arms Training Strategy
CBI	China-Burma-India
CBRN	chemical, biological, radiological, and nuclear
CBRNE	chemical, biological, radiological, nuclear, and explosives
CCATT	Critical Care Air Transport Team
CCP	casualty collection point
CCS	casualty clearing station
CENTCOM	Central Command
CERTX	certifying training exercise
CESC	Combat Extremity Surgery Course
CJSOTF-A	Combined Joint Special Operations Task Force-Afghanistan
CJSOTF-North	Combined Joint Special Operations Task Force-North
CJSOTF-South	Combined Joint Special Operations Task Force-South
CMF	Contingency Medical Force
CND	Council on National Defense
CNS	central nervous system
COIN	counterinsurgency operations
COL	colonel
CONUS	continental United States
COS	Contingency Operating Station
CPG	Clinical Practice Guideline
CPT	captain
CRASH 2	Clinical Randomization of an Antifibrinolytic in Significant Hemorrhage 2
CRTS	Casualty Receiving and Treatment Ship
CSH	combat support hospital
C-STARS	Center for the Sustainment of Trauma and Readiness Skills
CT	computed tomography
CTE	culminating training event
CTSC	Combat Trauma Surgical Committee
CTT	Common Task Training
CWCP	Civilian War Casualty Program
DCR	damage control resuscitation
DCRF	Defense CBRN Response Force
DDS	4-4-diaminodiphenylsulfone
DEPMEDS	deployable medical systems
DIC	disseminated intravascular coagulopathy
DoD	Department of Defense
DOW	died of wounds
DRB	Defense Readiness Brigade
EMEDS	Expeditionary Medical Support

ETO	European Theater of Operations
FAST	Forward Airborne Surgical Team
FEMA	Federal Emergency Management Agency
FM	field manual
FST	forward surgical team
GEN	general
GMC	General Motors Corporation
GRF	Global Response Force
HMMWV	high-mobility multipurpose wheeled vehicle
IV	intravenous
JCCP	joint casualty collection point
JTF-B	Joint Task Force-Bravo
KIA	killed in action
LDH	lactate dehydrogenase
LTC	lieutenant colonel
LTG	lieutenant general
LST	landing ship, tank
LTG	lieutenant general
MA	mobile Army
MACV	Military Assistance Command, Vietnam
MAJ	major
MASF	mobile aeromedical staging facility
MASH	mobile Army surgical hospital
MAST	Military Assistance to Safety in Traffic
MEDCAP	Medical Civic Action Program
MFSS	Medical Field Service School
MG	major general
MILPHAP	Military Provincial Health Assistance Program
MST	mobile surgical team
MUST	medical unit self-contained transportable
NATO	North Atlantic Treaty Organization
NCO	noncommissioned officer
NGO	nongovernmental organization
NRC	National Research Council
NVA	North Vietnamese Army
POW	prisoner of war
PROFIS	Professional Filler System
PSH	portable surgical hospital
RA	Regular Army
RAMC	Royal Army Medical Corps
RVN	Republic of Vietnam
SGOT	serum glutamic-oxaloacetic transaminase
SGPT	serum glutamic-pyruvic transaminase

STEPPS	Team Strategies and Tools to Enhance Performance and Patient Safety
TB	technical bulletin
TBA	Table of Basic Allowance
TDA	Table of Distribution and Allowances
TO&E	Table of Organization and Equipment
UN	United Nations
USARV	US Army, Republic of Vietnam
USNORTHCOM	US Northern Command
USSOUTHCOM	US Southern Command
VE	Victory in Europe
WIA	wounded in action
WRAIR	Walter Reed Army Institute of Research

Index

A
Adams, John, 34
Adams, John Quincy, 46
Adams-Onis Treaty of 1819, 46
Advanced surgical center, 221
AEF. *See* American Expeditionary Forces
Aerosol antibiotics, 313
Afghanistan, 357–370
Agency for International Development, 307
Agramonte, Dr Aristides, 126
AHLTA. *See* Armed Forces Health Longitudinal Technology Application
Ainsworth, Dr Fred, 119–120, 122
Airborne forward surgical teams, 333, 359–363, 378–381
AK-47 rifles, 12
AK-74 rifles, 12
Albumin, 130
Albumin volume
burn care, 383–384
Alcohol
    abuse of, 53
    medical use in Civil War, 93, 97
    spirits as anesthesia, 54
Allgood, Lieutenant Colonel Brian, 414
Allopathic physicians, 93
Alpha echelon, 433, 434
Ambulance Americaine, 149–152
Ambulance Corps, 77, 80–82, 84, 87–88, 93
Ambulance Corps Act, 77
Ambulances
    Ambulance Corps, 77, 80–82, 87–88
    ambulance trains, 83, 93–94
    Confederate Ambulance Corps, 91
    Korean War, 280
    Letterman ambulance, 77, 80–81, 93, 132–133
    World War I, 155, 161–162
American Ambulance, 149–152

American Ambulance Field Service, 149
American Continental Army, 4–5
American Expeditionary Forces, 116–117, 144
American Hospital, 149
American Hospital Board, 149
American Northern Army, 7–8
American Pharmaceutical Association, 43
American Red Cross, 151, 159
American Volunteer Motor-Ambulance Corps, 149
Amputations
    during Civil War, 83, 84–85
    frostbite, 122
Anaconda Plan, 66
Anderson, Major Robert, 66
Andrew, A Piatt, 149
Anesthesia
    alcohol spirits, 54
    chloroform, 54
    Civil War era, 97–98
    equipment, 402
    ether, 53–54
    sulfuric ether, 54
    World War II advances, 224–228
Anti-Comintern Pact, 174
Antibiotics
    aerosol, 313
    sulfa drugs, 231
    use during Vietnam War, 310–312
Antietam, Battle of, 67–68
Antiseptics, 98, 128–129, 150, 153
Apel, Dr Otto F, Jr, 252, 263, 269, 282
Apothecaries Act, 43
Apothecary General, 42–43, 45, 46
Apprenticeships, 54
Area support medical companies, 435, 437
Armed Forces Health Longitudinal Technology Application, 406
Armen, Major Scott, 445

Armstrong, John, Jr, 36, 37, 40
Armstrong, Surgeon General George F, 250, 260
Army Medical Department
    adaptation of civilian advances, 130–131
    challenges and new technology during
        Spanish-American War, 131–135
    establishment of, 45
    during the Indian Wars, 46–47
    involvement outside medicine, 61
    Medical and Surgical History of the War of
        the Rebellion, 1861-1865, 108
    start of World War II, 175
    status after War of 1812, 45–46
    World War I medical assets, 153–161
Army Medical Service Graduate School, 269, 277
Army of the West, 57
Army Role 2 surgical unit, 356
Army Specialized Training Program, 176
Army techniques publications, 408
Army Training Evaluation Program, 407–408
Army Trauma Training Course, 413
Arnold, General Benedict, 5, 9
ARTEP. *See* Army Training Evaluation Program
Artillery, 102, 165
Artz, Major Curtis P, 277, 280
ASMCs. *See* Area support medical companies
Astor, John Jacob, 37
Atlanta Campaign, 68
Autenrieth Wagon, 95
Auto-chir, 152, 155
Auxiliary surgical groups, 205–207

B
Bacon, Robert, 149
Baetjer, Frederick Henry, 135
Baker, Major Janice L, 390
Balfour, Lord Arthur, 151
Balkan Wars, 142
Baltimore Shock Trauma Center, 410
Bandages, 98
Barnes, Surgeon General Joseph K, 89, 108,
    110–111, 129
Barton, Clara, 99
Base hospitals, 159–161, 162–164
Bataan Death March, 180
Battalion aid stations, 154
Battle of Little Bighorn, 122
Battlefield Health and Trauma Research Institute, 405
Battlefield surgery
    amputations, 83, 84–85
    during Civil War, 69–70

Baxter, Surgeon General Jedediah, 112
Beadling, Colonel Charles, 443
Beaumont, Dr William, 37–38, 51–53
Becker, Major Tyson, 371
Becker, Surgeon General Quinn H, 349
Beecher, Henry, 224, 226
Beitler, Colonel Alan L, 366
Belgium
    World War II battles, 212–215
Bell, Alexander Graham, 129
Bell H-13 helicopters, 247, 295
Bellamy, Colonel Ronald F, 331, 397
Bellows, Henry W, 72
Bickerdyke, Mary A, 99
Billings, Dr John Shaw, 61, 104
Bini, Major John K, 395
Bischoff, Second Lieutenant Kristy, 441
Bishop, Maurice, 325
Black Hawk War, 46–47
Blackbourne, Colonel Lorne, 390
Blackwell, Dr Elizabeth, 99
Blair, Major Kelly, 437
Blanck, Surgeon General Ronald R, 350
Blease, Lieutenant Colonel Robert, 388
Bliss, Surgeon General Raymond W, 244
Blood collection equipment, 402
Blood products, 399–400
Blood program, 308–309
Blood transfusions
    Vietnam War, 308–309
    World War I, 168–169
    World War II, 227–228
Blue Spoon plan, 335
Boerhaave, Hermann, 14–15
Bone fractures, 54
Bosnia and Herzegovina, 347
Boston, Massachusetts, 2
Boston Tea Party, 2
Boxer Rebellion, 128
Boyer, First Lieutenant Matthew, 445
Brady, Major Patrick, 300
Bragg, General Braxton, 59, 102–103
Brandywine, Battle of, 8, 21
Brannon, Lieutenant Colonel Robert, 336
Bravo echelon, 433, 434
Breech-loading rifles, 100–101
Brevet ranks, 109
Brigade Surgeons Course, 414–415
Brinton, Dr John, 99
British Expeditionary Force, 188
British Medical Service, 12–14
Brock, General Sir Issac, 36, 38

Brodie, Alexander, 118
Brown, Major Lorrie, 430–431
Buckner, Lieutenant General Simon, 69
Bull Run, First Battle of, 67, 70
Buna Campaign, 196–199
Burgoyne, General John, 7–8
Burlingame, Major Brian S, 359
Burma
    China-Burma-India Theater, 182–184
    use of portable surgical hospitals, 199–200
Burn Center, 413
Burn treatment, 231–232, 313
Burns, Staff Sergeant Robert, 379
Burnside, Major General Ambrose, 82
Burr, Aaron, 29
Bush, George HW, 335

C
C-STARS. *See* Centers for the Sustainment of Trauma and Readiness Skills
Calomel, 43
Camp Adder, 383, 384
Camp Furlong, New Mexico, 136
Campbell, Dr Eldridge, 266–267
Canada. *See also* War of 1812
    Revolutionary War battle, 5
Canestrini, Lieutenant Colonel Ken, 376
Cannons, 102
Carlsson, Captain Glen, 379
Carranza, Venustiano, 136
Carrel, Dr Alexis, 150
Carrel-Dakin solution, 150, 153
Carroll, Colonel Percy J, 193
Carroll, Dr James, 126
Carroll, Lieutenant Colonel Francis L, 260
Casualty clearing stations, 152–153
Casualty collection points, 327
Casualty rates
    Civil War, 71, 90, 107
    Revolutionary War, 11
    Vietnam War, 288
    World War I, 141
    World War II, 173, 180, 181
Casualty receiving and treatment ship, 357
Caventou, Joseph, 43, 44
CBI. *See* China-Burma-India Theater
CBRN. *See* Chemical, biological, radiological, and nuclear response force
CCATTs. *See* Critical care air transport teams
CCP. *See* Casualty collection points
CCS. *See* Casualty clearing stations
Center and School Capabilities Development Integration Directorate, 450
Center and School Lessons Learned Division, 450
Center for Disaster and Humanitarian Assistance Medicine, 443
Centers for the Sustainment of Trauma and Readiness Skills, 410
Central Blood Bank, 308–309
Central Highlands description, 285
Central Lowlands description, 285–286
Chancellorsville, Battle of, 68
Charlie Med, 434
Chattanooga Campaign, 68
Chemical, biological, radiological, and nuclear response force, 435–438
Chennault, Claire, 186
Chiang Kai-shek, 186
Chickamauga, Battle of, 68, 102
China
    Boxer Rebellion, 128
China-Burma-India Theater, 182–184
Chindits, 182
Chloroform, 54, 97
Choi, Major Young, 365
Cholera, 44, 46–47, 53, 109–110
Chotek, Sophie, 142
Chovanes, Major John, 395
Church, Dr Benjamin, 17–18
Churchill, Colonel Edward D, 228
Churchill, Winston, 174
Civil War
    Ambulance Corps, 77, 80–82, 84, 87–88, 93
    anesthesia, 97–98
    battlefield amputations, 83, 84–85
    casualty rates, 71, 90, 107
    Confederate Ambulance Corps, 91
    Confederate Medical Services, 89–92
    contributions of Jonathan Letterman, 77–82, 83, 84, 86–88
    diet, 92
    end of, 103
    events leading up to war, 65–66
    female nurses and physicians, 98–100
    hospitals, 73, 87, 91, 95–96
    importance to military medicine, 71–82
    inexperience of soldiers and surgeons, 70–71
    introduction of female nurses and physicians, 98–100
    Letterman ambulance, 77, 80–81
    main battles of, 66–69
    medical care advances, 95–100

medical care at Battle of Gettysburg, 83–88
medical evacuation, 93–95
medical outcomes, 103–104
medications, 92–93
mortality rate in prisoner-of-war hospitals, 90
post-war developments, 108–110
post-war international issues, 107–108
railroad hospitals, 93–94
Sanitary Commission, 72–74, 82
status of medical care prior to war, 61
surgeons and their training, 75–76
Surgeons General during post-war period, 110–117
Surgeons General during war, 88–89
surgery, 69–70, 98
vaccinations, 92
volunteer units, 107
weapons, 100–102
wounds and diseases, 95–97, 100–102
Civilian War Casualty Program, 306, 307
CJSOFT-A. See Combined Joint Special Operations Task Force-Afghanistan
Clark, General Mark C, 188–189, 215, 259
Clark, Maurine, 271
Clay, Henry, 55, 66
Claymore mines, 315
Cleveland, Grover, 130–131
CND. See Council on National Defense
Cochran, Dr John, 12, 23
Cockburn, Admiral George, 39, 40
Codeine, 44
Coercive Acts, 1–2
Collins, Major General Glenn J, 306
Combat application tourniquets, 398
Combat Extremity Surgery Course, 413
Combat Gauze, 399
Combat Ready Clamp, 399
Combat support hospitals
    Afghanistan, 365–367
    Iraq, 376–378
Combat Trauma Surgical Committee, 410
Combined Joint Special Operations Task Force-Afghanistan, 359, 364
Combined Joint Task Force 120, 326
Comintern, 174
Commanders Course, 414
Committee on Tactical Combat Casualty Care, 398, 400, 406
Common Task Training, 407
Company aid stations, 154
Compromise of 1850, 66

Concord, Massachusetts, 2
Confederate Ambulance Corps, 91
Confederate Medical Services, 89–92
Confederate States of America, 71
Connolly, Lieutenant Colonel Maurice R, 255
Constitutional Convention, 28
Continental Army
    creation of, 4–5
    Medical Department, 11
    organization of medical departments, 15–17
Continental Congress, 4
Continental Line, 2
Contingency Operation Base Basrah, 384
Contingency Operation Station Gary Owen, 382–383
Contingency operations
    foreign operations, 443–448
    foreign surgical elements, 448–449
    future directions, 449–452
    Global Response Force, 431–435
    Hurricane Katrina, 435–440
    Operation Lifeline, 440–441
    Operation Nobel Eagle, 430–431
    Operation Unified Response, 442–443
    roles of military medical care, 432
    Task Force 212, 440–441
Convalescent facilities, 307
Corbusier, Dr William Henry, 75, 76, 93, 101, 104, 109, 117
Cornell, Colonel WS, 264, 266
Cornwallis, General Charles, 6, 10
Corps of Invalids, 26
Council on National Defense, 151
Counihan, Colonel Timothy, 382
Coviello, Major Lisa, 446
Cowpens, Battle of, 10
Crain, Corporal Bob, 257
Crandall, Major Albert, 207–208
Crane, Surgeon General Charles H, 111
Creek Indians, 41, 46, 47
Crile, Brigadier General George, 146–148, 150, 162, 163, 166
Critical care air transport teams, 357
Crook, Captain Samuel L, 252
Crook, General George, 120
CRTS. See Casualty receiving and treatment ship
CSA. See Confederate States of America
CSH. See Combat support hospitals
Cuba
    tropical diseases and sanitation problems, 125–126

Cubano, Captain Miguel, 443
Cullen, Dr John, 12
Cullen, Dr William, 15, 21
Cushing, Dr Harvey, 134–135, 145–147, 150–151, 158, 162–163, 166
Cutler, Brigadier General Elliott C, 232, 233, 291
CWCP. See Civilian War Casualty Program

D
Dade, Major Francis, 47
Dakin-Carrel solution, 150, 153
Damage control resuscitation, 399–400
Damage control surgery, 402
Davis, First Lieutenant Frank, 208, 209
Davis, Jefferson, 120–121
DCRF. See Defense CBRN Response Force
DD form, 4–6
Dearborn, Major General Henry, 36–37
Debridement, 307–308
Declaration of Independence, 4
Defense Appropriations Act of 1916, 151–152
Defense Casualty Analysis System, 11
Defense CBRN Response Force, 435–438
Defense Medical Readiness Training Institute, 412
Defense Readiness Brigade, 378
DeLaney, First Lieutenant RE, 261
Deleon, Dr David C, 72, 90
Delvigne, Captain Henri-Gustave, 100
Democratic Republicans, 34
Dengue fever, 44
Dennis, Dr Frank M, 94
Deployable medical systems, 343
DEPMEDS. See Deployable medical systems
Detro, Major John, 436
Devine, Major John, 379
Dewey, Brigadier General Lawerence E, 260
Diet, Civil War soldiers, 92
Disseminated intravascular coagulopathy, 310
Division Readiness Brigade, 431
Division Surgeons Course, 414
Dix, Dorothea, 99
Dodge Commission, 125
Dogs, military working, 389–391
Dominguez, Colonel Marie, 446, 448
Doniphan, Colonel Alexander, 56, 57–58
Dovell, Colonel Chauncey E, 245
Dover's powder, 43
Doyle, Chaplain Thomas L, 265
Dressing stations, 154–155
Dressings, 98
Dust off helicopters, 289, 300
Dysentery treatments, 43

E
Eagle Dust Off units, 291
Earthquake response, 128, 440–443, 446–448
Eaton, John, 46
Eichelberger, Major General Robert, 198
Eiseman, Dr Ben, 291
Eisenberg, Captain Louis, 274, 280
Eisenhower, General Dwight D, 188, 190
Ellison, Colonel Richard, 443
Embedded unexploded ordnances, 392–397
EMEDS. See Expeditionary medical support teams
Emergency War Surgery Course, 412
EOD. See Explosive ordnance disposal
Ether anesthesia, 53, 97
European Continent operations, 190–191
Eustis, William, 36
Evacuation. See Medical evacuation
Evacuation hospitals
    World War I, 155, 159–161
    World War II, 203–205
Everett, Josiah, 46, 47
Ewing, Captain Charles B, 123
Exercise Tiger, 210–211
Expeditionary medical support teams, 357, 362
Explosive ordnance disposal, 392

F
Falklands War, 322–324
Fallen Timbers, Battle of, 29
Farpell, Airman First Class Peter J, 265
FAST. See Forward Airborne Surgical Teams
Federal Emergency Management Agency, 430, 437
Federalist Party, 34
FEMA. See Federal Emergency Management Agency
Fencibles, 36
Ferdinand, Archduke Franz, 142
Field hospitals
    World War I, 155, 159
    World War II, 201–202
Field medical card, 4–6
Fillmore, Millard, 59
Finley, Surgeon General Clement A, 59, 61, 73, 88, 166
First Battle of Ypres, 143
First Continental Congress, 4

First Seminole War, 46
Flak jackets, 312
Flint, Colonel JM, 156
Florey, Sir Howard, 231
Flying ambulances, 69
Ford Motor Company, 161–162
Fort Sumter, 67
Fort Ticonderoga, 7
Forward Airborne Surgical Teams, 333, 359–363, 378–381
Forward resuscitative surgical systems, 357, 375, 415
Forward surgical elements, 344, 356
Forward surgical teams
    advantages of, 321–322
    airborne, 333, 359–363, 378–381
    anesthesia equipment, 402
    blood collection equipment, 402
    blood products use, 399–400
    care for military working dogs, 389–391
    damage control resuscitation, 399–400
    damage control surgery, 402
    evolution of medical planning in the mid-1980s, 331–334
    Falklands War, 322–324
    formal establishment of, 347–348
    Global War on Terrorism and, 355–357
    hemostasis, 398–399
    hemostatic pharmacologics, 400
    hypothermia management, 401
    injured and fallen providers, 386–388
    Institute of Surgical Research, 404–405
    Joint Trauma System, 404–405
    medical evacuation, 402–404
    missions, 415–416
    Operation Enduring Freedom, 357–370
    Operation Iraqi Freedom, 370–385
    Operation Just Cause, 334–342
    Operation Urgent Fury, 324–331
    pain management, 401–402
    patient medical records, 405–406
    Persian Gulf War, 342–345
    radiography, 402
    Surgeons General contributions, 385–386
    tactical combat casualty care, 397–398
    training and readiness, 406–415
    transition to formal team designation, 345–348
    unexploded ordnance embedded in patients, 392–397
    US Army airborne teams and locations, 432

Forwood, Surgeon General William H, 114–115
Foust, Colonel Jerome, 335, 340
Fox, William F, 71
Fox Indians, 46
Fractures. *See* Bone fractures
France
    influence on Western medicine, 69
    Quasi-War with, 34
    triage system, 148
    World War I medical assets, 152
    World War II battles, 212–215
Fredendall, Major General Lloyd, 215
Fredericksburg Campaign, 82
Frontier Indian Wars, 120–123
Frostbite, 122
FRSS. *See* Forward resuscitative surgical systems
FSE. *See* Forward surgical elements
FST. *See* Forward surgical teams
FST Commanders Course, 414
Fullerton, Sergeant First Class Luke, 379
Funston, Brigadier General Frederick, 128

G
Gallatin, Albert, 37
Garfield, James A, 129
Gas gangrene, 148
General Motors Corporation, 162
Gennari, Lieutenant Commander James, 396
Germ theory, 128–129
Germany
    Schlieffen Plan, 143
    Stosstruppen, 144
    World War II forward surgery, 220–221
Geronimo, 120–121
Gettysburg, Battle of, 68, 83–88
Ginn, Brigadier General L Holmes, Jr, 259–261
Girard, Captain Alfred C, 129
Girard, Stephen, 37
Glidewell, Captain Jennifer, 430–431
Global Response Force
Global Response Force mission, 378, 431–435
Global War on Terrorism
    injured and fallen forward surgical providers, 386–388
    Operation Enduring Freedom, 357–370
    Operation Iraqi Freedom, 370–385
    Surgeons General contributions, 385–386
    use of forward surgical teams, 355–357
Goldsworth, Specialist William, 379
Gorgas, Surgeon General William C, 115–116, 125, 135, 151, 162, 165
Grant, General Ulysses S, 69, 103, 120, 122

Great Britain. *See also* War of 1812
    British Medical Service, 12–14
    Royal Army Medical Corps, 151
    World War I medical assets, 152–153
    World War II forward surgery, 220–221
Great Sioux War of 1876 to 1877, 122
Greater East Asia Co-Prosperity Sphere, 182
Greenleaf, Colonel Charles, 123
Grenada invasion, 324–331
GRF. *See* Global Response Force
Griffiths, Colonel Harold, 308
Grindlay, Captain John, 184, 185
Groupe complimentaire, 152, 156
Guild, Dr Lafayette, 86
Gunshot wounds
    Civil War, 100–102
    World War I, 165
    World War II, 230
GWOT. *See* Global War on Terrorism

H
Haiti
    humanitarian assistance, 348
    Operation Unified Response, 442–443, 446–448
Hales ventilators, 26
Hall, Captain "Blinker," 136
Halsted, Dr William Stewart, 129–130, 145–146, 147
Hammond, Surgeon General William A, 73, 86, 87, 88–89, 104
Hampton Roads Conference, 108
Handguns, 101
Handy, Lieutenant Colonel Robert, 364
Hardin, John, 55
Harding, Major General Edwin, 196, 197
Harjes, H Herman, 149
Harris, Dr Elisha, 72
Harrison, Dr William Henry, 29
Hawkins, Captain Michael, 395
Hawley, Major General Paul R, 232
Hays, Surgeon General Silas B, 315–316
Head wounds, 168
Heaton, Surgeon General Leonard D, 292, 316
Helicopter Ambulance, 289
Helicopters
    air-evacuation system, 300
    Bell H-13 Sioux, 247, 295
    dust off helicopters, 289
    Jungle Canopy Platform System, 298
    Korean War, 247, 265, 273, 281
    Personal Rescue Hoist, 298
    Sikorsky H-5, 265, 295
    Sikorsky H-19, 273, 281
    UH-1, 289, 296, 298, 305
    Vietnam War, 289, 295–296, 298–300, 302, 305
Helmick, Lieutenant General Frank, 382
Hely, Captain Joseph W, 247
Hemostasis technology, 398–399
Hemostatic pharmacologics, 400
Hessian troops, 6–7
Hetz, Colonel Stephen P, 395
High-velocity projectile wounds, 314–315
Highly mobile military wheeled vehicles, 379
Hills, Dr Henry M, 213
HMMWVs. *See* Highly mobile military wheeled vehicles
Ho Chi Minh, 286–287
Holmes, Dr Oliver Wendell, 93
Homeland Defense
    future directions, 449–452
    Operation Nobel Eagle, 430–431
    US Northern Command, 435–438
Homeopathic physicians, 93
Honoré, Lieutenant General Russel, 438
Hopkins, Opie, 99
Hornberger, Dr Richard, 245–246
Horoho, Surgeon General Patricia D, 386
Horwitz, Dr Mel, 261, 263–264
Hospital Corps, 110, 123
Hospital ships, 94–95
Hospitals
    Ambulance Americaine, 149–152
    base hospitals, 159–161, 162–164
    Civil War, 73, 87, 91, 95–96
    evacuation hospitals, 155, 159–161, 203–205
    field hospitals, 155, 159, 201–202
    full-sized surgical hospitals in combat environments, 191
    hospital ships, 94–95
    Medical Unit, Self-Contained, Transportable units, 289–297
    mobile hospitals, 155–158, 232
    portable surgical hospitals, 191–201, 202–203, 232
    railroad hospitals, 93–94, 150
    Revolutionary War, 15–17
    Spanish-American War, 127, 132
    Sternberg Hospital, 127, 132
    World War I, 162–164
Howard, Captain, 261
Howard Air Force Base, 336–337, 339

Howe, General Sir William, 5–6
Huerta, Victoriano, 136
Hueys, 289, 296, 298, 305
Hull, Brigadier General William, 36
Hunnewell, HH, 119
Hunter, Dr John, 12, 13, 22, 27
Hunter, Dr William, 12, 22
Hurricane Katrina, 435–440
Hussein, Saddam, 342–343
Hypothermia management, 401

I
Ideus, Colonel Eldon, 344
India
    China-Burma-India Theater, 182–184
Indian Confederacy, 38
Indian conflicts, 29
Indian Removal Act, 46
Indian Wars
    Battle at Wounded Knee, 123
    Battle of Little Bighorn, 122
    Black Hawk War, 46–47
    First Seminole War, 46
    Great Sioux War of 1876 to 1877, 122
    Red River War, 122
    Second Seminole War, 47
    Third Seminole War, 47
    Wood's role, 120–123
Influenza
    World War I pandemic, 166–167
Institute of Surgical Research, 404–405, 413
Internists
    assignment to Vietnam, 306–307
Intolerable Acts, 1–2
Ipecac, 93
Iraq, 342–345
Ireland, Surgeon General Meritte, 116–117, 165–166
ISR. See Institute of Surgical Research
Italy
    World War II battles, 188–190

J
Jackson, Andrew, 38, 41, 46
Jackson, Colonel Joseph, 326–327, 329, 331
Janney, Captain Steve, 333
Jay Treaty, 34
JCCP. See Joint casualty collection points
Jennings, Surgeon General Hal B, 316
Johns Hopkins School of Medicine, 129–130
Joint casualty collection points, 336–339
Joint En-route Care Course, 404

Joint Operations Access Exercise, 433–435
Joint Task Force-Bravo, 446–447
Joint Task Force South, 335, 339–340
Joint Theater Trauma System, 405
Joint Trauma System, 404–405
Jones, Dr John, 17
Jones, Dr Joseph, 90
JTS. See Joint Trauma System
JTTS. See Joint Theater Trauma System
Junctional Emergency Treatment Tool, 399
Jungle Canopy Platform System, 298

K
Kasserine Withdrawal, 215
Kean, Colonel Jefferson, 155
Kean, Dr William W, 104
Kearny, General Stephen, 56, 57
Keller, Colonel William, 166
Kelly, Major Charles, 289
Kembro, Major Ronald, 384
Kennedy, John F, 289
Kerr, Robert E, 47
Kesselring, Field Marshal Albert, 189
Kiley, Surgeon General Kevin C, 385
King, Benjamin, 48
King George III, 2, 4
Kirk, Surgeon General Norman T, 223
Knisely, Major Tom, 441
Knox, Major General Henry, 28
Koch, Robert, 129
Korean War
    events leading up to war, 244–245
    Medical Field Service School, 243
    Mobile Army Surgical Hospitals, 239–242
    Mobile Army Surgical Hospitals, 1950, 245–249
    Mobile Army Surgical Hospitals, 1951, 249–259
    Mobile Army Surgical Hospitals, 1952, 259–272
    Mobile Army Surgical Hospitals, 1953, 272–276
    Renal Insufficiency Team, 276
    Surgical Research Teams, 276–282
Kosovo, 347

L
Ladies Aid Society, 99
Lafitte, Jean, 41
Lakota Indians, 123
LaNoue, Surgeon General Alcide M, 350
Larrey, Dr Dominque Jean, 42, 69

Laux, Captain Suzan, 371
Lava Bed Wars, 122
Lawson, Surgeon General Thomas, 48, 50, 53, 58, 60, 61, 71, 88
Lawton, Captain Henry, 121, 122, 125
Lazear, Dr Jesse, 126
Lead poisoning, 53
League of Nations, 145
Ledford, Surgeon General Frank F, Jr, 349–350
Lee, General Robert E, 59, 69, 79, 83, 103
Leedham, Colonel Charles L, 282
Lend-Lease Program, 190, 194
Letterman, Dr Jonathan, 77–82, 83, 84, 86–88
Letterman ambulance, 77, 80–81, 93, 132–133
Lexington, Massachusetts, 2
Lincoln, Abraham, 55, 66, 67, 74, 108
Lincoln, Major General Benjamin, 9
Lister, Joseph, 128–129
Litters
    Civil War, 84
    Indian Wars, 54, 121
    Korean War, 247, 253, 254, 262, 265
    Spanish-American War, 134
    Vietnam War, 295–296, 298
    War of 1812, 39
    World War I, 154
    World War II, 192, 199, 208, 209, 221
The Louisiana Maneuvers, 176
Lounsbury, Colonel Dave E, 395
Lovell, Dr James, 37
Lovell, Surgeon General Joseph, 46, 48, 49
Lynn, Major David, 436

M

MacArthur, General Douglas, 179–180, 197–198
MacGregor, Major Jacob, 371
Macomb, Brigadier General Alexander, 40
Madero, Francisco, 136
Madison, James, 33, 34, 35, 40
Magee, Surgeon General James C, 222–223
Malaria
    during Revolutionary War, 25, 26
    during Spanish-American War, 132
    during Vietnam War, 307
    during War of 1812, 44
    during World War II, 180, 198
Malish, Major Richard, 379, 447
Mann, Dr James, 37
Marine Corps Role 2 surgical unit, 357
Market-Garden Operation, 212
Marne, Battle of the, 143
Marshall, General George, 179–180

Marshall Islands, 200
Martin, Dr Jerry, 289, 293–294
MASF. *See* Mobile aeromedical staging facilities
MASH. *See* Mobile Army Surgical Hospitals
McAllister, Lieutenant Colonel Robert W, 364
McClellan, Major General George, 66, 67, 73, 77
McClimans, Captain Joshua M, 388
McCorey, Lieutenant Colonel Thomas, 374
McGowan, Colonel Frank, 200–201, 223–224, 227
McKee, Captain Willis P, 208, 210
McKinley, Ida Sexton, 123, 125
McKinley, William, 118, 123, 125
McParlin, Dr Thomas A, 87
MEDCAP. *See* Medical Civic Action Program
Medical and Surgical History of the War of the Rebellion, 1861-1865, 108
Medical Civic Action Program, 306
Medical Communications for Combat Casualty Care, 405
Medical Corps, 108
Medical Department. *See also* Army Medical Department
    Continental Army Medical Department, 4–5, 11, 15–17
    in the Indian Wars, 46–47
    status after War of 1812, 45–46
    Medical education
    apprenticeships, 54
    examination requirements, 54
    quality of education for Civil War surgeons, 75–76
Medical emergency response team, 404
Medical evacuation
    Afghanistan, 402–404
    Ambulance Corps, 77, 80–82, 87–88
    ambulance trains, 83, 93–94, 150
    Civil War, 84, 93–95
    Indian Wars, 54, 121–122
    Iraq, 402–404
    Korean War, 247, 253, 254, 265, 273, 281
    Letterman ambulance, 77, 80–81, 93
    Mexican-American War, 54
    Spanish-American War, 134
    Vietnam War, 289, 295–296, 298–302, 305
    War of 1812, 39
    World War I, 154, 169
    World War II, 192, 199, 208, 209, 221
Medical Field Service School, 176, 243, 264
Medical proficiency training program, 408–409

Medical records, 405–406
Medical Reengineering Initiative, 365
Medical Reserve Corps, 151
Medical Service Corps, 263
Medical Unit, Self-Contained, Transportable units, 289–297
Medications
    Civil War, 92–93
    War of 1812, 43–44
    World War II, 230–231
Mediterranean
    World War II battles, 215–216
Meiers, Lieutenant Junior Grade Bruce, 257
Mekong Delta, 285–286
Merrill, Brigadier General Frank D, 187–188
Merrill's Marauders, 187–188
MERT. *See* Medical emergency response team
Metabolic diseases, 309–310
Metcalf, Vice Admiral Joseph, III, 326
Mexican-American War
    anesthesia methods, 54–55
    Doniphan's success, 57–58
    events leading up to war, 55–56
    medical care during war, 59–61
    Missouri Volunteers, 57–58
    Scott's move toward Mexico City, 58–59
    start of, 55–56
    status of medical care prior to war, 53–54
    strategies and goals for, 56
    Taylor's forces, 56–57
    transportation of wounded, 54
    views concerning, 55
Meyer, Albert, 61
MFSS. *See* Medical Field Service School
MFST. *See* Mobile field surgical teams
Middle East, 342–345
Midway, Battle of, 180–181
Miketinac, Colonel Bruce T, 333
Miles, General Nelson A, 120–121, 122, 123
Military medical care roles, 432
Military Medical Manual, 192–193
Military Provincial Health Assistance Program, 306, 307
Military working dogs, 389–391
MILPHAP. *See* Military Provincial Health Assistance Program
Mines, Claymore, 315
Minié, Captain Claude-Etienne, 100
Minié ball rifles, 84, 85, 100, 101–102
Missouri Compromise of 1820, 66
Missouri Volunteers, 57–58
Mitchell, Dr S Weir, 103–104

Mittemeyer, Surgeon General Bernhard T, 348–349
Mobile aeromedical staging facilities, 339
Mobile Army Surgical Hospitals
    Iraq, 376
    Korean War, 1950, 245–249
    Korean War, 1951, 249–259
    Korean War, 1952, 259–272
    Korean War, 1953, 272–276
    in Middle East, 343–345
    Mobile Striking Force, 242
    moves by year, 239, 240
    nomenclature, 243
    numerical designations, 243
    in Panama, 338
    patient statistics by unit and year, 278–279
    replacement with MUST in Vietnam War, 291
    table of organization review, 242
    units during interwar years of 1948-1950, 241–242
    World War II, 202, 240–241
Mobile field surgical teams, 356
Mobile hospitals, 155–158, 191–203, 232
Mobile Striking Force, 242
Modoc Wars, 122
Molotov-Ribbentrop Pact, 173
Monmouth Court House, Battle of, 9–10
Monro, Major General David C, 232
Mons, Battle of, 143
Montgomery, General Richard, 5
Moore, Dr Samuel Preston, 72, 90–91
Moore, Surgeon General John, 112
Morgan, Dr John, 12, 18–19, 21
Morgan, General Daniel, 10
Morgan-Harjes *Ambulance Mobile de Premiers Secours*, 149
Morley-Fletcher, Sir Walter, 150–151
Morphine, 44
Moss, Private Channing, 394
Mothershead, Lieutenant Colonel John L, 252
Mudd, Dr Samuel, 109
Muench, Lieutenant Colonel Alan, 333, 344
Murray, Surgeon General Robert, 111, 129
MUST. *See* Medical Unit, Self-Contained, Transportable units
MWDs. *See* Military working dogs

N

Nashville, Battle of, 69
National Defense Authorization Act, 410
National Research Council, 151

Navigation Acts, 1–2
Navy Role 2 surgical unit, 357
Neel, Major General Spurgeon, 306
Nessen, Major Shawn, 395, 438
Neurosurgery, 168
New England Trade and Fisheries Act, 2
New Orleans, Battle of, 41
New Orleans Charity Hospital, 440
Nightingale, Florence, 70, 99
Non-Importation Act of 1811, 35
Noriega, Manuel, 334–335
Normandy Invasion, 211–212
North African Campaign, 188–190, 215
Northwest Ordnance of 1787, 66
Norton, Richard, 149
Novak, Sergeant First Class Robert, 379
NRC. *See* National Research Council
Nurses
    beginnings of nursing profession, 70
    Civil War, 98–100

O

Officer Reserve Corps, 151
Oh, Major John S, 394
O'Hara, Captain Donald H, 184
Olmsted, Frederick Law, 73
Onis, Luis de, 46
Operation Allied Force, 347
Operation Anaconda, 361
Operation Anvil, 212
Operation Big Switch, 274
Operation Continue Hope, 345–346
Operation Continuing Promise, 447
Operation Desert Shield, 342–345
Operation Desert Storm, 342–345
Operation Enduring Freedom
    48th Combat Support Hospital, 366–367
    339th Combat Support Hospital, 365–366
    250th Forward Surgical Team (Airborne), 362–363
    274th Forward Surgical Team (Airborne), 359–362
    102nd Forward Surgical Team, 364
    555th Forward Surgical Team, 365
    909th Forward Surgical Team, 364–365
    947th Forward Surgical Team, 364–365
    1980th Forward Surgical Team, 364
    implementation of military action, 357–359
    Role 2 and Role 3 expansion, 367–370
Operation Iraqi Freedom, 370–385
Operation Joint Endeavor, 347
Operation Joint Guardian, 347
Operation Just Cause, 334–342
Operation Lifeline, 440–441
Operation Little Switch, 274
Operation New Dawn, 382
Operation Nobel Eagle, 430–431
Operation Overlord, 205, 210–212
Operation Pacific Partnership, 447
Operation Promote Liberty, 339–340
Operation Restore Hope, 345–346
Operation Torch, 188, 215
Operation Unified Response, 442–443, 446–447
Operation Uphold Democracy, 348
Operation Urgent Fury, 324–331
Opium, 44
Orders-in-Council, 35
Ordinance of Secession, 66–67
O'Reilly, Surgeon General Robert M, 115
Osceola, 47
Osler, Second Lieutenant Edward Revere, 163
Osler, Sir William, 150–151, 163
Overlord Invasion, 205, 210–212

P

Pacific Theater, 178–182
Page, Colonel Thomas N, 249, 251, 253, 259, 260
Pain management, 401–402
Pakistan
    Operation Lifeline, 440–441
Panama invasion, 334–342
Parish, David, 37
Parker, Lieutenant John, 125
Pasteur, Louis, 129
Patch, Major General Alexander, 181
Patient medical records, 405–406
Patton, General George, 215
Peake, Surgeon General James B, 385, 414
Pearl Harbor attack, 174, 179
Pediatricians
    assignment to Vietnam, 306–307
Pellatier, Pierre, 43, 44
Pelvic Binder, 399
Penicillin, 231, 310
Peninsula Campaign, 77–80
Percy, Dr Pierre Francois, 69
Perez, Corporal Winder, 396
Perry, Commodore Oliver Hazard, 38
Pershing, Brigadier General John J, 136, 144, 165–166
Persian Gulf War, 342–345
Personal Rescue Hoist, 298

Petersburg, Battle of, 69
Petit, Jean Louis, 27
Phelan, Dr Henry du R, 128
Philippine Insurrection, 127–128
Philippines
    disease prevention efforts of Dr Leonard Wood, 126–128
    Philippine War, 127–128
    Sternberg Hospital, 127, 132
    use of portable surgical hospitals, 200–201
Pierce, Franklin, 61
Pistols, 101
Placket, Major Timothy, 384
Plastic surgery, 168, 231–232
Pneumonia
    during Civil War, 96
Polk, James K, 55–56
Portable surgical hospitals
    creation of, 191–193
    organization of, 193–195
    staffing of, 196
    table of organization and equipment, 195
    use during the Buna Campaign, 196–199
    use in Burma, 199–200
    use in New Guinea, 202–203
    use in the Pacific Islands, 200
Porter, Dr Henry, 119, 122
Porter, Lieutenant Colonel Clifford, 362
Posse Comitatus Act, 437
Post, Lieutenant Colonel James C, 366
Posttraumatic renal insufficiency, 312
Predeployment trauma training, 409–412
Prevost, Lieutenant General Sir George, 36, 40
Prisoners of war
    mortality rate in prison hospitals during Civil War, 90
Professional Filler System, 333, 408
PROFIS. *See* Professional Filler System
Projectiles, 101–102
Prussians
    contributions to wartime surgical treatment, 70
Pryor, Major John P, 387, 395
PSH. *See* Portable surgical hospitals
Puerto Rico invasion, 133–134
Punji stakes, 315

Q
Quasi-War, 34
Quebec, Canada
    Revolutionary War battle, 5
Queenston Heights, Battle of, 38
Quinine, 43–44, 92–93

R
Radiography
    forward surgical teams, 362, 402
    Spanish-American War, 134–135
    World War I, 168
Railroads
    ambulance trains, 83, 93–94
    railroad hospitals, 93–94, 150
Rainbow-5, 174
RAMC. *See* Royal Army Medical Corps
Reagan, Ronald, 325
Recombinant Factor VIIa, 400
Red Cross, 151, 159
Red River War, 122
Redman, Dr John, 20
Reed, Major Walter, 125–126, 134
Regimental aid stations, 154
Regular Medical Corps, 176
Renal Insufficiency Team, 276
Repeating rifles, 100–101
Research and Material Command, 450
Respiratory diseases, 309–310
Restraining Act, 2
Revolutionary War
    advances resulting from, 27
    American Continental Army creation, 4–5
    American medical system, 14–26
    American soldiers, 24–26
    Bennington, Battle of, 7–8
    Brandywine, Battle of, 8, 21
    British medical system, 12–14
    Canadian battle, 5
    casualties, 11
    clothing, 24–25
    Continental Army's Medical Department, 11
    Cowpens, Battle of, 10
    diseases, 25, 26
    early conflict, 1–7
    end of, 26–27, 28
    First Continental Congress, 4
    Fort Ticonderoga capture, 7
    hospitals, 15–17
    medical system during, 14–26
    medications, 26
    Monmouth Court House, Battle of, 9–10
    naval battles, 9
    post-war threats, 28–29

rations, 24
Saratoga, Battle of, 8–9
smallpox epidemic, 16–17, 25, 26
surgeons and physicians, 17–24
Washington's successes and failures, 4, 5–7
Yorktown, Siege of, 10
Reynolds, Surgeon General Charles Ranson, 221–222
Richmond Ambulance Committee, 91
Ridgway, General Matthew, 249–250
Rifles
    Minié ball rifles, 84, 85, 100
    rifle-muskets, 100–101
    Spencer and Henry breech-loading repeating rifles, 100–101
Rivera, Major David, 333
Rob, Dr Charles, 433
Robinson, Brigadier General Paul I, 272
Roentgen, Wilhelm, 134
Role 2 surgical unit, 356
Role 3 surgical unit, 367–370
Role 4 surgical unit, 367–370
Roosevelt, Franklin D, 174, 179–180
Roosevelt, Theodore, 118, 123, 125
Rosenburg, Sergeant Matthew, 431
Rough Riders, 118, 125
Royal Army Medical Corps, 151, 152
Rumbaugh, Major General James, 334
Rush, Dr Benjamin, 11, 15, 19–22, 24
Russell, Richard, 292
Ryder Trauma Center, 410–411

S
Sac Indians, 46
Salerno, Battle of, 188–189
SAM Junctional Splint, 399
SAM Sling, 399
Sams, Brigadier General Crawford F, 263
San Francisco earthquake, 1906, 128
Sanitary Commission, 72–74, 82, 86
Saratoga, Battle of, 8–9
Saudi Arabia, 342–345
Savo Island, Battle of, 181
Schlieffen Plan, 143
Schoomaker, Surgeon General Eric B, 386
Schuyler, General Philip, 16
Schwarzkopf, General Norman, 342–343
Scott, First Lieutenant, 261
Scott, Lieutenant General Winfield, 39, 42, 46, 47, 56, 58–61, 66, 73
Scurvy
    Civil War era, 96
    War of 1812 era, 44–45, 53
Seagrave, Lieutenant Colonel Gordon S, 182–184
Seagrave Unit, 182–184
Second Battle of Ypres, 143, 150
Second Seminole War, 47
Seery, Major Jason, 436
Selective Training and Service Act of 1940, 176
Seminole Wars
    First, 46
    Second, 47
    Third, 47
Serum enzymes, 310
Seward, William, 108
Shackelford, Sergeant Keith, 371
Shambora, Brigadier General William E, 203, 260
Shaw, Lieutenant Colonel William J, 202–203
Sheaffe, General Sir Roger, 38
Shell shock, 167
Sheridan, General Philip, 120, 122
Shiloh, Battle of, 67
Shippen, Dr William, 12, 19, 21, 22–23
Ships, hospital, 94–95
Shock, treatment of, 227–228, 310
Sibley, Brigadier General Henry, 87
Sicily
    World War II battles, 188–190, 215–216
Signal Corps, 61
Sikorsky H-5 helicopters, 265, 295
Sikorsky H-19 helicopters, 273, 281
Slim, Lieutenant General Sir William, 183, 185
Small portable expeditionary aeromedical rapid response teams, 356–357
Smallpox
    Civil War era, 96–97
    Civil War vaccination, 92
    post-Civil War, 109
    Revolutionary War epidemic, 16–17, 25, 26
    War of 1812 vaccination, 42–43
Smarz, First Lieutenant Marie, 257
Smith, Corporal James, 399
Smith, Dr Charles H, 90
Smith, Lieutenant General Kirby, 69
Smith, Major Kim, 374
Smith anterior splint, 92
Snakeroot, 96
Society of Apothecaries, 43
Solomon Pacific Islands, 200
Somalia operations, 345–346

Somme, Battle of the, 141, 143
Spanish-American War
    events leading up to war, 123–125
    medical challenges and new technology, 131–135
    Philippine Insurrection, 127–128
    Puerto Rico invasion, 133–134
    Rough Riders, 118, 125
Sternberg Hospital, 127, 132
Spanish Civil War, 220
SPEARR. *See* Small portable expeditionary aeromedical rapid response teams
Special Operations forces tactical tourniquets, 398
Spencer, Major James H, Jr, 225
Spencer and Henry rifles, 100–101
Spino, Staff Sergeant Ronald J, 387–388
Splints
    splint boards, 167
    Thomas splints, 148, 167
SSTP. *See* Surgical shock trauma platoon
St Clair, Arthur, 29
St Martin, Alexis, 51
Standlee, Brigadier General Earl E, 260
Staten Island Peace Conference, 5
Stephens, Alexander Hamilton, 108
Sternberg, Surgeon General George M, 109–110, 113–114, 123–126, 131
Sternberg Hospital, 127, 132
Stilwell, General Joseph "Vinegar Joe," 183–188
Stinger, Lieutenant Colonel Harry, 378–379
Stojadinovic, Lieutenant Colonel Alexander, 374
Stosstruppen, 144
Streit, Colonel Paul, 202
Stringer, Dr Samuel, 18, 19
Sulfa drugs, 231
Sulfuric ether, 54
Sully, Brigadier General Alfred, 87
Surgeons General
    Civil War, 88–89
    creation of post, 45
    during interwar period, 1818-1861, 48–50
    during period from 1865 to 1917, 110–117
    during post-Vietnam Era, 348–350
    Vietnam War, 315–317
    World War I, 165–166
    World War II, 221–223
Surgical Research Teams, 276–282, 309, 313
Surgical shock trauma platoon, 357
Sutherland, Surgeon General Charles, 113
Swan, Colonel Kenneth, 317
Swann, Lieutenant Colonel Steve, 414
Swieten, Baron Gerhard Von, 13
Sylvester, Major Cleve, 371

T

T-POD, 399
Tactical combat casualty care, 358, 368, 397–398
Task Force 212, 440–441
Task Force Falcon, 347
Task Force Hawk, 347
Tavarez, Staff Sergeant Abel, 379
Taylor, Brigadier General Zachary, 56–57, 60–61
Taylor, Dr Wesley M, 390
Taylor, General Maxwell, 272
Taylor, Major Mark D, 387
Taylor, Surgeon General Richard R, 316–317
TCCC Card, 4–6
Tecumseh, 35, 38
Tenskwatawa, 35
Teperman, Dr Sheldon, 430
Terreri, Lieutenant Colonel Anthony, 395
Terrorism. *See* Global War on Terrorism; Homeland Defense
Tet Offensive, 288
Tetanus antitoxin, 154
Third Battle of Ypres, 163
Third Seminole War, 47
Thomas, Major General John, 16
Thomas splints, 148, 167
Thoracic surgery, 228–230
Tilton, Dr James, 38
Tingey, Captain Thomas, 40
Tissue adhesives, 313
Tompkins, Sally, 100
Torney, Surgeon General George H, 115
Tourniquets, 398–399
Tovell, Colonel Ralph M, 202
Trains
    ambulance trains, 83, 93–94
    railroad hospitals, 93–94, 150
Tranexamic acid, 400
Transfusions
    Vietnam War, 308–309
    World War I, 168–169
    World War II, 227–228
Travois, 121
Treaty of Amity and Commerce, 9
Treaty of Fort Jackson, 41
Treaty of Ghent, 33, 41
Treaty of Guadalupe Hidalgo, 60
Treaty of Paris, 27
Treaty of Versailles, 142, 144–145

Triage system, 148
Tripler, Dr Charles, 77, 78–79
Trist, Nicholas, 55, 60
Trobaugh, Major General Edward L, 327
Typhoid fever, 44, 132

U
UH-1 helicopters, 289, 296, 298, 305
Unexploded ordnances, 392–397
Uniformed Services University of Health Sciences, 443
Union Army Medical Service, 95
United Nations
    intervention in the Former Republic of Yugoslavia, 346–347
United States Volunteer Cavalry, 125
Universal Protective Dressing, 313
US Army Ambulance Service, 161
US Army Institute of Surgical Research, 404–405
US Army Medical Corps, 71
US Army Medical Department
    adaptation of civilian advances, 130–131
    challenges and new technology during Spanish-American War, 131–135
    establishment of, 45
    during the Indian Wars, 46–47
    involvement outside medicine, 61
    Medical and Surgical History of the War of the Rebellion, 1861-1865, 108
    start of World War II, 175
    status after War of 1812, 45–46
    World War I medical assets, 153–161
US Christian Commission, 86
US Department of Defense Role 2 surgical unit, 356
US Navy Trauma Training Center, 410
US Northern Command, 435–438
US Province Senior Advisors, 307
US Sanitary Commission, 72–74, 82, 86
UXO. *See* Unexploded ordnances

V
Vaccinations
    Civil War, 92–93
    smallpox, 42–43, 92
    War of 1812, 42–43
Van Buskirk, Colonel Kryder, 247–248, 252, 282
Van Fleet, Lieutenant General James A, 250
Van Rensselaer, Major General Stephen, 36, 38
Vanasse, Major William, 433
Vandergrift, Major General Alexander, 181
Vascular surgery, 227, 314

Verdun, Battle of, 143–144
Vietnam War
    casualty rates, 288
    Central Highlands description, 285
    Central Lowlands description, 285–286
    combat medicine, 301–306
    events leading up to war, 286–289
    high-velocity projectile wounds, 314–315
    medical evacuation, 295–301
    Medical Unit, Self-Contained, Transportable units, 289–297
    Mekong Delta description, 285–286
    military blood program, 308–309
    Mobile Army Surgical Hospitals, 291
    programs supported by medical assets, 306–307
    Surgeons General, 315–317
    surgical and medical care advances, 307–314
Villa, Francisco "Pancho," 136
von Moltke, General Helmuth, 143

W
Wainwright, Lieutenant General Jonathan, 180
Walker, Dr Mary, 100
Walter Reed Army Institute of Research, 309–311, 313
War neurosis, 167
War of 1812
    Canadian invasion attempt, 36–37, 39
    events leading up to war, 34–35
    post-war status of Army Medical Department, 45–46
    state of medicine and surgery, 42
    status of disease and medications at end of war, 42–45
    strategies and goals for, 35–41
    views concerning, 33–34
Warren, Dr John, 43
Warren, Dr Joseph, 2, 3
Washington, General George, 4, 5–7
Wassner, Colonel Dirk, 365
Watie, Brigadier General Stand, 69
Wayne, Major General Anthony, 29
Websites
    list of casualty clearing stations in Flanders and France, 153
Webster, Daniel, 66
Welch, Dr William Henry, 129, 131
West, Major Brad, 379
Western Sanitary Commission, 95
Westmoreland, General William, 287

Whig Party, 56, 60
White, Lieutenant Colonel William, 411
Whitman, Walt, 74
Wilderness, Battle of, 68
Wilkinson, Commanding General James, 29
Williams, Colonel Robert, 183–185, 201, 205
Wilsey, Captain John J, 257
Wilson, Lieutenant Colonel Edward B, 326
Wilson, Woodrow, 136, 144–145
Wilson's Fourteen Points, 144–145
Wingate, Major General Orde, 182
Women's Central Association of Relief, 72–73
Wood, Dr Leonard
    activities during period before Spanish-American War, 123–125
    disease prevention in the Philippines, 126–128
    early military career during Frontier Indian Wars, 120–123
    efforts to control sanitation problems and tropical diseases in Cuba, 125–126
    Medal of Honor, 122
    medical education, 117–119
    medical training, 119–120
Wood, Surgeon General Robert C, 73
World War I
    Ambulance Americaine concept, 149–152
    ambulances, 161–162
    American medical assets, 153–161
    British medical assets, 152–153
    chronology of war, 142–145
    events leading up to war, 135–137, 141
    French medical assets, 152
    gunshot wounds, 165
    hospitals, 162–164
    influenza pandemic, 166–167
    leaders of medical effort, 145–148
    medical advances, 167–169
    organization of medical assets in theater, 149–161
    Surgeons General, 165–166
    treatment philosophy, 148–149
World War II
    auxiliary surgical groups, 205–207
    beginning of, 173–175
    China-Burma-India Theater of operations, 182–184
    deployment of medical assets, 177–178
    end of, 233
    European Continent operations, 190–191
    evacuation hospitals, 203–205
    field hospitals, 201–202
    forward surgery in combat theaters, 210–221
    France/Belgium combat, 212–215
    full-sized surgical hospitals in combat environments, 191
    Italian operations, 188–190
    levels of care, 201–207
    major combat theaters, 178–191
    medical advances, 223–232
    medical officer training, 175–177
    Mobile Army Surgical Hospitals, 202, 240–241
    North African Campaign, 188–190, 215
    Operation Overlord, 205, 210–212
    other militaries' experiences, 216–221
    Pacific Theater, 178–182
    physicians' experience, 207–210
    portable surgical hospitals, 191–201, 202–203, 232
    Sicily and Mediterranean battles, 188–190, 215–216
    start of war for Army Medical Department, 175
    structure of forward surgery, 191–201
    Surgeons General, 221–223
Worth, Major General William, 58
Wounded Knee, Battle at, 123
Wounds. *See specific injury type*
WRAIR. *See* Walter Reed Army Institute of Research
Wyman, Lieutenant Colonel Isaac, 2

Y

Yaffee, Lieutenant Colonel Michael, 409
Yellow fever
    during post-Civil War period, 109–110
    during Spanish-American War, 125–126, 132
    during War of 1812, 44
Yellow Fever Commission, 125–126
Yorktown, Siege of, 10
Ypres, Belgium
    First Battle of, 143
    Second Battle of, 143, 150
    Third Battle of, 163
Yugoslavia, the Former Republic of
    United Nations intervention in, 346–347

Z

Zarzabal, Lieutenant Colonel Esmeralso, 446
Zollinger, Major Robert, 232